Springer

Tokyo
Berlin
Heidelberg
New York
Barcelona
Budapest
Hong Kong
London
Milan
Paris
Santa Clara
Singapore

F. Hanyu · K. Takasaki (Eds.)

Pancreato-
duodenectomy

With 191 Figures, Including 1 in Color

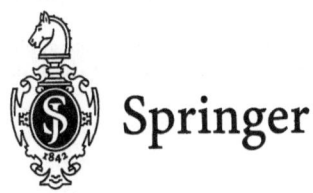

Springer

Fujio Hanyu, M.D., Ph.D.
Professor Emeritus
Tokyo Women's Medical College
8-1 Kawada-cho, Shinjuku-ku, Tokyo 162, Japan

Ken Takasaki, M.D., Ph.D.
Professor and Chairman, Department of Surgery
Institute of Gastroenterology
Tokyo Women's Medical College
8-1 Kawada-cho, Shinjuku-ku, Tokyo 162, Japan

ISBN 978-4-431-68543-2   ISBN 978-4-431-68541-8 (eBook)
DOI 10.1007/ 978-4-431-68541-8

Library of Congress Cataloging-in-Publication Data

Pancreatoduodenectomy / F. Hanyu, K. Takasaki (eds.).
    p.   cm.
    Based on the International Symposium on Pancreatoduodenectomy, held
in Tokyo, in Nov. 1995.
    Includes bibliographical references and index.

    1. Pancreaticoduodenectomy—Congresses. I. Hanyu, F. (Fujio),
1930– . II. Takasaki, K. (Ken), 1940– . III. International
Symposium on Pancreatoduodenectomy (1995 : Tokyo, Japan)
    [DNLM: 1. Pancreaticoduodenectomy—methods—congresses. WI 830
P188 1997]
RD546.P37 1997
617.5'57—dc21
DNLM/DLC
for Library of Congress   97-16186

Printed on acid-free paper

© Springer-Verlag Tokyo 1997
Softcover reprint of the hardcover 1st edition 1997

Typesetting: Best-set Typesetter Ltd., Hong Kong

Preface

Alessandro Condivilla of Bologna first attempted a resection of the head of the pancreas in 1898, but several decades of further trial-and-error attempts ensued before the prototype procedure of pancreatoduodenectomy (PD) was established by Whipple in 1935. In the half-century following that landmark, refinements of surgical technique, including pancreatico- and bilio-entero anastomosis as well as development of new technology to support perioperative management and patient care have contributed to the decrease in mortality and morbidity rates for obstructive jaundice and pancreatic fistula.

The improvement in mortality and morbidity rates associated with PD has led to an increase in the number of patients undergoing the procedure and in the number of institutions performing it. Indications for PD have also been expanded. In the early years after PD was established as a viable procedure, periampullary carcinoma was the most common indication; now PD is indicated for a number of benign and malignant diseases. Some surgeons believe that PD is the procedure of choice for certain types of chronic pancreatitis, pancreatico-biliary maljunction, and pancreatic and duodenal trauma. Other surgeons have reported the necessity of PD for lymph node dissection of gallbladder carcinoma. Consequently, the basic procedure has been greatly modified to accommodate the specific conditions of each disease. For patients with malignancy, extended procedures have been developed to improve the curative resection rate and ensure complete lymph node dissection. These procedures may entail concurrent resection of potentially involved hepatic blood vessels such as the portal vein and hepatic artery, concomitant with hepatic resection for some patients with gallbladder carcinoma. For selected patients with benign or low-grade malignancy, less invasive procedures have been indicated.

As widely accepted procedures have rapidly evolved for PD, new sets of problems have arisen. In a period of 30 years under the direction of Professor Hanyu, PD was carried out in more than 1000 patients at our institution. To commemorate that achievement, we organized an international symposium in 1995 to bring together surgeons from around the world who are experts in PD. The meeting provided an opportunity for these renowned practitioners from 24 countries to focus on current problems involved in PD. This volume presents papers from the symposium, providing a wealth of information and expertise from specialists in the field. We believe that the book will serve as a valuable reference for surgeons and all others who are concerned with diseases for which PD is indicated.

We are grateful to our secretaries and other staff members for their assistance in the symposium and in preparation of the manuscripts. Our special thanks go to the staff of Springer-Verlag Tokyo who assisted in editing all chapters to ensure consistent grammatical style. The content of the book was edited and completed with the cooperation of Prof. T. Takada, Prof. T. Imaizumi, Prof. T. Yoshikawa, Dr. T. Nakasako, Dr. T. Araida, and other colleagues at our institute.

No matter how expertly PD is performed, for the patient to do well requires intensive, expert perioperative surgical care and nursing. Fortunately for our patients, we have an abundance of outstanding surgical staff members, nurses, and paramedical co-workers. To them we owe all our ultimate achievements, and to all of them, this book is dedicated.

KEN TAKASAKI

Contents

Historical Aspects

One Thousand Pancreatoduodenectomies

Pancreatoduodenectomy for Benign Disease
Indications and Results

Pancreatoduodenectomy for Cancer Indications and Results

Techniques for Extended Pancreatoduodenectomy

Duodenum-Preserving Pancreatoduodenectomy

Reconstruction after Pancreatoduodenectomy

Quality of Life After Pancreatoduodenectomy

Experience of Pancreatoduodenectomy in Various Countries

List of Contributors

Addresses are given at the beginning of the respective contribution.

Historical Aspects

Historical Aspects and the Future of Pancreatoduodenectomy*

JOHN M. HOWARD

Key words. Pancreatic carcinoma—Pancreatoduodenectomy—History of pancreatic resection—Allen O. Whipple

Introduction

Allen Oldfather Whipple was born in 1881, in Persia (Iran) of American missionary parents. He received his undergraduate degree from Princeton University, then graduated in medicine in 1908 from the College of Physicians and Surgeons of Columbia University. After internship, he returned to his alma mater. Thirteen years after graduation from medical school, he became Professor of Surgery and Director of the Surgical Service of Presbyterian Hospital [1].

Development of the Two-stage Pancreatoduodenectomy (Carcinoma of the Ampulla of Vater)

March 16, 1934, Presbyterian Hospital, New York City. The patient was a 60-year-old woman with painless jaundice; serum bilirubin 6.8 mg%; her disease was carcinoma of the ampulla of Vater. A first-stage operation consisted of cholecystostomy and anastomosis of the common duct to the duodenum. Her jaundice cleared. Seven weeks later, the second stage included resection of the duodenum around and including the ampullary carcinoma and the adjacent pancreas. The remnant pancreas was sutured to the duodenal opening created by the resection of the ampulla. The patient died 30 h after operation from leakage of the duodenal anastomosis [2], which had been created with catgut sutures [3]. As Whipple subsequently pointed out, catgut dissolves rapidly in this environment.

Medical College of Ohio, PO Box 10008, Toledo, OH 43699, U.S.A.
* This chapter first appeared as an article in the *Journal of Hepato-Biliary-Pancreatic Surgery* (1996) 3:149–153.

There then followed two successful (two- or three-stage) resections in 1934 and 1935, the respective patients dying 8 and 25 months after operation [2,4]. Having learned from their initial failure, a silk technique was utilized in the latter two patients. Whipple had decided that pancreatointestinal anastomosis was too hazardous and it was not employed.

As he described later [4], ". . . in February 1935, the writer [Whipple] performed a two-stage operation for carcinoma of the ampulla, consisting in the first stage of a cholecystojejunostomy and in the second stage, . . . a total duodenectomy with a large portion of the head of the pancreas. The lower end of the common duct and the pancreatic duct were ligated." Dr. Whipple stated that this was the first recorded total duodenectomy in man, although Dragstead et al. [5] had shown that dogs and pigs could survive after total duodenectomy.

These operations have been universally credited with spurring the development of pancreatic surgery. They apparently were not, however, the first such operations.

The One-Stage Pancreatoduodenectomy

The time now shifts about 5 years, to early 1940. The patient was a 33-year-old woman, with epigastric pain and weight loss. She was not jaundiced. An erroneous diagnosis of carcinoma of the gastric antrum had been made. On March 6, 1940, Dr. Whipple found a benign gastric ulcer and a mass in the head of the pancreas. Dr. Purdy Stout, the father of surgical pathology, stated that the tumor in the head of the pancreas was an islet cell carcinoma. As reported by Dr. Whipple, the first recorded one-stage removal of the entire head of the pancreas and the entire duodenum with occlusion of the pancreas was then performed (Fig. 1). Silk sutures were used. The patient survived, to die of metastasis 9 years later.

Reporting the case, as a 5-year follow-up in 1945, Dr. Whipple stated that ". . . I condemn the two-stage procedure and advocate the one-stage procedure with choledochojejunostomy and implantation of the pancreatic duct into the jejunum as the procedure of choice." By 1945 he had performed eight two-stage resections, with a mortality rate of 38%, and 19 one-stage operations, with a mortality of 31% [6].

In 1942, Dr. Whipple closed his remarks to the Boston Surgical Society as follows: "Many more cases with 5-year survival will be required before valid claims can be made for the operation as done at present. But, it must be remembered that those patients untreated have an average of 6 months' survival from onset of symptoms until death. . . . The considerable risk of 30%–35% is justified if they can be made comfortable for even a year or two [1]."

The Whipple Era—His Peers

Whipple was not working in a surgical vacuum. Indeed, there was a ferment in pancreatic surgery, led largely by American surgeons. Only a few weeks after Whipple had performed the first one-stage resection for neuroendocrine carcinoma (1940), Trimble et al. [7] performed the first one-stage radical resection of carcinoma of the ampulla of Vater. After Whipple's 1934 two-stage resections, Brunschwig (1937) [8] had been the first to perform successfully a radical two-stage resection for carcinoma of the head of the pancreas.

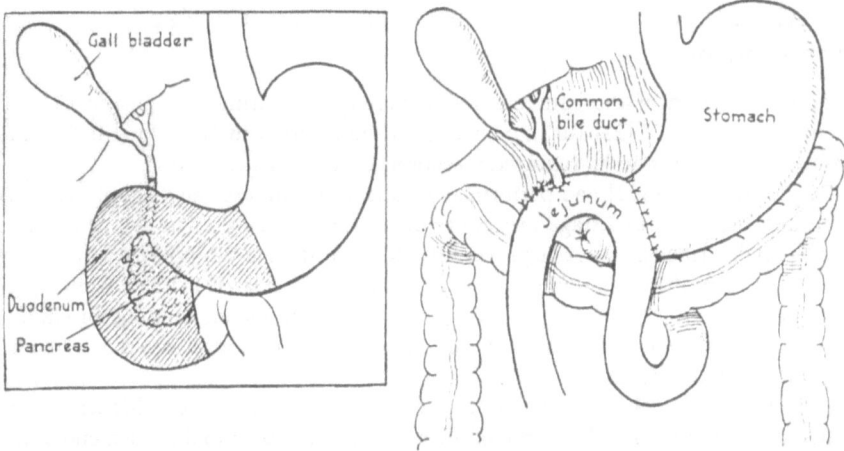

FIG. 1. Dr. Allen Whipple's first (1940) one-stage pancreaticoduodenectomy. Resection of an islet cell carcinoma of the head of the pancreas. Note the ligation of the pancreatic (duct) remnant. From [6], with permission

Earlier Building Blocks Preceding and Leading to Pancreatoduodenectomy

Praderi [9] credits Alexander von Winiwarter (1848–1917) [10], a student of Billroth's, as the first surgeon (1882) to anastomose the gallbladder to the intestine in a patient with obstructive jaundice due to cancer of the head of the pancreas, a procedure actually requiring six operations.

Five years later (1887), Oddi [11] ligated the distal common bile duct in three dogs; he then anastomosed the gallbladder to the stomach. The dogs remained metabolically healthy.

Kappeler [12] successfully performed a cholecystojejunostomy in a patient in 1889. A decade later, in 1897, Roux utilized what we know as the Roux-en-Y principle [13]. Köcher described mobilization of the duodenum in 1903 [14].

Meanwhile, Courvoisier (1890) [15] had written of his findings, proposing the principle which became known as Courvoisier's law.

Surgical Exploration and Local Resection of the Papilla of Vater

Pancreatoduodenectomy was built on experiences with "papillectomy," the local excision of lesions of the ampulla of Vater. Charles MacBerney [16], in 1878, successfully performed duodenotomy for removal of a papillary calculus. Köcher [17] followed with a larger series in 1895. Thus, most of the progress in this period was coming from central Europe.

In North America, Halsted (1899) had been the first to locally resect a tumor of the ampulla of Vater [18]. Other surgeons followed: local resection of ampullary carcinomas was performed via duodenotomy. Cordua (1906) [19] and Hirschel (1914) [20] added gastroenterostomy as a safety vent following transduodenal papillectomy.

Pre-Whipple Approaches Toward Resection of the Head of the Pancreas

The first resection of the pancreas was apparently performed by Johann Conrad Brunner (1653–1727) [21] (of duodenal gland fame) who, in 1683, long before the introduction of anesthesia, reported resections of the pancreas in dogs.

Desjardins (1907) [22] had performed a radical resection of the head of pancreas and duodenum as a two-stage procedure on a human cadaver. The following year, Sauvé [23] described a one-stage procedure, but, according to Whipple [4], apparently did not perform the operation on a human. Another year later, in 1909, Coffey [24] took the problem to the dog laboratory, performing, and recommending for clinical application, resection with reimplantation of the pancreatic stump into the distal end of the resected duodenum.

Kausch [25], in 1909, had carried out a successful partial pancreaticoduodenectomy in two stages, implanting the stump of the resected pancreas into the distal end of the resected duodenum (the Coffey canine operation). The patient remained in good condition for 9 months before dying of acute cholangitis.

In 1914, Hirschel [20] performed a partial pancreaticoduodenectomy as a one-stage procedure for carcinoma of the ampulla of Vater. A rubber tube was used to bridge the gap between the transected common duct and the duodenum. The patient lived for approximately 1 year.

Tenani [26] successfully performed a partial pancreaticoduodenectomy in two stages for carcinoma of the ampulla in 1922. His operation consisted of a gastro-jejunostomy and a choledochoduodenostomy, followed a month later by resection of the ampullary carcinoma and the adjacent duodenum. The transected pancreas was anastomosed to the transected end of the distal duodenum. The patient was living and considered cured by the surgeon 3 years after resection.

In 1907, Desjardins [22] had written that Berns had removed the head of the pancreas in 1881, but the operation may not have included resection of the duodenum.

According to Sauvé [23], the first en bloc resection of the head of the pancreas and duodenum had been performed in 1898 by Alessandro Codivilla [27] of Bologna. The tumor was a carcinoma of the head of the pancreas; the patient died 24 days postoperatively.

The Discovery of Vitamin K and Insulin

The discovery of vitamin K by Dam [28] in 1929 was a fundamental prerequisite to the development of radical surgery in the jaundiced patient. Also of importance had been the 1922 discovery of insulin by Banting and Best [29].

Progress Since the Whipple Era

Reducing the Morbidity and Mortality of Resection

Hemorrhage, shock, and renal failure were the frequent causes of death in the immediate postoperative period after pancreaticoduodenectomy. As the standards of care improved throughout the surgical world these causes of mortality abated. As experience was gained, the one-stage resection became the accepted norm, leading Lord

Rodney Smith (1995) [30] to reiterate the validity of his statement of a quarter of a century earlier: "The view held today is that radical pancreaticoduodenectomy should be performed in one stage unless there is some very good reason for preferring a two-stage procedure. It is doubtful if a one-stage operation should be rejected on the score of the age or infirmity of the patient . . ."

Leakage of the pancreatoenteric anastomosis continused to be a major cause of mortality. Cattell (1948) [31] described the clinical technique of end-to-side pancreaticojejunostomy, utilizing the mucosa-to-mucosa technique. A few years ago, Warren [32] noted that experimental studies "confirmed a longstanding, unalterable and probably unreasonable insistence on my part that mucosa-to-mucosa anastomosis, carefully done, is a superior method . . . that an end-to-side anastomosis can be performed with any size duct and in the presence of any degree of friability of the pancreas." Utilizing a similar technique with non-absorbable or slowly absorbable sutures, this author (JMH) has not had a recognizable pancreatic fistula in the last 52 anastomoses [33], an experience paralleling that of Walsh and associates [34].

The postoperative mortality rate after the Whipple resection remained in the range of 25%–35% until Howard [35] (in 1968) reported 41 consecutive resections without a hospital mortality, a series subsequently extended to 72 patients [36]. The lower mortality rate was attributed to the concentration of experience in the hands of a single surgeon, supported by a specialized team, including residents and intensive care nurses. A recommendation was made for the development of specialized centers for such treatment. Since that time, evolving centers have reported mortality rates in the 0%–5% range, including major reports by Trede et al. [37] and Cameron and associates [38].

Other Modifications of the Whipple Operation

According to Leger and Brehant [39], there have been at least 68 modifications of the Whipple resection, 20 of which were outlined diagrammatically by Jordan [40], including the pyloric-preserving resection, as described by Traverso and Longmire [41].

Improving Long-Term Survival

Survival rates following Whipple resection for carcinoma of the head of the pancreas have been slowly improving, but it is difficult to know to what degree, since many authors have recently expressed their survival rates as projected rates, estimates being calculated by the Kaplan-Meier method.

Baumel et al. (1994) [42], reporting the French experience of 555 resections, projected a 5-year survival of 15%; Wade et al. (1994) [43] in a United States series of 327 patients noted a projected 5-year survival rate of 12%. Cameron (Yeo et al.) [44] and Trede and associates [45] have reported estimated 5-year survivals of selected patients at significantly higher rates.

Nevertheless, most survivors of resection ultimately die of recurrent carcinoma; most, therefore, have micrometastasis at the time of "curative" resection. Dare we project the future modality by which improvement in survival will result? Our current options include:

(a) Earlier diagnosis, which is slowly evolving, utilizing the techniques made possible by ERCP, computerized tomography, improvements in ultrasound, and collection of malignant cells for cytologic and immunohistochemical studies.

In multi-institutional reviews in Japan, Satake and colleagues [46] and Tsuchiya and associates [47] demonstrated the encouraging results of resection of cancers identified while still quite small.

(b) Will improvement result through the development of more effective adjuvant therapy regimens? So far I have never seen an unequivocal response to chemotherapy or to irradiation therapy of an established pancreatic exocrine carcinoma; yet our tools are improving [48–50], and, hopefully, we are building the blocks for adjuvant therapy as the early surgeons built for resection.

(c) At an international symposium held in June 1989, under the honorary sponsorship of former United States President Jimmy Carter, whose family had experienced a very high incidence of pancreatic cancer, Manabe et al. [51], Ozaki et al. [52], and Hiraoka et al. [53] representing three different Japanese surgical teams, reported a 25%–35% projected 5-year survival of selected patients following radical resection with or without adjuvant therapy; a different approach from that utilized by Fortner [54], who had extended the field of resection in patients with advanced cancer.

Meanwhile, Saitoh and his many Japanese colleagues initiated the Japanese Pancreatic Cancer Registry, an organ of historic significance in permitting the more rapid collection and analysis of data.

Any objective survey of the literature of the past decade cannot but recognize the dominant leadership of Japanese surgeons and their colleagues in the field of pancreatic cancer.

Finally, I should like to acknowledge, with keen appreciation, the remarkable contributions being presented in the evaluation of extension of the Whipple resection by Prof. Hanyu [55].

May we judge our current efforts with charity, the results with keen analysis and, when successful, with heartfelt appreciation on behalf of our patients, for today's contributions are tomorrow's historical landmarks.

References

1. Cheever D (1942) Presentation of the (Bigelow) medal. New Engl J Med 226:514–515
2. Whipple AO, Parsons WB, Mullins CR (1935) Treatment of carcinoma of the ampulla of Vater. Ann Surg 102:763–779
3. Peters JH, Carey LC (1991) Historical review of pancreaticoduodenectomy. Am J Surg 161:219–225
4. Whipple AO (1960) A historical sketch of the pancreas. In: Howard JM, Jordan GL Jr (eds) Surgical disease of the pancreas. JB Lippincott, Philadelphia
5. Dragstead LR, Dragstead C, McClintock JT, Chase CS (1918) Extirpation of the duodenum. Am J Physiol 46:584–590
6. Whipple AO (1945) Pancreaticoduodenectomy for islet carcinoma. Ann Surg 121:847–852
7. Trimble JR, Parsons JW, Sherman C (1941) One-stage operation for cure of carcinoma of ampulla of Vater and of head of pancreas. Surg Gynecol Obstet 73:711–722
8. Brunschwig A (1937) Resection of head of pancreas and duodenum for carcinoma-pancreatoduodenectomy. Surg Gynecol Obstet 65:681–684
9. Praderi RC (1993) History of pancreatic surgery. In: Trede M, Carter DC (eds) Surgery of the pancreas, chapter 1. Churchill Livingstone, Edinburgh
10. von Winiwarter A (1882) Ein Fall von Gallenretention betingt durch Impermeabilitat des Ductus choledochus, Anlegung einer Gallenblasen-Darmfistel, Heilung. Prager Med Wochenschr 7:201

11. Oddi R (1887) D'une disposition a sphincter speciale de l'ouverture du canal choledoque. Arch Ital Biol 8:317
12. Kappeler A (1889) Die einzietige Cholecystenterostomie. Korrespondenzbelatt fur Schweizerische Artze 17:513
13. Roux C (1897) De la gastro-enterostomie. Rev Gynecol Chir Abdomin 1:67
14. Köcher T (1903) Mobilisierung des Duodenum und gesteroduodenostomie. Zentralblatt für Chirurgie n.2. Sonnabend, den 10 Januar. Writing from Bern
15. Courvousier LG (1890) Casuistisch-Statistische Beitrage zur Patholgie und Chirurgie der Gallenwege. Vogel, Leipzig
16. MacBurney CH (1878) Removal of biliary calculi from the common duct by the duodenal route. Ann Surg 28:481
17. Kocher T (1895) Ein Fall von Choledochoduodenostomia interna wegen Gallenstein. Korrespondenzblatt für schweizerische arzte. I:193
18. Halsted WS (1899) Contributions to the surgery of the bile passages, especially of the common bile duct. Boston Med Surg J 141:645–654
19. Cordua (1906) Cited by: Praderi, Carcinom der Papilla duodenalis. Munchener Med Wochensch 53:2324
20. Hirschel G (1914) Die Resektion des Duodenums mit der Papilla wegen Karzinoms. Münvhrn. Med Exhnschr 6:1728
21. Brunner JC (1683) Experimenta nova circa pancreas. Wetstenius. Amsterdam
22. Desjardins A (1907) Technique de la pancreatectomie. J Rev Chir 35:945–973
23. Sauvé L (1908) Des pancreatectomies et specialement de la pancreatectomie cephalique. J Rev Chir 37:113,335
24. Coffey RC (1909) Pancreatoenterostomy and pancreatectomy. Ann Surg 50:1238–1264
25. Kausch W (1912) Das Carcinom der Papilla duodeni und seine radikale Entfernung. Zentralbe Chir 1909; 39:1350
26. Tenani O (1922) Contributo alla chirurgia della papilla del Vater. Policlinico 29:291
27. Codivilla A (1898) Rend stat seq. Chir Ospe d'Imala (Italy)
28. Dam H (1939) Biochem J 215:468
29. Banting FG, Best CH (1922) The internal secretion of the pancreas. J Lab Clin Med 7:251
30. Smith R Personal communication (1995) Quoted by: Maingot R (1974) Pancreatic tumors and periampullary carcinomas. In: Maingot R (ed) Abdominal operations, 6th ed. Appleton-Century-Crofts, New York
31. Cattell RB (1948) A technique for pancreaticoduodenal resection. Surg Clin North Am 28:761–775
32. Warren K. Discussion of paper by Greene BS, Loubeau JM, Peoples JB, Elliott DW (1991) Are pancreatoenteric anastomoses improved by duct-to-mucosa sutures? Am J Surg 161:45–49
33. Howard JM. Discussion of paper by Yeo CJ, Cameron JL, Maher MM (1995) A prospective randomized trial of pancreaticogastrostomy versus pancreaticojejunostomy after pancreaticoduodenectomy. Ann Surg 222:580–592
34. Walsh DB, Eckhauser FE, Cronenwett JL, Turcotte JG, Lindenauer SM (1982) Adenocarcinoma of the ampulla of Vater. Diagnosis and treatment. Ann Surg 195:152–157
35. Howard JM (1968) Pancreaticoduodenectomy: 41 consecutive Whipple resections without an operative mortality. Ann Surg 168:629
36. Howard JM (1981) Benign and malignant disease of the pancreas. J R Coll Surg Edinb 26:206 (62 patients reported at that time)
37. Trede M, Schwall G, Saeger HD (1990) Survival after pancreaticoduodenectomy: 118 consecutive cases without operative mortality. Ann Surg 211:447–458
38. Cameron JL, Pitt HA, Yeo CJ, Lillemoe KD, Kaufman HS, Coleman J (1993) One hundred forty-five consecutive pancreaticoduodenectomies without mortality. Ann Surg 217:430–435
39. Leger L, Brehant J (1956) Chirurgie du pancreas. Masson, Paris

40. Jordan GL Jr (1987) Pancreatic resection for pancreatic cancer. In: Howard JM, Jordan GL Jr (eds) Surgical diseases of the pancreas. Lea and Febinger, Philadelphia. Modified from Maingot R (1974) Abdominal operations, 6th ed. Appleton-Century Crofts, New York

41. Traverso LW, Longmire WP Jr (1978) Preservation of the pylorus in pancreaticoduodenectomy. Surg Gynecol Obstet 146:959–962

42. Baumel H, Huguier M, Manderscheid JC, Fabre JM, Houry S, Fagot H (1994) Results of resection for cancer of the exocrine pancreas: A study from the French Association of Surgery. Br J Surg 81:102–107

43. Wade TP, Radford DM, Virgo KS, Johnson FE (1994) Complications and outcomes in the treatment of pancreatic adenocarcinoma in the United States veteran. J Am Coll Surg 179:38–48

44. Yeo CJ, Cameron JL, Lillemoe KD, Sitzmann JV, Hruban RH, Goodman SN, Dooley WC, Coleman J, Pitt HA (1995) Pancreaticoduodenectomy for cancer of the head of the pancreas-201 patients. Ann surg 221:721–733

45. Trede M (1995) Address to the American College of Surgeons. Chicago; April

46. Satake K, Nishiwake H, Yokomatsu H, Kawazoe Y, Kim K, Haku A, Umeyama K, Miyazaki I (1992) Surgical curability and prognosis for standard versus extended resection for Ti carcinoma of the pancreas. Surg Gynecol Ostet 175:259–265

47. Tsuchiya R, Noda T, Harada N, Miyamoto T, Tomioka T, Yamamoto K, Yamaguchi T, Izawa K (1986) Collective review of small carcinomas of the pancreas. Ann Surg 203:77–81

48. Magnani JL, Steplewski Z, Koprowski H, Ginsburg V (1983) Identification of the gastrointestinal and pancreatic cancer-associated antigen detected by monoclonal antibody 19-9 in the sera of patients as a mucin. Cancer Res 43:5489–5492

49. Tian F, Appert HE, Myles J, Howard JM (1992) Prognostic value of serum Ca 19-9 levels in pancreatic adenocarcinoma. Ann Surg 215:350–355

50. Abe M, Arakawa M (1967) Fundamental studies on surgical irradiation during laparotomy of dogs. J Jpn Cancer Ther 2:271

51. Manabe T, Ohshio G, Baba N, Tobe T (1990) Factors influencing prognosis and indications for curative pancreatectomy for ductal adenocarecinoma for head of the pancreas. Int J Pancreatol 7:187–194

52. Osaki H, Kinoshita T, Kosute T, Egawa S, Kishi K (1990) Effectiveness of multimodality treatment for resectable pancreatic cancer. Int J Pancreatol 7:195–200

53. Hiraoka T, Uchino R, Kanemitsu M, Toyonaga M, Saitoh N, Nakamura I, Tashiro S, Miyauchi Y (1990) Combination of intraoperative radiation with resection of cancer of the pancreas. Int J Pancreatol 7:201–208

54. Fortner JG (1984) Regional pancreatectomy for cancer of the pancreas, ampulla and other related sites. Tumor staging and results. Ann Surg 199:418–425

55. Hanyu F, Suzuki T (1993) Whipple operation for pancreatic carcinoma: Japanese experience. In: Beger HG, Büchler M, Malfertheiner P (eds) Standards of pancreatic surgery. Springer, Berlin Heidelberg New York Tokyo, pp 646–653

One Thousand Pancreatoduodenectomies

One Thousand
Pancreaticoduodenectomies

One Thousand Pancreatoduodenectomies at a Single Institution

Fujio Hanyu

Summary. This chapter discusses our experience of 1000 pancreatoduodenectomies at a single institution. Supported by progress in both diagnostic and operative techniques, various types of pancreatoduodenectomy were carried out by several authors. Our retrospective study revealed that it was possible to indicate the pylorus-preserving Whipple procedure for 90% and more of patients with periampullary malignancy and gallbladder cancer when there was no direct invasion of the duodenal bulb or the antrum of the stomach. We performed pancreatoduodenectomy not only for malignant disease but also for benign disease. Of 1060 pancreatoduodenectomies, 861 operations were performed for malignant diseases and 199 for benign diseases. We aggressively performed pancreatoduodenectomy for chronic pancreatitis to relieve the intractable abdominal pain caused by inflammation of the pancreatic parenchyma and the spreading of this inflammation to surrounding tissues. Although morbidity rates did not change in all the periods, mortality has decreased remarkably as the result of progress in operative techniques and postoperative management by using computed tomography (CT) scan or interventional radiology. On the other hand, morbidity and hospital mortality after pancreatoduodenectomy with hepatectomy were strongly related to the extent of hepatic resection, and 70% of hospital deaths were caused by postoperative hepatic failure. This is the greatest problem in decreasing hospital mortality after pancreatoduodenectomy with massive hepatectomy in future. However, it is considered that pancreatoduodenectomy is indicated as one of the fundamental operations for various diseases of the upper abdomen.

Key words. Pancreatoduodenectomy—Pancreatoduodenectomy with hepatectomy—Hepatoligamentpancreatoduodenectomy

Introduction

Pancreatoduodenectomy has been considered to be the fundamental procedure for periampullary diseases since 1935 when Whipple [1] performed pancreatoduodenectomy for pancreatic cancer. In Japan, Kuru performed pancreato-

Department of Gastroenterological Surgery, Tokyo Women's Medical College, Shinjuku-ku, Tokyo 162, Japan.

duodenectomy for the first time in 1946. Supported by progress in both diagnostic and operative techniques, various types of pancreatoduodenectomy have been reported, such as the pylorus-preserving procedure in 1978 by Traverso [2] and pancreatoduodenectomy with hepatectomy in 1979 by Takasaki [3]. In August 1995, we had achieved 1000 pancreatoduodenectomies at a single institution. In this chapter, we present our concept of pancreatoduodenectomy based on our experience of 1000 operations.

History of Pancreatoduodenectomy at Our Institution

In 1967, the Institute of Gastroenterology, Tokyo Women's Medical College, was established; it has been 28 years since the founding of our institution. The first pancreatoduodenectomy was undergone by Professor Komei Nakayama in April 1968 for chronic pancreatitis. Between 1968 and August 1995, 1000 pancreatoduodenectomies were carried out in our institution (Table 1).

The distribution of pancreatoduodenectomy by year is shown in Fig. 1. After introduction of various pancreaticocholedocho diagnostic examinations such as percutaneous transhepatic cholangiography (PTC), endoscopic retrograde cholangiopancreatography (ERCP), and PTC drainage (PTCD), the number of pancreatoduodenectomies increased. By March 1979, 100 pancreatoduodenectomies had been performed; that is, about 10 years passed after the first pancreatoduodenectomy before 100 procedures were accomplished. Total pancreatectomy was performed for pancreatic cancer in 1971, and an extended radical Whipple

TABLE 1. History of pancreatoduodenectomy in our institution

1967. 12. 2.	Foundation of our institution
1968. 4. 27.	1st case of PD (chronic pancreatitis)
1971. 7. 2.	1st case of TP (pancreatic head cancer)
1972. 6. 8.	PD + PV + HA (pancreatic head cancer)
1978. 3. 14.	TP + SMA + SMV (pancreatic head cancer)
1979. 3. 13	1st case of HPD (gallbladder cancer)
1979. 3. 18.	100th case of PD
1981. 9. 10.	200th case of PD
1983. 10. 20.	300th case of PD
1984. 7. 1.	1st case of PpPD (anomalous arrangement of pancreatobiliary system)
1985. 8. 20.	400th case of PD
1986. 5. 13.	1st case of HLPD (gallbladder cancer)
1987. 3. 27.	500th case of PD
1989. 2. 17.	600th case of PD
1990. 11. 20.	700th case of PD
1992. 10. 15.	800th case of PD
1994. 3. 3.	900th case of PD
1995. 8. 24.	1000th case of PD
1995. 12. 26.	1024th case of PD

PD, Whipple operation; PpPD, pylorus-preserving Whipple operation; TP, total pancreatectomy; HPD, pancreatoduodenectomy with hepatectomy; HLPD, hepato-ligament-pancreatoduodenectomy; PV, resection of the portal vein; HA, resection of the hepatic artery; SMA, resection of the superior mesenteric artery; SMV resection of the superior mesenteric vein.

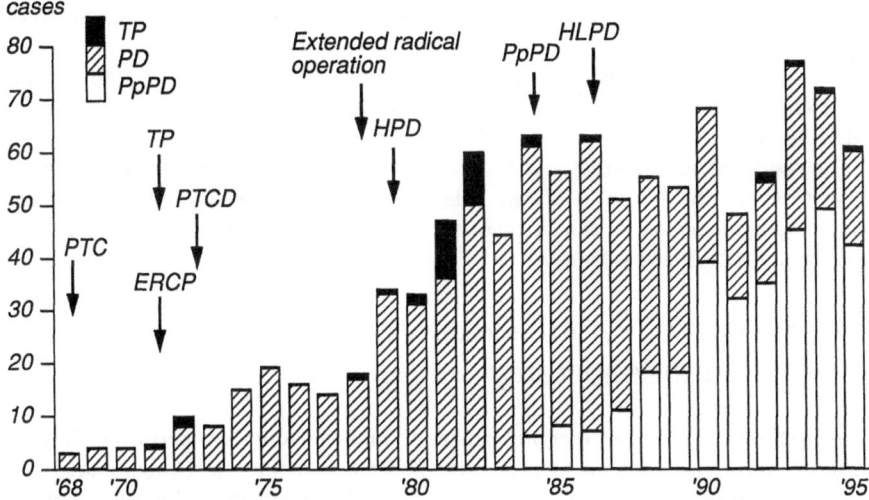

FIG. 1. Distribution of pancreatoduodenectomies by year (X-axis), January 1968 through December 1995. *TP*, total pancreatoduodenectomy (*black bars*); *PD*, Whipple procedure (*shaded bars*); *PpPD*, pylorus-preserving Whipple procedure (*white bars*); *PTC*, percutaneous transhepatic cholangiography; *ERCP*, endoscopic retrograde cholangiopancreatography; *PTCD*, PTC drainage; *HPD*, pancreatoduodenectomy with hepatectomy; *HLPD*, hepato–ligament-pancreatoduodenectomy

operation with portal vein resection and hepatic arterial reconstruction was carried out in 1972.

In 1968 a famous paper titled "Pancreaticoduodenectomy: forty-nine consecutive Whipple resections without an operative mortality" was published by Professor John Howard. We remember that we read this paper from beginning to end many times and we were deeply impressed. Another famous paper written by Dr. Fortner [4], titled "Regional pancreatectomy," also strongly influenced us and changed our ideas about pancreatoduodenectomy. We then indicated extended radical resection for pancreatic and biliary cancer. In March 1979, we experienced the Whipple resection with right hepatectomy for advanced gallbladder cancer without operative death.

Our standard procedure of extended radical pancreatoduodenectomy is composed of portal vein resection, with wide lymph node dissection around the celiac artery and hepatic, splenic, and superior mesenteric arteries; the right kidney, inferior vena cava, and abdominal aorta are exposed completely for lymph node and retroperitoneal tissue dissection. We would say that skeletonization with radical lymph node and perineural tissue dissection in the upper abdomen is the operation of choice for pancreatic cancer. Only extended radical pancreatoduodenectomy offers a curative operation for patients with pancreatic cancer, and has resulted in 11 patients who have survived longer than 5 years postoperatively.

We show an interesting case, a 50-year-old woman with advanced gallbladder cancer. The preoperative examination showed massive tumor invasion to the hepatoduodenal ligamentum and the head of the pancreas. Extended radical pancreatoduodenectomy with right hepatectomy was performed without major postoperative complications, and this patient is still alive 11 years postoperatively.

Again, it took 10 years to experience 100 pancreatoduodenectomies since the first one was performed. Since 1980, the number of pancreatoduodenectomies has increased remarkably; 200 patients underwent pancreatoduodenectomy in 1981, 300 in 1983, and 500 by March 1987. We have performed 900 pancreatoduodenectomies within the last 15 years.

The results of 500 pancreatoduodenectomies were reported at the American Pancreas Club in Chicago in 1987; the title of the presentation was "Five hundred pancreatoduodenectomies at a single institute." After the presentation, we were congratulated by Professor J. Howard.

Introduction of Pylorus-Preserving Pancreatoduodenectomy

In 1984, the first pylorus-preserving pancreatoduodenectomy was performed in our institute. We chose the pylorus-preserving procedure mainly for benign disease to maintain postoperative gastrointestinal function. However, the pylorus-preserving procedure has been the operation of choice not only for benign disease but also for malignant disease without losing radicality. We investigated retrospectively 202 patients who underwent pancreatoduodenectomy with gastric resection for periampullary malignancy and gallbladder cancer. In the cases without direct invasion to the duodenal bulb or antrum of the stomach, positive lymph node metastases around the stomach were detected in 8.7% of cases of pancreatic head cancer and in 3.7% of cases of carcinoma of the ampulla of Vater; there were no lymph node metastases around the stomach in distal bile duct carcinoma, gallbladder cancer, or duodenal cancer.

It was concluded that pylorus-preserving pancreatoduodenectomy could be indicated for 90% and more of periampullary malignancy and gallbladder cancer cases without losing curability, because if tumor invades to the duodenal bulb or the antrum of the stomach, it is necessary to resect the distal stomach (Table 2). In this way, in the past 10 years the incidence of pancreatoduodenectomy with gastrectomy has decreased, and 70% and 80% of patients have received a pylorus-preserving pancreatoduodenectomy.

On the other hand, we have indicated extended radical pancreatoduodenectomy or a superextended radical operation to obtain further curability. We had another interesting case, a 50-year-old woman with massive tumor invasion to the hepatoduodenal

TABLE 2. Pylorus-preserving pancreatoduodenectomy for periampullary malignancy and gallbladder cancer in cases of no direct invasion to the duoddenal bulb or antrum of the stomach

	Lymph node metastasis surrounding the stomach	
	Positive (%)	Negative (%)
Pancreatic head cancer ($n = 92$)	8.7	91.3
Carcinoma of the ampulla of Vater ($n = 54$)	3.7	96.3
Distal bile duct cancer ($n = 34$)	0.0	100
Gallbladder cancer ($n = 16$)	0.0	100
Duodenal cancer ($n = 6$)	0.0	100

ligamentum, the right and left hepatic duct, and the right hepatic artery. Extended radical pancreatoduodenectomy with right hepatectomy and total resection of the hepatoduodenal ligamentum, called hepato–ligament–pancreatoduodenectomy (HLPD) [5], was carried out for this patient.

Various Types of Pancreatic Head Resection

Various types of operations for resection of the head of the pancreas have been reported. The standard Whipple operation was first performed in 1935 [1]. In 1978, Dr. Traverso reported his new operation, pylorus-preserving pancreato-duodenectomy [2]. Dr. Beger [6] demonstrated duodenum-preserving resection of the head of the pancreas in 1980. We performed duodenum-preserving total pancreatic head resection (DpPHR) in 1989 as the most minimized resection of the head of the pancreas [7].

In the last 5 years, various types of procedures of resection of the head of the pancreas have been performed. About 70 pancreatoduodenectomies were performed in 1 year (see Fig. 1). The one-thousandth case of pancreatoduodenectomy was done on August 24, 1995 (see Table 1).

Indication for Pancreatoduodenectomy

We performed pancreatoduodenectomy not only for malignant disease but also for benign disease. Figure 2 demonstrates the indications for pancreatoduodenectomy. Of 1060 pancreatoduodenectomies, 861 operations were performed for malignant diseases. Pancreatic cancer was the indication for the operation in 370 patients, bile

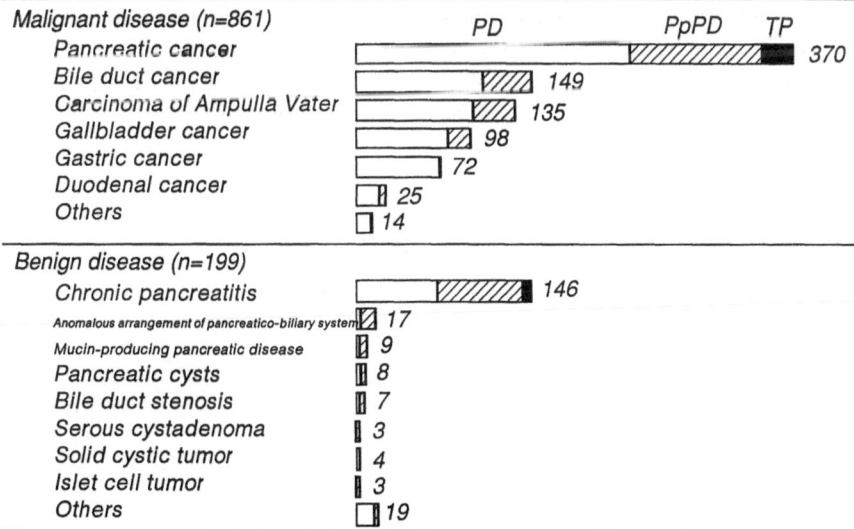

FIG. 2. Indications for pancreatoduodenectomy, January 1968 through December 1995 ($n = 1060$). PD, *white bars*; PpPD, *shaded bars*; TP, *black bars*. Duplicate cases were included

duct cancer in 149, ampulla of Vater cancer in 135, and gallbladder cancer in 98; the remainder were other diseases. Of the 199 patients who underwent pancreatoduodenectomy for benign disease, 146 patients had chronic pancreatitis, 17 had an anomalous arrangement of the pancreatobiliary system, and the others had other diseases.

Of the 321 operations for chronic pancreatitis, 277 cases (86%) were direct surgery to the pancreas, and we chose pancreatoduodenectomy in 50% of these 277 cases (Fig. 3). We consider the cause of the persistent abdominal pain caused by chronic pancreatitis to be not simply a rise in pressure inside the pancreatic duct but also inflammation of the pancreatic parenchyma and the spreading of this inflammation to surrounding tissues, such as other researchers have reported. As a result, we aggressively performed pancreatoduodenectomy for such benign diseases, so it is not an overstatement to say that we have achieved 1000 pancreatoduodenectomies.

Mortality and Morbidity After Pancreaticoduodenectomy

Although morbidity rates did not change in all time periods, mortality has decreased from 11% to 1% (Fig. 4). Mortality and morbidity caused by leakage of the pancreaticojejunostomy after pancreaticoduodenectomy decreased remarkably (Fig. 5). We consider this improvement of the results after pancreaticoduodenectomy was the result not only of progress in our operative techniques but also was aided by introduction of computed tomogrpahy (CT) and interventional radiology, because it was possible to diagnose and drain the abdominal abscess after operation by CT scan; also, we could stop massive abdominal bleeding from the arterial aneurysm caused by leakage of the pancreaticojejunostomy using the techniques of interventional radiology.

On the other hand, the morbidity rate after pancreaticoduodenectomy with hepatectomy was 34% in patients with hepatectomy of less than two segments, 71% in patients with more than two segments of hepatectomy, and 80% in patients undergomg HLPD; the hospital mortality rates were 5%, 42%, and 47%, respectively. Morbidity and hospital mortality were strongly related to the extent of hepatic resection (Table 3).

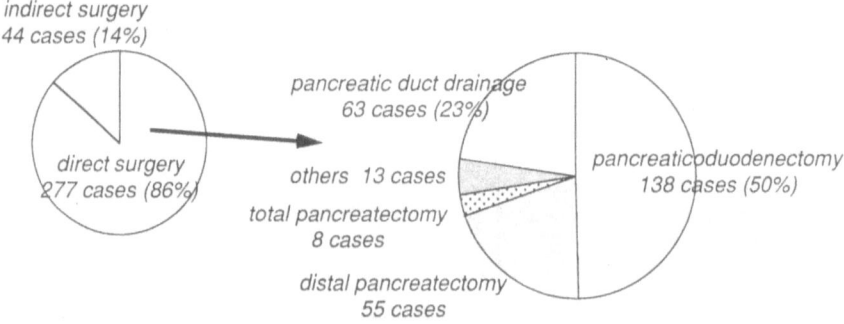

FIG. 3. Surgical management for chronic pancreatitis, January 1968 through December 1995 ($n = 321$)

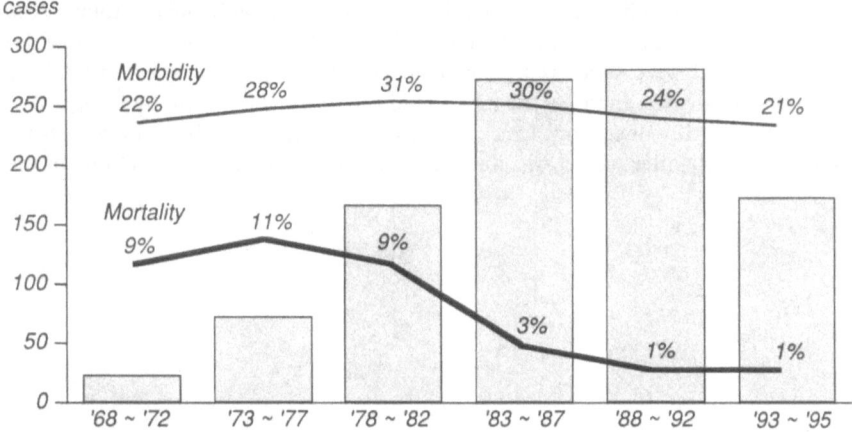

FIG. 4. Morbidity and mortality after pancreatoduodenectomy, January 1968 through December 1995 ($n = 895$). Cases of pancreatoduodenectomy with hepatectomy were excluded

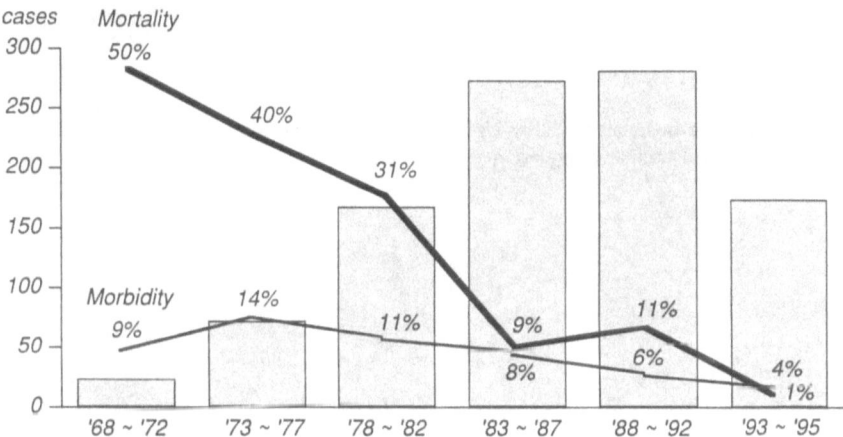

FIG. 5. Morbidity and mortality caused by leakage of pancreaticojejunostomy, January 1968 through December 1995 ($n = 895$). Cases of pancreatoduodenectomy with hepatectomy were excluded

TABLE 3. Morbidity and mortality after pancreaticoduodenectomy with hepatectomy, January 1968 through December 1995

Extent of liver resection	Morbidity	Hospital mortality
Less than two segments ($n = 64$)	34% ⌝* ⌝**	5% ⌝* ⌝*
More than two segments ($n = 24$)	71% ⌟	42% ⌟
HLPD ($n = 15$)	80% ⌟	47% ⌟
Total ($n = 103$)	50%	19%

HLPD, hepato–ligament–pancreatoduodenectomy.
*, $P < .05$; **, $P < .01$.

Of 20 hospital deaths after pancreaticoduodenectomy with hepatectomy, 70% were caused by postoperative hepatic failure (Fig. 6). We have tried to improve the mortality rate of percutaneous transhepatic portal vein embolization (PTPE) by resecting lobes so as to increase the function of the residual liver and by using active blood bypass during operation. However, this is the greatest problem in decreasing hospital mortality after pancreaticoduodenectomy with massive hepatectomy in the future.

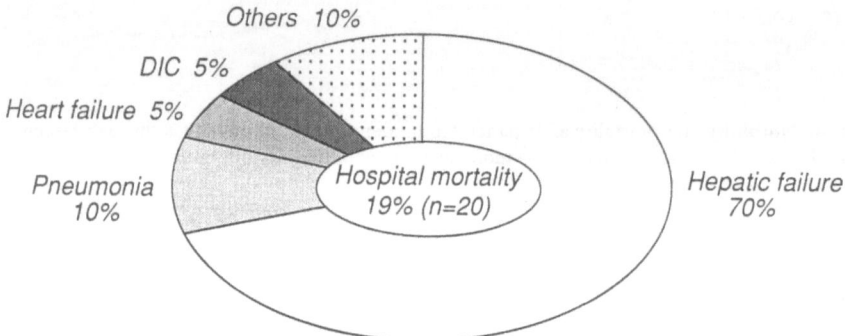

FIG. 6. Causes of hospital mortality after pancreatoduodenectomy with hepatectomy. *DIC*, disseminated intravascular coagulation

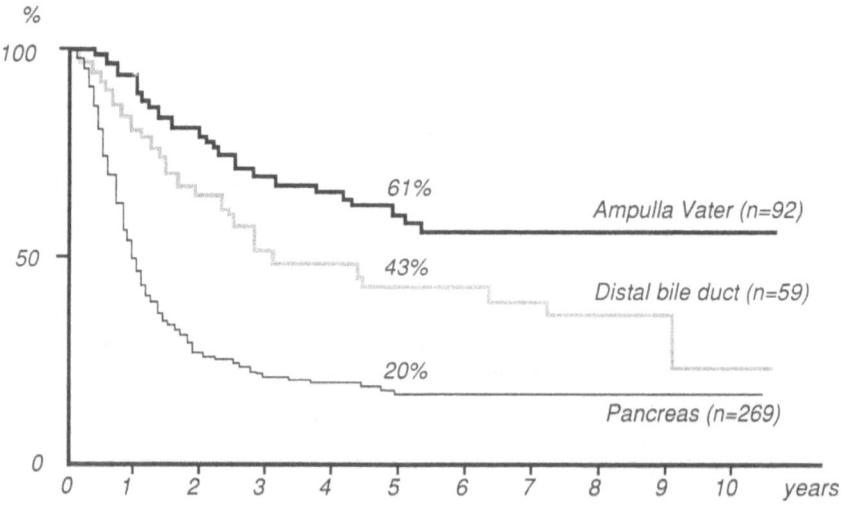

FIG. 7. Survival rates after pancreatoduodenectomy for periampullary cancer, January 1968 through December 1995

Postoperative Survival Rates After Pancreatoduodenectomy

Finally, we demonstrate the postoperative survival curves after pancre-atoduodenectomy for periampullary cancer in Fig. 7. The 5-year survival rate was 61% in patients with carcinoma of the ampulla of Vater, 43% in cases of distal bile duct cancer, and 20% in pancreatic cancer.

Conclusion

We conclude, briefly, that pancreatoduodenectomy is indicated as one of the fundamental operations for various diseases of the upper abdomen.

References

1. Whipple AO, Parsons WB, Mullins CR (1935) Treatment of carcinoma of the ampulla of Vater. Ann Surg 102:736–779
2. Traverso LW, Longmire WP (1978) Presevation of the pylorus in pancre-aticoduodenectomy. Surg Gynecol Obstet 117:959–962
3. Takasaki K, Kobayashi S, Mutoh H, et al (1980) Our experiences (5 cases) of extended right lobectomy combined with pancreatoduodenectomy for the carcinoma of the gall-bladder (in Japanese). Tan to Sui (J Bil Panc) 1:923–932
4. Fortner JG (1973) Regional resection of cancer of the pancreas. A new surgical approach. Surgery (St Louis) 73:307–320
5. Hanyu F, Nakamura M, Yoshikawa T (1988) Hepato-ligament-pancreatoduodenectomy (in Japanese). Gekachiryo (Surg Ther) 59:12–21
6. Beger HG, Witte CH, Krautzbeger W, et al (1980) Wrfahrung mit einer das Duodenumer hartenden Pankreaskopfresektion bei chronischer Pankreatitis. Chirurg 51:303–307
7. Imaizumi T, Hanyu F, Suzuki M, et al (1990) A new procedure of duodenum-preserving total resection of the head of the pancreas with pancreatico and choledocho-duodenostomy (in Japanese). Tan to Sui (J Bil Panc) 11:621–626

Pancreatoduodenectomy for Benign Disease Indications and Results

Pylorus-Preserving Pancreatoduodenectomy with a Newly Devised Reconstruction of the Alimentary Tract

Hidemi Yamauchi and Mikio Imamura

Summary. Experiences with pancreatoduodenectomy (PD) with Child's reconstruction method have led us to devise a new method of alimentary tract reconstruction: the remaining stomach is anastomosed to the oral stump of the jejunum, and a short segment of the midportion of the small intestine is interposed between the pancreatic and bile ducts and the upper jejunum. Based on satisfactory results in experiments using dogs, we first applied the reconstruction method to 4 patients undergoing PD, then to 13 patients undergoing pylorus-preserving pancreatoduodenectomy (PPPD). In PPPD, the pyloric branch of the anterior vagal nerve was preserved in most cases. It took longer for patients undergoing PPPD to take a liquid meal compared to those undergoing PD (mean, 9.9 vs. 5.6 days, $P < .01$). Body weight increased gradually after discharge, and returned to or exceeded preoperative values at time of follow-up in most patients undergoing PPPD. Gastric acid output showed normoacidity both before and after surgery except in 2 cases suffering from bleeding gastric ulcers. Pancreatic exocrine function maintained above 75% in the pancreatic function diagnostant (PFD) test after PPPD. At follow-up, an upper gastrointestinal barium study showed a good coordination of the movement of the upper gastrointestinal tract, and only slight reflux of barium into the interposed intestine was observed. Three patients died, 2 of recurrence of cancer and 1 of lung sarcoma. The remaining 10 patients have been in good condition for a follow-up period from 6 months to more than 5 years. In conclusion, it is considered that our method of reconstruction of the alimentary tract after PPPD (or PD) brings about a good nutritional state because the upper jejunum is used efficiently and both pancreatic juice and bile are mixed with ingested food at a location close to the stomach.

Key words. Pylorus-preserving   pancreatoduodenectomy—Pancreatoduodenectomy—Alimentary tract reconstruction—Nutritional state—Follow-up study

Department of Surgery, National Sendai Hospital, Miyagino-ku, Sendai, Miyagi 983, Japan.

Introduction

Nowadays, pancreatoduodenectomy (PD) or pylorus-preserving pancreatoduo-denectomy (PPPD) is widely performed with low morbidity and low mortality. Although it seems that the use of PPPD overcame several sequelae resulting mainly from gastric resection, there may still be serious complications such as gastric stasis or peptic ulcer. Moreover, new complications relating to the reconstruction method of the alimentary tract such as reflux cholangitis may arise with PPPD. Through follow-up studies of patients undergoing PD accompanied by Child's reconstruction method, we found that the release of several gastrointestinal hormones such as gastrin, gastric inhibitory polypeptide (GIP), and insulin was diminished after surgery, accompanied by anacidity, disturbance of glucose metabolism, body weight loss, etc. [1,2].

It was assumed that these sequelae were brought about by the massive resection of the upper gastrointestinal tract with the pancreatic head, so we devised a new method of alimentary tract reconstruction after PD. When we performed experimental studies using dogs, we obtained satisfactory results: in the group of dogs undergoing our devised reconstruction method, loss of body weight was much less than for Child's method, and the increase of plasma triglyceride and both cholecystokinin (CCK) and secretin levels after ingestion of butter were greater in the former group than in the latter [3]. We therefore applied this new reconstruction method to patients undergoing PD. Around that time, PPPD, which had been devised by Watson in 1994 [4], was introduced by Traverso and Longmire [5]. Because of nutritional improvement solving troublesome steatorrhea, which was usually observed after PD, many surgeons were quick to follow this procedure. As we were confident about the postoperative course of those patients undergoing PD with our reconstruction method [6], we applied it also to patients undergoing PPPD.

In the present study, we examined the postoperative outcomes of patients who underwent PPPD with our method of alimentary tract reconstruction and further compared them with those of patients undergoing the classical Whipple's procedure.

Subjects and Methods

As shown in Table 1, 13 patients underwent PPPD with reconstruction of the alimentary tract using our method. Briefly, the whole stomach and the duodenal bulb, about 4 cm in length, were preserved, and both the right gastric artery and the pyloric branch of the anterior vagal nerve were also preserved in most cases. The oral stump of the jejunum was anastomosed to the duodenal bulb in an end-to-end fashion so as not to form a blind loop, that is, to facilitate efficient contact between the upper jejunum and ingested food. A short intestinal segment, 20 cm long, was interposed between the pancreatic and bile ducts and the upper jejunum to prevent reflux of intestinal contents into the pancreatic and bile ducts. As for the interposed intestine, a midportion of the small intestine was used. Both pancreatic juice and bile were allowed to flow into the upper jejunum, that is, the "new duodenum" (Fig. 1).

In these patients, body weight was measured before surgery, at discharge, and at follow-up, and postoperative gastric function was evaluated by the length of fasting period. Also, the following studies were done before surgery and about 4 weeks after surgery: (1) a gastric juice study using synthesized gastrin (Amogastrin, 4 μg/kg, i.m.) and (2) the pancreatic function diagnostant (PFD) test using p-amino-benzoic acid

TABLE 1. Our series undergoing intestinal interposition PPPD

Case	Age (yr)	Sex	Diagnosis	Stage	Follow-up period (yr, mo)	Prognosis
1. S.O.	80	M	Lower bile duct cancer	II	3,4	Died of lung sarcoma
2. H.W.	71	F	Pancreatic head cancer	IV	0,5	Died of recurrence
3. A.M.	62	F	Lower bile duct cancer	I	5,4	
4. T.W.	52	M	Cancer of papilla Vateri	I	2,7	Died of recurrence
5. S.K.	67	M	Cancer of papilla Vateri	I	4,4	
6. S.K.	54	M	Chronic pancreatitis		2,10	
7. T.S.	64	F	Localized stricture of pancreatic duct		2,8	
8. N.Y.	26	F	Solid cystic tumor		2,6	
9. K.C.	70	M	Lower bile duct cancer	II	2,2	
10. S.H.	45	M	Chronic pancreatitis (groove pancreatitis)		2,0	
11. A.F.	75	F	Mucin-producing tumor		1,11	
12. T.I.	73	M	Lower bile duct cancer		1,0	
13. H.T.	67	F	Serous cystadenoma		0,6	

PPPD, pylorus-preserving pancreatoduodenectomy.

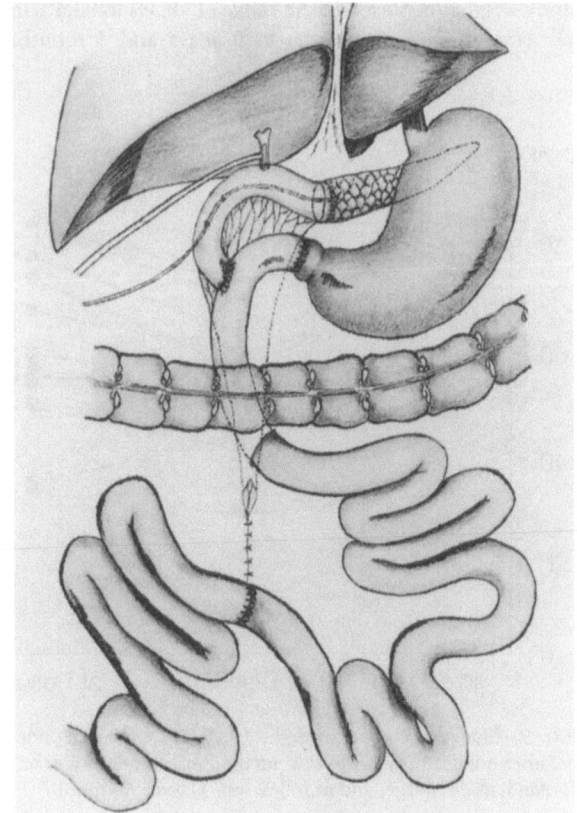

FIG. 1. Our method devised for alimentary tract reconstruction using an interposed midintestine following whole stomach- and duodenal bulb-preserving pancreatoduodenectomy. End-to-end duodenojejunostomy, end-to-end pancreatoenterostomy by the "dunking" method, end-to-side hepaticoenterostomy, end-to-side enterojejunostomy, and end-to-end enteroenterostomy are performed. The length of interposed midintestine is 20 cm. The pancreatic duct tube is led extracorporeally through the interposed intestine. The bile duct tube is also led extracorporeally

(PABA). At follow-up, upper gastrointestinal series were performed to observe the movements of the upper gastrointestinal tract and the regurgitation of barium into the interposed intestine. Control data for the period of postoperative fasting, gastric juice study, and PFD test were obtained from patients who underwent the classical Whipple's procedure.

Analysis of Data

All values were expressed as mean ± standard error of the mean (SEM). Student's t-test was used for statistical analysis of data. Statistical significance was accepted at the 5% level.

Results

Postoperative Gastric Function

Patients undergoing PPPD were fed a liquid meal starting at 9.9 ± .6 (range, 9–14) postoperative days, while patients undergoing the Whipple procedure started feeding at 5.6 ± .2 (range, 5–7) postoperative days ($P < .01$).

Body Weight

Body weight decreased in the range of −8.3% to −3.4% in all patients at discharge (Fig. 2). At follow-up, 6 months to 5 years and 4 months after surgery, body weight

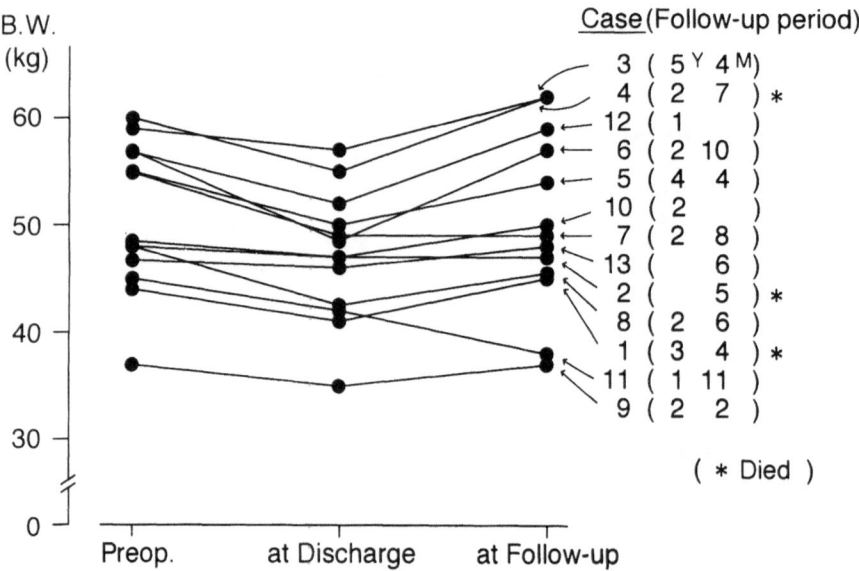

FIG. 2. Changes in body weight (*B.W.*) of patients undergoing pylorus-preserving pancreatoduodenectomy with our method of alimentary tract reconstruction: before surgery (*preop.*), at discharge, and at follow-up. Y, year; M, month

FIG. 3. Gastric acid output in response to tetragastrin (4 μg/kg, i.m.). *Open columns and open circles,* preoperative values; *hatched columns and hatched circles,* postoperative values (about 4 weeks after surgery). BAO, basal acid output, *left*; MAO, maximum acid output, *right*; values are mean ± SEM; *, P < .05. *ii PPPD,* intestinal interposition pylorus-preserving pancreatoduodenectomy

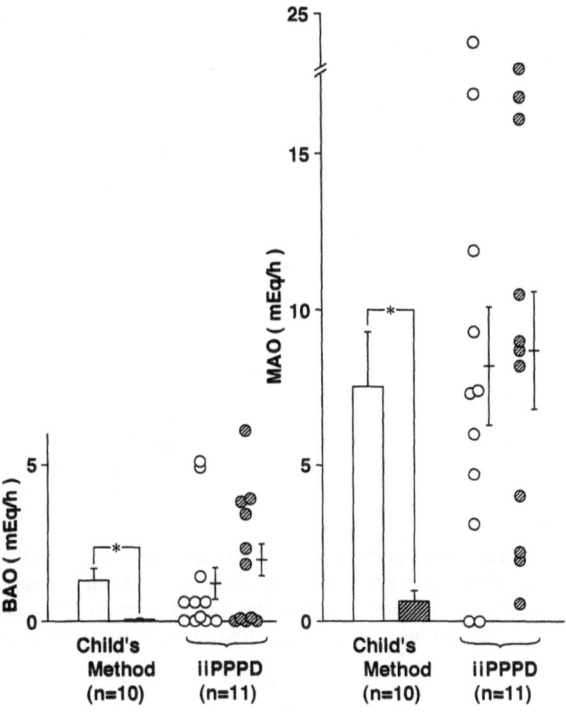

exceeded preoperative value by 2.3%–5.1% in six cases. In four other cases, body weight returned to preoperative values, and in three cases still remains below preoperative values.

Gastric Juice Study and Peptic Ulcer

Both basal acid output (BAO) and maximum acid output (MAO) were reduced significantly and approached anacidity in patients undergoing Whipple's procedure (Fig. 3). On the other hand, patients undergoing PPPD with our alimentary tract reconstruction method showed normoacidity in terms of BAO and MAO. Among them, two patients, however, showed hyperacidity preoperatively as well as postoperatively and developed a bleeding gastric lesion; one (case 4) suffered from acute gastric mucosal lesion (AGML) and another (case 6) from gastric ulcer. Case 4 was treated medically, while case 6 needed surgical treatment.

Pancreatic Exocrine Function

The value of the PFD test remained unchanged after PPPD with our reconstruction method; that is, 75.9% ± 5.1% before surgery and 77.1% ± 5.7% about 4 weeks after surgery. On the other hand, the value decreased after surgery in the group of Child's method; that is, 76.1% ± 2.8% before surgery and 64.9% ± 2.8% after surgery, although the difference was not significant.

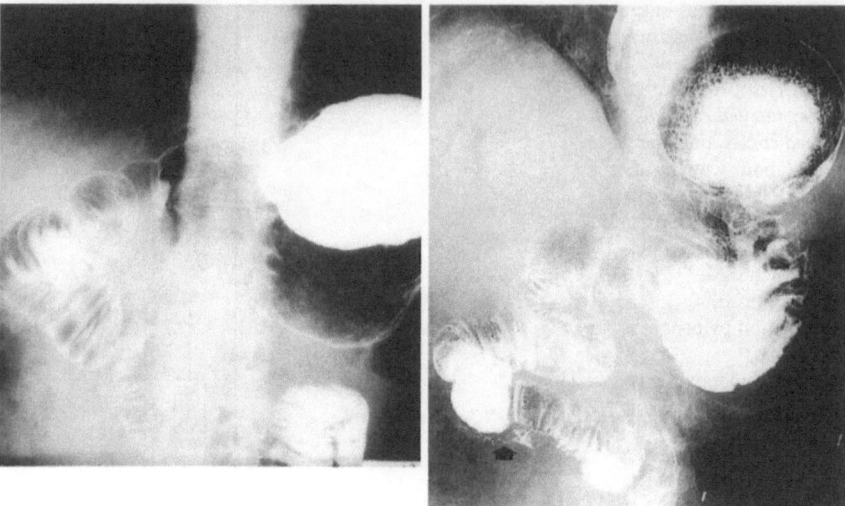

Fig. 4a,b. Upper gastrointestinal barium study demonstrates good coordination of the movement of the antrum, pyloric ring, duodenal bulb, and upper jejunum. a Case 5 (*left*): reflux of barium into the interposed intestine was not observed. b Case 7 (*right*): only a small amount of barium flowed back to the interposed small intestine (*arrow*)

Prognosis and Follow-Up Study

As shown in Table 1, 3 of 13 patients who underwent PPPD with our method of alimentary tract reconstruction died. Case 1 had surgery when he was 80 years old, and was in good condition for about 3 years after surgery, but died of lung sarcoma. Case 2, with far-advanced cancer of the pancreatic head, underwent a palliative PPPD hoping for a better quality of life. She died of growth of the remaining tumor. Case 4 was in excellent condition for more than 2 years after surgery, but the cancer recurred locally and also metastasized to the liver. Case 7 suffered from reflux cholangitis and acute pancreatitis, but responded well to medical treatment. Case 10 continued to drink alcohol after surgery and suffered from acute necrotizing pancreatitis, which needed surgical treatment. The remaining 8 cases have been well for the observation period of 6 months to more than 5 years.

Figure 4 shows the upper gastrointestinal series of cases 5 and 7 at 1 year after PPPD with our reconstruction method, denoting a cooperative movement of the gastric antrum, pyloric ring, duodenal bulb, and proximal part of the jejunum. Reflux of barium into the interposed intestine could barely be seen. Similar findings were observed on the upper gastrointestinal series in other cases.

Discussion

In the classical Child's method, the whole length of the duodenum is resected together with the oral portion of the jejunum, which has a very important role in the absorption of nutrients as well as in the release of several gastrointestinal hormones such as CCK and secretin. Therefore, it seems desirable to use the remaining upper jejunum as the food pathway instead of leaving it as a kind of blind loop as with Child's reconstruction method. Moreover, in our previous studies on reconstruction of the biliary tract, it was shown that jejunal interposition hepaticoduodenostomy is a more advantageous procedure than the Roux-en-Y-hepaticojejunostomy from the standpoint of gastric acid secretion and the release of gastrointestinal hormones [7–9]. These are the main grounds upon which we devised a new method of reconstruction of the alimentary tract after PD. Here, a short length of the midintestine is used for the interposition procedure, because a long interposed segment results in stasis of bile and intestinal contents [8] and because the ileum, especially the distal portion, is important for the enterohepatic circulation of bile [10] and also for the release of several gastrointestinal hormones such as enteroglucagon, peptide YY, and neurotensin [11–13], not to mention the importance of the remaining jejunum.

In 1960, Imanaga [14] devised a new reconstruction method of the alimentary tract after PD: the remaining stomach was anastomosed to the oral stump of the jejunum, and both the pancreatic and bile ducts were anastomosed directly to the upper jejunum in an end-to-side fashion. This procedure subsequently became common in Japan, and good pancreatic and liver function are expected after surgery. There have been, however, several reports of pyogenic cholangitis and liver abscess following this procedure [15]. To resolve those problems we used an interposed intestinal segment with a short length between the pancreatic and bile ducts and the upper jejunum. As shown in the upper gastrointestinal series, reflux of barium from the upper jejunum into the interposed segment was very slight. Although one patient suffered from mild reflux cholangitis, a biliary scintigram using ^{99m}Tc-PMT (pyridoxyl-5-methyl-tryptophan) revealed no delay of excretion of the radioisotope from the liver when her liver function recovered.

As shown in our series, PPPD brought about a good nutritional state, which was apparent from the increase of body weight in most cases at follow-up time. Still, there are several serious complications induced by PPPD, such as gastric stasis [16–18] and peptic ulcer [19–21]. In regard to gastric stasis, Warshaw and Torchiana [16] first reported a significantly increased gastric dysfunction during the early postoperative period. They emphasized the impairment of gastric muscular tone and peristalsis, rather than anastomotic obstruction or mechanical block, as the reason for delayed gastric emptying after PPPD. We usually administer H$_2$-blocker for a period after PPPD and observe the volume of gastric juice from the nasogastric tube. As mentioned previously, it took a significantly longer period for patients undergoing PPPD to start a liquid meal than for those undergoing PD with Child's method. In our procedure, both the antral and pyloric branches are preserved in most cases, so it is believed that the disturbances of propagation of movement over the anastomotic site (i.e., the duodenojejunostomy) would cause gastric stasis during the early period after surgery. Furthermore, it is known that hypersecretion of gastric acid inhibits both the interdigestive migration of contractions and gastric emptying [22,23]. Accordingly, it appears prudent to aspirate gastric juice sufficiently in addition to administration of H$_2$-receptor antagonist for a slightly longer period after PPPD.

Another point that should be taken into consideration is the presence of diabetes mellitus, especially in cases of pancreatic cancer or chronic pancreatitis. Kawagishi et al. [24] reported that the frequency of antroduodenal coordination was significantly reduced in patients with diabetes. Horowitz and Fraser [25] also reported retarded gastric emptying in about 50% of diabetic patients. In our series, case 2, who had pancreatic head cancer with diabetes, suffered from severe gastric stasis after PPPD and no gastrokinetic drugs were effective. Cancer of the pancreatic head is often accompanied by chronic pancreatitis and glucose intolerance. This indicates that prominent gastric stasis may occur postoperatively in patients with pancreatic head cancer as well as chronic pancreatitis. Case 8 (Table 1) was another patient who had severe gastric stasis; she was very thin, having a marked gastroptosis, and suffered from gastric motor dysfunction for a long period after PPPD in spite of administration of H_2-blocker and gastrokinetic drugs.

Another complication that should be considered in PPPD is the occurrence of stomal ulcer. In PPPD, especially when the duodenal bulb is preserved together with the whole stomach, this complication is lessened [19]. In this regard, in 1960 Anderson [26] first postulated the existence of a specific inhibitory mechanism for acid secretion in the duodenal bulb. In fact, Pearlman et al. [27] and Kim et al. [28] reported that gastric acid secretion did not change significantly after the PPPD procedure, which preserved the duodenal bulb. In our series, mean values of gastric acid secretion in terms of basal and gastrin-stimulated maximum secretion were not altered after PPPD. Moreover, pancreatic exocrine function, which was evaluated by the PFD test in the present study, was maintained in good condition after PPPD. Presumably, an adequate amount of bicarbonate could participate in neutralizing acid in the duodenal bulb and also in the "new" duodenum.

On the other hand, although Nishikawa et al. [19] reported a low incidence of peptic ulceration after PPPD, they also pointed out that the holding time of pH above 3–4 was shorter during the night, and that gastric acidity tended to increase after PPPD. In fact, in the series of Gebhardt et al. [20], 7 of 18 patients (39%) developed peptic ulcer. Tsao et al. [21] also reported a relatively high incidence of peptic ulcer after PPPD: marginal ulcer in 7% and bleeding gastritis in 2%. In our series of 13 patients, 2 had gastric bleeding from AGML or ulcer. Those two cases had hyperacidity even before surgery. Therefore, it should be considered that proximal selective vagotomy would be necessary for cases of hyperacidity if PPPD is indicated.

References

1. Sato T, Imamura M, Matsuno S, Sasaki I, Ohneda A (1986) Gastric acid secretion and gut hormone release in patients undergoing pancreaticoduodenectomy. Surgery 99:728–734
2. Matsuno S, Imamura M, Takeda K, Miyashita E, Miyagawa K, Sato T (1987) Pathophysiology and rehabilitation after pancreaticoduodenectomy (in Japanese). Nippon Shokakigeka Zasshi (Jpn J Gastroenterol Surg) 20:904–908
3. Imamura M, Yamauchi H, Kakizaki K (1991) Alimentary tract reconstruction following pancreatoduodenectomy: A new method with improvements in the nutritional state and gastrointestinal hormone release in dogs. Tohoku J Exp Med 164:111–123
4. Watson K (1944) Carcinoma of ampulla of Vater. Successful radical resection. Br J Surg 31:368–373
5. Traverso LW, Longmire WP (1978) Preservation of the pylorus in pancreaticoduodenectomy. Surg Gynecol Obstet 146:959–962
6. Imamura M, Yamauchi H, Kakizaki K (1991) Two cases undergoing a new reconstruction method of the alimentary tract after pancreatoduodenectomy (in Japanese with English abstract). Suizou (J Jpn Pancreas Soc) 6:90–97
7. Sato T, Imamura M, Sasaki I, Kameyama J (1982) Effect of biliary reconstruction on gastric acid secretion. Am J Surg 144:549–553

8. Imamura M, Kamayama J, Ohneda A, Sato T (1982) Effect of various reconstructions of the biliary tract upon the secretion of gastric acid and gastrointestinal hormones in dogs. Surg Gastroenterol 1:105–114
9. Sato T, Imamura M, Sasaki I, Kameyama J (1983) Gastric acid secretion and gastrointestinal hormone release after biliary tract reconstruction procedures. Am J Surg 146:245–249
10. Dietschy JM (1968) Mechanisms for the intestinal absorption of bile acids. J Lipid Res 9:297–309
11. Ghatei MA, Bloom SR (1981) Enteroglucagon in man. In: Bloom SR, Polak JM (eds) Gut hormones. Churchill Livingstone, London, pp 332–338
12. Adrian TE, Ferri G-L, Bacarese-Hamilton AJ, Fuessl HS, Polak JM, Bloom SR (1985) Human distribution and release of a putative new gut hormone, peptide YY. Gastroenterology 89:1070–1077
13. Doyle H, Greeley GH Jr, Mate L, Sakamoto T, Townsent CM Jr, Tompson JC (1985) Distribution of neurotensin in the canine gastrointestinal tract. Surgery 97:337–341
14. Imanaga H (1960) A new method of pancreaticoduodenectomy designed to preserve liver and pancreatic function. Surgery 47:577–586
15. Miyaishi S, Sato C, Nakamura H, Miyaishi M, Morimoto T (1992) Clinical and pathological analysis on status during 25 years after pancreaticoduodenectomy. Autopsy report of an 87-year-old female case (in Japanese). Tan To Sui (J Biliary Pancr) 13:307–314
16. Warshaw AL, Torchiana DL (1985) Delayed gastric emptying after pylorus-preserving pancreaticoduodenectomy. Surg Gynecol Obstet 160:1–4
17. Braasch JW, Rossi RL, Watkins E Jr, Deziel DJ, Winter PF (1986) Pyloric and gastric preserving pancreatic resection. Experience with 87 patients. Ann Surg 204:411–418
18. Itani KMF, Colemen RE, Akwari OE, Meyers WC (1986) Pylorus-preserving pancreatoduodenectomy. A clinical and physiologic appraisal. Ann Surg 204:655–664
19. Nishikawa M, Tangoku A, Hamanaka Y, Suzuki T, Rayford PL (1994) Gastric pH monitoring after pylorus-preserving pancreaticoduodenectomy with Billroth 1 type reconstruction. J Am Coll Surg 179:129–134
20. Gebhardt VC, Gall FP, Rosch W, Schackert HK (1982) Anastomosenulkus nach Whipplescher operation mit magenerhaltung. Zentralbl Chir 107:952–958
21. Tsao JI, Rossi RL, Lowell JA (1994) Pylorus-preserving pancreatoduodenectomy. Is it an adequate cancer operation? Arch Surg 129:405–412
22. Hayashi N, Mizumoto A, Itoh Z (1991) Inhibition of gastric acid secretion normalizes interdigestive motor activity in the stomach in dogs (in Japanese with English abstract). Nippon Shokakibyo Gakkai Zasshi (Jpn J Gastroenterol) 88:1168–1176
23. Dubois A, Castell DO (1981) Abnormal gastric emptying response to pentagastrin in duodenal ulcer disease. Dig Dis Sci 26:292–296
24. Kawagishi T, Nishizawa Y, Okuno Y, Shimada H, Inaba M, Konishi T, Morii H (1994) Antroduodenal motility and transpyloric fluid movement in patients with diabetes studied using duplex sonography. Gastroenterology 107:403–409
25. Horowitz M, Fraser R (1994) Disordered gastric motor function in diabetes mellitus. Diabetologia 37:543–551
26. Anderson S (1960) Inhibitory effects of hydrochloric acid in antrum and duodenum on gastric secretory responses to test meal in Pavlov and Heidenhain pouch dogs. Acta Physiol Scand 49:231–241
27. Pearlman NW, Stiegmann GV, Ahnen DJ, Schultz AL, Fink LM (1986) Acid and gastrin levels following pyloric-preserving pancreaticoduodenectomy. Arch Surg 121:661–664
28. Kim H-C, Suzuki T, Kajiwara T, Miyashita T, Imamura M, Tobe T (1987) Exocrine and endocrine stomach after gastrobulbar preserving pancreatoduodenectomy. Ann Surg 206:717–727

Pancreaticoduodenectomy for Benign Pancreatic Diseases: Surgical Management of Chronic Pancreatitis

Masao Kobari[1], Jan Axelson[2], and Seiki Matsuno[1]

Summary. The incidence of operative complications and mortality rate were studied in patients who underwent pancreaticoduodenectomy (PD) for benign pancreatic disease. Survival curves according to type of operation were compared in patients with alcoholic pancreatitis. From 1972 to 1994, 38 PD were done for a total of 365 patients with benign pancreatic diseases. The incidence of anastomotic leakage from the pancreaticojejunostomy was less in the patients with chronic pancreatitis (9%). Operative death occurred in 4 patients (2.4%) of 164 PD for malignant pancreatic diseases, but mortality was zero for patients with benign pancreatic diseases. In survival curves according to type of operation for patients with alcoholic pancreatitis, a statistical difference was not detected. The 20-year survival rate for patients who underwent PD was about 60%. Therefore, PD can be one procedure of choice in surgical management for chronic pancreatitis.

Key words. Pancreaticoduodenectomy—Pancreaticojejunostomy—Chronic pancreatitis

Introduction

Pancreaticoduodenectomy has been a standard method of surgical management for periampullary malignancies. Even though the operation can now be done with fewer complications, the outcomes of these complications are still severe, and this point is most important for surgeons. In this study, results of pancreaticoduodenectomy (PD) for benign pancreatic disease, especially focusing on chronic pancreatitis, are investigated.

Patients and Methods

From 1972 to 1994, 245 PD were performed for 580 patients with malignant pancreatic disease; the total resection rate was 42%. In 272 patients with pancreatic head cancer,

[1] First Department of Surgery, Tohoku University School of Medicine, Sendai, Miyagi 980-77, Japan.
[2] Department of Surgery, Lund University, Lund, Sweden.

TABLE 1. Number of patients undergoing pancreaticoduodenectomy (PD) for malignant disease

Disease	n	PD	Resection rate (%)
Cancer of the pancreatic head	272	73	27
Cancer of the papilla of Vater	84	63	75
Bile duct cancer	120	85	71
Duodenal cancer	15	5	33
Mucin-producing pancreatic tumor	21	10	48
Islet cell tumor	68	9	13
Total	580	245	42

From Tohoku University School of Medicine.

73 PD were performed, a resection rate of 27%. In patients with cancer of the papilla of Vater or lower bile duct cancer, the rates were 75% or 71%, respectively. Because half of mucin-producing pancreatic tumors were located in the body or tail of the pancreas, the number of patients who underwent PD for this disease was about half. Because most islet cell tumors were treated by enucleation or distal pancreatectomy, this rate for PD was only 13% (Table 1).

For a total of 365 patients with benign pancreatic diseases, 38 PD were done; the rate was only 10%. In patients with chronic pancreatitis, 27 PD were performed among 226 patients, a rate of 12%. For patients with benign pancreatic cysts, PD was done in only 5% of patients. For patients with trauma, the rate was 19% (Table 2).

For these patients with malignant or benign pancreatic disease who underwent PD, the incidence of operative complications or mortality rate was compared. Also, the results of surgical management for 215 patients with chronic pancreatitis were analyzed.

Results

Complications and Operative Death in Patients Undergoing PD

Leakage from the pancreaticojejunostomy (P-J), a major complication after PD, occurred in 5 of 47 (11%) patients who underwent PD for pancreatic head cancer; for 21 patients with chronic pancreatitis, the leakage rate was 9%. P-J leakage was more than 20% in patients with cancer of papilla of Vater (23%), bile duct cancer (21%), or mucin-producing pancreatic cancer (20%), and these rates were significantly higher compared with the rate in patients with chronic pancreatitis. P-J leakage occurred in more than half of patients with pancreatic trauma (54%). The operative death rate in this series was about 2%, and the mortality of patients with benign pancreatic diseases was zero.

Surgical Management for Patients with Chronic Pancreatitis

The causes of chronic pancreatitis among 215 patients were alcoholism (120 patients), idiopathy (53 patients), and gallstone (18 patients). A drainage operation for pancreatic duct was done 90 times. These operations included 43 Partingtons, 28 Puestows, and 7 Frey's operations. Pancreatic resections included 37 distal pancreatectomies, 22

TABLE 2. Number of patients undergoing pancreaticoduodenectomy (PD) for benign disease

Disease	n	PD	Resection rate (%)
Chronic pancreatitis	226	27	12
Pancreatic cysts	108	5	5
Pseudocysts	92	3	3
True cysts	16	2	13
Trauma	31	6	19
Total	365	38	10

From Tohoku University School of Medicine.

PDs, 5 pylorus-preserving PDs (PPPD), and 3 Berger's operations. In patients with alcoholic pancreatitis, 48 drainage operations and 45 pancreatic resections were done; 20 patients underwent PD. In patients with idiopathic pancreatitis, 25 drainage operations and 14 pancreatic resections including 6 PDs were performed.

Of 18 patients with alcoholic pancreatitis, PD was performed on the suspicion of pancreatic head cancer in 9. Indication for the drainage operation was intractable pain in 34 patients of 37. In half of the patients with idiopathic pancreatitis, distal pancreatectomy (DP) or PD was performed for suspected pancreatic cancer. Again, the indication for a drainage operation was pain. Overall, DP was done for complications or suspected cancer in half of the patients, and PD was selected for suspected cancer in more than half. Drainage operations were performed to relieve patients from pain.

Effect of Operations for Relief of Pain

In 83 patients who underwent drainage operations, the pain disappeared in 60 patients and was lessened in 21. In 98% of patients, the effect of pain relief was obtained by the operation. Similar results were found in pancreatic resections.

Effects of Operations on Diabetes Mellitus (DM)

In 14 patients with alcoholic pancreatitis who underwent DP, the diabetic state deteriorated or was not changed in 86%. This rate was 77% for 17 patients who underwent PD and 79% for 38 patients undergoing drainage operations. In patients with idiopathic pancreatitis, these rates were a little lower. Collectively, the diabetic state was not improved in 80% of patients who underwent DP, in 67% undergoing PD, and 72% with drainage operations.

Effects of Operations on the Quality of Life of Patients with Chronic Pancreatitis

In patients with alcoholic pancreatitis, DP improved the quality of life (QOL) of 67% of patients; PD improved the QOL in 68% of patients and drainage operations in 56%. In patients with idiopathic pancreatitis, drainage operations improved patient QOL in 84%. As a whole, both pancreatic resections and drainage operations improved patient QOL in more than 60% of patients.

Causes of Death

Of 6 deaths in 23 patients with alcoholic pancreatitis who underwent DP, 2 were caused by apoplexy, 2 by liver disease, 1 by cardiovascular disease, and 1 by an unknown cause. In the patients who underwent PD, 4 deaths were caused by DM. In 17 deaths in the patients who underwent drainage operations, 9 were caused by DM, 2 by apoplexy, and 4 by other causes, including unknown causes. As a whole, patients who underwent DP died of various causes, and half of patients who underwent PD or drainage operations died of DM.

Survival According to Type of Operation

No statistical difference was detected among survival curves of patients who underwent drainage operations, those who underwent PD, and those who underwent DP. The 20-year survival rates of patients who underwent one of these three types of operations was about 60%. However, the survival of patients who underwent PD became lower during the interval from 5 years to 15 years after their operation compared with survival rates of patients who underwent other types of operations.

In patients with alcoholic pancreatitis, no statistical difference was detected among the three types of operations. However, the survival of patients who underwent drainage operations dropped to 40% at 20 years after operation compared with 60% in the patients who underwent PD or DP.

At 15 years after operation, the survival curve of patients with idiopathic pancreatitis who underwent a drainage operation was 83% and was statistically higher than the survival curves of patients who underwent PD (30%) or DP (33%).

Discussion

Pancreaticojejunostomy is the method of choice for surgical treatment of pain in chronic pancreatitis in the case of ductal dilatation [1,2]. The study of effects of the drainage operation on abdominal pain and follow-up results showed exellent maintenance of operative benefit [1]. Residual pancreatic stones, however, are considered to be one of the causes of progression of the inflammatory process after a drainage operation because later results of surgical management for patients with pancreatic stones are worse than those for patients without pancreatic stones [3]. In this context, resective operations are thought to be better than simple drainage operations to suppress inflammation. In the present study, both drainage operations and PD could control pain effectively. Late results of both types of operation were good in more than 60% of patients undergoing the operations. No difference in survival curves between patients who underwent drainage operations and patients who underwent PD was detected. The incidence of leakage from the pancreaticojejunostomy was less in patients with chronic pancreatitis. Operative death from PD occurred in 2% of patients with malignant pancreatic disease but did not occur in patients with chronic pancreatitis. Many reports have indicated that PD provides excellent results in the relief of the pain of chronic pancreatitis [4]. Although resection of pancreatic tissue diminishes pancreatic function, the metabolic deficits are partially compensated by the better nutritional status resulting from pain relief and discontinuation of narcotics [4]. Also, PD for severe complications of chronic pancreatitis in the pancreatic head is reported to be a safe and effective operation leaving few gastrointestinal sequelae [5]. Therefore, PD can be one selection in surgical management for chronic pancreatitis.

On the other hand, such operative procedures as duodenum-preserving resection of the head of the pancreas reported by Beger [6] or local resection of the head of the pancreas combined with longitudinal pancreaticojejunostomy by Frey [7] have recently been introduced to avoid the disadvantages of PD, which necessitates resection of the stomach, the duodenum, and extrahepatic biliary tree. It has been shown that both techniques are equally safe and effective with regard to pain relief, improvement of QOL, and definitive control of complications [8]. Therefore, we have begun to perform Frey's operation instead of PD or the simple drainage operation and to analyze the effect of this new surgical management for patients with chronic pancreatitis.

References

1. Sato T, Miyashita E, Matsuno S, Yamauchi H (1986) The role of surgical treatment for chronic pancreatitis. Ann Surg 203:266–271
2. Ihse I, Borch K, Larsson J (1990) Chronic pancreatitis: results of operations for relief of pain. World J Surg 14:53–58
3. Matsuno S, Kobari M (1991) Surgical treatment for pancreatic stones. Mon Book Gastroenterol 1:67–73
4. Howard JM, Zhang Z (1990) Pancreaticoduodenectomy (Whipple resection) in the treatment of chronic pancreatitis. World J Surg 14:77–82
5. Traverso LW, Kozarek RA (1993) The Whipple procedure for severe complications of chronic pancreatitis. Arch Surg 128:1047–1053
6. Beger HG, Büchler M (1990) Duodenum-preserving resection of the head of the pancreas in chronic pancreatitis with inflammatory mass in the head. World J Surg 14:83–87
7. Frey CF, Amikura K (1994) Local resection of the head of the pancreas combined with longitudinal pancreaticojejunostomy in the management of patients with chronic pancreatitis. Ann Surg 220:492–507
8. Izbicki JR, Bloechle C, Knoefel WT, Kuechler T, Binmoeller KF, Broelsch CE (1995) Duodenum-preserving resection of the head of the pancreas in chronic pancreatitis. Ann Surg 221:350–358

Long-Term Follow-Up Study After Pancreatoduodenectomy for Benign Periampullary Disease

Mamoru Suzuki, Fujio Hanyu, and Toshihide Imaizumi

Summary. From 1968 to 1995, 196 patients underwent pancreatoduodenectomy for benign diseases. Of these, ninety-nine underwent standard pancreatoduodenectomy with gastrectomy and 97 underwent pylorus-preserving methods. Late postoperative complications developed in 35 patients: 19 patients had postoperative cholangitis, 8 had acute inflammation of the residual pancreas, and 6 had postoperative peptic ulcers. Reoperations were required in seven patients with cholangitis, in four with acute pancreatitis, and in three with peptic ulcers. The incidence of patients who required insulin injection was 28% at 10 years in patients with chronic pancreatitis, but 8% in those without chronic pancreatitis. Postoperative survival rates at 10 years were 55% in patients with chronic pancreatitis and 90% in those without chronic pancreatitis.

Key words. Pancreatoduodenectomy—Benign disease—Postoperative complication —Diabetes—Survival rate

Introduction

Traditionally, pancreatoduodenectomy has been associated with high mortality and morbidity rates. However, recent reports suggest that the mortality rates and morbidity rates for this operation have decreased. This decrease of postoperative mortality and morbidity rates has provided further indication for the use of pancreatoduodenectomy for benign periampullary diseases, including chronic pancreatitis, benign pancreatic tumor, and cystic disease of the pancreas as well. Whether pancreatoduodenectomy is indicated for benign diseases must be decided not only by early postoperative results but also by the long-term results. The aim of this study was to evaluate both early and late postoperative results after pancreatoduodenectomy to determine the indication of pancreatoduodenectomy for benign periampullary disease.

Department of Gastroenterological Surgery, Tokyo Women's Medical College, Shinjuku-ku, Tokyo 162, Japan.

TABLE 1. Surgical indications of pancreatoduodenectomy for Benign periampullary
disease

Condition	Patients (n)
Chronic pancreatitis	133
Pancreaticobilliary maljunction	17
Benign pancreatic tumor	16
Pancreatic true cyst	8
Benign bile duct stenosis	7
Others	15
Total	196

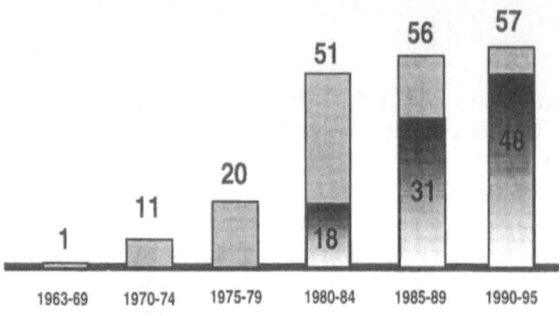

FIG. 1. Distribution by year of 196 pancreatoduodenectomies (PD) for benign periampullary
disease. *Lighter shaded bars,* PD (*n* = 99); *darker shaded bars,* PPPD (pylorus-preserving
pancreatoduodenectomies) (*n* = 97)

Materials and Methods

From 1968 to 1995, 196 patients underwent pancreatoduodenectomy at our hospital.
Indications for this operation were chronic pancreatitis in 133 and pancreaticobiliary
maljunction in 17; 16 patients had this operation for benign pancreatic tumor, including 8 islet cell tumors and 4 benign cystic lesions of the pancreas. True pancreatic cyst
was seen in 8 patients, benign bile duct stenosis in 7, and other diseases in 15 (Table
1). The number of pancreatoduodenectomies has been increasing year by year. The
first pancreatoduodenectomy was performed in our hospital in April of 1968. After
1980, the number of patients has increased remarkably. In 1984, the first pylorus-
preserving pancreatoduodenectomy was indicated for a young patient with pancreaticobiliary maljunction.

Since the introduction of pylorus-preserving pancreatoduodenectomy, the incidence of this procedure has increased. Between 1990 and 1995, of 57 pancreatoduodenectomies, only 8 patients underwent pancreatoduodenectomy with
gastrectomy. Among the 196 pancreatoduodenectomies for benign disease, 99 had
a standard pancreatoduodenectomy with gastrectomy and 97 had the pylorus-
preserving methods (Fig. 1). Two types of gastrointestinal reconstruction have been
performed in our hospital; 118 patients underwent gastropancreaticocholedoco-
jejunostomy and 75 had pancreaticocholedocogastrostomy. Gastrointestinal reconstruction after pylorus-preserving pancreatoduodenectomy was carried out with

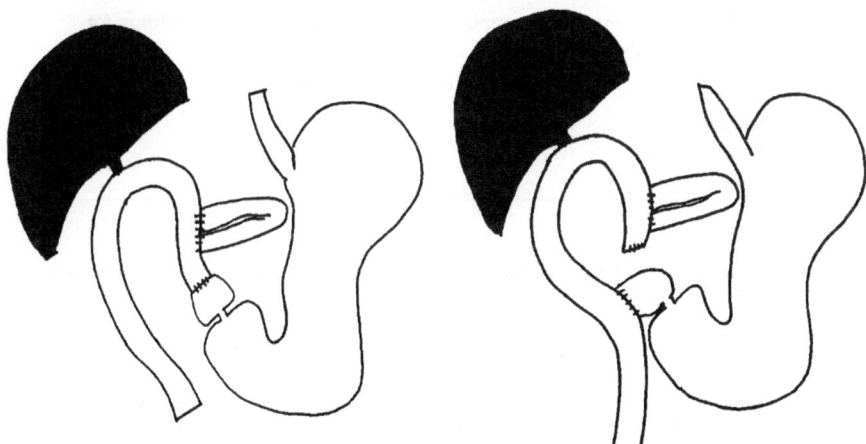

FIG. 2. Gastrointestinal reconstructions after pancreatoduodenectomy for benign ampullary disease. *Left*, gastropancreaticoholedocojejunostomy, $n = 118$; *right*, pancreaticocholedocogastroejejunostomy, $n = 75$ (other types, $n = 3$; not shown)

TABLE 2. Early postoperative results after pancreatoduodenectomy for benign periampullary disease

Result	Patients (n)	Percent
Operative death	0	
Hospital death	9	4
Major postoperative complications		
Massive hemorrhage	4	2
Major anastomosis leakage		
Pancreas	7	3
Bile duct	4	2

duodenopancreaticocholedocojejunostomy   or   pancreaticocholedocoduodenojejunostomy (Fig. 2).

Results

Operative mortality was 0, and 9 patients died before discharge from the hospital. Major postoperative complications occurred in 15 patients, including massive intraabdominal hemorrhage in 4 and major anastomosis leakage in 11 patients, from the pancreatoduodenectomy in 7, and from biliary anastomosis in 4 (Table 2). Late postoperative complications developed in 35 patients; 19 patients had postoperative cholangitis and 8 had acute inflammation in the residual pancreas. Postoperative peptic ulcer occurred in 6 patients who had received the pylorus-preserving procedure. Reoperation for late complications was indicated in 7 patients with cholangitis, 4 with acute pancreatitis, and 3 with a peptic ulcer (Table 3). Eight patients showed stricture of the choledochojejunal anastomosis. Bowel stasis in the jejunal loop or poor bowel movement were the cause of cholangitis in 6 patients, but the cause of cholangitis was unknown in 5 patients. Of the 8 patients with stricture of

TABLE 3. Late postoperative complications after pancreatoduodenectomy for benign periampullary disease

Complication	Number of patients	Patients requiring reoperation
Cholangitis	19	7
Acute pancreatitis	8	4
Peptic ulcer	6	3

TABLE 4. Cause of postoperative cholangitis after pancreatoduodenectomy for benign periampullary disease

Complication	Number of patients	Patients requiring reoperation
Stricture of choledoco jejunal anastomosis	8	5
Bowel stasis in jejunal loop	6	2
Unknown	5	0

TABLE 5. Cause of postoperative acute pancreatitis after pancreatoduodenectomy for benign periampullary disease

Complication	Number of patients	Patients requiring reoperation
Mechanical trouble of stent tube	3	2
Stricture of choledoco jejunal anastomosis	2	2
Unknown	3	0

choledocojejunostomy, 5 had reanastomosis; all 5 patients who underwent reanastomosis have been well. Two patients had segmental resection of the jejunum because of bowel stasis in the jejunal loop; these 2 patients also are well postoperatively (Table 4).

Among eight patients who developed acute inflammation in the residual pancreas, the cause of inflammation was mechanical trouble with the stent tube in three, stricture of the pancreaticojejunal anastomosis in two, and unknown in three patients. Reanastomosis of the pancreaticojejunostomy was carried out in four patients, and their postoperative courses after reoperation have been satisfactory (Table 5). The incidence of patients who required insulin injection was 12% preoperatively among patients with chronic pancreatitis; it increased to 17% at 3 years, 20% at 5 years, and 28% at 10 years postoperatively. On the other hand, the incidence was 4% at 3 years, 6% at 5 years, and 8% at 10 years in patients without chronic pancreatitis (Fig. 3).

Postoperative survival rates after pancreatoduodenectomy differed between patients with chronic pancreatitis and patients without chronic pancreatitis; the 5-year survival rate was 92% in patients without chronic pancreatitis and 80% with chronic pancreatitis. At 10 years, the survival rate was still high in patients without chronic pancreatitis but was about 55% in patients with chronic pancreatitis (Fig. 4).

Discussion

Because of the technical difficulty of pancreatoduodenectomy, many surgeons do not prefer this procedure for treatment of patients with benign periampullary diseases. In the past, the reported mortality rate after pancreatoduodenectomy was from 10% to

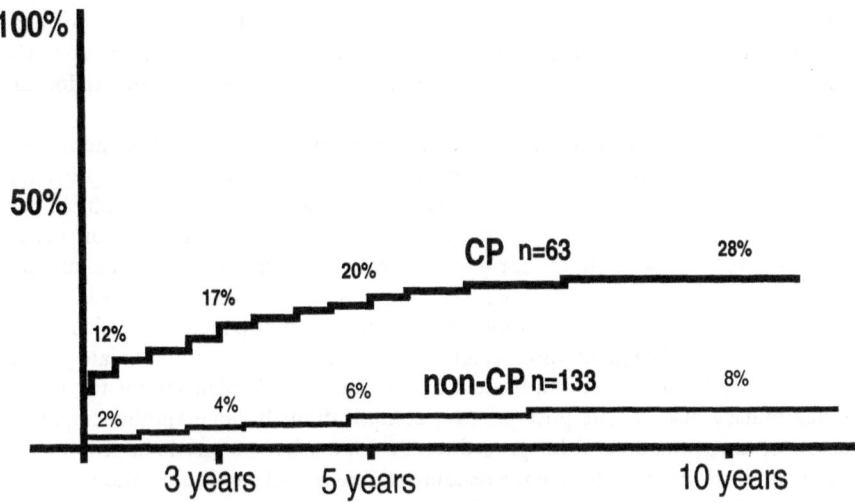

FIG. 3. Postoperative diabetes after pancreatoduodenectomy for benign periampullary disease. *CP*, chronic pancreatitis ($n = 63$); *non-CP*, other benign diseases ($n = 133$)

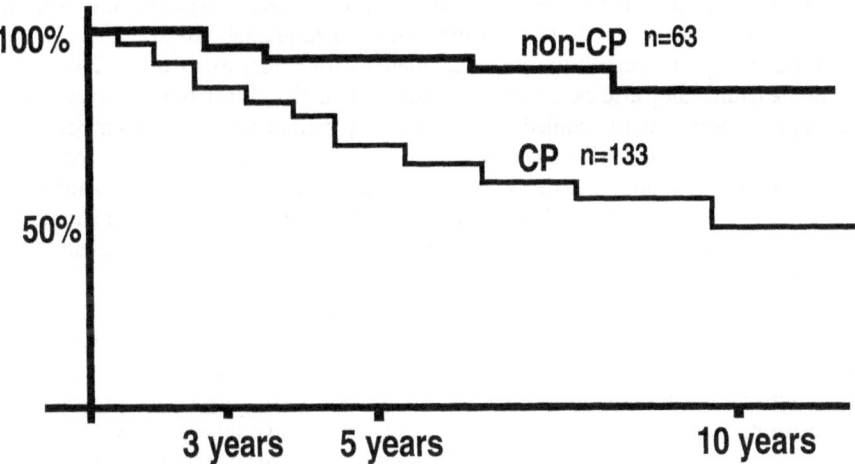

FIG. 4. Postoperative survival curves after pancreatoduodenectomy for benign periampullary disease. *Non-CP*, $n = 63$; *CP*, $n = 133$

15%. High mortality rates have limited this procedure to only periampullary malignant diseases. With advances in operative technique and postoperative management, the mortality and morbidity rates for this operation have decreased.

Recent reports suggest that mortality and morbidity after pancreatoduodenectomy are now less than 5% and 15%, respectively [1,2]. The reason for decreased early postoperative mortality was not only advances in operative technique but adequate management for early postoperative fatal complications, including leakage from the pancreaticojejunostomy or intraabdominal hemorrhage. A computed tomography (CT) scan is useful for diagnosis of intraabdominal abscess formation, and early drainage of the infected focus can be done. Rupture of the stump of the gastroduodenal artery is a serious postoperative complication and is the main cause of early operative death after pancreatoduodenectomy. Interventional radiotherapy with transarterial embolization has been useful in management of intraabdominal hemorrhage.

Decrease of postoperative mortality and morbidity rates provided further indication of pancreatoduodenectomy for benign periampullary diseases. This procedure has been used in the management of chronic pancreatitis with good results in pain relief [3,4]. In our series, indications of pancreatoduodenectomy for benign periampullary disease included chronic pancreatitis, pancreaticobiliary maljunction, benign pancreatic tumor, pancreatic true cyst, and benign bile duct stenosis.

Because there have been so few long-term survivors after pancreatoduodenectomy for periampullary malignant disease, few surgeons have paid attention to late postoperative complications. After introduction of pancreatoduodenectomy for benign periampullary disease, late postoperative complications became another important factor for determination of this procedure. Postoperative retrograde infection of the bile duct, acute inflammation of the residual pancreas, and peptic ulceration occurred in some patients between 1 and several years after pancreatoduodenectomy.

Postoperative retrograde cholangitis is the most common late complication after pancreatoduodenectomy [5], occurring 3 or more years postoperatively. Repeated unknown temperature rise with abdominal pain is a symptom of postoperative cholangitis, and its main cause is stricture of the choledochojejunostomy. Among patients who develop leakage from choledochojejunal anastomosis early-postoperatively, stricture of the choledochojejunostomy may easily occur. Bowel stasis in the jejunal loop also causes postoperative cholangitis. Weak bowel movement of the jejunal loop near the choledochojejunostomy cannot transport discharged bile adequately; bile juice with bacteria then causes retrograde infection from the choledochojejunostomy. Reanastomosis is required for patients whose cholangitis is caused by stricture of the choledochojejunostomy. Jejunal loop resection should be done in patients who develop retrograde cholangitis because of weak movement of the jejunum.

Postoperative acute inflammation of the residual pancreas was not a common complication. The cause of postoperative acute inflammation of the residual pancreas was related to insufficient drainage of the pancreatic juice at the pancreaticojejunal anastomosis. Mechanical trouble of the stent tube or stricture of the pancreatico-jejunostomy are the main reasons for acute postoperative inflammation of the residual pancreas. Reanastomosis or an additional side-to-side pancreaticojejunostomy must be performed for patients who do not obtain pain relief by conservative treatment.

The incidence of postoperative ulceration was reported to be 6%–10% [6]. Warrren showed that the original Whipple procedure with resection of the partial stomach was associated with a 17% incidence of anastomotic ulceration [7]. In our series, six patients developed severe symptomatic postoperative peptic ulcer. All six underwent pylorus-preserving pancreatoduodenectomy; peptic ulcer occurred 2–3 months postoperatively. Of the six patients, three required partial gastric resection because of intolerable symptoms. After introduction of the H_2-blocker, few patients suffered from severe symptoms of peptic ulcer.

Postoperative diabetes after pancreatoduodenectomy occurs in 20%–40% of patients with chronic pancreatitis [2,8]. Both massive resection of parenchyma of the head of the pancreas and severe fibrosis with poorly survived islet cells in the residual pancreas cause development of postoperative diabetes and sometimes cause nutritional disturbance. Diabetes is one of the most common causes of death after pancreatoduodenectomy. In our series, 20% of the patients who received pancreatoduodenectomy for chronic pancreatitis required insulin injection at 5 years postoperatively; the incidence increased to 28% at 10 years. Among patients without chronic pancreatitis, the incidence of diabetes requiring insulin injection was very low: 6% at 5 years and 8% at 10 years. From these data, resection of the head of the pancreas itself is not always the cause of diabetes postoperatively.

Postoperative survival after pancreatoduodenectomy also differs between patients with and patients without chronic pancreatitis. In our series, the 5-year survival rate was 80% in patients with chronic pancreatitis and 92% in patients without chronic pancreatitis. The postoperative survival rate decreased to 55% in patients with chronic pancreatitis at 10 years. This survival rate is almost the same as that of patients who received side-to-side pancreaticojejunostomy for chronic pancreatitis in our hospital and does not differ from data from other reports [1,2,9].

Pancreatoduodenectomy can be done safely for patients with benign disease and can provide fairly good postoperative results. However, it should be considered very carefully for patients with chronic pancreatitis to prevent late death as the result of diabetes and nutritional disturbance.

References

1. Moreaux J (1984) Long-term follow-up study of 50 patients with pancreato-duodenectomy for chronic pancreatitis. World J Surg 8:346–353
2. Rossi RI, Rothschld J, Braasch JW, et al (1987) Pancreatoduodenectomy in the management of chronic pancreatitis. Arch Surg 122:416–420
3. Traverso LW, Longmire WP (1978) Preservation of the pylorus in pancreato-duodenectomy. Surg Gynecol Obstet 146:959–962
4. Hanyu F, Suzuki M, Imaizumi T (1990) Resection of the head of the pancreas in the treatment of chronic pancreatitis. In: Beger (ed) Chronic pancreatitis. Springer, Berlin Heidelberg New York
5. Frey CF, Child CG, Fry W (1976) Pancreatectomy for chronic pancreatitis. Ann Surg 154:403–412
6. Grant CS, van Heerden JA (1979) Anastomotic ulceration following subtotal and total pancreatectomy. Ann Surg 190:1–12
7. Warren KW (1969) Surgical management of chronic relapsing pancreatitis. Am J Surg 117:24–32
8. Gall FP, Gebhardt C, Zisngibl H (1982) Chronic pancreatitis—results in 116 consecutive, partial duodenopancreatectomies combined with pancreatic duct occlusion. Hepato-Gastroenterology 28:115–120
9. Frey CF, Bodai B (1984) Surgery in chronic pancreatitis. Clin Gastroenterol 13:913–940

The Role of Pancreatoduodenectomy in the Management of Complex Pancreatic Trauma

Jake Krige[1], Philippus C. Bornman[1], and John Terblanche[2]

Summary. Major injuries to the head of the pancreas are uncommon but may result in considerable morbidity and mortality because of the magnitude of associated trauma or underestimation of the extent of the injury with consequent inappropriate treatment. Prognosis is determined by the cause and extent of the pancreatic injury, the amount of blood loss, duration of shock, and rapidity of resuscitation and surgical intervention. Early mortality results from uncontrolled or massive bleeding from associated vascular and large organ injuries. Late mortality is a consequence of infection and multiple organ failure. Neglect of major duct injury may lead to life-threatening complications including pancreatitis, pseudocyst, fistula, sepsis, and secondary hemorrhage.

Pancreatoduodenectomy is reserved for maximal injuries to the head of pancreas and duodenum in which salvage or reconstruction is not feasible. The need for resection is usually obvious when there is massive destruction with gross devitalization or pancreatobiliary, duodenal, and ampullary disruption requiring debridement that results in a near-complete pancreatoduodenectomy. With less severe trauma to the head of the pancreas, in particular penetrating injuries, the decision whether to resect or to adopt a more conservative approach is more difficult and requires the assistance of an experienced pancreatic surgeon. The success of the treatment of complex injuries to the head of the pancreas depends largely on the initial correct assessment and appropriate treatment. The management of severe injuries to the head of the pancreas remains one of the most difficult challenges in abdominal trauma surgery.

Key words. Pancreas—Surgery—Resection—Pancreatoduodenectomy

[1] Surgical Gastroenterology and Department of Surgery and [2] Department of Surgery, University of Cape Town and Groote Schuur Hospital, Cape Town 7925, South Africa.

Introduction

The principles of management of pancreatic injuries include the need for the early diagnosis and accurate definition of the nature and extent of injury to facilitate optimal surgical strategy [1–6]. Failure to accomplish these fundamental tenets may result in serious sequelae if the injury is underestimated or inappropriately treated [7]. The management of combined injuries to the pancreas and duodenum may be complex, especially if there is devitalized tissue and associated damage to contiguous vital structures including the bile duct, portal vein, vena cava, aorta, or colon [1,3,4,8]. Major complications including pancreatic fistula, pseudocyst, abscess, or hemorrhage occur in one-third of surviving patients [1,4,6,9–11]. The gravity of major pancreatic injuries and the potentially serious complications necessitate a comprehensive and multidisciplinary approach [1]. This review addresses the evaluation and management of severe injuries to the head of the pancreas with special reference to the role of pancreatoduodenectomy, based on our own experience and reported series.

Incidence

Trauma to the pancreas is uncommon, accounting for 1%–4% of severe abdominal injuries [7,8]. Recent data, however, indicate an increasing incidence of pancreatic trauma resulting from more frequent high-speed automobile accidents and an escalation in civil violence associated with increasingly dangerous weapons. In North American cities, penetrating abdominal injuries from gunshot wounds are the most common cause of pancreatic trauma, while in Western Europe and the U.K. the cause is usually road traffic accidents [1,6]. This geographic difference in etiology results in considerable variation in the reported incidence and severity of pancreatic injury [6].

Associated Injuries

Isolated injuries to the pancreas are infrequent. The incidence of associated injuries ranges from 50% to 90% and the mean number of organs injured in the same patient is 3.5 [4,12]. These associated injuries cause most of the morbidity and mortality linked with pancreatic trauma. The organs most commonly injured are the liver (42%), stomach (40%), major vessels (35%), thorax (31%), colon and small bowel (29%), central nervous system, skeleton, and extremities (25%), and duodenum (18%). Colonic injuries are more common after penetrating than blunt trauma and are associated with an increased incidence of postoperative sepsis [6,8]. Penetrating injuries also result in damage to retroperitoneal vessels in one-third of cases [3,4,8].

Mechanism of Injury

The unique anatomical features of the pancreas influence the site and type of injury. The proximity to major vascular structures and surrounding viscera adds to the complexity of injuries. The leakage of pancreatic exocrine secretions with duct disruption exacerbates the mechanical effects of pancreatic injury with consequent surrounding edema and tissue necrosis [3]. The nature and consequence of *penetrating* injuries depend on the type and kinetic energy of the wounding force. Penetrating injuries with adjacent contusions occur in single-fragment missile wounds, while severe fragmentation occurs with shotgun wounds. High-velocity missiles produce devastating and often lethal abdominal injuries. *Blunt* trauma to the pancreas and duodenum is usually the result of a direct blow to the upper abdomen caused by assault, pedestrian road traffic accidents, or torso deceleration against unyielding surfaces or steering wheels in unrestrained drivers or passengers without seat belts [1,3,6].

The mechanism of injury in blunt trauma relates to the direction of the impact force and the retroperitoneal position of the pancreas closely applied to the lumbar spine. Blunt upper-abdominal midline trauma results in posterior compression of the anterior abdominal wall against the spine, with injury to the pancreas over or to the left of the portal vein and superior mesenteric vessels. Impact forces concentrated to the right produce crush injuries of the pancreatic head and duodenum against the spine. Serious associated injuries including liver lacerations, and avulsions of the common bile duct and gastroduodenal, right, and middle colic vessels, compound the trauma [3,8,13].

Classification of Injuries

Comparisons between various forms of treatment are often difficult to interpret because isolated pancreatic injuries are infrequent, experience in most centers is limited, and there is no universally acceptable injury classification system. Several classifications have been applied to pancreatic injuries. The system proposed by Lucas [5] is the most widely used (Table 1).

Diagnosis

The retroperitoneal location of the pancreas contributes to delay in diagnosis because clinical signs may be subtle and late in onset. Blunt trauma to the pancreas may be clinically occult, and parenchymal and duct injury may go unrecognized during initial evaluation or during surgery. Awareness of these factors and recognition of the mechanism of injury should lead to a high index of suspicion. Delay in diagnosis and intervention is the most important cause of increased morbidity and mortality.

Serum amylase levels correlate poorly with the presence or absence of pancreatic trauma. Amylase levels may be normal in severe pancreatic damage or may be elevated when no demonstrable injury to the gland has occurred. Measuring serum isoamylase levels has also yielded disappointing results [6]. The incidence of hyperamylasemia in patients with proven blunt pancreatic trauma ranges from 25%

TABLE 1. Classification of pancreatic injury (from [5], with permission)

Class 1.	Simple superficial contusion or peripheral laceration with minimal parenchymal damage. Any portion of the pancreas can be affected, but the main pancreatic duct is intact
Class 2.	Deep laceration, perforation, or transection of the neck, body, or tail of the pancreas with or without pancreatic duct injury
Class 3.	Severe crush, perforation, or transection of the head of the pancreas with or without ductal injury
Class 4.	Combined pancreaticoduodenal injuries, subdivided into: (a) Minor pancreatic injury (b) Severe pancreatic injury and duct disruption

to 75%. Conversely, in patients with hyperamylasemia after blunt abdominal trauma, the pancreas has been found to be injured in 10%–90% of patients.

Plain Radiographs

A plain radiograph of the abdomen may raise the suspicion of pancreatic trauma, especially when associated with duodenal trauma. Gas bubbles in the retroperitoneum, adjacent to the right psoas muscle, around the kidneys, or anterior to the upper lumbar vertebrae seen on frontal or cross-table radiographs may indicate duodenal injury [4,8]. Free intraperitoneal gas may be present. Fractures of the transverse processes of the lumbar vertebrae are collateral evidence of forceful retroperitoneal trauma. Other indirect signs of pancreatic injury are displacement of the stomach or transverse colon or a general "ground-glass" appearance [4,5]. A gastrografin meal may demonstrate a duodenal leak with or without distortion of the duodenal C-loop.

Computerized Tomography

Computerized tomography (CT) is uniquely suited to the evaluation of pancreatic trauma. The main indications for CT are in hemodynamically stable patients with abdominal pain or tenderness after trauma who have suspected pancreatic injury and in the late complications of pancreatic trauma. Dynamic incremental bolus CT provides the optimal contrast enhancement of the pancreas necessary to identify subtle fractures. The CT findings of post-traumatic pancreatitis are time dependent and may not be evident on scans performed immediately after injury. The features of posttraumatic pancreatitis are edema and infiltration of the peripancreatic soft tissues, thickening of the anterior pararenal fascia, and focal or diffuse pancreatic enlargement [1].

Endoscopic Retrograde Cholangiopancreatography (ERCP)

ERCP is the most accurate method of detecting pancreatic ductal injury. The concept of preoperative endoscopic pancreatography is appealing as it avoids opening the duodenum and performing difficult operative cannulation of the papilla during laparotomy when a pancreatic duct injury is suspected. However, even in centers with the necessary expertise, the often impractical logistics involved in arranging ERCP outweigh the potential benefits. Preoperative ERCP is seldom feasible in acute pancreatic trauma because most patients require urgent laparotomy for bleeding or associated injuries. ERCP after blunt trauma to the pancreatic head or neck may be technically difficult because of distortion of recognizable landmarks, including the papilla, in the medial wall of the duodenum caused by intramural hematoma or surrounding peripancreatic edema. In addition, the patient's supine position, the need for high-quality X-ray facilities, and the necessity for complete vizualization of the pancreatic duct add to the technical difficulties.

Management

Operative Strategy

A long midline incision provides optimal exposure. In the presence of shock and a hemoperitoneum, the first priority is to identify the source of bleeding. Immediate survival is dependent on successful control and repair of major vascular injuries. The inaccessable retropancreatic position of the superior mesenteric, splenic, and portal veins make proximal and distal clamping or circumferential control of individual vessels impractical during massive bleeding. Rapid initial control is best obtained by surgical packing or digital pressure. Early duodenal mobilization and bimanual compression of the bleeding site is helpful if there is suspicion of a major portal or superior mesenteric vein injury. Vigorous resuscitation with blood and blood components should continue until bleeding has been staunched and normovolemia achieved. Thereafter, attention is directed to other priority visceral injuries before coping with the pancreatic trauma.

Intraoperative Evaluation

In most patients, the diagnosis of pancreatic injury is made at laparotomy. Determining the presence and extent of a pancreatic injury intraoperatively requires recognition of the features that indicate a potential pancreatic injury, adequate exposure of the pancreas, definition of the integrity of the pancreatic parenchyma, and determination of the status of the major pancreatic duct. This may be complicated by the extent and severity of associated injuries. A critical step in the evaluation is recognition of a disruption injury involving the ampulla, bile duct, and pancreatic duct. Gross inspection and palpation of the pancreas alone can be misleading as retroperitoneal or subcapsular hematoma and peripancreatic edema may mask major parenchymal and duct injuries.

Clues suggesting that a pancreatic injury is present include retroperitoneal bile staining or hematoma overlying the pancreas at the base of the transverse mesocolon or visible through the gastrohepatic ligament. Metastatic fat necrosis may be present if there has been undue delay before laparotomy. With such findings, complete visualization of the gland and accurate determination of the integrity of the pancreatic duct are crucial. Failure to recognize a major pancreatic duct injury is the principal cause of pancreatic injury-related postoperative morbidity.

The lesser sac is entered through the gastrocolic omentum outside the gastroepiploic arcade and, by retracting the transverse colon downward and the stomach upward, exposure of the anterior surface and the superior and inferior borders of the body and tail of the pancreas is obtained. Surrounding hematoma may complicate adequate assessment of the tail, and further detailed evaluation may require division of the lateral peritoneal attachments. For full inspection of the pancreatic head and uncinate process, the Kocher maneuver is necessary to mobilize the second part of the duodenum medially toward the superior mesenteric vessels. The dissection and downward reflection of the hepatic flexure of the colon and the mesocolon further improve exposure of the second portion of the duodenum and uncinate process [14]. All penetrating wounds should be traced through their entire intra-abdominal course to exclude pancreatic or other visceral injury.

Operative Pancreatography

Several radiological methods of intraoperative pancreatography to delineate the pancreatic duct have been recommended by other authors [3,6,8]. We have not found this to be technically feasible or practical. In the presence of an associated open duodenal injury, the papilla may be conveniently accessible and should be located. A firm squeeze of the gallbladder helps to identify the papillary opening by producing bile in the lumen. A fine lacrimal probe passed through the papilla into the pancreatic duct may provide sufficient information by demonstrating the position of an intact duct beyond the site of the injury. A skilled endoscopist may be of assistance in performing an intraoperative ERCP if logistics permit.

Treatment

Injuries to the head of the pancreas that do not involve the main pancreatic duct are best managed by simple external drainage. A controlled fistula thus created either settles spontaneously or may later require elective internal drainage after definition of the exact site of duct leakage. Techniques describing onlay Roux-en-Y loop anastomoses to incorporate injured areas in the head of the pancreas are not advisable because of the difficulty in assuring the integrity of the anastomosis in the acute event [3,6].

In determining the best option for patients with combined injuries, it is crucial to define the integrity of the common bile duct, pancreatic duct, and ampulla and the viability of the duodenum. If the existing injury is in the second part of the duodenum, careful retraction of the edges of the wound or extension of the laceration in the direction of the papilla may provide adequate exposure of the papilla. Gentle passage of a probe through the ampulla up the bile duct is generally sufficient to exclude injury to the bile duct and ampulla. Alternatively, a cholangiogram performed through the gallbladder or bile duct may provide the same information. If there is unobstructed flow of contrast into the duodenum without extravasation, the common bile duct and ampulla are likely to be intact. The presence of bile staining in the retroperitoneum or around the lower bile duct in the hepatoduodenal ligament raises suspicion of a bile duct injury or ampullary avulsion. If the duodenal injury involves the third or fourth part, which is remote from the ampulla, and there is concern about ductal integrity, a duodenotomy opposite the papilla is helpful to adequately evaluate the ductal system.

If the common bile duct and ampulla are shown to be intact, the duodenal laceration is repaired and the pancreatic injury treated according to the site of the injury. Penetrating injury in the pancreatic head without devitalization is best treated by careful drainage of the area. Localized ischemia at the site of the duodenal injury should be debrided before primary duodenal closure, and if there is concern about the integrity of the duodenum, decompression using a carefully placed nasogastric tube is useful.

With severe injury to the duodenum in association with a lesser pancreatic head injury, some authors advise diversion of gastric and biliary contents away from the duodenal repair [3,6,8]. Several complex and innovative techniques have been described to deal with this situation. Diversion can be accomplished by a duodenal "diverticulization" procedure that employs primary closure of the duodenal wound, a vagotomy, an antrectomy with an end-to-side gastrojejunostomy, a T-tube common bile duct drainage, and a tube duodenostomy. The aim is to convert a potentially uncontrolled lateral duodenal fistula into a controlled end-fistula by diversion of gastric and biliary contents away from the duodenal injury, while making provision for early enteral nutrition via a gastrojejunostomy.

An alternative option avoiding a vagotomy and antrectomy is the "pyloric exclusion" procedure. The pylorus is closed with an absorbable suture performed through a gastrotomy, and a side-to-side gastrojejunostomy provides temporary diversion of gastric flow away from the duodenum while the duodenal and pancreatic injuries heal. The pylorus opens when the sutures dissolve 3 or 4 weeks later, or the sutures can be removed endoscopically after an intact duodenum has been confirmed. In selected patients, pyloric exclusion has been reported to be useful in managing severe duodenal injuries combined with pancreatic head injuries in which a Whipple procedure is not justified [2–4,6,8]. We believe that the same objectives can be achieved by less complex procedures and in this situation we use primary duodenal closure, external catheter drainage near the site of the repair, a diverting gastrojejunostomy without closure of the pylorus, and a fine-bore silastic nasojejunal or percutaneous jejunal feeding tube.

Reconstruction may not be possible in combined injuries of the proximal duodenum and head of the pancreas with devitalization, complete disruption of the ampulla involving the proximal pancreatic duct and distal common bile duct, or avulsion of the duodenum from the pancreas. In this situation, the only rational option is Whipple's resection. Specific indications that have been proposed for pancreatoduodenectomy for trauma are (1) extensive devitalization of the head of the pancreas and duodenum so that reconstruction is not possible; (2) ductal disruption of the pancreatic head in association with injuries to the duodenum and distal common bile duct; (3) injury to the ampulla of Vater, with disruption of the main pancreatic duct from the duodenum; (4) uncontrollable bleeding from vessels in the head of the pancreas; and (5) inaccessible exsanguinating retropancreatic portal or superior mesenteric vein injury [15,16].

The technical procedure of emergency pancreatoduodenectomy is essentially similar to the elective operation. However, in cases in which there is penetrating injury to the retropancreatic portal mesenteric venous system with exsanguinating hemorrhage, the steps of the procedure change and are directed toward rapid exposure and control of the site of hemorrhage [17]. The duodenum and head of the pancreas are rapidly mobilized medially by the Kocher maneuver and the portal mesenteric venous system is compressed manually between the surgeon's thumb on the anterior aspect of the pancreas and his second and third fingers, which have been inserted through the foramen of Winslow, posterior to the pancreas and portal vein. This usually controls the bleeding. The lesser sac is then opened, the stomach retracted superiorly, the hepatic flexure of the colon mobilized inferiorly, and the neck of the pancreas divided to gain direct access to the site of injury. Once exposure of the portal–mesenteric–splenic venous confluence has been achieved, the vascular injuries can be identified and repaired [17].

Associated vena caval lacerations are best repaired by direct suture techniques. It is possible to repair the vena cava both anteriorly and posteriorly without mobilizing and clamping the vessel proximally and distally. Digital or stick sponge pressure above and below the rent controls bleeding while the defects are closed. A small posterior caval defect often can be sutured through an anterior rent without rotating the vessel. This is helpful when the wound in the vena cava is at the level of the renal veins. If a posterior rent cannot be visualized in this area, the kidney is mobilized and elevated medially, thereby exposing the junction of renal vein and vena cava [18].

Pancreatoduodenectomy may be necessary in 1%–3% of pancreatic injuries and in as many as 10% of combined pancreaticoduodenal injuries [2,17,52]. Pancreatoduodenectomy for trauma has been reported in 61 publications, involving 205 patients with an overall mortality of 34% (Table 2). Three series have treated 10 or

TABLE 2. Pancreatoduodenectomy for trauma

Author	Year	No. of patients	Survivors	Mortality (%)
Thal [19]	1964	2	1	50
Thompson [20]	1966	2	1	50
Walters [21]	1966	1	1	0
Salyer [22]	1967	1	1	0
Wilson [23]	1967	4	3	25
Brawley [24]	1968	3	1	67
Werschky [25]	1968	1	0	100
Foley [26]	1969	3	3	0
Halgrimson [27]	1969	3	3	0
Pantazelos [28]	1969	1	1	0
Gibbs [29]	1970	1	1	0
Bach [15]	1971	5	1	20
Nance [30]	1971	5	3	40
Smith [31]	1971	5	3	40
Roman [32]	1971	3	2	33
Jones [33]	1971	3	3	0
Salam [34]	1972	4	3	25
White [35]	1972	5	5	0
Owens [36]	1973	3	2	33
Steele [37]	1973	3	0	100
Anderson [38]	1973	2	1	50
Sturm [39]	1973	5	2	60
Anane-Sefah [40]	1975	6	6	0
Chambers [18]	1975	3	3	0
Yellin [17]	1975	10	4	60
Lucas [41]	1975	4	3	25
Balasegaram [42]	1976	8	3	62
Heyse-Moore [43]	1976	1	1	0
Heitsch [44]	1976	2	0	100
Karl [45]	1977	1	0	100
Lowe [16]	1977	6	6	0
Hagan [46]	1978	2	0	100
Graham [47]	1979	6	4	33
Majeski [48]	1980	1	1	0
Flint [49]	1980	3	1	33
Stone [12]	1981	3	0	100
Cogbill [50]	1982	1	1	0
Henarejos [51]	1983	3	1	67
Fabian [52]	1984	1	0	100
Moore [53]	1984	1	1	0
Oreskovich [54]	1984	10	10	0
Sims [55]	1984	2	2	0
Hassan [56]	1984	1	1	0
Levison [57]	1984	2	1	50
Adkins [58]	1984	5	4	20
Ivatury [59]	1985	7	4	43
Jones [13]	1985	8	5	38
Smego [10]	1985	1	1	0
Wynn [60]	1985	3	1	67
Hendel [61]	1985	1	1	0
Walker [62]	1986	1	1	0
Feliciano [2]	1987	13	7	46
Melissas [63]	1987	1	1	0

TABLE 2. *Continued*

Author	Year	No. of patients	Survivors	Mortality (%)
McKone [64]	1988	5	5	0
Eastlick [65]	1990	1	1	0
Ivatury [66]	1990	6	4	33
Heimansohn [67]	1990	6	6	0
Gentillo [68]	1991	6	2	67
Delcore [69]	1994	4	4	0
Mistry [70]	1996	1	1	0
Krige [1]	1995	9	7	22
Total		220	145	34

more patients [2,17,54]. Ten patients underwent pancreatoduodenectomy for either gunshot (8) or blunt trauma (2) to the pancreas at the Los Angeles County–University of Southern California Medical Center [17]. Seven patients had a standard resection and 3 underwent total pancreatectomy; 4 of the 10 patients survived. Of 117 patients with pancreatic injuries treated in a 6-year period in Seattle, 10 underwent pancreatoduodenectomy for nonreconstructible injury to the ampulla or severe combined pancreatoduodenal injuries [54]. Seven injuries were caused by gunshot wounds and 3 by blunt trauma. Ninety percent of the patients had associated intraabdominal injuries with an average of 3.4 organ systems involved. All 10 patients survived. In Houston (Texas, U.S.A.), 13 of 129 patients with pancreatoduodenal injuries treated during an 18-year period underwent pancreatoduodenectomy for complex trauma [2]. Ten had a standard resection and 3 total pancreatectomy; 6 of the 13 patients died. In a further ten series totaling 1554 patients with pancreatoduodenal injuries, 57 (3.6%) required a pancreatoduodenectomy (Table 3).

Nine patients underwent a Whipple resection for trauma in our hospital during a 60-month period. All patients were men, of median age 24 years (range, 14–40 years). Six had sustained gunshot wounds involving the head of the pancreas and three had blunt trauma to the abdomen; eight of the nine patients were shocked on admission to the trauma unit. The median delay between injury and definitive operation was 4h (range, 2–88h). The mean number of associated injuries was 3.4, and six patients had associated inferior vena cava (IVC) injuries. Seven underwent a pylorus-preserving pancreatoduodenectomy and two a standard Whipple resection because injury extending to involve the pylorus precluded a pylorus-preserving resection. The median intraoperative blood replacement was 12 units (range, 8–32 units). The median duration of surgery was 5h and 35min (range, 4h and 20min to 6h and 45min). Two patients died postoperatively of multiorgan failure. Five patients developed anastomotic leaks caused by pancreatic (two), biliary (two), or duodenojejunal (one) fistulas. Two patients had delayed gastric emptying and three required percutaneous catheter drainage of intraabdominal fluid collections. Two patients had late complications; one developed alcohol-induced pancreatitis and the other malabsorption, which resolved with pancreatic enzyme replacement therapy. The factors complicating surgery were the presence of shock on admission, the number of associated injuries, coagulopathy, hypothermia, gross bowel edema, and traumatic pancreatitis.

Technical problems arise in the reconstruction of pancreatic and biliary anastomoses because of the small size of the ducts and the soft and friable consistency of the

TABLE 3. Frequeny of pancreatoduodenectomy (PD) in patients with pancreatoduodenal trauma (from [69], with permission)

Author	Year published	Study period	No. of patients with pancreatoduodenal injuries	No. of patients requiring PD (and %)
Stone [12]	1981	1950–1980	283	3 (1)
Sims [55]	1984	1972–1979	54	2 (4)
Adkins [58]	1985	1973–1983	56	5 (9)
Jones [13]	1985	1950–1985	500	12 (2)
Smego [10]	1985	1976–1982	72	1 (1)
Wynn [60]	1985	1970–1983	84	3 (3)
Feliciano [2]	1987	1969–1985	129	13 (10)
Mansour [71]	1989	1977–1989	62	4 (7)
Cogbill [72]	1990	1983–1988	164	5 (3)
Krige [1]	1995	1986–1995	150	9 (6)
Total			1554	57 (3.6)

pancreatic parenchyma. For the pancreatic anastomosis, invagination of the end of the pancreas into a Roux-en-Y jejunal loop is the most widely used technique. We however have used a pancreatogastrostomy in this situation with minimal morbidity. In an acutely injured patient with severe associated injuries, pancreatogastrostomy offers several advantages over pancreatojejunostomy. Enterokinase is present in the small bowel but not the stomach, and the active form, trypsin, requires an alkaline environment to function. Pancreatogastrostomy avoids the creation of a long jejunal loop, and the anatomical proximity of the posterior stomach wall to the pancreas allows a tension-free anastomosis. The thick stomach wall holds sutures well and is less likely to develop ischemic complications than a jejunal loop, the vascular supply of which is most tenuous at its distal end and may be compromised during mobilization [69]. Biliary-enteric continuity is usually restored with a side-to-side choledochojejunostomy or hepaticojejunostomy using a high bile duct reconstruction technique with preplaced sutures.

Because major vascular injuries are frequent, massive blood loss, coagulopathy, and hypothermia are often present by the time the pancreatic repair is undertaken. Gross bowel edema and localized pancreatitis may aggravate the technical aspects of the pancreaticoduodenectomy and jeopardize the anastomosis. In unstable patients with serious associated injuries, simple controlled drainage and delayed reconstruction may be the most judicious and appropriate procedure [73].

Postoperative Care

The principles of postoperative care in patients undergoing resection for complex pancreatic injuries are similar to those in patients with other major abdominal injuries. Attention is paid to ventilatory status, fluid balance, renal function, intestinal ileus, and nasogastric tube losses. Meticulous charting of drain content and volume is important. Prolonged ileus and pancreatic complications may preclude normal oral intake in severely injured patients. A catheter jejunostomy using a submucosal needle technique or a fine-bore silastic nasogastric tube with a weighted tip placed at the initial operation in all complex pancreatic injuries allows the option of early postoperative enteral feeding rather than total parenteral nutrition. The enteral route is more efficient for nitrogen utilization and may be more effective in restoring immunocompetence. In addition, the morbidity and cost of enteral nutrition are considerably less than for parenteral nutrition.

The most common specific complication is a pancreatic fistula, which occurs in 10%–20% of major injuries to the pancreas. The majority of fistulas are minor and resolve spontaneously within 1 or 2 weeks of the injury, provided that adequate external drainage has been established. High-output fistulas (>700 ml/day) usually indicate major pancreatic duct or anastomotic disruption. A careful limited gastrografin meal is useful to establish the cause and site of the fistula as well as to plan further therapy if a high-output fistula fails to progressively decrease in volume or persists more than 10 days. Nutritional support should be provided throughout this period. Somatostatin has been used with variable results.

Peripancreatic, subhepatic, and subphrenic fluid collections are common, and the diagnosis is confirmed on ultrasound or CT. Clinical evidence of intraabdominal sepsis mandates guided aspiration to obtain fluid for bacteriology and amylase content. Empiric broad-spectrum parenteral antibiotic therapy should be instituted to cover the full bacterial spectrum until definitive culture results become available. Percutaneous aspiration or catheter drainage is usually effective in patients with accessible unilocular collections and no evidence of pancreatic necrosis. The presence of necrotic pancreatic tissue generally mandates surgery with debridement of nonviable tissue and generous external catheter drainage, although percutaneous insertion of large-bore drainage catheters may be beneficial in selected cases. Secondary hemorrhage from the pancreatic bed or surrounding vessels as a consequence of infected devitalized tissue and retroperitoneal autodigestion from uncontrolled pancreatic drainage is an uncommon but formidable complication after pancreatic trauma. Failing control by angiographic embolization, operative exposure and packing with abdominal swabs may be life saving.

References

1. Krige JEJ, Bornman PC, Beningfield SJ, Funnell IC (1995) Pancreatic trauma. In: Pitt H, Carr-Locke D, Ferrucci J (eds) Hepatobiliary and pancreatic disease. Little, Brown, Philadelphia, pp 421–435
2. Feliciano DV, Martin TD, Cruse PA, Graham JM, Burch JM, Mattox KL, Bitondo CG, Jordan GL (1987) Management of combined pancreatoduodenal injuries. Ann Surg 205:673–680
3. Frey CF, Wardell JW (1993) Injuries to the pancreas. In: Trede M, Carter DC (eds) Surgery of the pancreas. Churchill Livingstone, Edinburgh, pp 565–589
4. Jurkovich GJ, Carrico CJ (1990) Pancreatic trauma. Surg Clin North Am 70:575–593
5. Lucas CE (1977) Diagnosis and treatment of pancreatic and duodenal injury. Surg Clin North Am 57:49–65
6. Wilson RH, Moorehead RJ (1991) Current management of trauma to the pancreas. Br J Surg 78:1196–1202
7. Lewis G, Krige JEJ, Bornman PC, Terblanche J (1993) Traumatic pancreatic pseudocysts. Br J Surg 80:89–93
8. Glancy KE (1989) Review of pancreatic trauma. West J Med 151:45–51
9. Funnell IC, Bornman PC, Krige JEJ, Beningfield SJ, Terblanche J (1994) Endoscopic drainage of traumatic pancreatic pseudocysts. Br J Surg 81:879–881
10. Smego DR, Richardson JD, Flint LM (1985) Determinants of outcome in pancreatic trauma. J Trauma 25:771–776

11. Wisner DH, Wold RL, Frey CF (1990) Diagnosis and treatment of pancreatic injuries. An analysis of management principles. Arch Surg 125:1109–1113
12. Stone HH, Fabian TC, Satiani B, Turkleson ML (1981) Experiences in the management of pancreatic trauma. J Trauma 21:257–262
13. Jones RC (1985) Management of pancreatic trauma. Am J Surg 150:698–704
14. Sawyers JL, Carlisle BB, Sawyers JE (1967) Management of pancreatic injuries. South Med J 60:382–386
15. Bach RD, Frey CF (1971) Diagnosis and treatment of pancreatic trauma. Am J Surg 121:20–29
16. Lowe RJ, Saletta JD, Moss GS (1977) Pancreaticoduodenectomy for penetrating pancreatic trauma. J Trauma 17:732–741
17. Yellin AE, Rosoff L (1975) Pancreatoduodenectomy for combined pancreatoduodenal injuries. Arch Surg 110:1117–1183
18. Chambers RT, Norton L, Hinchey EJ (1975) Massive right upper quadrant intra-abdominal injury requiring pancreaticoduodenectomy and partial hepatectomy. J Trauma 15:714–719
19. Thal AP, Wilson RF (1964) A pattern of severe blunt trauma to the region of the pancreas. Surg Gynecol Obstet 119:773–778
20. Thompson RJ, Hindshaw DB (1966) Pancreatic trauma. Ann Surg 163:153–160
21. Walters RL, Gaspard DJ, Germann TD (1966) Traumatic pancreatitis. Am J Surg 111:364–368
22. Salyer K, McClelland RN (1967) Pancreatoduodenectomy for trauma. Arch Surg 95:636–639
23. Wilson RF, Tagett JP, Pucelik JP (1967) Pancreatic trauma. J Trauma 7:643–651
24. Brawley RK, Cameron JL, Zuidema G (1968) Severe upper abdominal injuries treated by pancreaticoduodenectomy. Surg Gynecol Obstet 126:516–522
25. Werschky LR, Jordan GL (1968) Surgical management of traumatic injuries to the pancreas. Am J Surg 116:768–772
26. Foley WJ, Gaines RD, Fry WJ (1969) Pancreaticoduodenectomy for severe trauma to the head of the pancreas and associated structures. Ann Surg 170:759–765
27. Halgrimson CG, Trimble C, Gale S, Waddell WR (1969) Pancreaticoduodenectomy for traumatic lesions. Am J Surg 118:877–882
28. Pantazelos HH, Kerhulas AA, Byrne JJ (1969) Total pancreaticoduodenectomy for trauma. Ann Surg 170:1016–1020
29. Gibbs BF, Crow JL, Rupnik EJ (1971) Pancreaticoduodenectomy for blunt pancreaticoduodenal injury. J Trauma 10:702–705
30. Nance FC, DeLoach DH (1971) Pancreaticoduodenectomy following abdominal trauma. J Trauma 11:577–782
31. Smith AD, Woolverton WC, Weichert RF, Drapanas T (1971) Operative management of pancreatic and duodenal injuries. J Trauma 14:570–579
32. Roman E, Silva YJ, Lucas C (1971) Management of blunt duodenal injury. Surg Gynecol Obstet 129:7–14
33. Jones RC, Shires GT (1971) Pancreatic trauma. Arch Surg 102:424–430
34. Salam A, Warren WD, Kalser M, Laguna V (1972) Pancreatoduodenectomy for trauma: clinical and metabolic studies. Ann Surg 175:663–672
35. White PH, Benfield JR (1972) Amylase in the management of pancreatic trauma. Arch Surg 105:158–163
36. Owens MP, Wolfman EF (1973) Pancreatic trauma: management and presentation of a new technique. Surgery (St Louis) 73:881–886
37. Steele M, Sheldon GF, Blaisdell FW (1973) Pancreatic injuries. Arch Surg 106:544–549
38. Anderson CB, Weisz D, Rodger MR, Tucker GL (1973) Combined pancreaticoduodenal trauma. Am J Surg 125:530–534
39. Sturm JT, Quattlebaum FW, Mowlem A, Perry JF (1973) Patterns of injury requiring pancreatoduodenectomy. Surg Gynecol Obstet 132:629–632
40. Anane-Sefah J, Norton LW, Eiseman B (1975) Operative choice and technique following pancreatic injury. Arch Surg 110:161–166

41. Lucas CE, Ledgerwood AM (1975) Factors influencing outcome after blunt duodenal injury. J Trauma 15:839–446
42. Balasegaram M (1976) Surgical management of pancreatic trauma. Am J Surg 131:536–540
43. Heyse-Moore GH (1976) Blunt pancreatic and pancreaticoduodenal trauma. Br J Surg 63:226–228
44. Heitsch RC, Knutson CO, Fulton RL, Jones CE (1976) Delineation of critical factors in the treatment of pancreatic trauma surgery. Surgery (St Louis) 80:523–529
45. Karl HW, Chandler JG (1977) Mortality and morbidity of pancreatic injury. Am J Surg 134:549–554
46. Hagan WV, Urdaneta LF, Stephenson SE (1978) Pancreatic injury. South Med J 171:892–894
47. Graham JM, Mattox KL, Vaughan GD, Jordan GL (1979) Combined pancreatoduodenal injuries. J Trauma 19:340–346
48. Majeski JA, Tyler G (1980) Pancreatic trauma. Am Surg 46:593–596
49. Flint LM, McCoy M, Richardson D, Polk H (1980) Duodenal injury. Analysis of common misconceptions in diagnosis and treatment Ann Surg 191:697–702
50. Cogbill TH, Moore EE, Kashuk JL (1982) Changing trends in the management of pancreatic trauma. Arch Surg 117:722–728
51. Henarejos A, Cohen DM, Moosa AR (1983) Management of pancreatic trauma. Ann R Coll Surg Engl 65:297–300
52. Fabian TC, Mangiante EC, Millis M (1984) Duodenal rupture due to blunt trauma: a problem in diagnosis. South Med J 77:1078–1082
53. Moore JB, Moore EE (1984) Changing trends in the management of combined pancreatoduodenal injuries. World J Surg 8:791–797
54. Oreskovich MR, Carrico CJ (1984) Pancreaticoduodenectomy for trauma: a viable option? Am J Surg 147:618–623
55. Sims EH, Mandal AU, Schlatter T (1984) Factors affecting outcomes in pancreatic trauma. J Trauma 24:125–128
56. Hassan JE, Stern D, Moss GS (1984) Penetrating duodenal trauma. J Trauma 24:471–474
57. Levison MA, Petersen SR, Sheldon GF, Trunkey DD (1984) Duodenal trauma: experience of a trauma center J Trauma 24:475–480
58. Adkins RB, Keyser JE (1984) Recent experiences with duodenal trauma. Am Surg 5:121–131
59. Ivatury RR, Nallathambi M, Gaudino J (1985) Penetrating duodenal injuries: analysis of 100 consecutive cases. Am Surg 2:153–158
60. Wynn M, Hill DM, Miller DR, Waxman K, Eisner ME, Gazzaniga AB (1985) Management of pancreatic and duodenal trauma. Am J Surg 150:327–332
61. Hendel R, Rusnak CH (1985) Management of pancreatic trauma. Can J Surg 28:359–361
62. Walker ML (1986) Management of pancreatic trauma: concepts and controversy. J Natl Med Assoc 78:1177–1183
63. Melissas J, Baart GD, Mannell A (1987) Pancreaticoduodenectomy for pancreatic trauma. S Afr Med J 71:323–324
64. McKone TK, Bursch LR, Scholten DJ (1988) Pancreaticoduodenectomy for trauma: a life-saving procedure. Am Surg 54:361–364
65. Eastlick L, Fogler RJ, Shaftan GW (1990) Pancreaticoduodenectomy for trauma: delayed reconstruction. J Trauma 30:503–505
66. Ivatury RR, Nallathambi M, Rao P, Stahl WM (1990) Penetrating pancreatic injuries. Analysis of 103 consecutive cases. Am Surg 56:90–95
67. Heimansohn DA, Canal DF, McCarthy MC, Yaw PB, Madura JA, Broadie TA (1990) The role of pancreaticoduodenectomy in the management of traumatic injuries to the pancreas and duodenum. Am Surg 56:511–514
68. Gentillo LM, Cortes V, Buechter KJ, Gomez GA, Castro M, Zeppa R (1991) Whipple procedure for trauma: is duct ligation a safe alternative to pancreaticojejunostomy? J Trauma 31:661–668

69. Delcore R, Stauffer JS, Thomas JH, Pierce GE (1994) The role of pancreatogastrostomy following pancreatoduodenectomy for trauma. J Trauma 37:395–399
70. Mistry BM, Durham RM (1996) Delayed pancreatoduodenectomy followed by delayed reconstruction for trauma. Br J Surg 83:527
71. Mansour MA, Moore JB, Moore EE (1989) Conservative management of combined pancreatoduodenal injuries. Am J Surg 158:531–536
72. Cogbill TW, Moore EE, Feliciano DV (1990) Conservative management of duodenal trauma: a multicenter perspective. J Trauma 30:1469–1475
73. Hirshberg A, Mattox KL (1993) Damage control in trauma surgery. Br J Surg 80:1501–1502

Long-Term Results Following Pylorus-Preserving Pancreatoduodenectomy for Chronic Pancreatitis

RONALD F. MARTIN[1] and RICARDO L. ROSSI[2]

Summary. A retrospective review of the medical records of all patients who had pylorus-preserving pancreatoduodenectomy (PPPD) for chronic pancreatitis at Lahey Clinic (Burlington, MA, U.S.A.) was performed to assess their long-term outcome. Mean follow-up period was 63 months (range, 1 month to 13.7 years). All patients who were alive were contacted by telephone. In cases in which the patient had died, information was gathered from family members and hospital records. Forty-five patients underwent PPPD for disabling chronic pancreatitis. The mean preoperative duration of pain was 50 months, with 70% of patients requiring daily narcotic. One resection required resection of the portal vein. One patient died within 30 days of the operation. Ninety-two percent had improvement of pain at 5 years. The mean pain score (0–10 scale) was 9.2 preoperatively and 1.5, .8, 1.1, 1.1, and .9 at 6 months, 1 year, 2 years, 5 years, and 10 years, respectively. Seventy-four percent of patients had a postoperative weight gain to an average of 92% of their preillness weight. Diabetes (of new onset) occurred in 14% of patients by 6 months and 46% by 5 years. Hypoglycemia was the cause of death in 1 patient who underwent total pancreatectomy. Four patients died from causes unrelated to PPPD, marginal ulcers occurred in 10% of patients, and 9 patients required late operations. We concluded that, in selected patients, resection of the head of the pancreas achieves long-term pain improvement in more than 90% of cases. The early development of diabetes mellitus is low but over longer follow-up reaches prevalence rates similar to those described in patients who have not undergone resection. Weight gain in this group was superior to that previously reported for our patients who underwent the "standard Whipple" operation for chronic pancreatitis.

Key words. Pancreas—Cancer—Pancreatectomy—Pancreatitis—Diabetes

---

[1] Division of General Surgery, Maine Medical Center and Mercy Hospitals, Portland, ME 04102, U.S.A. and University of Vermont, Burlington, VT 05405, U.S.A.
[2] Department of General Surgery, Hospital Clinico, Facultad de Medicina, and Pontificia Universidad Catolica de Chile, Santiago, Chile (formerly Department of General Surgery, Lahey Clinic Medical Center, Burlington, MA 01805, U.S.A. and Harvard Medical School, Boston, MA 02110, U.S.A.

Introduction

The management of the patient with chronic pancreatitis represents a challenge to physicians and surgeons of many specialties. The leading indication for surgical intervention is to relieve pain. Historically there has been a shift in favored technique from attempts to perform ductal decompression procedures to resection of the distal pancreas and most recently to resection of the head of the pancreas [1–7]. Even within the group of authors who favor resection of the head of the pancreas there is a difference in opinion as to whether pancreatoduodenectomy should be performed with or without preservation of the pylorus. Most recently, resection of the head of the pancreas with preservation of the duodenum has been championed by Beger and his colleagues with excellent results [8–10].

While procedures that resect the head of the pancreas seem to provide fairly comparable results for pain relief, there has been extensive discussion of which operations have less deleterious side effects, such as nutritional problems, dumping, gastric stasis, ulcer formation, and other problems. In 1996 we published a report of a group of 45 patients who underwent PPPD for chronic pancreatitis at Lahey Clinic [11]. These patients and a review of the literature serve as the basis for this discussion.

The Lahey Clinic Series

The medical records of all patients who were treated surgically for chronic pancreatitis between January 1, 1980, and July 1, 1994, at the Lahey Clinic Medical Center were reviewed retrospectively. Those patients who were treated with pylorus-preserving pancreatoduodenectomy (PPPD) as a primary or subsequent procedure were identified as the group for study. In cases in which the patient had died, the appropriate medical information was obtained from the facility at which the patient died (if other than Lahey Clinic) and from spouses and other family members when appropriate. Forty-five patients were ultimately identified as subjects for that report.

Of the 45 patients who had undergone PPPD for chronic pancreatitis, 28 (62%) were men and 17 (38%) were women. Their mean age at time of operation was 47.5 ± 11.3 years (range, 26–72 years). The mean follow-up interval was 63.1 ± 52.9 months (range, 1 month to 13.7 years). The duration of symptoms of pain averaged 49.9 ± 44.6 months (range, 8 months to 15 years). Preoperative pain score was obtained from 37 patients. The mean preoperative pain score was 9.24 ± 2.2 (with a scale of 0 equaling no pain and 10 equaling the highest level of pain). Thirty-seven of 45 patients (70%) had a documented use of narcotic drugs. Twenty-six patients required narcotic drugs on a daily or more frequent basis for extended periods of time preoperatively; 15 required injectable narcotics and 11 required oral narcotics only.

Six patients had obstructed biliary systems at the time of operation and 1 had a past history of bile duct obstruction that was treated without resection of head of the pancreas. No patient had cholangitis or gastric outlet obstruction at the time of operation. Eleven patients had preoperative cholangiopancreatograms; of these 11 patients, 8 had stricture or obstruction of the pancreatic duct. One patient had a dilated common bile duct, 1 had a pancreatic duct stone, and 1 had pancreas divisum.

Identifiable risk factors for pancreatitis were present in 30 of 45 patients (66%) (Table 1). The remaining 15 patients had no identifiable risk factors. Sixteen patients had a total of 20 pancreatic operations and 16 patients underwent a total of 23 biliary procedures before pancreatoduodenectomy. Eleven of the 15 prior cholecystectomies were performed remote to the onset of development of symptoms related to the pancreatitis. A summary of past prior pancreaticobiliary operations is included in Table 2. Eighteen patients (38%) had significant comorbidity; 12 had chronic obstructive pulmonary disease assoiciated with tobacco abuse, 1 was hemophilic, 1 had idiopathic hypertrophic subaortic stenosis, 2 had seizure disorders, 1 was morbidly obese, and 6 had severe atherosclerotic coronary artery disease.

All patients underwent a PPPD. The technique of reconstruction included a two-layered pancreaticojejunostomy, single-layered choledochojejunostomy, and an end-to-side duodenojejunostomy. The perioperative data are summarized in Table 3. Mean nasogastric tube duration was 9.1 ± 7.0 days (range, 0–40 days). Only 11 patients (23%) required more than 10 days of nasogastric decompression. Other complications included delayed gastric emptying in 3 patients, wound infection in 2 patients, myocardial infarction in 1 patient, subphrenic abscess in 1 patient, severe depression in 1 patient, narcotic withdrawal in 1 patient, an infected abdominal aortic graft in 1 patient with associated duodenal stump blowout associated with death on postoperative day 20, and unrelenting fungal sepsis and multisystem organ failure resulted in death for 1 patient on postoperative day 79.

A marked and sustained reduction of pain was seen immediately postoperatively. A reduction of pain score to 1.5 from a preoperative level of 9.2 was seen by 6 months. Subsequent pain scores of .8, 1.1, 1.1, and .9 were seen at 1, 2, 5, and 10 years, respectively (Fig. 1). Only four patients (11%) and two patients (5%) had pain scores greater than 5 at postoperative intervals of 6 months and 1 year, respectively, and only

TABLE 1. Risk factors for pancreatitis

Factor	n
Ethanol abuse	24 (51%)
Biliary calculi	5 (11%)
Pancreas divisum	1 (2%)
Total:	30 (64%)

TABLE 2. Prior pancreaticobiliary operations

Procedure	Number of patients
Distal pancreatectomy	9
Autotransplantation	4
Modified Puestow	4
Pseudocystenterostomy	3
Sphincterotomy	3
Cholecystectomy	15
Cholecystoenterostomy	1
Choledochoenterostomy	2
Common bile duct exploration	2

TABLE 3. Perioperative data for pylorus-preserving pancreatoduodenectomy ($n = 45$)

Blood transfusion (mean)	3.2 ± 2.6 units (range, 0–10)
Portal vein resection	1
In-hospital death	2 (4.4%)
30-Day mortality	1 (2.2%)
Pancreatic fistula	3 (6.6%)
Biliary fistula	2 (4.4%)
Nasogastric tube duration (mean)	9.1 ± 7.0 days (range, 0–40)
Hospital stay (mean)	23.1 ± 12.5 days (range, 12–79)

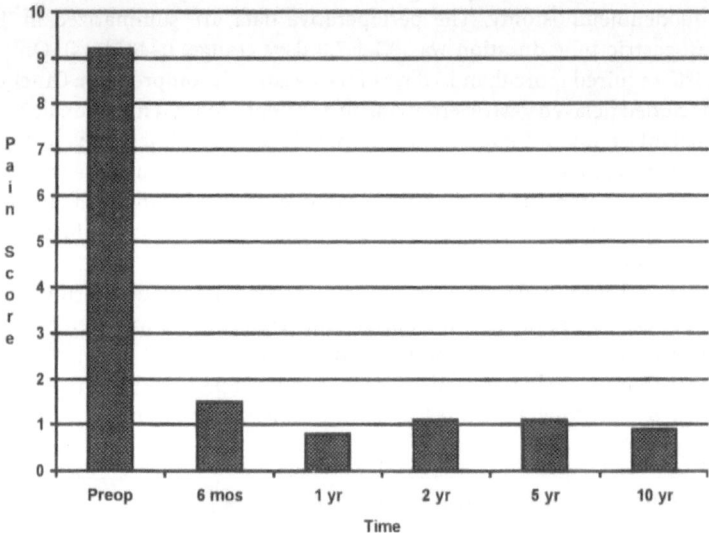

FIG. 1. Pain scores of Lahey Clinic patients undergoing pylorus-preserving pancreatoduodenectomy (PPPD) comparing preoperative levels to reduction in pain 6 months to 10 years after surgery

one patient had no resolution of pain whatsoever. One patient who had recurrence of pain symptoms at a later date underwent completion pancreatectomy with subsequent resolution of pain.

Seven of the original 45 patients had insulin-dependent diabetes mellitus at the time of operation. No patient with diabetes mellitus at the time of operation became free of insulin requirement. All patients who developed postoperative diabetes mellitus required insulin. Overall prevalence rates of insulin-dependent diabetes mellitus are shown in Fig. 2. A final 5-year prevalence rate of 47% was observed.

Exocrine insufficiency was treated with pancreatic enzyme replacement. The prevalence rates of pancreatic enzyme replacement are shown in Fig. 3. A final rate of 80.6% was observed. All but one of the patients who ultimately required pancreatic enzyme replacement were started on pancreatic enzyme supplements before 6 months postoperatively.

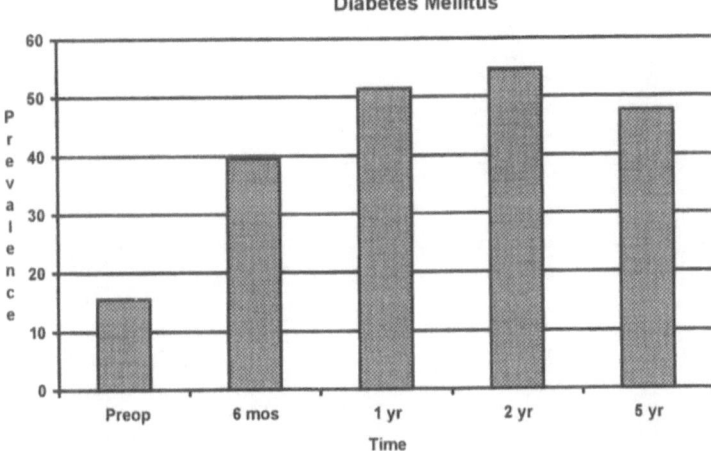

FIG. 2. Prevalence of insulin-dependent diabetes mellitus (%) comparing patients of series from time of surgery to 5 years after surgery

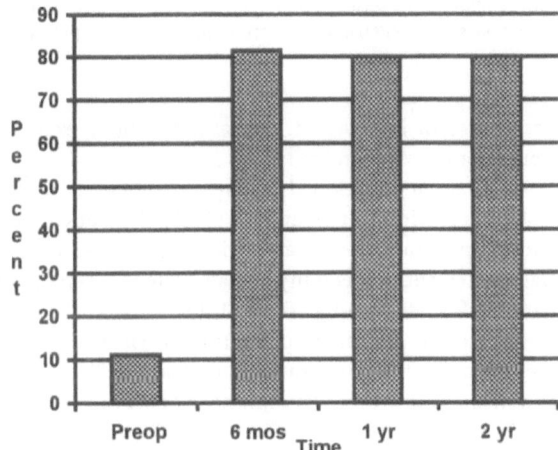

FIG. 3. Prevalence of pancreatic enzyme replacement
treatment from before surgery
until 2 years after surgery.
Note that most patients
required supplementation by 6
months postoperatively

Weights of all patients were recorded at the time of operation and postoperatively. Preillness weights were either derived from recorded weights of patients from prior medical records or as the best estimate of the patient. To avoid comparing people of significantly different body mass to one another, the weights of each patient at measured intervals were standardized as a fraction of their preillness weight. By definition each patient's preillness relative weight, therefore, becomes 1.00. Calculated relative weights measured at intervals of 6 months, 1 year, 2 years, 5 years, and 10 years are shown in Fig. 4. Approximately 15% weight loss was experienced by the group by the time of operation. At longest follow-up for each individual patient there had been an increase in weight of approximately one-third of the preoperative loss. However, those patients who were at postoperative interval of 10 years had regained a larger

Relative Weight History

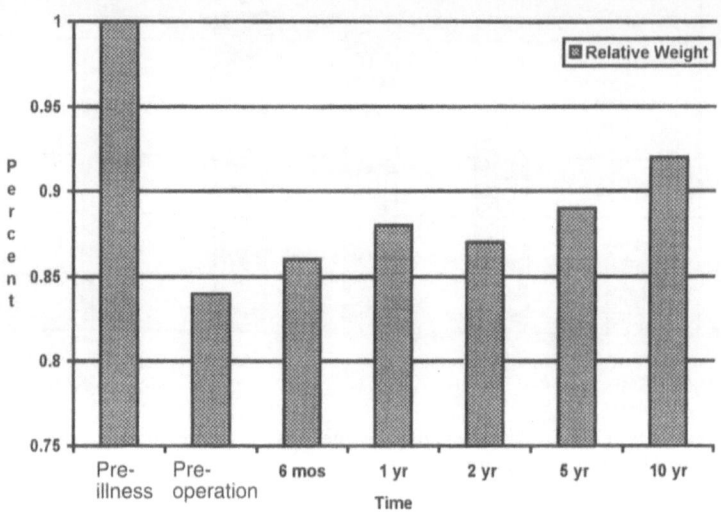

FIG. 4. Weights of series patients recorded before illness, at time of surgery, and postoperatively to 10 years after PPDD. Values are relative for each patient

percentage of lost weight. Of patients whose weights were known, 74% had a net weight gain postoperatively.

Two patients developed postoperative gastric outlet obstruction requiring operative intervention. Five patients (11%) developed marginal ulcers as diagnosed by endoscopy. Four were treated with histamine-2 receptor antagonists alone, and one was treated with vagectomy and antrectomy. Ten operations were performed on nine patients for late complications (Table 4).

Seven of the original 45 patients died. The causes of their deaths are listed as well as the interval between operation and death in Table 5. An actual survival rate of 84.4% at a mean follow-up of 63 months is observed.

Discussion

The technique of pylorus preservation during resection of the head of the pancreas and duodenum was first described by Traverso and Longmire for use in patients with chronic pancreatitis [12]. Since then it has also gained popularity for use in pancreatoduodenectomy for periampullary neoplasms as well. Debate over the physiological and nutritional benefits of this technique versus pancreatoduodenectomy with hemigastrectomy has been ardent since its inception. Very few controlled trials of these techniques exist, and as such the debate continues [13].

The main indication for operative management in chronic pancreatitis is pain. Numerous mechanisms for the development of pain with chronic pancreatitis have been put forth [1–5]. Perineural inflammation, chronic ischemia, pancreatic ductal obstruction, and increased pancreatic ductal pressure, as well as secretion of the pain neurotransmitters substance P and calcitonin gene-related peptide, have been pro-

TABLE 4. Operations for late complications

Procedure	n
Total gastrectomy	2
Vagectomy/Bilroth II	1
Completion pancreatectomy	1
Ligation pseudoaneurysm	1
Incisional hernia	1
Lysis of adhesions for small bowel obstruction	1
Abscess drainage (thigh autotransplant)	1
Removal infected autotransplant (thigh)	1

TABLE 5. Deaths

Patient number	Cause of death	Months postoperative
1	Pneumonia	24
2	Tylenol overdose	132
3	Sepsis/multisystem organ failure	1
4	Hypoglycemia/stroke	60
5	Trauma/motor vehicle accident	24
6	Cholangiocarcinoma	96
7	Multisystem organ failure	3

posed as wholly or partly causative in the development of the debilitating pain that these patients experience [10]. Pain control was fairly impressive in the group studied in this report. A reduction of pain score from 9.2 to 1.5 was seen within 6 months. This reduction was then maintained in groups studied to 5 years or longer. At intervals of more than 1 year, fewer than 6% of patients had pain scores of greater than 5. Furthermore, no patient required narcotic on a dialy basis. In many other reports, pain control characterized as "good" or "excellent" was seen in 73%–96% of patients [1,2,5,14–18]. We believe that a pain score offers a more objective approach and allows the patient to represent his own control for comparison. Our data seem comparable to those reported in the literature and are better than we had previously reported for PPPD with hemigastrectomy for long-term pain control of approximately 61% at 5 years [5].

Nutritional status following resection of head of the pancreas has also been an area of contention. There have been concerns over gastric stasis with preservation of the pylorus. In one report the rate of gastric stasis was as high as 14% [1]. Proponents of pylorus preservation cite the theoretical benefit of more controlled emptying of both liquids and solids, which may improve fat absorption [19] and glucose tolerance [20]. Only two patients in this series (4.4%) developed sufficiently poor gastric emptying to require operative intervention. Only three patients required nasogastric decompression for more than 14 days. One patient developed dumping following gastrectomy for poor gastric emptying. We did not find gastric retention to be a major concern in this group.

Our main determinant of long-term nutritional capacity was ability to gain weight. Again, each patient's weight was standardized against his own preillness weight to establish a self control. By 5 years an average gain of one-third the preoperatively lost weight was seen, and by 10 years nearly one-half the lost weight was regained. Overall,

92% of patients were able to gain weight postoperatively. A prospective series reported by Kozuschek et al. [13] also showed a weight gain for patients undergoing the pylorus-sparing procedure compared to those who underwent the "standard" Whipple operation.

Serum gastrin and gastric acid level have been shown to be reduced in "standard" Whipple operations and to remain normal in patients who undergo PPPD [21]. As such, the PPPD is theoretically a more ulcerogenic operation. It should not, however, be a more ulcerogenic anatomical configuration than in control subjects unless the alkaline secretions of the pancreas and duodenum are diverted away from the duodenojejunostomy. We saw five patients with marginal ulceration (11%), only one of whom required operative intervention; this intervention was for hemorrhage.

One patient died of a metabolic complication directly related to pancreatic resection, hypoglycemia. The overall issue of glucose tolerance in this group is complicated to analyze because many patients had varying degrees of pancreatic resection or multiple pancreatic operations, and some had autotransplantation of pancreas tissue. Nine patients had prior distal resection of the pancreas, and 3 others underwent total pancreatectomy at the time of PPPD for a total of 12 patients with no remaining orthotopic pancreas tissue. Five of these patients had autotransplantation of pancreas, 4 before PPPD and 1 at PPPD. While all 4 patients who had prior distal pancreatectomy and autotransplantation were not diabetic at the time of PPPD, 3 required insulin immediately following PPPD. Doses of insulin in this group, however, were fairly low, at 10–15 units of neutral protamine Hagedorn (NPH) insulin daily. Patients without autotransplantation and total pancreatectomy had higher insulin requirements and more episodes of hypoglycemia.

It is not clear from our data what the current role for segmental autotransplantation of the pancreas should be. While we are no longer using the technique routinely, a specific circumstance in which it may be useful is in the patient who has undergone previous resection of the head of the pancreas and requires completion pancreatectomy. The one patient who died of hypoglycemia had undergone a PPPD with total pancreatectomy. When preoperative diabetes mellitus prevalence is corrected for, nearly 30% of patients are diabetic at 6 months and almost half are diabetic by 5 years. This number is comparable with the approximately 45% of patients in whom diabetes develops without surgical intervention [22].

Exocrine insufficiency in this group is difficult to comment upon with confidence. Many of the patients were placed on pancreatic enzyme replacement as a matter of course and never displayed symptoms of pancreatic insufficiency. Although there were seven deaths overall in the group, only one late death was directly related to consequences of pancreatitis. Two deaths were in the postoperative period and four of the five late deaths were from unrelated causes. This finding has been borne out in other series [1,5,6].

In summary, 45 patients underwent PPPD for chronic pancreatitis. Long-term pain control was excellent and compared favorably with previously reported studies. The long-term prevalence of diabetes was similar to that of groups of patients who do not undergo surgery. The majority of patients were able to halt their trend of weight loss and regain a substantial protion of their weight that was lost preoperatively. Perioperative mortality was low. In selected patients, PPPD can be used for excellent pain relief with few complications and compares favorably to the standard pancreatoduodenectomy in our experience.

References

1. Traverso LW, Kozarek RA (1993) The Whipple procedure for severe complications of chronic pancreatitis. Arch Surg 128:1047–1053
2. Howard JM, Zhang Z (1990) Pancreaticoduodenectomy (Whipple resection) in the treatment of chronic pancreatitis. World J Surg 14:77–82
3. Easter DW, Cuschiere A (1991) Total pancreatectomy with preservation of the duodenum and pylorus for chronic pancreatitis. Ann Surg 214:575–580
4. Wilker DK, Izbicki JR, Knoefel W-T, Geissler K, Schweiberer L (1990) Duodenum-preserving resection of the head of the pancreas in treatment of chronic pancreatitis. Am J Gastroenterol 85:1000–1004
5. Rossi RL, Rothschild J, Braasch JW, Munson JL, ReMine SG (1987) Pancreatoduodenectomy in the management of chronic pancreatitis. Arch Surg 122:416–420
6. Braasch JW, Deziel DJ, Rossi RL, Watkins E Jr, Winter PF (1986) Pyloric and gastric preserving pancreatic resection: experience with 87 patients. Ann Surg 204: 411–418
7. Martin RF, Rossi RL. Pancreatoduodenectomy with or without pylorus preservation for chronic pancreatitis. In: Beger HG, Warshaw AL, Carr-Locke DL, Russell RCG, Buchler M, Neoptolemos JP, Saar MG (eds) The pancreas—a clinical textbook. Blackwell, London, (in press)
8. Beger HG, Buchler M (1990) Duodenum-preserving resection of the head of pancreas in chronic pancreatitis with inflammatory mass in the head. World J Surg 14:83–87
9. Beger HG, Buchler M, Bittner R, Uhl W (1990) Duodenum-preserving resection of the head of the pancreas: an alternative to Whipple's procedure in chronic pancreatitis. Hepato-Gastroenterology 37:283–289
10. Buchler M, Friess H, Jseumann R, Bittner R, Beger HG (1993) Duodenum-preserving resection of the head of the pancreas: the Ulm experience. In: Beger HG, Buchler M, Malfertheiner P (eds) Standards in pancreatic surgery. Springer, Berlin Heidelberg New York, pp 436–449
11. Martin RF, Rossi RL, Leslie KA (1996) Long-term results following pylorus-preserving pancreatoduodenectomy for chronic pancreatitis. Arch Surg 131:247–252
12. Traverso LW, Longmire WP (1978) Preservation of the pylorus during pancreaticoduodenectomy. Surg Gynecol Obstet 146:959–962
13. Kozuschek W, Reith HB, Waleczek H, Haarmann W, Edelmann M, Sonntag D (1994) A comparison of long-term results of the standard Whipple procedure and the pylorus-preserving pancreatoduodenectomy. J Am Coll Surg 178:443–458
14. Moreaux J (1984) Long-term follow-up study of 50 patients with pancreaticoduodenectomy for chronic pancreatitis. World J Surg 8:346–353
15. Hanyu F, Nakamura M, Suzuki M (1985) Surgical treatment of chronic pancreatitis: with special reference to pancreatectomy. In: Soto T, Yamauchi H (eds) Pancreatitis: its pathophysiology and clinical aspects. University of Tokyo Press, Tokyo, pp 425–431
16. Sato T, Yamauci H, Miyashita E, Matsuno S (1985) Long-term follow-up study on surgical treatment for chronic pancreatitis. In: Soto T, Yamauchi H (eds) Pancreatitis: its pathophysiology and clinical aspects. University of Tokyo Press, Tokyo, pp 415–421
17. Stone WM, Sarr MG, Nagorney DM, McIlrath DC (1988) Chronic pancreatitis: results of Whipple's resection and total pancreatectomy. Arch Surg 123:815–819
18. Gall FP, Gebhardt C, Meister R, Zirngibl H, Schneider MU (1989) Severe chronic cephalic pancreatitis: use of partial duodenopancreatectomy with occlusion of the pancreatic duct in 289 patients. World J Surg 13:809–817
19. Doty JE, Meyer JH (1987) Vagotomy and antrectomy impairs absorption of fat from solid, but not liquid dietary sources (abstract). Gastroenterology 97(5 pt 2):1374
20. Hongo M, Satake K, Sanoyama K, Lin YF, Ujiie H, Toyota T, Goto Y (1987) Regulation of insulin demand by gastric emptying in diabetics (abstract). Gastroenterology 92(5 pt 2):1440

21. Pearlman NW, Steigman GV, Ahnen DJ, Schultz AL, Fink LM (1986) Acid and gastrin levels following pyloric-preserving pancreaticoduodenectomy. Arch Surg 121:661–664

22. Ammann RW, Akovbiantz A, Largiader F, Scheuler G (1984) Course and outcome of chronic pancreatitis: a longitudinal study of a mixed medical-surgical series of 245 patients. Gastroenterology 86:820–828

Pancreatoduodenectomy for Benign Disease: Indication and Results

H.G. Beger[1], N. Harada[1,2], M. Siech[1], and F. Treitschke[1]

Summary. In benign lesions of the periampullary region, several modifications of pancreaticoduodenectomy have been developed to avoid major surgical resection. The pylorus-preserving pancreatic head resection provides the advantage of preservation of the stomach and the first segment of the postpyloric duodenum, whereas the duodenum-preserving head resection is a limited surgical procedure that leads to a local resection of the lesion with complete conservation of stomach and duodenum and, in most instances, spares the hepatobiliary extrahepatic tree. The ampullectomy results in a complete excision of the ampulla of Vater as a local excision of the wall of the duodenum with some parts of the head of the pancreas. In 478 patients with benign lesions in the periampullary region, a resection was carried out with a total hospital mortality of 0.6%. An indication for a limited resection exists in cases of benign adenoma of the papilla, in an endocrine tumor of the head of the pancreas, in a cystadenoma of the head of the pancreas, in pancreas divisum with an inflammatory process in the head of the pancreas, and in chronic pancreatitis with an inflammatory tumor in the head of the pancreas. The duodenum-preserving pancreatic head resection is indicated in benign, serous, or mucinous cystadenoma of the head of the pancreas and in large endocrine tumors located in the head. In chronic pancreatitis with an inflammatory mass in the head, the duodenum-preserving resection is the procedure of choice.

Key words. Adenoma of the papilla—Benign tumor in the pancreatic head—Cystadenoma—Duodenum-preserving pancreatic head resection—Pylorus-preserving pancreatic head resection

Introduction

Partial duodenopancreatectomy was introduced into clinical surgery by W. Kausch who, between 1909 and 1912, successfully performed a partial resection of duodenum and head of the pancreas in three patients with periampullary cancer [1].

[1] Department of General Surgery, University of Ulm, 89075 Ulm, Germany.
[2] Department of Surgery, Institute of Gastroenterology, Tokyo Women's Medical College, Shinjuku-ku, Tokyo 162, Japan.

Duodenopancreatectomy for malignant lesions is performed according to oncologic principles of surgical treatment, including wide excision of the cancer lesion, lymph tissue dissection, and peritumorous tissue clearance. However, in benign lesions of the periampullary region the application of pancreatoduodenectomy tends to be a limited excision of the lesion to avoid any removal of histologically and functionally normal tissue.

To avoid major surgical resection in benign lesions, several modifications of pancreatoduodenectomy have been developed. The pylorus-preserving pancreatic head resection was introduced in 1944 by Watson [2]; the duodenum-preserving pancreatic head resection for a benign inflammatory mass in the head of the pancreas in chronic pancreatitis was introduced in 1972 by Beger et al. [3]. Ampullectomy, which results in a complete excision of the ampulla of Vater, is a local excision of the wall of the duodenum with some parts of the head of the pancreas including the ampullary segment of the common bile duct and the confluence segment of the pancreatic main duct. A segmental resection of the peripapillary duodenum offers the possibility of resection of the head of the pancreas with conservation of 80% of the duodenum. In benign diseases of the periampullary region, the application of oncologic principles of surgery must be avoided.

Indications for Pancreaticoduodenectomy in Benign Lesions

Inflammatory and benign neoplastic lesions of the papilla are treated with a pancreaticoduodenal resection. Indications for pancreaticoduodencetomy are adenoma of the papilla with severe dysplasia, cystadenoma of the head of the pancreas, and endocrine tumor located in the head of the pancreas. In terms of inflammatory diseases, chronic pancreatitis with an inflammatory mass in the head and pancreas divisum are treated using the duodenum-preserving pancreatic head resection (Table 1). Use of the pancreaticoduodenal resection for a benign disease results, in most series, in low mortality and morbidity rates. Although published series usually cover small groups of patients, hospital mortality figures are between 0% and 1%.

Adenoma of the Papilla of Vater

On the basis of histomorphological criteria, adenoma of the papilla appears in 30% of cases as a papillary adenoma, in 20% as a tubular adenoma, and in 50% as a tubulovillous adenoma [4]. In papillary or tubular adenoma of the papilla, the surgical

TABLE 1. Pancreatoduodenectomy for benign lesion: Ulm experience[a]

Lesion	Patients (n)	Hospital mortality (%)
Adenoma of the papilla	36[b]	0
Cystadenoma of the pancreas head	10	0
Endocrine tumor of the pancreas head	1	0
Chronic pancreatitis	420	.7
Pancreas divisum	11	0
Totals:	478	.6

[a] 5/1982–9/1995, Department of General Surgery, University of Ulm.
[b] Of 36 patients, 32 underwent ampullectomy.

procedure of choice is a transduodenal papillectomy resulting in a wide excision of the adenoma and resection of the roof of the papilla; the entrance of the common bile duct and the pancreatic main duct are preserved. In patients with a villous adenoma, an ampullectomy with reinsertion of the common bile duct and the pancreatic main duct is the surgical treatment of choice (Fig. 1). However, in patients with a large villous adenoma and severe dysplasia or an additional carcinoma in situ, a pancreaticoduodenectomy has to be carried out with local lymph tissue dissection. Most of these patients had an endoscopic papillotomy or sphincterotomy with objectivation of an intraductal extension of the villous adenoma; in the past a Kausch–Whipple pancreaticoduodenectomy has been carried out. The standard surgical resection today is the pylorus-preserving pancreatic head resection. About 80% of patients with an adenoma of the papilla undergo resection of the papilla or an ampullectomy; 20% of the patients are candidates for a pancreaticoduodenectomy, the pylorus-preserving type of reconstruction being today the surgical procedure of choice (Table 2).

Cystadenoma of the Pancreatic Head

Cystadenomas of the pancreas are frequently localized in the pancreatic head. In terms of pathomorphology they are serous or mucinous cystadenomas; the risk of malignant disease is increased because mucinous cystadenoma has been observed to develop into pancreatic cancer [12]. About 40% of patients with the diagnosis

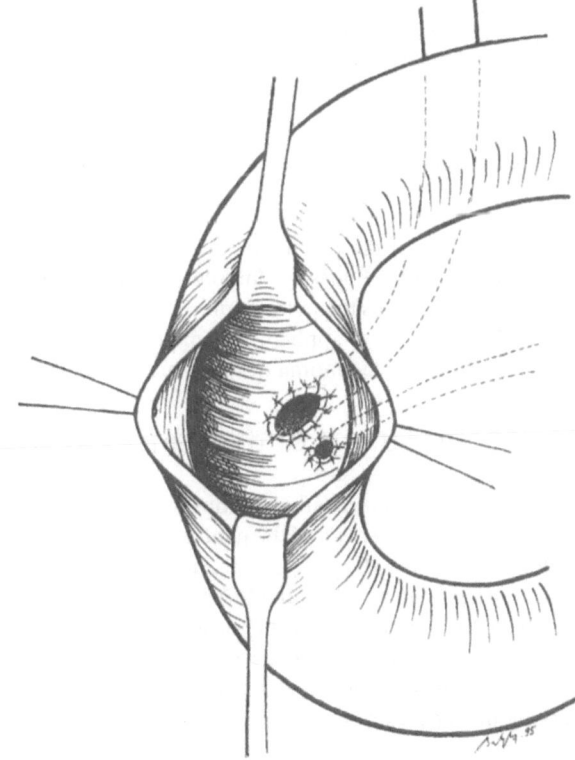

FIG. 1. Ampullectomy. In cases with villous adenoma plus severe dysplasia, a resection of the papilla has to be carried out. Reinsertion of the common bile duct and the pancreatic main duct is mandatory

TABLE 2. Pancreatoduodenectomy for benign lesion: adenoma of the papilla of Vater

Source	Patients (n)	Ampullectomy (n)[a]	PPPR (n)	Kausch Whipple (n)[b]	Hospital mortality
Ryan et al. [5] (1985)	12	5	—	7	None
Jones et al. [6] (1985)	7	4	—	3	None
Rosenberg et al. [7] (1985)	6	5	—	1	None
Pratschke et al. [8] (1988)	8	8	—	—	None
Koch et al. [9] (1991)	9	9	—	—	None
Seifert et al. [10] (1992)	7	7	—	—	None
Asbun et al. [11] (1993)	11	8	—	3	1/3
Ulm (1995)	36	32	4[b]	—	None
Totals:	96	81%	4%	15%	<1%

PPPR, Pylorus-preserving pancreatic resection.
[a] Tubulovillous adenoma in 59/71 cases.
[b] Villous adenoma with carcinoma in situ, large villous adenoma.

TABLE 3. Pancreatoduodenectomy for benign lesion: cystadenoma of the pancreatic head

Source	Patients (n)	PPPR/DPPHR (n)	Kausch–Whipple (n)	Hospital mortality (%)
Pyke et al. [13] (1992)	40	—	11	10
Bergmann et al. [14] (1992)	5	—	1	0
De Jong et al. [15] (1993)	31	18	—	?
Schneider et al. [16] (1993)	15	—	4	6.7
Danilov et al. [17] (1994)	33	—	5	9.1
Saint-Marseille et al. [18] (1994)	36	—	19	8
Machado et al. [19] (1994)	24	—	14	0
Ulm (1995)	17	10	—	0
Total:	201	82 (pPD)		5.5

DPPHR, Duodenum-preserving resection of the head of the pancreas.

of cystadenoma of the pancreatic head are treated surgically with a head resection. In most series the Kausch–Whipple pancreaticoduodenectomy was applied, and only very recently has the pylorus-preserving or the duodenum-preserving pancreatic head resection been applied. Hospital mortality increased after duodenopancreatectomy for cystadenoma of the pancreatic head (Table 3).

Endocrine Tumor of the Pancreatic Head

An endocrine tumour mostly develops in the body and tail of the pancreas; location of an insulinoma in the head of the pancreas is rarely seen. Because of the location of the endocrine tumor in the pancreas, in most cases a surgical enucleation or a limited left resection has been carried out. More than 80% of endocrine tumours are insulinomas, and only 10% are located in the head. Large endocrine tumours in the head of the pancreas (>2 cm) have to be treated surgically by pancreaticoduodenectomy; in the past a Kausch–Whipple resection was used. Very recently, however, a pylorus-preserving or duodenum-preserving pancreatic head resection has been used. Hospital mortality after surgical resection of an endocrine tumor is less than 1% (Table 4). The application of duodenopancreatectomy for large endocrine tumors in the head of the pancreas results in a low hospital morbidity.

Pancreaticoduodenectomy for Chronic Pancreatitis

In patients with alcohol-induced chronic pancreatitis and a small-duct disease with pancreatic head enlargement, the Kausch–Whipple procedure has been applied in the past. However, follow-up investigations after Kausch–Whipple resection in chronic pancreatitis revealed major disadvantages in regard to hospital mortality and late morbidity. In recently published series, the pylorus-preserving head resection has been used in chronic pancreatitis with a remarkably low hospital mortality. A major advantage for patients with chronic pancreatitis and an inflammatory mass in the head of the pancreas is offered by the duodenum-preserving head resection technique [25]. The duodenum-preserving head resection in chronic pancreatitis with an inflammatory mass did not result in a deterioration of glucose metabolism and insulin secretion even in the early postoperative course; furthermore it avoids the risk of cholangitis by preserving the extrahepatic biliary system. The surgical experience using duodenum-preserving head resection in chronic pancreatitis appears in the chapter by H. G. Beger "Duodenum-Preserving Head Resection: A Standard Operation for Chronic pancreatitis" (this volume).

Duodenum-Preserving Pancreatic Head Resection in Pancreas Divisum

In about 6% of all patients undergoing endoscopic retrograde cholangiopancreatography (ERCP), a pancreas divisum has been observed as the cause of pancreatitis. In patients with a pancreas divisum, the pancreatic juice outflow barrier in the prepapillary duct segments is effective. Any medical or endoscopic treatment including endoscopic sphincteroplasty, dilatation of the minor papilla, and papillotomy with stenting of the accessory pancreatic duct has been disappointing. In 11 patients with pancreatitis and pancreas divisum, a duodenum-preserving head resection has been carried out; 1 patient suffered from recurrent attacks of acute pancreatitis, and 10 patients had long-lasting chronic pancreatitis. The postoperative pain control was 100% with a mean follow-up time of 2.5 years. An oral glucose

TABLE 4. Pancreatoduodenectomy for benign lesion: endocrine tumor of the pancreatic head

Source	Patients (n)	Kausch–Whipple (n)	Left resection (n)	Enucleation (n)	Hospital mortality (%)	Late diabetes mellitus (n)
Demeure et al. [20] (1991)	7	—	5	2	0	1
Rösch et al. [21] (1992)	37	?	?	?	0	?
Mitrakou et al. [22] (1993)	6	—	—	6	0	—
Udelsman et al. [23] (1993)	12	12	—	—	0	?
Geoghegan et al. [24] (1994)	34	—	13	18	0	?
Ulm (1995)	9	1	3	5	0	0

Insulinoma, >80% of the endocrine tumors.

TABLE 5. Duodenum-preserving pancreatic head resection in pancreas divisum in 11 patients[a]

Disease	Patients (n)	Post-operative pain control[b]	Post-operative disease control[b]	Post-operative OGTT, normal/ restricted	Postoperative PLT, normal/ restricted	Hospital mortality (%)	Late mortality (%)[b]
Pancreas divisum[c]	1/11	100%	91%	11/0	2/9	0	0
Acute/chronic pancreatitis	1/10						

OGTT, Oral glucose tolerance test; PLT.
[a] 2/1989–9/1995, Department of General Surgery, University of Ulm.
[b] Postoperative follow-up, 30.4 months (median); chronic pancreatitis, 32.7 months; acute pancreatitis, 9.0 months.
[c] One patient after a second operation with duct revision pain and disease controlled; 10 patients with advanced chronic pancreatitis.

tolerance test demonstrated that none of the patients had deteriorated glucose metabolism late postoperatively. However, the deteriorated exocrine function could not be improved by the surgical treatment. Hospital and late mortality were 0 in this series (Table 5).

Pylorus-Preserving Pancreatic Head Resection or Whipple Resection in Benign Lesions of the Papilla and Pancreatic Head?

The Kausch–Whipple pancreaticoduodenectomy is used for surgical treatment of malignant lesions of the periampullary region. It includes hemigastrectomy, resection of the extrahepatic bile ducts, resection of the duodenojejunal segment of the upper small intestine, and a 50% resection of the pancreatic head as well as a tissue dissection of the surroundings of the pancreatic head. Clearly in benign lesions there is no indication for this type of pancreaticoduodenectomy. The use of the more limited pancreaticoduodenal resection using pylorus-preserving or duodenum-preserving resection implies major advantages for the early and late outcome of the patients. Decreasing morbidity and mortality rates were observed after pylorus- or duodenum-preserving pancreatic head resection, as compared to the Kausch–Whipple resection.

It has been demonstrated in animal experiments and by human data that the pylorus-preserving pancreatic head resection maintains the normal gastric acid secretion and the normal status of duodenal hormone interaction. Gastric emptying in patients after pylorus-preserving resection was found to be normal in 90%; in 10% there was a delay of solid food emptying in the first 2–3 postoperative weeks. Dumping complaints occur in 20% of patients after Kausch–Whipple resection, but dumping is rarely observed after pylorus-preserving resection. As summarized in Table 6, pylorus-preserving pancreatic head resection is superior to the Kausch–Whipple resection regarding the degree of impairment of the upper gastrointestinal tract physiology and in terms of early and late postoperative morbidity. The duodenum-

TABLE 6. Pylorus-preserving pancreatic head resection or Kausch–Whipple resection in benign lesion?

Postoperative complaint/Source	Pylorus-preserving pancreatic head resection	Kausch–Whipple procedure
Gastric acid secretion [26]	Normal	Decreased
Gastroduodenal hormones [26,27]	Normal	Decreased
Gastric emptying (Kunz et al., unpublished data)	Normal, 90%	Normal, 80%
	Delayed, 10%	Delayed, 10%
		Enhanced, 10%
Marginal ulceration [28]	5%–15%	5%–10%
Dumping complaints (Kunz, unpublished)	Absent	20%
Food intake after second postoperative week (Kunz, unpublished)	Normal	Restricted
Body weight increase [26]	>90%	≈30%

TABLE 7. Pancreatoduodenectomy for benign lesion: Surgical techniques[a]

Technique	Patients (n)	Patients (%)	Hospital mortality (%)
Kausch–Whipple resection	9	2	0
Pylorus-preserving head resection	49	10	0
Duodenum-preserving head resection	387	80	0.7
Ampullectomy	32	7	0
Duodenal segment resection	1	0.2	0
Totals:	478		0.6

[a] 5/1982–9/1995, Department of General Surgery, University of Ulm; 478 patients.

preserving pancreatic head resection applied in benign diseases of the pancreatic head offers a further major advantage, because the biliary tree and the duodenum are completely preserved and there is no risk of impairment of the endocrine functions of the pancreas. This is the major advantage in comparison to the pylorus-preserving pancreatic head resection. Therefore, as demonstrated in Table 7, duodenum-preserving head resection should be considered as the surgical technique of choice whenever the localized benign lesion in the head of the pancreas demands resection of the pancreatic head. In patients in whom the disease is caused by a cystadenoma or a large endocrine tumor or an inherited anomaly of the ductal system in the head of the pancreas, a duodenum-preserving head resection instead of a pylorus-preserving resection is recommended. In patients with a villous adenoma and a T_1 cancer, the surgical treatment of choice should be the pylorus-preserving pancreatic head resection, including oncologic lymph tissue dissection.

Conclusions

In benign lesions of the periampullary region, a local resection is the adequate surgical treatment, using papillectomy or ampullectomy in small adenomas of the papilla. In small endocrine tumors in the head of the pancreas, an enucleation should be performed.

In large villous adenomas of the papilla and in cystadenomas of the head of the pancreas suspected to be malignant, a pylorus-preserving pancreatic head resection is recommended. Duodenum-preserving pancreatic head resection is indicated in benign serous or mucinous cystadenoma of the head of the pancreas and in large endocrine tumors located in the pancreatic head. In chronic pancreatitis with an inflammatory mass in the head of the pancreas, the duodenum-preserving head resection is the procedure of choice.

Pylorus- and duodenum-preserving head resection are the appropriate surgical procedures for large benign tumours of the periampullary region and in chronic pancreatitis with an inflammatory mass in the head of the pancreas, respectively. The Kausch–Whipple operation should be avoided in benign diseases of the periampullary region because of substantial early and late postoperative disadvantages.

References

1. Kausch W (1912) Das Carcinom der Papilla duodeni und seine radikale Entfernung. Beitr Klin Chir 78:439–486
2. Watson K (1944) Carcinoma of ampulla of Vater: successful radical resection. Br J Surg 31:368
3. Beger HG, Witte C, Krautzberger W, Bittner R (1980) Erfahrung mit einer das Duodenum erhaltenden Pankreaskopfresektion bei chronischer Pankreatitis. Chirurg 51:303
4. Yamanake Y, Friess H, Kobrin MS, Büchler M, Kunz J, Beger HG, Korc M (1993) Overexpression of HER2/neu oncogene in human pancreatic carcinoma. Hum Pathol 24:1127–1134
5. Ryan PR, Schapiro RH, Warshaw AL (1986) Villous tumors of the duodenum. Ann Surg 203:301–306
6. Jones BA, Langer B, Taylor BR, Girotti M (1985) Periampullary tumors: which ones should be resected? Am J Surg 150:46–52
7. Rosenberg J, Welch JP, Pyrtek LJ, Walker M, Trowbridge P (1986) Benign villous adenomas of the ampulla of Vater. Cancer (Phila) 58:1563–1568
8. Pratschke E, Grab J, Krämling HJ, Günther B (1988) Zur operativen Behandlung von Papillenadenomen durch transduodenale submucöse Excision der Papilla Vateri. Chirurg 59:845–847
9. Koch B, Hildebrandt U, Schüder G, Seitz G, Feifel G (1991) Eingeschränkte chirurgische Radikalität beim okkulten Karzinom der Papilla Vateri. Langenbecks Arch Chir 376:195–198
10. Seifert E, Schulte F, Stolte M (1992) Adenoma and carcinoma of the duodenum and papilla of Vater: a clinicopathologic study. Am J Gastroenterol 87:37–42
11. Asbun HJ, Rossi RL, Munson JL (1993) Local resection for ampullary tumors. Arch Surg 128:515–520
12. Klöppel G, Maillet B (1991) Histological typing of pancreatic and periampullary carcinoma. Eur J Surg Oncol 17:139–152
13. Pyke CM, van Heerden JA, Colby TV, Sarr MG, Weaver AL (1992) The spectrum of serous cystadenoma of the pancreas. Clinical, pathologic and surgical aspects. Ann Surg 215:132–139
14. Bergmann LS, Russell JC, Gladstone A, Devers T (1992) Cystadenomas of the pancreas. Am Surg 58:65–71
15. De Jong SA, Pickleman J, Rainsford K (1993) Nonductal tumors of the pancreas. The importance of laparotomy. Arch Surg 128:730–734
16. Schneider C, Reck T, Greskotter KR, Köckerling F, Gall FP (1993) Zystische Pankreastumoren. Langenbecks Arch Chir 378:281–287
17. Danilov MB, Vikhorev AV, Buriev IM, Karmazanovskii GG, Savvina TV, Shiriaeva SV (1994) Cystic tumors of the pancreas. Khirurgiya (Mosc) 1994:10–14

18. Saint-Marseille S, Lapointe R, Roy A, Dagenais M, Gagnon J, Lavoie P (1994) Cystic tumors of the pancreas: apropos of 36 cases. Ann Chir 48:697–702
19. Machado MC, Montagnini AL, Machado MA, Falzoni R, Volpe P, Jukemura J, Abdo EE, Penteado S, Bacchella T, Monteiro-Cunha JE, et al. (1994) Cystic neoplasm of the pancreas: analysis of 24 cases. Rev Hosp Clin Fac Med Sao Paulo 49:208–212
20. Demeure J, Klonoff DC, Karam JH, Duh QY, Clark OH (1991) Insulinomas associated with multiple endocrine neoplasia type I: the need for a different surgical approach. Surgery (St Louis) 110:998–1004
21. Rösch TH, Lightdale CJ, Botet JF, Boyce GA, Sivak MV, Yasuda K, Heyder N, Palazzo L, Dancygier H, Schusdziarra V, Classen M (1992) Localization of pancreatic endocrine tumors by endoscopic ultrasonography. N Engl J Med 326:1721–1726
22. Mitrakou A, Fanelli C, Veneman T, Perriello G, Calderone S, Platanisiotis D, Rambotti A, Raptis S, Brunetti P, Cryer P, Gerich J, Bolli G (1993) Reversibility of unawareness of hypoglycemia in patients with insulinomas. N Engl J Med 329:834–839
23. Udelsman R, Yeo CJ, Hruban RH, Pitt HA (1993) Pancreaticoduodenectomy for selected pancreatic endocrine tumors. Surg Gynecol Obstet 177:269–278
24. Geoghegan JG, Jackson JE, Lewis MP, Owen ER, Bloom SR, Lynn JA, Williamson RC (1994) Localization and surgical management of insulinoma. Br J Surg 81:1025–1028
25. Beger HG, Büchler M, Bittner R (1990) The duodenum-preserving resection of the head of the pancreas (DPRHP) in patients with chronic pancreatitis and an inflammatory mass in the head. Acta Chir Scand 156:309–315
26. Braasch JW (1988) Pancreatoduodenal resection. Curr Probl Surg 25:5
27. Takada T (1993) Pylorus-preserving pancreatoduodenectomy: technique and indications. Hepato-Gastroenterology 40:422–425
28. Grant CS, van Heerden JA (1979) Anastomotic ulceration following subtotal and total pancreatectomy. Ann Surg 190:1–5

Pancreatoduodenectomy for Cancer Indications and Results

Pancreatectomy for Small Carcinoma of the Head of the Pancreas

Tadao Manabe[1], Keiji Mashita[1], Hiromitsu Takeyama[1],
Moritsugu Tanaka[1], Yuji Okada[1], and Masayuki Imamura[2]

Summary. The clinical and pathological characteristics of 25 small carcinomas (less than 2 cm in diameter) in the head of the pancreas are reviewed. At the time of initial surgery, lymph node metastases were found in 32% of the cases, capsular invasion in 20%, retroperitoneal invasion in 24%, and portal system involvement in 28%. Nine patients had Stage I disease, three had Stage II, seven had Stage III, and six had Stage IV. Pancreaticoduodenectomy or total pancreatectomy with or without combined resection of the portal vein and/or hepatic artery was performed. The cumulative 5-year survival rate for all patients was 28%. For nine Stage I patients, the 5-year survival rate was 56%. With the other stages there were no survivors after 4 years. The main recurrence sites in patients who died of carcinomas after surgery were the liver, peritonium, and local region. From the present findings we conclude that small, localized lesions, without any extratumoral extension, can be resected with a reasonable chance of a cure.

Key words. Small carcinoma of the pancreas—Pancreatectomy—Lymph node metastasis—Capsular invasion—Rotroperitoneal invasion

Introduction

The prognosis of carcinoma of the pancreas is very poor even after radical pancreatectomy. This pessimistic assessment follows from the fact that almost all carcinomas of the pancreas are advanced, often demonstrating lymph node metastasis, capsular invasion, and involvement of the adjacent vessels and neurons. En bloc extended pancreatectomy with resection of the associated vascular structure is considered to be indispensable to achieve a curative operation [1,2]. However, even this radical approach has failed to obtain a significant improvement in long-term survival of patients, and the discouraging findings point to the necessity for early diagnosis [3–5]. In this study the clinical and pathological characteristics of 25 small

---

[1] First Department of Surgery, Nagoya City University Medical School, Mizuho-ku, Nagoya, Aichi 467, Japan.
[2] First Department of Surgery, Faculty of Medicine, Kyoto University, Kyoto 606, Japan.

carcinomas of the head of the pancreas were reviewed to clarify what might be the most important prognostic factors for such surgically managed cases.

Patients and Methods

Twenty-six patients with small pancreatic carcinomas, less than 2 cm in largest diameter, were treated in either Nagoya City University Hospital or Kyoto University Hospital during the past 28 years. Twenty-five of the lesions were located in the head and 1 in the body of the pancreas. In this study, 25 patients with carcinoma of the head of the pancreas were evaluated; 20 men and 5 women aged 38 to 76 years, with a mean of 62 years. Surgical treatment was pancreaticoduodenectomy in 20 patients, including 1 with preservation of the pylorus and 5 with combined resection of the adjacent portal system.

Total pancreatectomy was performed on five patients, including two whose adjacent portal system and hepatic artery were removed. The pathological parameters examined included the size of the tumor, microscopic findings for the primary lesion, metastasis to the lymph nodes, capsular invasion, retroperitoneal invasion, and invasion of the adjacent portal system.

Results

The size of the tumor ranged from 1 to 2 cm, with a mean of 1.7 cm in largest diameter. Microscopic examination revealed tubular adenocarcinoma in 19 patients (well-differentiad type in 14, modenately differentiated type in 4, and poorly differentiated type in 1), papillary adenocarcinoma in 2 patients, an adenosquamous carcinoma in 1, an acinar cell carcinoma in 1, a cystadenocarcinoma in 1, and an islet cell carcinoma in 1. Lymph node metastases were found in 32% (8 of 25) of the patients, capsular invasion in 20% (5 of 25), retroperitoneal invasion in 24% (6 of 25), and portal system

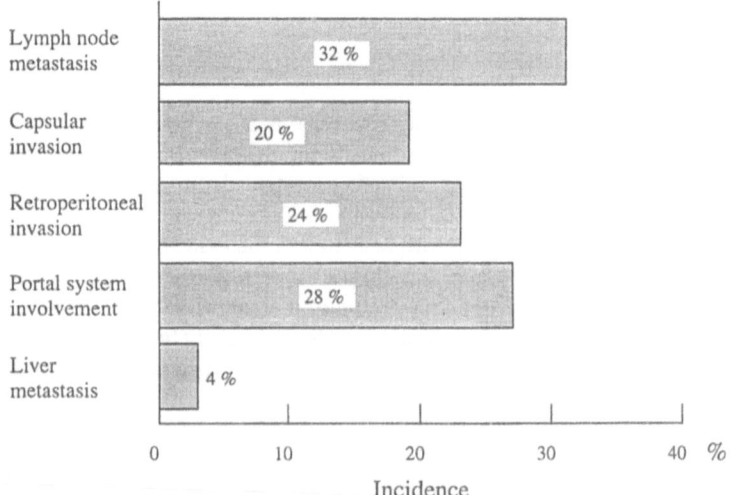

FIG. 1. Pathological findings (%) in 25 patients with small carcinoma of the head of the pancreas

involvement in 28% (7 of 25). One patient had a metastatic lesion in the liver (Fig. 1). According to the stage as classified by the Japanese Pancreatic Society [6], 9 patients had a stage I lesion (size of the tumor was 2 cm or less without regional lymph node metastasis, capsular invasion, retroperitoneal invasion, or involvement of the portal system) and 3 had a stage II lesion (primary group lymph node metastasis close to the tumor without capsular invasion, retroperitoneal invasion, or involvement of the portal system). Seven patients had a stage III lesion (lymph node metastasis to the secondary group, located between the primary and tertiary groups, suspected capsular invasion, suspected retroperitoneal invasion, or supected involvement of the portal system), and 6 patients had stage IV lesions (lymph node metastasis to the tertiary group defined as juxtaregional, or lymph node metastasis to the secondary group with suspected capsular invasion, suspected retroperitoneal invasion, or suspected involvement of the portal system). Only 9 of the 25 patients had a stage I, or early carcinoma of the pancreas.

Many different groups of lymph nodes around the pancreas were dissected en bloc with the pancreatectomy. One or more lymph nodes positive for metastasis were found in 32% of the patients (9 of 25). The posterosuperior pancreaticoduodenal, posteroinferior pancreaticoduodenal, superior mesenteric, common hepatic, and hepatoduodenal ligament lymph nodes were all involved in 12% (3 of 25). Anterosuperior pancreaticoduodenal and subpyloric lymph node metastases were found in 8% (2 of 25). No metastases were detected in the anteroinferior pancreaticoduodenal, cardiac, gastric, celiac axis, splenic, middle colic, superior or inferior pancreatic (tail of pancreas), or paraaortic lymph nodes (Fig. 2).

The postoperative mortality rate was zero. Twenty-one of the 25 patients died within 2–54 months after surgery, and 4 are still alive after more than 5 years. Among the nine stage I patients, 3 who underwent pancreaticoduodenectomy and 1 who

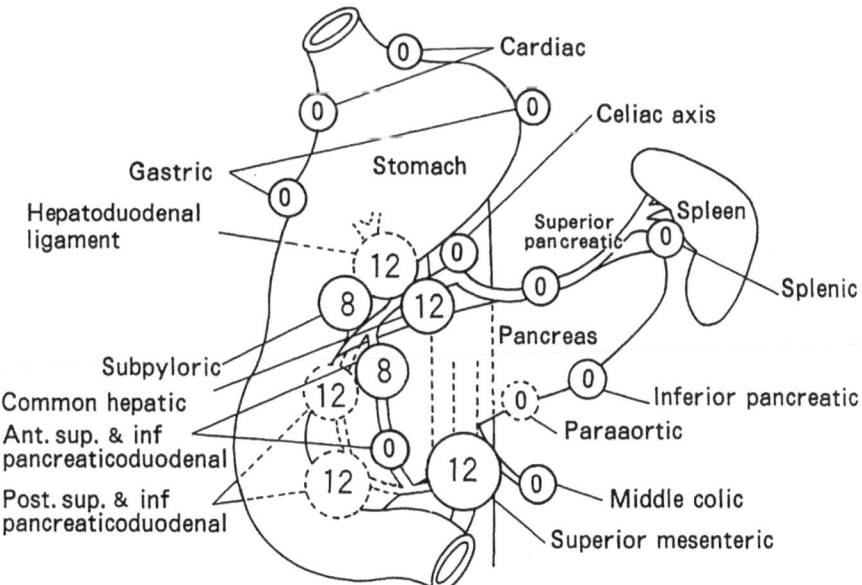

FIG. 2. Percentage (*circled numbers*) of metastases of lymph node per number of cases resected

underwent pancreaticoduodenectomy combined with portal vein resection died of recurrence at 13, 14, 17, and 43 months, respectively, after surgery. One patient who underwent total pancreatectomy died of a hepatic abscess of unknown cause 54 months after surgery. Two patients who underwent pancreaticoduodenectomy and 1 patient who underwent pylorus-preserving pancreaticoduodenectomy had demonstrated no recurrence more than 5 years later. The other patient who underwent pancreaticoduodenectomy for acinar cell carcinoma of the pancreas suffered recurrence of the tumor in the abdominal cavity after 1 year and 11 months and again after 3 year and 9 months, suggesting dissemination of the original carcinoma. However, the lesions could be removed surgically each time, and the patient is still alive 5 years after pancreatectomy.

Of the three stage II patients, two patients underwent panreaticoduodenectomy and died of recurrence 5.6 months and 42 months, respectively, after surgery. One patient who underwent total pancreatectomy died of septic shock of unknown cause after 2 months.

Of seven stage III patients, four patients underwent pancreaticoduodenectomy, one dying of septic shock after 3 months and three of recurrence after 9–19 months. Of the others, two died of recurrence 13 months after total pancreatectomy or total pancreatectomy with combined resection of portal vein, and one of apoplexy 25 months after combined resection of the hepatic artery.

Among the six stage IV patients, two underwent pancreaticoduodenectomy: one died of recurrence after 17 months and the other of unknown disease after 22 months. The other four, who underwent pancreaticoduodenectomy with portal vein resection, died of recurrence 7, 10, 29, and 35 months, respectively, after surgery.

Tumor recurrence sites in the 15 patients who died of carcinoma were the liver in 8 (54%), peritoneum in 4 (27%), the lung in 1 (7%), and local region in 6 (40%) (Fig. 3).

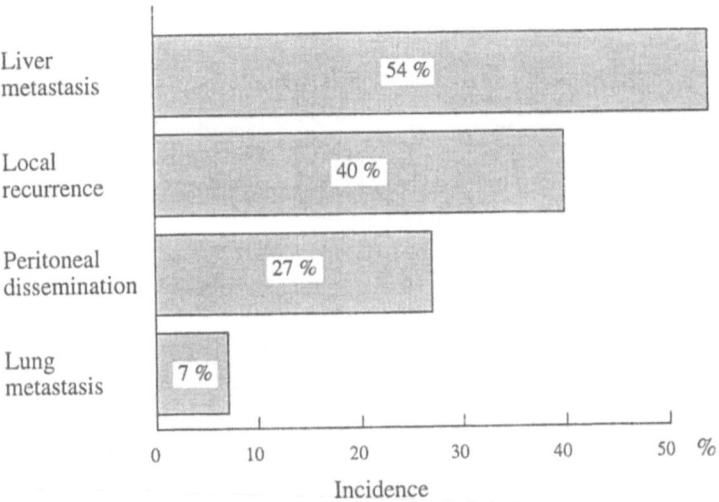

FIG. 3. Tumor recurrence sites in the 15 patients who died of carcinoma of the pancreas

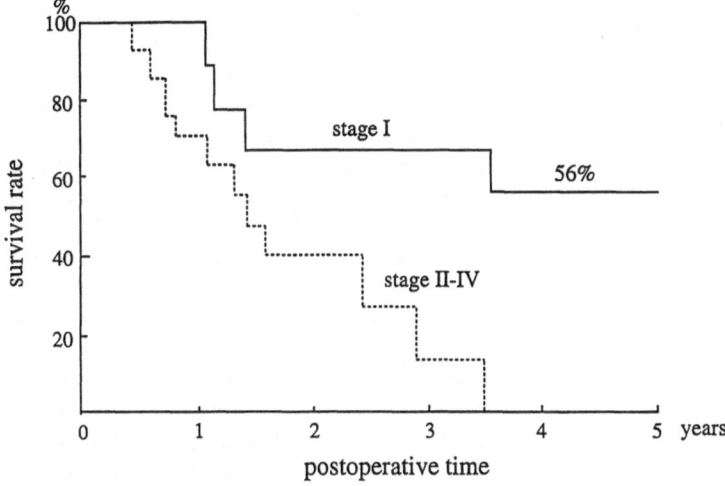

FIG. 4. Cumulative survival curve after pancreatectomy for small carcinoma of the pancreas with stage I (9 patients, *solid line*) or stage II–IV (16 patients, *dotted line*)

The cumulative 1-, 3-, and 5-year survival rates for all patients after surgery were 83%, 40%, and 28%, respectively; for the nine stage I patients, cumulative 1-, 3-, and 5-year survival rates were 100%, 67%, and 56%. The respective figures for those with stage II–IV were 71%, 40%, and 0% (Fig. 4).

Discussion

With solid carcinomas, small lesions are considered to have a better prognosis because the smaller the tumor, the earlier the stage of the disease. Unfortunately, however, small carcinomas of the pancreas are not always early carcinomas. This chapter describes retrospective clinical results of patients with small carcinoma of the head of the pancreas.

Radical pancreatectomy has been advocated as a curative approach for resectable lesions, but the prognosis still remains poor. In many cases of pancreatic carcinomas, the tumors extend to the outer margin of the origin and involve the capsule, lymphatic vessels, and nodes, as well as the adjacent vessels and neural network. Even if these lesions appear to be completely resected in the course of pancreatectomy, there are often overlooked remnants. Extensive procedures in the form of en bloc radical pancreatectomy for advanced pancreatic carcinoma have been developed allowing the resection rate to be improved, but the results have so far been discouraging [1–3,7–9]. The possibility that microscopic lesions might be left behind can never be precluded. Thus, to achieve a better prognosis, early diagnosis of pancreatic carcinoma is indispensable.

The size of the tumor is clearly one of the most important factors [10]. However, clinical diagnosis is often difficult because the symptoms of small carcinoma of the pancreas are frequently vague and nonspecific. Fortunately, in our series jaundice was an initial symptom in almost all patients in which the lesion was located close to the common bile duct. Patients with jaundice have an approximately ninefold greater chance of having a resectable tumor [11]. Recent advances in sophisticated imaging approaches such as ultrasonography (US), computerized tomography (CT), and endoscopic retrograde cholangiopancreatography have allowed relatively good sensitivity in detecting pancreatic carcinomas [12,13]. In our patients, US and CT were applied to make an accurate diagnosis and assess the operability of the tumors.

In this series, 24 of the 25 patients with small carcinomas underwent curative-type operations, the one exception having metastasis to the liver. The 5-year cumulative survival rate of 28% achieved in our series is better than that generally reported for pancreatic carcinomas [4,11]. However, this basically was true only for those with stage I lesions, where the survival rate was in fact 56%, and few of the patients with stage II, III, or IV were alive after 4 years despite extended pancreatectomy with combined resection of adjacent vessels.

In our series, lymph node metastasis, capsular invasion, retroperitoneal invasion, and involvement of the portal system were correlated with a poor prognosis irrespective of the histological pattern of the carcinoma. While all appeared to be completely resected macroscopically, the fact of more extensive spread was obvious from the eventual outcome. Nagai et al. [14] earlier reported the precise extent of lymphatic and local spread of small and localized carcinomas of the pancreas. Microscopic metastases were found in grossly negative lymph nodes, and in 50% of the examined patients there were a few metastatic foci in the paraaortic regions. In their study, all of eight patients had carcinoma infiltration within the lymphatic vessels, nerves, or connective tissues, and this was particularly pronounced in those with lymph node metastasis; interstitial invasion was almost invariably present in the regions where lymph node metastases were found.

The fact that the main sites of recurrence in our series of 15 patients who died of carcinoma were the liver and peritoneum strongly suggests that many small carcinomas of the pancreas disseminate extensively through the extratumoral lymphatic, venous, and neural networks at an early stage. However, this is not always the case, and some carcinomas less than 1 cm in size have a limited extension [7]. There are therefore grounds for optimism that advances in our ability to make an early diagnosis will eventually allow a much higher cure rate to be achieved for carcinomas of the pancreas.

References

1. Fortner JG (1981) Surgical principles for pancreatic cancer: regional total and subtotal pancreatectomy. Cancer (Phila) 47:1712–1718
2. Manabe T, Suzuki T, Tobe T (1985) Evalutation of *en bloc* radical pancreatectomy for carcinoma of the head of the pancreas involving the adjacent vessels. Dig Surg 2:27–30
3. Manabe T, Ohshio G, Baba N, et al (1989) Radical pancreatectomy for ductal cell carcinoma of the head of the pancreas. Cancer (Phila) 64:1132–1137
4. Lerut JP, Gianello PR, Otte JB, et al (1984) Pancreaticoduodenal resection: surgical experience and evaluation of risk factors in 103 patients. Ann Surg 199:432–437
5. Fortner JG (1984) Regional pancreatectomy for cancer of the pancreas, ampulla, and other related sites. Ann Surg 199:418–425
6. Japanese Pancreatic Society (1993) General rules for surgical and pathological studies on cancer of the pancreas, 4th edn (in Japanese). Kanehara, Tokyo
7. Fortner JG (1973) Regional resection of cancer of the pancreas: a new surgical approach. Surgery (St Louis) 73:303–320

8. Nagakawa J, Kurachi M, Konishi K, et al (1982) Translateral retroperitoneal approach in radical surgery for pancreatic carcinoma. Jpn J Surg 12:229–233
9. Fortner JG, Kim DK, Cubilla A, et al (1977) Radical pancreatectomy: *en bloc* pancreatic, portal vein and lymph node resection. Ann Surg 186:42–50
10. Tsuchiya R, Tomioka T, Izawa K, et al (1986) Collective review of small carcinomas of the pancreas. Ann Surg 203:77–81
11. Kalser MH, Barkin J, McIntyre JM (1985) Pancreatic cancer: assessment of prognosis by clinical presentation. Cancer (Phila) 56:397–402
12. Hessel SJ, Siegelman SS, McNeil BJ, et al (1982) A prospective evaluation of computed tomography and ultrasound of the pancreas. Radiology 143:129–133
13. Freeny PC, Marks WM, Ball TJ (1982) Impact of high-resolution computed tomography of the pancreas on utilization of endoscopic retrograde cholangiopancreatography and angiography. Radiology 142:35–39
14. Nagai H, Kuroda A, Morioka Y (1986) Lymphatic and local spread of T1 and T2 pancreatic cancer: a study of autopsy material. Ann Surg 204:65–71

Surgical Results of Pancreatoduodenectomy for Disease in the Pancreatic Head Region

Toshimichi Nakayama, Hisafumi Kinoshita, Hideki Saitsu,
Hiroyasu Imayama, Kouji Okuda, Masao Hara,
Shuichi Fukuda, and Naoyuki Saitoh

Summary. Between January 1965 and September 1995, 330 patients underwent pancreatoduodenectomy in our institution. In 249 cases, we performed the Child method of reconstruction after pancreatoduodenectomy. Of these patients, 299 underwent pancreatoduodenectomy because of malignant disease and 19 died in the hospital after the operation; the mortality rate was 5.8%. We must be aware of certain complications after pancreatoduodenectomy, especially anastomotic leakage of the pancreatiocojejunostomy. It 16 cases of pancreatic fistula, 7 patients died of this complication. Five-year survival rates of patients with carcinoma of the pancreas, bile duct, and papilla of Vater were 17.3%, 19.7%, and 56.2%, respectively. In cases of carcinoma of the papilla of Vater with no lymph node involvement, the 5-year survival rate was 64.9%; for cases with lymph node involvement, it was 40.0%. Many more strategies must be developed to obtain a better outcome in cases of carcinoma of the pancreas and bile duct. The most important need is to prevent metastasis of carcinoma to the liver in these patients.

Key words. Pancreatoduodenectomy—Complications—Surgical results

Introduction

Diseases in the region of the head of the pancreas are increasing in frequency, and recent advances in diagnostic techniques have contributed to the diagnosis of malignant disease in the early stage. Surgical resection is the only possibility of cure for patients with malignant disease of the pancreatic head region, and other methods of treatment, including chemotherapy and radiation therapy, have been of little benefit. However, surgical results in these patients are still poor, in spite of advances in operation technique and perioperative management. This study was undertaken to document the surgical results of patients who underwent pancreatoduodenectomy (PD) in our institution and to discuss some problems of this operation.

Second Department of Surgery, Kurume University School of Medicine, Kurume, Fukuoka 830, Japan.

TABLE 1. Pancreatoduodenectomy[a]

Disease	Cases	Hospital deaths
Malignant		
Cancer of the papilla of Vater	98	5
Cancer of the bile duct	85	7
Cancer of the head of the pancreas	90	5
Cancer of the duodenum	13	
Cancer of the stomach	3	
Cancer of the gallbladder	5	
Cancer of the colon	1	
Carcinoid of the papilla of Vater	3	2
Carcinoid of the pancreas	1	
Benign		
Chronic pancreatitis	21	
Adenoma of the papilla of Vater	2	
Giant ulcer of the duodenum	1	
Pancreatic cyst	2	
Solid cystic tumor of the pancreas	1	
Benign biliary stricture	2	
Papillitis of Vater	2	
Total	330	19

[a] From the Second Department of Surgery, Kurume University Hospital, January 1965 to July 1995; mortality rate was 5.8%.

TABLE 2. Reconstruction procedure[a]

Method	Cases
Whipple	58
Child	249
P-loop Child	8
Child Roux-Y	5
Pylorus-preserving pancreatoduodenectomy	8
Pancreatogastrostomy	2
Total	330

[a] From the Second Department of Surgery, Kurume University Hospital, January 1965 to July 1995.

Clinical Materials

The hospital records of 330 patients who underwent PD at the Second Department of Surgery, Kurume University Hospital, between January 1965 and September 1995 were reviewed. Of these patients, 299 underwent PD because of malignant disease (Table 1): 98 patients were found to have carcinoma of the papilla of Vater, 90 had carcinoma of the head of the pancreas, and 85 had carcinoma of the bile duct. Carcinoma of the duodenum was found in 13 patients, and 13 other patients underwent PD for reasons of other malignant disease (Table 1). Thirty-one patients underwent surgery for nonmalignant disease, and chronic pancreatitis was the indication for PD in 21 patients (5%) (Table 1).

Of 330 patients, 249 (76%) underwent Child's method of reconstruction after PD. Pylorus-preserving pancreatoduodenectomy was applied for 8 cases of early malignant disease (Table 2).

Results

Nineteen of 330 patients died in the hospital, which was an overall operative mortality of 5.8% for the 30-year period (see Table 1). Complications after PD are shown in Table 3. Anastomotic leakage of the pancreaticojejunostomy was found in 16 of 330 patients, and 7 died in the hospital. The leakage occurred at the

TABLE 3. Complications after pancreatoduodenectomy[a]

Complication	Number	Hospital deaths
Anastomotic leakage		
Pancreaticojejunostomy	16	7
Choledocojejunostomy	14	2
Gastrojejunostomy	3	
Hemorrhage		
Intraperitoneal space	7	2
Gastrointestinal tract	11	1
Rupture of a pseudoaneurysm	3	1
Abscess		
Intraperitoneal space	21	
Wound	7	
Liver	2	
Ileus	19	
Pulmonary complication	5	
Postoperative pancreatitis	3	
Cholangitis	3	
Diarrhea	11	
Hepatic insufficiency	14	2
Biliary peritonitis	2	
Other	11	4

[a] From the Second Department of Surgery, Kurume University Hospital, January 1965 to July 1995.

TABLE 4. Anastomotic leakage of pancreaticojejunostomy in pancreatoduodenectomy[a]

Disease	Cases	Hospital deaths
Cancer of the bile duct	6	2
Cancer of the papilla of Vater	5	2
Cancer of the head of the pancreas	2	2
Cancer of the gallbladder	1	1
Chronic pancreatitis	1	
Papillitis	1	
Total	16 (7)	

[a] From the Second Department of Surgery, Kurume University Hospital, January 1965 to July 1995.

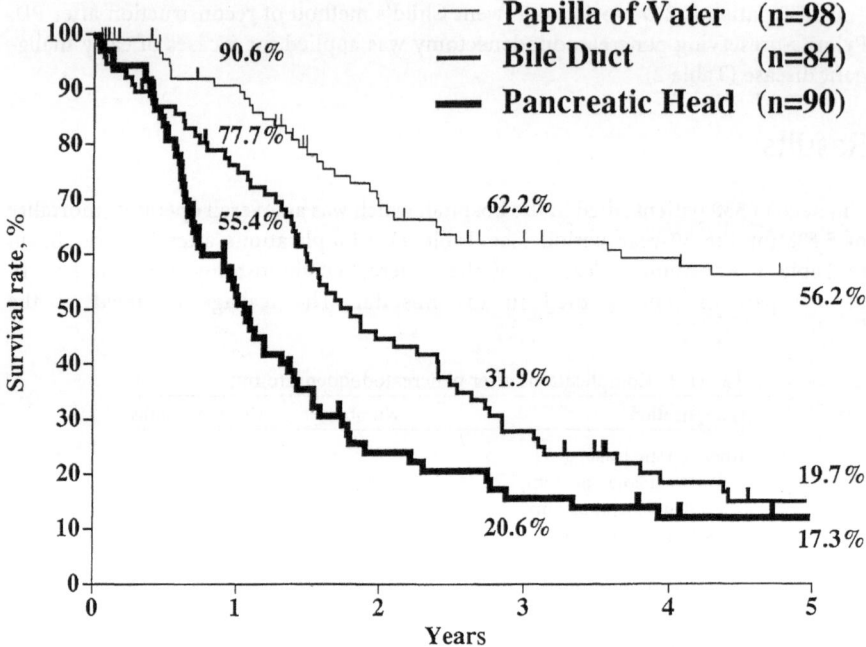

Fig. 1. Cumulative survival rate of disease in pancreatic head region after pancreatoduodenectomy (Second Department of Surgery, Kurume University Hospital, January 1965–July 1995)

choledocojejunostomy in 14 patients, and abscess formation in the intraperitoneal space was found in 21 patients. Four of the 19 deaths were associated with hemorrhage, and 2 patients died of postoperative hepatic insufficiency.

Basal diseases of the cases with pancreatic fistula are shown in Table 4. Six patients of 16 (37.5%) had carcinoma of the bile duct, and 5 (31.3%) had carcinoma of the papilla of Vater. The actual survival rate for patients with adenocarcinoma of the papilla of Vater was 56.2% at 5 years. The actual 5-year survival rate for patients with carcinoma of the bile duct was 19.7%, and for carcinoma of the pancreas it was 17.3% (Fig. 1). In the cases of carcinoma of the papilla of Vater with no lymph node involvement, the 5-year survival rate was 64.9%, but for cases with lymph node involvement the rate was 40.0% (Fig. 2).

Comments

In this report the mortality was 5.8% among 330 patients who underwent pancreatoduodenectomy between 1965 and 1995. During the past 20 years, several investigators have reported their experiences with PD. Analysis of these reports suggests a decrease in operative mortality during this period [1–3]. An improvement in operative morbidity has also been reported, and recent reports suggest that only 20%–30% of patients undergoing PD may develop a major postoperative complication [4]. Thus, PD, which is the only means of treatment offering the possibility of cure for

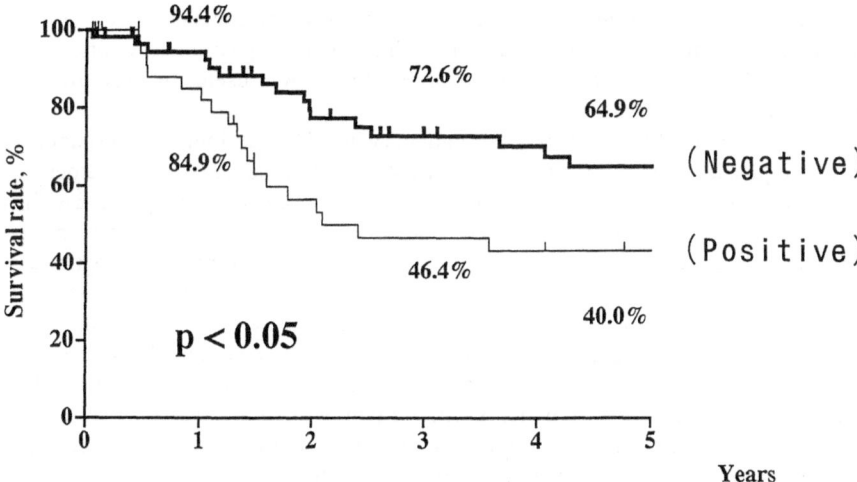

FIG. 2. Cumulative survival rate of carcinoma of papilla of Vater after pancreatoduodenectomy. Negative (thick line), cases with no lymph node involvement; positive (thin line), cases with lymph node involvement (Second Department of Surgery, Kurume University Hospital, January 1965–July 1995)

patients with malignant disease of the pancreatic head region, carries an acceptable operative risk.

Anastomotic leakage of the pancreaticojejunostomy is the most common complication after PD. The reported incidence of this complication has varied from 3.6% to 18.5% [5,6]. In our institution, pancreatic fistula occurred in 16 of 330 patients, an incidence of 4.8%. It was not, in comparison with other reports, a high incidence, but we have to emphasize the clinical importance of pancreatic fistula, which is associated with mortality rates of 43%. The operative management of the pancreatic duct must be an important factor in the development of this complication. Stenting of the pancreatojejunal anastomosis by inserting a small tube into the pancreatic duct, which can drain pancreatic juice almost completely, has been recommended to prevent pancreatic fistula. Clinically, changes in volume, color, and transparency of pancreatic juice draining from the tube are important signs of the development of complications.

In an analysis of 16 patients who suffered from pancreatic fistula, 12 of 16 (75%) had no abnormal findings in the pancreas; there was no dilatation of the pancreatic duct, no increase in consistency, and no decreased exocrine function of the pancreas. In these patients, who had no pathological changes in the pancreas, delicate manipulation and suture technique should be required to perform the pancreaticojejunostomy. Other factors that affect the leakage of an anastomosis were infection and ischemia of the oral end of the jejunum. We also have to pay attention to the blood supply to the cut end of jejunum and to avoid intraabdominal infection by intestinal fluid.

Upper gastrointestinal hemorrhage, usually from erosive gastritis or ulceration, is also a major complication after PD. In an attempt to reduce the incidence of postoperative anastomotic ulceration, Scott et al. have recommended that truncal vagotomy be performed concomitantly with PD [7]. In our institution, however, we have not perfomed truncal vagotomy. Grace et al. reported that vagotomy did not decrease the incidence of postoperative upper gastrointestinal hemorrhage or anastomotic ulceration [4]. Perioperative administration of H_2-blocker was useful in prevention of gastrointestinal hemorrhage.

A survival rate of 17.3% at 5 years for patients with adenocarcinoma of the pancreas has reemphasized the poor long-term outlook for these patients. Improvement of operative management, including radical resection of regional lymph nodes, has contributed to a decrease in local recurrence of the carcinoma, which worsens the prognosis for patients. One of the most important factors to improve the prognosis of these patients with carcinoma of the pancreas is the prevention of liver metastasis of the carcinoma. When we devise some effective way to prevent metastasis of the tumor to the liver, the clinical importance of surgical resection of he tumor will be increased markedly. In 98 patients with carcinoma of the papilla of Vater, the 5-year survival rate was 56.2%, and 64.9% in patients without lymph node involvement. This result can be improved clinically, and we want to emphasize the value of surgical management in patients with carcinoma of the papilla of Vater.

References

1. Newman KD, Braasch JW, Ross RL, O'Campo-Gonzales S (1983) Pyloric and gastric preservation with pancreatoduodenectomy. Am J Surg 145:152–156
2. Trede M (1985) The surgical treatment of pancreatic carcinoma. Surgery (St Louis) 97:28–35
3. Jones BA, Langer B, Taylor B, Girotti M (1985) Periampullary tumors. Which ones should be resected? Am J Surg 149:46–52
4. Grace PA, Pitt HA, Tompkins RK, DenBesten L, Longmire WP Jr (1986) Decreased morbidity and mortality after pancreatoduodenectomy. Am J Surg 151:141–149
5. Lerut JP, Gianello PR, Othe JB, Kestens PJ (1984) Pancreaticoduodenal resection. Ann Surg 199:432–437
6. Warshaw AL, Swanson RS (1988) What's new in general surgery—pancreatic cancer in 1988. Ann Surg 208:541–553
7. Scott WH, Dean RH, Parker T, Avant G (1980) The role of vagotomy in pancreaticoduodenectomy. Ann Surg 191:688–696

Indications for Extended Radical and Pylorus-Preserving Whipple Operation for Pancreatic Cancer

Toshiaki Nakasako, Fujio Hanyu, Ken Takasaki,
Toshihide Imaizumi, Nobuhiko Harada, Takashi Hatori,
and Akira Fukuda

Summary. The aim of this study was to evaluate whether both the extended radical Whipple operation and the pylorus-preserving Whipple operation are applicable to the treatment of patients with carcinoma of the head of the pancreas. This study included 273 patients who underwent the Whipple operation for carcinoma of the head of the pancreas. Our results show that many cases of pancreatic cancer are histologically advanced, and invasion to adjacent organs and tissues or lymphatic metastasis is often seen. Considering this mode of histological invasion, it is obvious that the extended radical Whipple operation is indicated for curative resection. We also emphasize that introduction of the extended radical Whipple operation allows increased resectability and curability without an increase in postoperative mortality and morbidity compared with the standard Whipple operation. However, we cannot confirm indication of the extended operation from the standpoint of cumulative survival rate because no differences were seen between patients who underwent the extended radical Whipple operation and the standard one. On the other hand, in our series of 106 patients who underwent the extended radical Whipple operation, the incidence of lymph node metastasis around the stomach and of direct invasion to the stomach or the duodenal bulb was only about 10%. Also, morbidity, mortality, and survival rates in patients with cancer of the head of the pancreas do not differ significantly between those who have undergone the extended radical Whipple operation and those who have undergone the pylorus-preserving Whipple operation. Therefore, the pylorus-preserving Whipple operation is as applicable to the treatment of many patients with carcinoma of the head of the pancreas as is the extended radical operation.

Key words. Whipple operation—Surgical treatment—Pylorus-preserving pancreaticoduodenectomy—Extended radical operation

Department of Gastroenterological Surgery, Tokyo Women's Medical College, Shinjuku-ku, Tokyo 162, Japan.

Introduction

Much effort has been expended in surgical therapy for pancreatic cancer following the success of pancreaticoduodenectomy by the Whipple procedure in 1935 to the extended operation represented by Fortner's regional pancreatectomy [1–4]. On the other hand, since Traverso reported the validity of the pylorus-preserving Whipple operation for benign periampullary diseases in 1978 [5], this surgical method has been widely practiced. More recently, some surgeons have aggressively adopted the pylorus-preserving Whipple operation as a treatment for malignant as well as benign diseases [6–8].

The aim of this study was to evaluated whether both the extended radical Whipple operation and the pylorus-preserving Whipple operation are applicable to the treatment of patients with carcinoma of the head of the pancreas.

Patients and Methods

From 1968 to August 1995, 314 patients underwent the Whipple operation for carcinoma of the head of the pancreas at the gastroenterological surgery department at Tokyo Women's Medical College. We excluded 41 patients who had a mucin-producing tumor or did not have other ductal adenocarcinoma; the remaining 273 patients were enrolled in this study.

Study I

The aim of study I was to evaluate whether the extended radical Whipple operation is applicable to the treatment of patients with carcinoma of the head of the pancreas. Modes of tumor invasion were examined by postoperative histopathological examination. The subjects were divided into two large groups according to the surgical period: those who underwent the standard Whipple operation from 1968 to 1977 ($n = 17$) and those who underwent mainly an extended radical Whipple operation from 1978 to August 1995 ($n = 256$). Resectability, mortality, and morbidity were investigated and compared in the two groups. The survival rate for patients who underwent the Whipple operation was compared in the extended radical Whipple operation ($n = 186$) and the standard Whipple operation ($n = 54$). Also, the survival rate for patients who underwent the extended radical Whipple operation was compared for curative resection ($n = 92$) and noncurative resection ($n = 94$).

Additionally, the survival rate for patients who underwent the extended radical Whipple operation was compared in two groups according to tumor invasion: those who had no marked invasion to the retroperitoneum and no invasion to the major arteries ($n = 121$), and those who had marked invasion to the retroperitoneum or positive invasion to the major arteries ($n = 44$).

Study II

The aim of study II was to evaluate whether the pylorus-preserving Whipple operation is applicable to the treatment of patients with carcinoma of the head of the pancreas. We evaluated the state of lymph node metastasis around the stomach and direct invasion to the stomach or the duodenal bulb in 106 patients who underwent the extended radical Whipple operation.

Mortality and morbidity were investigated in 57 patients who underwent the pylorus-preserving Whipple operation from 1984 to August 1995. Additionally, the survival rate for patients who underwent the Whipple operation was compared in the patients who underwent the pylorus-preserving Whipple operation ($n = 56$) and the patients who underwent the extended radical Whipple operation ($n = 141$).

Cumualtive survival rates were assessed by the Kaplan–Meier method. The χ^2 test and the generalized Wilcoxon test were used for statistical analysis, and a P value less than .05 was considered significant. Survival rate differences were assessed based on standard error.

Results

Study I

Ductal adenocarcinoma of the pancreas demonstrated severe tumor invasion to the adjacent organs and tissues. Of the patients, 50% presented with tumor invasion to the pancreatic capsule and 78% had retioperitoneal tissue invasion. Nerve plexus invasion was seen in 56% of the patients, portal vein invasion in 38%, duodenal invasion in 70%, and lymph node involvement in 82%. Also, invasion of the pancreatic cut end (Whipple resection line) was recognized in 13%. These results suggested that the extended radical Whipple operation could be indicated for about 90% of the patients with pancreatic cancer (Fig. 1).

After introduction of the extended radical Whipple operation in 1978, resectability improved from 20% to about 60%. The curability also improved, from 12% to about 50% (Fig. 2). Mortality after the standard Whipple operation was 11%; it improved to 3% even after the extended radical Whipple operation. No difference in morbidity was seen between the two operations (Table 1).

The 1-year survival rate after the standard Whipple operation was 41%, the 3-year survival rate was 11%, and the 5-year survival rate was 7%; only one patient survived more than 5 years after the standard Whipple operation, but the 1-year, 3-year, and 5-year survival rates in the patients who received the extended radical Whipple opera-

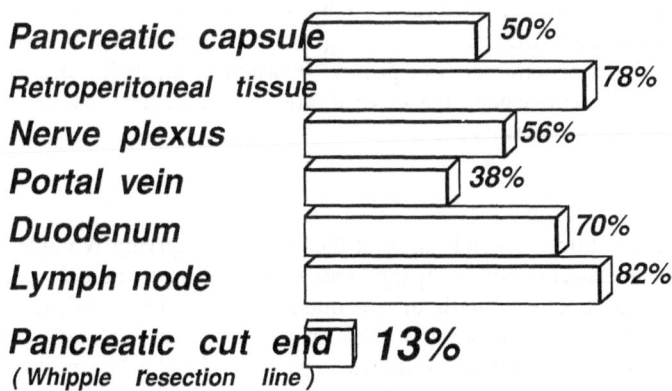

FIG. 1. Mode of tumor invasion

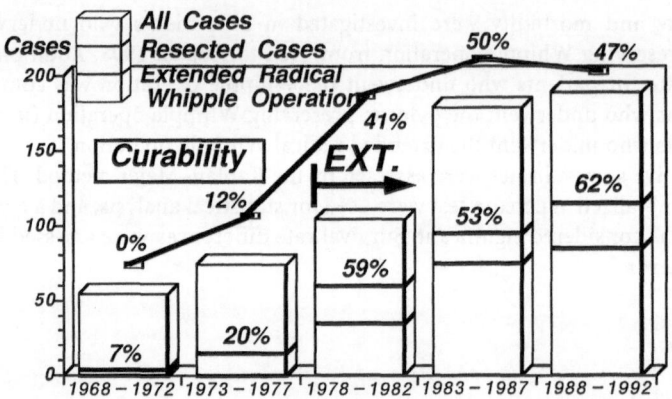

FIG. 2. Distribution by year of resectability and curability after extended radical Whipple operation

TABLE 1. Mortality and morbidity after standard and extended radical Whipple operation

Procedure	Mortality	Morbidity
Standard Whipple operation (1968–1977)	11%	26%
Extended radical Whipple operation (1978–1995)	3%	20%

tion were 43%, 9%, and 8%, respectively, and ten patients survived more than 5 years after this operation (Fig. 3).

The difference in survival between patients with curative resection and patients with noncurative resection after the extended radical Whipple operation was statistically significant. The survival rate in patients with curative resection was 54% at 1 year and was 14% at 5 years after the extended radical Whipple operation. Among patients with non-curative resection, however, the 1-year survival rate was 30%, the 3-year survival rate was 2%, and no patients survived more than 5 years after the operation. That is to say, even the extended radical Whipple operation could not produce long-term survival without curative resection (Fig. 4). If a patient had a tumor with marked invasion to the retroperitoneum or positive invasion to the major arterial wall, the prognosis was extremely poor; the survival rate was poorer than that of the patients without resection of the tumor (Fig. 5).

Study II

Histological conditions for indication of the pylorus-preserving Whipple operation are absolutely subject to both no lymph node metastasis around the stomach and no direct invasion to the stomach or the duodenal bulb. The incidence of lymph node metastasis was extremely low, 10%, in patients with pancreatic cancer. The incidence of direct invasion to the stomach or the duodenal bulb was also low, 13%, in patients with pancreatic cancer. These results suggested that preservation of the whole stomach and duodenal bulb could be indicated for about 90% of the patients

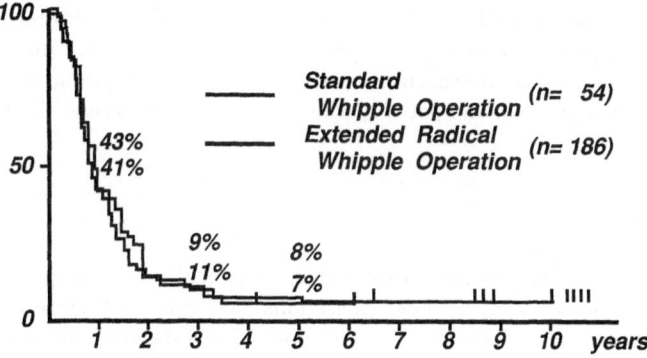

FIG. 3. Survival curves after standard and extended radical Whipple operation

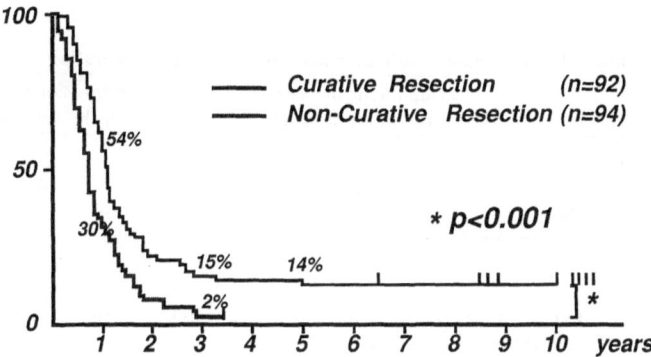

FIG. 4. Survival curves after extended radical Whipple operation for ductal adenocarcinoma of the pancreas

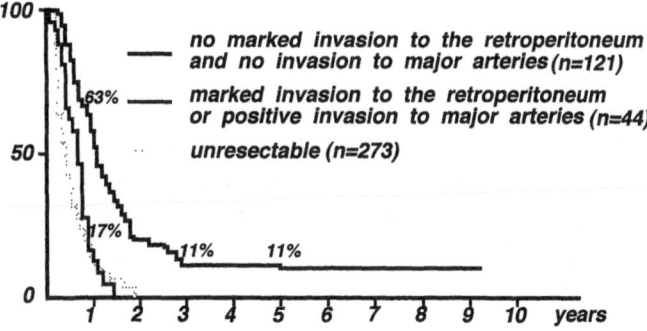

FIG. 5. Survival curves after extended radical Whipple operation

with pancreatic cancer (Table 2). The low mortality and morbidity also encouraged us to indicate the pylorus-preserving Whipple operation for pancreatic cancer (Table 3). No difference was seen in survival between patients undergoing the extended radical Whipple operation and patients with the pylorus-preserving Whipple operation (Fig. 6).

Discussion

Because many cases of pancreatic cancer that are considered for surgical treatment are in the advanced stages, extended operations have been tried since the 1970s to obtain long-term survival. However, in the United States the extended radical operation is no longer performed because the opinion is that it does not prolong life and improve the quality of life (QOL) [9,10]. Our results show that many cases of pancreatic cancer are histologically advanced and that invasion to the adjacent organs and tissues or lymphatic metastasis is frequently seen. Considering this mode of histologi-

TABLE 2. Histological retrospective study on conventional Whipple operation

Periampullary cancer	Lymph node metastasis around the stomach	Direct invasion to the stomach or the duodenal bulb
Pancreas ($n = 106$)	10%	13%
Ampulla of Vater ($n = 54$)	4%	0%
Distal bile duct ($n = 40$)	0%	15%

TABLE 3. Mortality and morbidity after pylorus-preserving Whipple operation

Site	Mortality	Morbidity
Pancreas ($n = 57$)	0%	19%
Ampulla of Vater ($n = 26$)	0%	27%
Distal bile duct ($n = 18$)	0%	17%
Total ($n = 109$)	0%	20%

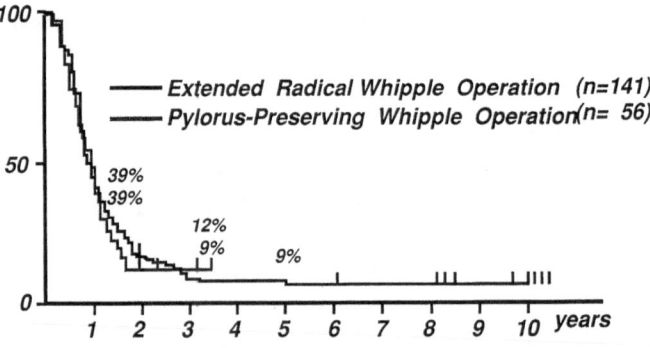

FIG. 6. Survival curves after extended radical and pylorus-preserving Whipple operation

cal invasion, it is obvious that the extended radical Whipple operation is indicated for curative resection. We also emphasize that introduction of the extended radical Whipple operation allows increased resectability and curability without increased postoperative mortality and morbidity compared with the standard Whipple operation.

However, we cannot confirm that the extended radical operation is indicated from the aspect of cumulative survival rate because no differences were seen between patients who underwent the extended radical Whipple operation and those undergoing the standard one. Moreover, patients with pancreatic cancer who underwent the extended radical Whipple operation with curative resection show a significantly better cumulative survival rate than those without curative resection. Also, no life-prolonging effect was seen in patients with massive invasion to the retroperitoneum or the major arteries. Both these facts suggest that we need to select patients for whom the extended radical Whipple operation is indicated.

On the other hand, whether the extent of resection for malignant disease, especially for carcinoma of the head of the pancreas, is adequate in the pylorus-preserving Whipple operation is a controversial issue. The only difference between the pylorus-preserving Whipple operation and the standard Whipple operation lies in the preservation of the distal stomach and the duodenal bulb with some blood vessels and lymphatics.

In our series of 106 patients who underwent the radical Whipple operation, the incidence of lymph node metastasis around the stomach and the incidence of direct invasion to the stomach or the duodenal bulb were about 10%. These results revealed that positive involvement of regional lymph nodes of the stomach and direct invasion to the stomach or the duodenal bulb were rare. Also, morbidity, mortality, and survival rates in patients with cancer of the head of the pancreas do not differ significantly between those who have undergone extended a radical Whipple operation and a pylorus-preserving Whipple operation. Therefore, the pylorus-preserving Whipple operation is applicable to the treatment of patients with carcinoma of the head of the pancreas.

References

1. Whipple AO, Parsons WB, Mullins CR (1935) Treatment of carcinoma of the ampulla of Vater. Ann Surg 102:763–769
2. Priestley JT, Comfort MW, Radlite J Jr (1944) Total pancreatectomy for hyperinsulinism due to an islet-cell adenoma: survival and cure at sixteen months after operation. Presentation of metabolic studies. Ann Surg 119:211–221
3. Fortner JG (1973) Regional resection of cancer of the panreas: a new surgical approach. Surgery (St Louis) 73:307–320
4. Imaizumi T, Hanyu F, Nakamura M, et al (1984) Extended operation for cancer in the head of the pancreas. With special reference to resection of the portal and superior mesenteric veins (in Japanese). Jpn J Gastroenterol Surg 17:615–623
5. Traverso LW, Longmire WP (1978) Preservation of the pylorus in pancreaticoduodenectomy. Surg Gynecol Obstet 146:959–962
6. Nakasako T, Hanyu F, Imaizumi T, et al (1990) Criteria for pylorus-preserving pancreaticoduodenectomy in patients with periampullary carcinoma. Histopathological study on 245 surgically resected cases (in Japanese). Jpn J Gastroenterol Surg 23:2532–2537
7. Grace PA, Pitt HA, Longmire WP (1990) Pylorus-preserving pancreatoduodenectomy: an overview. Br J Surg 77:968–974

8. Braasch JW, Gagner M (1991) Pylorus-preserving pancreaticoduodenectomy—technical aspects. Langenbecks Arch Chir 376:50–58
9. Fortner JG (1987) The rationale, technique, and results of treating pancreatic and peripancreatic cancer by regional pancreatectomy. Acta Gastro-Enterol Belg 40:121–127
10. Gudjonsson B (1987) Cancer of the pancrease: 50 years of surgery. Cancer (Phila) 60:2284–2303

Pylorus-Preserving Pancreatoduodenectomy for Cancer: Is It an Adequate Operation?

Ronald F. Martin[1] and Ricardo L. Rossi[2]

Summary. William S. Halsted published his report of local excision of a periampullary neoplasm in 1899. The patient subsequently died of metastatic disease. During the past nearly 100 years there have been tremendous advancements in the understanding of physiology, anesthetic and perioperative care, nutritional support, and surgical technique. These have served to improve short- and long-term survival for patients with these periampullary tumors. Despite the many advances in this arena there remains significant controversy as to how best approach these tumors. In this brief discussion we present the data from the most recent analysis of the experience with pylorus-preserving pancreatoduodenectomy (PPPD) for periampullary neoplasms and a rationale for this approach based on the experimental and clinical data that are available. On the basis of analysis of 106 patients who have undergone PPPD for cancer over a 13-year period and the rapidly expanding world experience with this operation, we conclude that PPPD is an adequate operation for periampullary carcinoma, but has not been proven to be a superior operation to the "standard Whipple" procedure in controlled trials.

Key words. Pancreatic cancer—Adult—Pancreatoduodenectomy—Pylorus—Surgery

Introduction

In 1978 Traverso and Longmire published a landmark article [1] describing the use of pylorus-preserving pancreatoduodenectomy (PPPD) for chronic pancreatitis. Shortly thereafter efforts for use of this procedure for benign as well as malignant disease were undertaken at the Lahey Clinic Medical Center. During this period of time there have been some minor refinements of the technical aspects of the operation, but the procedure remains essentially unchanged in our hands. Our institution and others

---

[1] Division of General Surgery, Maine Medical Center and Mercy Hospitals, Portland, ME 04102, U.S.A. and University of Vermont, Burlington, VT 05405, U.S.A.
[2] Department of General Surgery, Hospital Clinico, Facultad de Medicina and Pontificia Universidad Catolica de Chile, Santiago, Chile.

have reported several series on this technique [2–6]. During the past two decades an almost religious difference of opinion has evolved over the preference of PPPD or "standard Whipple" operation for the treatment of benign or malignant conditions. The origin of this difference in opinion stems from an argument that is akin to the "half-full or half-empty glass of water" that is best summarized by the titles of two articles that appeared in the *Archives of Surgery* during the past 2 years. In 1994 the *Archives of Surgery* published a report by Tsao et al. entitled "Pylorus-preserving pancreatoduodenectomy: is it an adequate cancer operation?" [6]. In 1995 a similar report from Patel et al. [7] entitled "Pylorus-preserving Whipple resection for pancreatic cancer: is it any better?" was published in the same journal. In our estimation it is the altered argument of adequacy versus superiority that fuels this ongoing debate. The remainder of this chapter attempts to describe our position on the status of PPPD as a cancer operation. We intend to also provide a rational basis for our conclusions about the adequacy and possible superiority of this procedure.

The functioning premise of those who favor the preservation of the pylorus during pancreatoduodenectomy for periampullary carcinoma or pancreatic ductal adenocarcinoma is that the duodenal margin and the gastric and pyloric nodes are rarely involved with disease [6]. Furthermore, if these structures were involved with tumor, the disease would be in very late stages and would be inappropriately treated with resection. In our opinion the relevant issues for increasing the successful management of these tumors are early diagnosis, advances in adjuvant therapy, and increase in knowledge of tumor biology. Additionally, we believe that a controlled randomized prospective trial of dissection of the early nodal basins should be conducted.

The Lahey Clinic Experience

The Lahey Clinic Medical Center experience with this operation was reviewed by Tsao and others in 1993 [6]. The purpose of this study was to determine the long-term survival, morbidity, and patient quality of life following PPPD. The records of all patients from November 1979 to June 1992 were reviewed for all patients who underwent resection for periampullary carcinoma or other primary carcinoma of the head of the pancreas. In total, 111 patients were identified; 106 patients underwent PPPD and 5 patients underwent "standard Whipple." The 5 patients who underwent pancreatoduodenectomy with hemigastrectomy did so for the following reasons: 2 had an ischemic pylorus, 2 had undergone prior distal gastrectomy for ulcer disease, and 1 had direct invasion of the tumor into the stomach. No patient was converted to "standard Whipple" for a positive duodenal margin. A total of 106 patients who had undergone PPPD served as the basis for this report.

The group was composed of 58 men and 48 women; their mean age was 60 years, with a range of 20–82 years. Presenting symptoms included jaundice in 48% of patients, weight loss in 44%, abdominal or back pain in 43%, and cholangitis in 7%. Preoperative diagnostic studies consisted mainly of computed tomography (CT) and endoscopic retrograde cholangiopancreatography (ERCP): 73 patients underwent CT that revealed a mass in 37 patients (51%), and 74 patients (70%) were studied with ERCP. Of these patients, 13 (18%) were found to have a "double-duct" sign, 7 (10%) had pancreatic ductal obstruction, and 40 (54%) had obstruction of the common bile duct. Prior biliary decompression was performed in 34 patients (32%); 15

TABLE 1. Procedure type according to primary tumor type

		Proximate pancreatectomy		Total pancreatectomy	
Cancer site	Number	Alone	With PVR	Alone	With PVR
Ampullary	34	31	0	3	0
Pancreatic	27	15	7	4	1
Bile duct	24	23	0	0	1
Duodenal	11	11	0	0	0
Islet cell	6	5	0	0	1
Cystadenoca	4	3	0	1	0
Total:	106	88	7	8	3

PVR, Portal vern resection.
From [6], with permission.

TABLE 2. Assessment of surgical margins by primary tumor type by examination of positive margins

Histology	Number	Duodenum	Bile duct	Pancreas[a]	Retroperitoneal	Vascular
Ampullary	34	0	0	1	3	0
Pancreatic	27	0	0	9	1	2
Bile duct	24	0	1	2	1	0
Duodenal	11	0	0	0	2	0
Islet cell	6	0	0	0	0	0
Cystadenocarcinoma	0	0	0	0	0	1
Total:	106	0	1	12	7	3

[a] All pancreatic neck margins were free of tumor.
From [6], with permission.

TABLE 3. Type and frequency of complications

Complication	Percentage
Pancreatic leak	15
Delayed gastric emptying	15
Abdominal sepsis	10
Pulmonary complications	7
Bile leak	5
Intraabdominal hemorrhage	4
Cardiac complications	3

had prior biliary enteric anastomosis, 7 had placement of a T-tube, 7 had percutaneous transhepatic decompression of the biliary system, and 5 had endoscopic decompression.

Anatomical site of tumor included ampullary carcinoma in 37 patients, pancreatic ductal adenocarcinoma in 26, distal common bile duct carcinoma in 22, duodenal adenocarcinoma in 11, islet cell tumors in 6, and pancreatic cystadenocarcinoma in 4 patients. Partial pancreatectomy with PPPD was performed in 95 of the 106 patients. Seven of these procedures required portal vein resection, and 11 patients had total pancreatectomy with 3 requiring portal vein resection. The specific breakdown of procedures by anatomical site of tumor is shown in Table 1. The pathological reports of all surgical margins are shown in Table 2. It is of note that all pancreatic neck margins, as well as all duodenal margins, were free of neoplasm. Perioperative mortality measured at 30 days was 2 patients (1.9%), and total hospital mortality was 6 patients (5.7%); 39 patients suffered perioperative morbidity. The specific complications are listed in Table 3.

Nodal metastasis and involvement of margins with tumor was statistically significant in association with decreased long-term survival following PPPD. Tumor size of greater than 2 cm was also shown to correlate with poorer survival in patients with pancreatic ductal adenocarcinoma. However, this was demonstrated by univariate analysis.

Postoperative weight gain was variable, with 30% of patients exceeding their preoperative weight. The median postoperative weight of this subset of patients was 105% of their preoperative weight; 44% of patients were within 10% of their preoperative weight, and 26 patients lost more than 10% of preoperative weight.

Discussion

Since William S. Halsted first published his account of local resection of a periampullary neoplasm in 1899 [8] there has been debate in the surgical literature about the best approach for resection of neoplasms of the duodenum and the head of the pancreas [1–7,9–13]. The technique of resection and approach to these tumors has changed remarkably throughout the first half of the twentieth century. A better understanding of physiology, including realization of the importance of vitamin K, and improvement in surgical technique markedly improved survival following the Whipple operation [5]. Despite these advances, the Whipple operation still carried a significant morbidity and mortality, so much so that in 1970 George Crile Jr. opined that "Although some of the unusual types of pancreatic carcinomas and some of the small ones of the ducts may be cured by a radical operation, the average patient with an adenocarcinoma of the head of the pancreas that is large enough to be palpated will live longer and more comfortably if no attempt is made to take a biopsy specimen or to remove it" [13].

Not all, however, subscribed to this belief. John Howard [12] and others [2–6,9,11] published reports demonstrating large numbers of these procedures performed with very low to no mortality and significantly decreased morbidity that have since reversed the course of this nihilism. While it is widely accepted that in expert hands resection of the head of the pancreas and duodenum can be performed safely, there still remains controversy as to which approach is best. This particular discussion concentrates on the measured and theoretical differences between PPPD and the "standard Whipple" operation.

Much attention has been given to the desired extent of resection to achieve adequate margins. In Traverso and Longmire's paper describing PPPD for chronic pancreatitis [1], there is even a caveat against using this procedure for malignancy. One of the reasons given for adding a hemigastrectomy to the pancreatoduodenectomy is to achieve a clear duodenal margin. No patient in our series had a positive duodenal margin. In our estimation, the margin of greatest concern is the retroperitoneal margin. Figure 1 shows the relationship of most commonly located resectable tumors of the head of the pancreas to the duodenum and surrounding

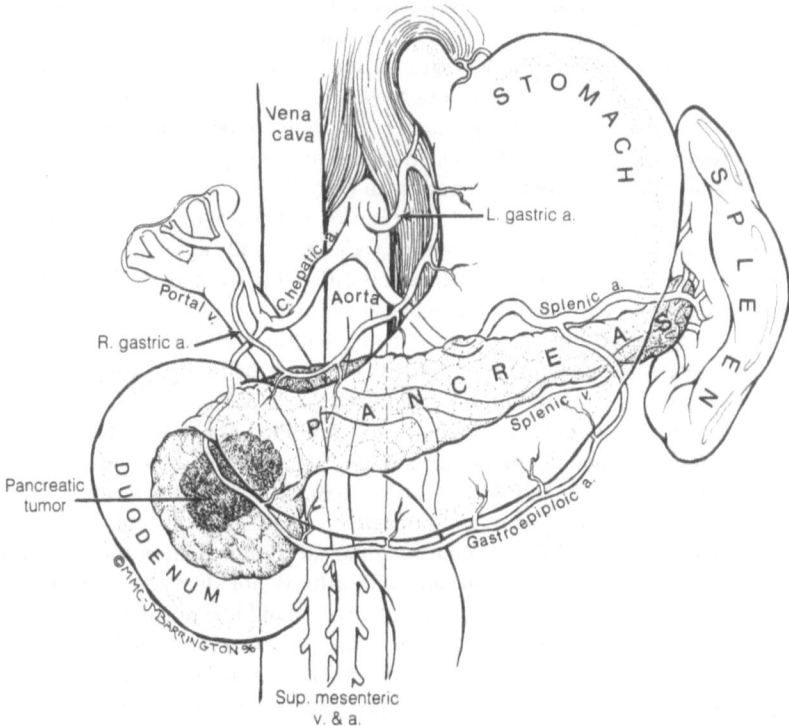

Fig. 1.

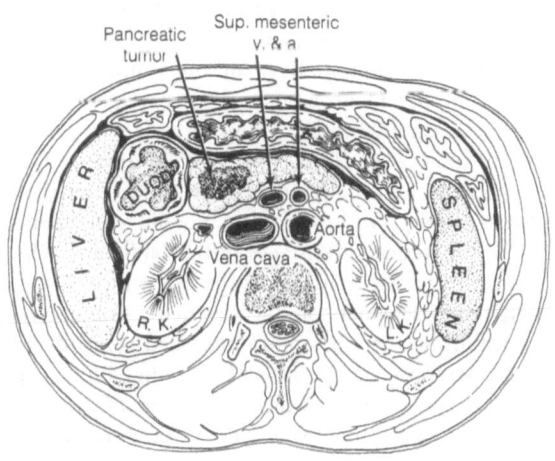

Fig. 2.

structures. It can easily be seen that the posterior margin and the superior mesenteric artery and portal vein are at greatest risk of compromise by neoplasm. Similarly, clearance of the nodal groups in the region of the proximal duodenum, pylorus, and distal stomach does add theoretical value to the operation. In a study performed by Cubilla et al. [14], nodes in these regions were not found to be involved with tumor in otherwise resectable patients. The posterior and anterior pancreatic nodal regions were most commonly involved with neoplasm (Fig. 2).

Gastric stasis is the single greatest criticism of PPPD by those who espouse the "standard Whipple" operation. We do not have a universally agreed-upon definition of what constitutes gastric stasis; therefore, it is difficult to compare series. Significant delay in return of gastric function is almost invariably related to pancreatic leak or infection. In one series, this complication was found in 14% of patients [15]. In the Lahey clinic series, the percentage of patients who have had long-term gastric stasis requiring operative intervention has ranged from 2% to 5%.

Marginal ulceration has also been a concern with PPPD. It has been suggested that PPPD is a more ulcerogenic operation than the "standard Whipple" operation. Patients who have undergone PPPD have normal basal acid output and normal stimulated acid output when compared to nonoperated control subjects [16]. The jejunum may be at a higher risk of developing marginal ulceration than is the duodenum. However, if the flow of bicarbonate and bile salts is not diverted from the duodenojejunostomy, the jejunal exposure to a low pH should be normal.

Preservation of the antropyloric mechanism has also been shown to have benefit in the regulation of fat and carbohydrate metabolism. Doty et al. [17] have shown that fat absorption remains normal when the antropyloric mechanism is maintained. Glucose absorption has also been shown to remain normal by increased glucose tolerance and decreased insulin requirement in patients in whom the antropyloric mechanism was preserved [2,18].

No perfect nutritional parameter to compare postoperative performance in patients who have undergone pancreatic resection has been found. The roughest overall estimate of nutritional performance has been the ability to gain or retain weight. In our series 74% of patients were able to maintain at least 90% of their preoperative weight or gain weight. In a comparative, although not randomized, series by Kozuschek et al. [9], an improvement in postoperative weight gain was shown in the PPPD group over the "standard Whipple" group.

The theoretical advantages of PPPD can be summarized as retention of antropyloric function, perhaps a better operation from a nutritional standpoint, avoidance of postgastrectomy syndromes, and possibly an operation technically easier to perform. The theoretical advantages of the "standard Whipple" operation include a lesser chance of gastric stasis, perhaps a technically easier operation to perform, and no nutritional detriment, and it is a "better" cancer operation. Despite all the foregoing possibilities, there are no randomized controlled studies to prove these claims of either operation. On the basis of the Lahey Clinic experience and the data that exist in the literature, we believe that PPPD is an *adequate* cancer operation. Complication rates and survival rates are comparable between patients who have had either operation. While data seem to be emerging that may support the idea that preservation of the pylorus confers a nutritional advantage, this remains to be proved. In response to the question posed by Drs. Patel, Reber, and colleagues, "Is it any better?", we do not think that this question can be answered with the existing information.

References

1. Traverso LW, Longmire WP (1978) Preservation of the pylorus during pancreaticoduodenectomy. Surg Gynecol Obstet 146:959–962
2. Braasch JW, Deziel DJ, Rossi RL, Watkins E Jr, Winter PF (1986) Pyloric and gastric preserving pancreatic resection: experience with 87 patients. Ann Surg 204:411–418
3. Newman KD, Braasch JW, Rossi RL, O'Campo-Gonzales S (1983) Pyloric and gastric preservation with pancreatoduodenectomy. Am J Surg 145:152–156
4. Grace PA, Pitt HA, Longmire WP Jr (1990) Preservation of the pylorus in pancreaticoduodenectomy: an overview. Br J Surg 77:968–974
5. Crist DW, Sitzmann JV, Cameron JL (1987) Improved hospital morbidity, mortality, and survival after the Whipple procedure. Ann Surg 206:358–365
6. Tsao JI, Rossi RL, Lowell JA (1994) Pylorus-preserving pancreatoduodenectomy: is it an adequate cancer operation? Arch Surg 129:405–412
7. Patel AG, Toyama MT, Kusske AM, Alexander P, Ashley SW, Reber HA (1995) Pylorus preserving Whipple resection for pancreatic cancer: is it any better? Arch Surg 838–843
8. Halsted WS (1899) Contributions to the surgery of bile passages, especially of the common bile duct. Boston Med Surg J 141:645–654
9. Kozuschek W, Reith HB, Waleczek H, Haarmann W, Edelmann M, Sonntag D (1994) A comparison of long-term results of the standard Whipple procedure and the pylorus-preserving pancreatoduodenectomy. J Am Coll Surg 178:443–458
10. Whipple AO, Parsons WB, Mullins CR (1935) Treatment of carcinoma of the ampulla of Vater. Ann Surg 181:763–779
11. Trede M, Schwall G, Saeger H-D (1990) Survival after pancreatoduodenectomy: 118 consecutive resections without an operative mortality. Ann Surg 211:447–548
12. Howard JM (1968) Pancreaticoduodenectomy: forty-one consecutive Whipple resections without an operative mortality. Ann Surg 168:629–640
13. Crile G Jr (1970) The advantages of bypass operations over radical pancreatoduodenectomy in the treatment of pancreatic carcinoma. Surg Gynecol Obstet 130(6):1049–1053
14. Cubilla AL, Fortner J, Fitzgerald PJ (1978) Lymph node involvement in carcinoma of the head of the pancreas area. Cancer (Phila) 41:880–887
15. Traverso LW, Kozarek RA (1993) The Whipple procedure for severe complications of chronic pancreatitis. Arch Surg 128:1047–1053
16. Pearlman NW, Steigman GV, Ahnen DJ, Schultz AL, Fink LM (1986) Acid and gastrin levels following pyloric-preserving pancreaticoduodenectomy. Arch Surg 121:661–664
17. Doty JE, Meyer JH (1987) Vagotomy and antrectomy impairs absorption of fat from solid, but not liquid dietary sources (abstract). Gastroenterology 97(5 pt 2):1374
18. Hongo M, Satake K, Sanoyama K, Lin YF, Ujiie H, Toyota T, Goto Y (1987) Regulation of insulin demand by gastric emptying in diabetics (abstract). Gastroenterology 92(5 pt 2):1440

The Oncological Approach of Pylorus-Preserving Pancreatoduodenectomy for Malignancies

Hans-Bernd Reith[1], Waldemar Kozuschek[2], Wilhelm Haarmann[2], and L. William Traverso[3]

Summary. There has been considerable debate about whether pylorus preservation significantly detracts from the radicality in a palliative procedure in which a conventional Whipple operation would have been curative. We know now that the extended radicality of the Whipple operation does not improve long-term survival rates. Our results of 81 pylorus-preserving pancreatoduodenectomy (PPPD) and 34 standard Whipple procedures in pancreas malignancies from 1985 to April 1995 showed the nutritional benefits for the PPPD group as compared to the standard Whipple group. The long-term survival rates of both groups and results reported in the literature are similar. The weakest aspect of the radical resection is addressing the retroperitoneal margin of the pancreas head and not the gastric resection. Considering all examination results, it is mandatory that the restricted organ loss in the Whipple procedure with pylorus preservation leaves the incretory capacity of the upper gastrointestinal tract almost unchanged. We doubt whether loss of radicality is a serious problem, because the majority of resections carried out for pancreatic cancer are in truth palliative rather than curative.

Key words. Pancreatic cancer—Pylorus preservation—Comparison to standard Whipple

Introduction

The removal of the head of the pancreas, the terminal bile duct, all of the duodenum, a portion of the proximal jejunum, and half of the stomach is a substantial operation. With improvements in medical understanding and technology, this procedure is being performed more often with an ever-decreasing morbidity and mortality rate. The nutritional aspect of the reconstructed gastrointestinal tract has stimulated much

[1] Department of Surgery, University Würzburg, D-97080 Würzburg, Germany.
[2] Department of Surgery, Ruhr-University Bochum, Knappschaftskrankenhaus, D-44892 Bochum, Germany.
[3] Department of Surgery, Virgina Mason Clinic, Seattle, WA 98111, U.S.A.

investigation [1]. The procedure has been modified to promote a return to normal nutrition in patients who are expected to have long-term survival. Also adding to our knowledge of nutrition in the postoperative period are the increasing numbers of patients undergoing the Whipple procedure for severe complications of benign disease: chronic pancreatitis. It is not a coincidence that the improvements in medical knowledge and technology applied to pancreaticoduodenectomy include preservation of the pylorus [2,3].

Various objective measurements of digestive function have been obtained following the Whipple procedure in animals and humans. These observations include gastric emptying, small bowel intestinal transport, and the serum levels of gut hormones. All these excellent approaches to the study of the physiological sequelae of the Whipple procedure have made contributions. Regardless of the long-term survival outcome and other objective tests, the most important aspect is the patient's ability to gain and then maintain weight postoperatively. In chronic pancreatitis, Traverso and Kozarek presented, in an average follow-up of 27 months after pylorus-preserving pancreaticoduodenectomy (PPPD), that 96% of these patients were able to gain weight postoperatively [2]. Unfortunately, in more than a dozen reports of the pylorus-preserving procedure, few authors have mentioned the ability to gain weight after surgery [3].

Material and Methods

From 1985 until April 1995 we operated on 81 patients with a malignant process of the head of pancreas, using PPPD, and compared it with a group of 34 patients operated in the same time period with a standard Whipple procedure for adenocarcinoma. The histological examination and the spread of tumor was compared to the tumor invasion at the surgical border on retroperitoneal margin, lymphatic, or perineuric spreading. The histological examination was carried out in the Department of Pathology, Ruhr-University Bochum.

In our study we have also compared the ability to regain body weight between patients receiving the pylorus-preserving Whipple porcedure versus the standard Whipple. We found that 88% of the patients were able to regain their preoperative weight after pylorus preservation but only 47% of the standard Whipple patients had done so within a 1-year period. Statistical analysis was done with Student's t-test or the chi-square test with $P < .05$.

Results

We have resected 115 patients with a malignant pancreas head tumor; our resection rate during this period was 115/209 (53.6%). Indications for the standard Whipple procedure are tumor size, previous operations, and the intraoperative decision that the tumor invasion comes near to the pylorus region (Table 1). The operation times for the two procedures showed significant differences: PPPD requires $3.6 \pm .8$ h versus the standard $5.1 \pm .9$ h ($P < .01$); mortality rates in the groups were 3.7% in the PPPD and 8.8% in the standard Whipple group. The Bochum survival data are convincing because no significant difference was found between patients with pancreatic adenocarcinoma recieving a pylorus-preserving Whipple and those undergoing the standard Whipple.

TABLE 1. Reasons for performing
the standard Whipple procedure in
the period 1985–April 1995

Reason	n
Previous operations	11
Hemigastrectomy	8
Bile duct anastomosis	3
Tumor staging	16
Previous diseases	7
Ulcer disease	5
Pylorus stenosis	2
Total:	34

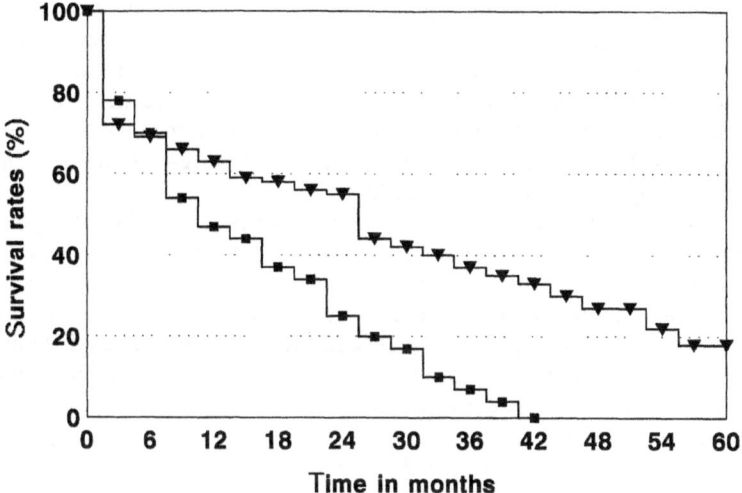

FIG. 1. Survival rates (%) of all patients with a pancreatic head resection in comparison to their kind of resection. R0, No tumor invasion or more than 5 mm to retroperitoneal margin, no perineuric or lymphatic invasion (*triangles*); R1, all other cases (*squares*)

The tumor node metastasis (TNM) classification and grading of the tumors showed no differences in the treatment groups. The patients with an adenocarcinoma of the head of the pancreas, 56 in the PPPD and 34 in the standard Whipple group, were compared as to tumor invasion. If we found tumor near the surgical margin or less than 5 mm from the margin, or a lymphatic, perineuric invasion, we classified this as an R1 resection. In the PPPD group, 24 were classified as R1 and 32 as R0; 16 of the standard Whipple group were classified as R1 resection and 18 were not. The survival rates of this groups (R1 and R0) showed significant differences (Fig. 1).

Discussion

Many oncologic surgeons have avoided pylorus preservation because the wide dissection to preserve the pylorus might interfere with en bloc resection, but has this changed survival [4]. The Bochum data provide convincing results. This is not new; in

1986 Grave et al. compared patients with pylorus preservation versus the standard Whipple and showed that the pylorus-preserving Whipple patients might have fared slightly better in long-term survival [5]. A report from the Netherlands led by Klinkenbijl and colleagues reported similar results [6]. Finally, Crist and Cameron in 1987 [7] showed that it really made no difference for survival whether a Whipple or a total pancreatectomy was performed. Therefore, the literature supports the conclusion that there is no difference in survival in patients with pancreatic cancer or periampullary tumors who receive a pancreatoduodenectomy whether without or with pylorus preservation. However, the latter patients have better nutrition as a result.

The results of other investigators have given us tactical clues to pursue why the results of the Whipple procedure are so poor when applied to pancreatic adenocarcinoma. The group in Boston led by Warshaw [8] investigated the matter of surgical margins after the Whipple procedure. It was not surprising that there were no 5-year survivors with positive surgical margins and a 22% 5-year survival rate with negative margins. Half the patients had positive margins, and the most common area was the retropancreatic soft tissue just posterior to the pancreatic head. This is the weak area for any Whipple procedure for clearance of tumor, not the area of the pylorus. It makes little sense to have a millimeter margin posteriorly and have centimeter-long margins on the stomach!

Crist showed that another important variable favoring survival was the presence of negative nodes [7]. This has most recently been confirmed with the new Japanese staging system. The results of extended nodal clearance from Germany and Japan allow us to examine some of the new resection classifications. The group in Mannheim, led by Trede, presented a 24% survival rate with standard Whipple and wide nodal clearance [9]. The Japanese groups, e.g., Ishikawa and colleagues [10], found better survival rates after extended radical surgery when applied to appropriately selected patients.

The study from Lund (Sweden, 1991) become very important to our understanding of why the Whipple procedure fails for pancreatic adenocarcinoma of the head of the pancreas, whether the radical or standard procedure, regardless of pylorus preservation or hemigastrectomy. Since 1958 they have performed an extended radical standard Whipple procedure with total pancreatectomy. Most recently, they have performed the same operation, excepting the tail of the pancreas to avoid diabetes. The 3-year survival rate was 2% and 6% in the first and second periods, respectively, and 25% in the latest period. Thus, their survival rate increased with a slightly less radical procedure and better patient selection. Despite radical resection, local recurrence was seen in approximately 90% of their patients in each of the three time periods reportd [11].

Conclusion

In conclusion, surgery alone is not the answer, whether it is a pylorus-preserving or an extended Whipple procedure. It is necessary to select patients by use of sensitive screening tests, resulting in early diagnosis, so that they will benefit from this operation. Aggressive chemoradiotherapy protocols in nonresectable patients will be one aspect of treatment, and also chemoradiotherapy protocols after resection provide another factor in increasing survival rate. However, the time of patient recovery is shorter with preservation of the pylorus because much of the function of the gastrointestinal (GI) tract as possible is retained and diabetes is avoided, so additional treatment can be started earlier. We would say the best operation is the pyloruspreserving Whipple procedure done radically with negative microscopic margins.

References

1. Traverso LW, Longmire WP (1978) Preservation of the pylorus during pancreaticoduodenectomy. Surg Gynecol Obstet 146:959–962
2. Traverso LW, Kozarek RA (1993) The Whipple procedure for severe complications of chronic pancreatitis. Arch Surg 128:1047–1053
3. Kozuschek W, Reith HB, Waleczek H, Haarmann W, Edelmann M, Sonntag D (1994) A comparision of long-term results of the standard Whipple procedure and the pylorus-preserving pancreatoduodenectomy. J Am Coll Surg 178:443–458
4. Carter D, Trede M, Beger HG, Roder JD, Siewert JR (1994) Hat die Pyloruserhaltung bei der Pankreatoduodenektomie wegen periampullären Karzinoms einen Stellenwert? Langenbecks Arch Chir 379:58–63
5. Grace PA, Pitt HA, Longmire WP (1986) Pancreaticoduodenectomy with pylorus preservation for adenocarcinoma of the head of the pancreas. Br J Surg 73:647–650
6. Klinkenbijl JHG, van der Schelling GP, Hop WCI, van Pel R, Bruining HA, Jeefel J (1992) The advantages of pylorus-preserving pancreatoduodenectomy in malignant disease of the pancreas and periampullary region. Ann Surg 216:142–145
7. Crist DW, Sitzmann JV, Cameron JL (1982) Improved hospital morbidity, mortality and survival after the Whipple procedure. Ann Surg 206:358–365
8. Willett CG, Lewandrowski K, Warshaw AL, Efird J, Compton CC (1993) Resection margins in carcinoma of the head of the pancreas: implication for radiation therapy. Ann Surg 217:144–148
9. Trede M, Schwall G, Saeger HD (1990) Survival after pancreaticoduodenectomy: 118 consecutive resections without an operative mortality. Ann Surg 211:447–458
10. Ishikawa O, Ohigashi H, Imaoka S, Furukawa H, Sasaki Y, Fujita M, Kuruda C, Iwanaga T (1992) Preoperative indications for extended pancreatectomy for locally advanced pancreas cancer involving the portal vein. Ann Surg 215:231–236
11. Andren-Sandberg A, Ahren B, Tranberg KG, Bengmark S (1991) Surgical treatment of pancreatic cancer. Int J Pancreatol 9:145–151

Techniques for Extended Pancreatoduodenectomy

Extended Resection Combined with Intraoperative Radiotherapy

Takehisa Hiraoka, Keiichiro Kanemitsu, and Tetsuro Morisaki

Summary. Since 1984, intraoperative radiotherapy (IORT) combined with extended resection for pancreatic cancer has been performed in our clinic to prevent local recurrence. Following extended resection, a dose of 30 Gy of 9–12 MeV electrons is administered to the operative field, including the paraaortic area from the diaphragm above to the inferior mesenteric artery below. The 5-year survival rate was 19.4% in all 33 cases, 26.6% in patients who had macroscopic tumor clearance, and 20.3% in patients with stage IVa tumor according to the Japanese classification. In autopsies of 7 patients who underwent the combined therapy, only 2 had local recurrence enclosed by thick, firm connective tissue. There was no local recurrence in 2 patients who underwent noncurative resection. Enhanced local control induced by the combined therapy, however, has only a limited impact on overall survival because of system disease progression, especially hepatic metastases. These results suggest that a combination of IORT and extended resection should be performed on selected patients to control local recurrence and that anticancer treatment for metastases of the liver must be established as soon as possible for the cure of pancreatic cancer.

Key words. Extended pancreatectomy—Intraoperative radiotherapy—Pancreatic cancer—Carcinoma

Introduction

Despite recent advances in diagnostic methods and surgical techniques, the long-term survival of patients following resection for pancreatic carcinoma remains poor. Radical resection for pancreatic carcinoma has not produced a discernible benefit, and even following such extensive surgery local recurrence at autopsy is seen in a high proportion of patients. Despite these results, surgery remains the mainstay for treating this disease and the only chance for cure.

Given the promising results of intraoperative radiotherapy (IORT) for pancreatic cancer, this therapy has been combined with resection at the Kumamoto University Medical School since 1976, but the results when combined with conventional surgery

First Department of Surgery, Kumamoto University School of Medicine, Kumamoto 860, Japan.

proved disappointing [1]. In 1982, extended radical resection was introduced as a means of improving local control of pancreatic cancer. Although the operative mortality and morbidity proved to be acceptable, the long-term results showed little improvement.

Since 1984, therefore, extended radical resection has been combined with extended IORT at our institute. Our results with this approach for cancer of the pancreas are presented here.

Patients and Methods

Patients and Type of Resection

From 1984 to February 1996, 33 patients with adenocarcinoma of the pancreas of duct cell origin apart from cystoadencarcinoma and intraductal mucinous adenocarcinoma underwent extended radical resection with IORT. This procedure included pancreatectomy with almost complete resection en bloc of the lymph nodes around the porta hepatis, the celiac axis, the origin of the superior mesenteric artery, and the aorta extending from the diaphragm above to the inferior mesenteric artery below. The inferior vena cava and aorta were also skeletonized, with all tissue being removed en bloc (Fig. 1). Of the 33 patients, 23 had cancer of the head of the pancreas and underwent pancreaticoduodenectomy. The remaining 10 had cancer of the pancreas body and/or tail; 7 underwent distal pancreatectomy, 2 total pancreatectomy, and 1 pancreaticoduodenectomy. The pancreatic segment of the portal vein was removed in 12 of the 33 patients. Of these 12, 1 with resection of the portal vein underwent resection of the common hepatic artery. Of the 33, 29 had

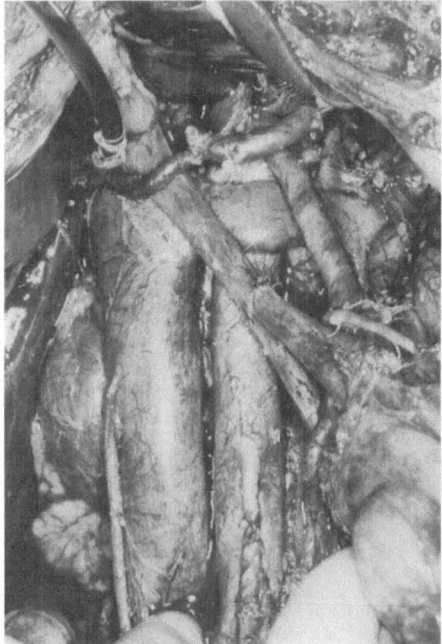

FIG. 1. Extent of dissection in extended radical resection of the pancreas. The inferior vena cava, aorta, mesenteric artery, and celiac axis are routinely skeletonized

TABLE 1. Stage classification proposed by the Japan Pancreas Society

T category (extent of tumor invasion)	P_0, H_0, M_0				$P_1 \lesseqgtr, H_1 \lesseqgtr$ or M_1
	N_0	N_1	N_2	N_3	
T_1a: size $\leqq 2$ cm	I	II	III		
$S_0 + RP_0 + PV_0 + A_0 + DU_0 + CH_{0,1}$				IV_a	
T_1b: size >2 cm	II	II	III		
$S_0 + RP_0 + PV_0 + A_0 + DU_0 + CH_{0,1}$					
T_2:	III	III	IV_a		
$S_1, RP_1, PV_1, A_1, Du_{1,2,3}, CH_{2,3}$ (any factor $\geqq 1$)					
T_3:	IV_a				IV_b
$S_{2,3}, RP_{2,3}, PV_{2,3}, A_{2,3}$ (any factor $\geqq 1$)					

P, peritoneal metastasis; H, liver metastasis; M, distant metastasis; N, lymph node metastasis; N_0, no evidence of lymph node metastasis; N_1, adjacent lymph node metastasis; N_2, regional lymph node metastasis; N_3, remote lymph node metastasis; S, invasion into the anterior pancreatic capsule; RP, invasion to the retroperitoneal tissue; PV, invasion to the portal venous system; A, invasion to the arterial system; DU, invasion to the duodenal wall; CH, invasion to the distal bile duct; 0, no evidence of invasion; 1, invasion suspected; 2, definite invasion; 3, marked invasion, but direct invasion to the adjacent viscera in S and RP factor.

TABLE 2. Tumor stage and tumor clearance in resected cases, $n = 33$

Tumor stage:	
I	0
II	1
III	5
IV_a	23
IV_b	4
Tumor clearance:	
Macroscopic	
Complete	29
Incomplete	4
Microscopic	
Complete	23
Incomplete	10

macroscopic tumor clearance, but 6 of the 29 had histologically incomplete tumor clearance.

The pancreatic cancers were staged in accordance with the classification of the Japan Pancreas Society [2] (Table 1). Tumor staging and the macroscopic and microscopic tumor clearance of the patients are summarized in Table 2.

Cumulative survival rates were calculated by the Kaplan–Meier method for each of the two treatment groups. Survival differences were calculated using log rank analysis.

Extended Electron Beam IORT

Following resection, including vascular reconstruction, a dose of 30 Gy of 9–12 MeV electrons was administered to the operative field, including the paraaortic area from the diaphragm above to the inferior mesenteric artery below, using a special applica-

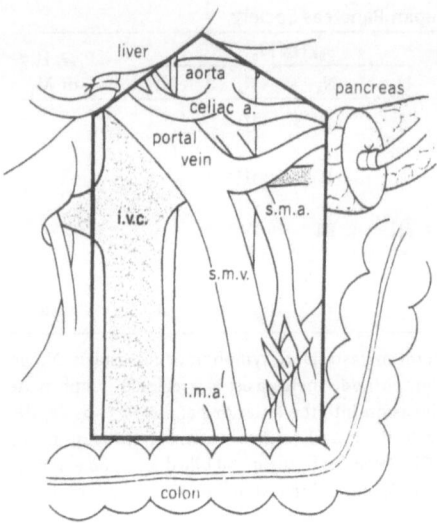

FIG. 2. Radiation field of extended intra-operative radiotherapy (IORT) combined with extended surgery. The pentagon indicates the borders of the radiation field. *i.v.c.*, Inferior vena cava; *celiac a.*, celiac axis; *s.m.a.*, superior mesenteric artery; *s.m.v.*, superior mesenteric vein; *i.m.a.*, inferior mesenteric artery

tor. For expansion of the IORT portal, a special applicator was used that could be varied in size to accommodate the operative field on an individual basis [3]. The pancreatic remnant and the bile duct were both kept outside the field of irradiation (Fig. 2).

Results

Patient Survival

Of these 33 patients, 3 died at the hospital in the postoperative period; 2 of these 3 patients died of anastomotic leakage from the pancreticojejunostomy. There were no other postoperative complications that could be attributed to IORT. All the patients who had extended radical resection, involving pancreaticoduodenectomy as well as total pancreatectomy, had poor postoperative nutritional status including watery diarrhea and fatty liver infiltration from 4 to 33 months postoperatively; however, patients who survived more than 3 years had a high quality of life. Of these 33 patients, 31 were treated successfully by administration of fatty emulsion or intravenous hyperalimentation. The other 2 patients had severe nutritional depletion and both eventually died of sepsis; however, there were no features of recurrent cancer at 8 months and 32 months after the resection and IORT, respectively, in these 2 cases.

At the present time, 10 patients who have had extended radical resection combined with IORT are still alive from 2 months to 11 years and 7 months postoperatively; 23 died of recurrence of cancer within 8 years and 2 months. Of 33 patients with extended resection combined with IORT, 18 died of recurrence of cancer.

The cumulative survival rates of all the cases are shown in Fig. 3; the 5-year survival rate of all 33 patients was 19.4%. The 5-year survival rate of 26 patients who had complete macroscopic clearance of all tumor in combination with IORT, excluding the 3 patients who died at the hospital, was 26.6% (Fig. 4). Of these 26 cases, 6 had histologically incomplete tumor clearance. The 5-year survival rates of 20 patients who had complete microscopic tumor clearance and 5 patients who had incomplete

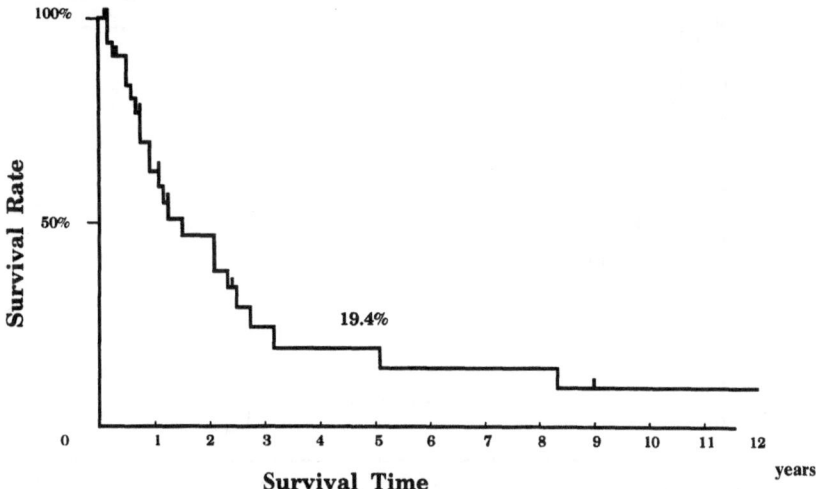

FIG. 3. Cumulative survival rates of patients who had extended resection in combination with IORT for cancer of the pancreas ($n = 33$, *thick line*), including operation-related deaths and noncuratively resected cases

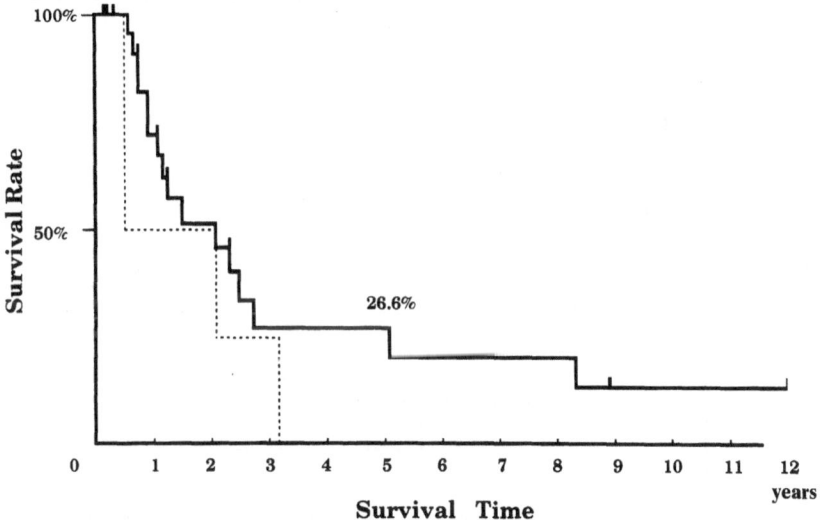

FIG. 4. Cumulative survival rates of patients who had extended resection for cancer of the pancreas. Incomplete macroscopic tumor clearance ($n = 4$, *hatched line*); complete macroscopic tumor clearance ($n = 26$, *thick line*). Three cases who died of operation-related complications are excluded

microscopic tumor clearance were 31.7% and 11.1%, respectively. One patient with stage II tumor is still alive more than 10 years after the operation, and 1 of 4 patients with stage III tumor is still alive after more than 2 years and 5 months. The 5-year survival rate of 22 cases with stage IVa tumor was 20.3%; 3 patients with stage IVb tumor died within 8 months (Fig. 5).

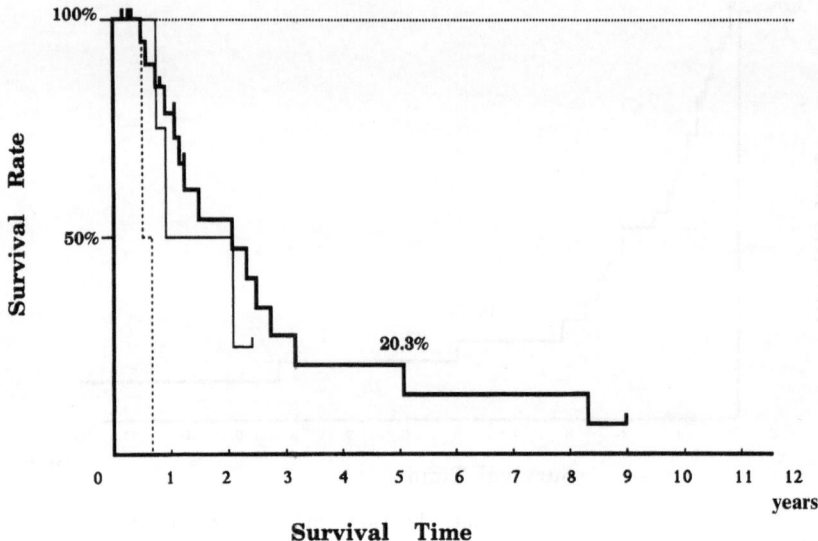

FIG. 5. Cumulative survival rate of patients who had extended resection for cancer of the pancreas according to histological tumor stage of Japanese classification, excluding operation-related deaths. Stage II (1), *small dashed line*; stage III (4), *thin line*; stage IVa (22), *thick line*; stage IVb (3), *large hatched line*

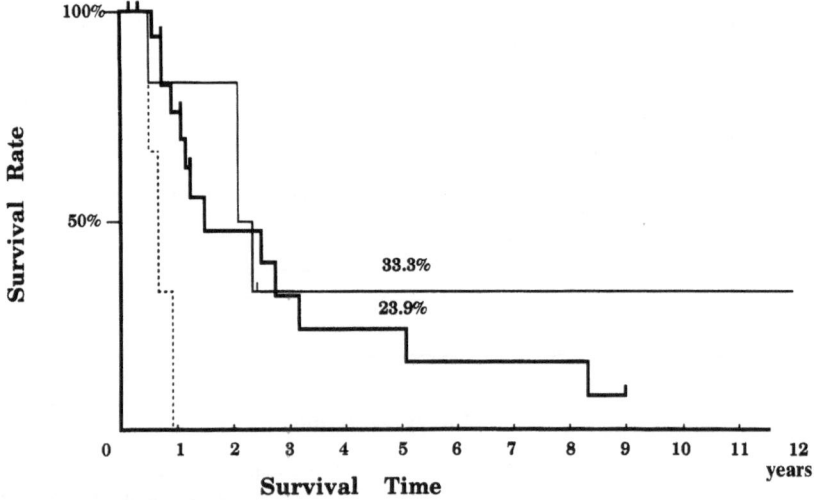

FIG. 6. Cumulative survival rate of patients who had extended resection for cancer of the pancreas according to classification of involvement of lymph node in Japanese classification, excluding operation-related deaths. Stage n0 (6), *thin line*; n1 (20), *thick line*; n2 (4), *hatched line*

TABLE 3. Results of treatment of 33 patients by extended resection combined with intraoperative radiotherapy (IORT)

Reason for death	n
Still alive	10
Dead (23):	
In hospital	3
Other disease	2
Tumor recurrence (18):	
Liver metastases	11
Carcinomatosis peritonei	4
Liver metastasis/ileal perforation	1
Recurrence in remnant of pancreas	1
Pleural/lung earcinomatosis	1

According to the degree of involvement of lymph nodes in the Japanese classification, the 5-year survival rates of six patients of n0 and 20 patients of n1 were 33.3% and 23.9%, respectively; four patients of n2 died within 1 year (Fig. 6). Four patients survived more than 5 years; three patients were stage IVa and one was stage II. Three of these four had involvement of lymph nodes.

Two of the 33 patients underwent resection of recurrent lesions after the combined therapy. One patient underwent partial resection of the liver for metastases two times, at 32.5 and 49.5 months postoperatively, and survived more than 4 years after the last operation. The other patient underwent partial resection of the liver and right lung 21 months after first operation and partial resection of the left lung 2 months later. This patient survived 7 months after the last operation.

Eighteen patients who had extended combined surgical and radiation therapy died of tumor recurrence within 8 years and 2 months after the operation. Eleven of the 18 cases died of liver metastases, 4 died of carcinomatosis peritonei, 1 died of ileal perforation associated with metastases, 1 died of recurrent tumor in the remnant pancreas, and the remaining patient died of pleural carcinomatosis (Table 3).

Pathological Findings at Autopsy of Patients Who Died During Follow-Up

Autopsies were performed in seven cases, excepting one case of operative death with autopsy. Five cases had no evidence of any local recurrence in the radiation field but peritoneal tumor seedlings were found in two cases and liver metastases in one case, respectively, of the seven. In the other two cases there was no evidence of any recurrence at autopsy; these two patients died of sepsis associated with severe nutritional disturbance. Two of the five cases without local recurrence had incomplete tumor clearance.

In the remaining two patients who were autopsied at 8 months and 5.1 years, respectively, following extended resection and IORT, local microscopic recurrence was found within the radiation field around the aorta just above the left renal artery in the patient with cancer of the body of the pancreas and around the aorta from the level of the celiac axis to the level of common iliac artery in the other patient who had cancer of the body of the pancreas. These microscopic findings showed sporadic cancer cells and cancer cell clumps in connective tissue, in the perineural space, and in small lymph nodes of 1 mm in diameter in the nervous plexus around the aorta.

Discussion

The prognosis for patients with resectable pancreatic cancer has consistently been poor; at best, resection offers a modest prolongation of life or temporary palliation of symptoms. The results of total pancreatectomy and regional pancreatectomy, including resection and reconstruction of the portal vein and/or superior mesenteric artery, have not been shown to be superior to lesser procedures in terms either of operative mortality or morbidity or of long-term survival [4–8]. One of the reasons for these disappointing results is local recurrence around the celiac axis, mesenteric vessels, and aorta. It is therefore apparent that involved lymphatics and lymph nodes and local micrometastases cannot normally be removed by the surgical procedure alone.

In an attempt to overcome this problem, the first approach adopted at Kumamoto University Medical School was the application of IORT to the celiac axis and mesenteric region following conventional pancreaticoduodenectomy [1]. Prolongation of survival, however, was not seen from this combined approach despite an improvement of control of local disease. Local recurrences were not frequently found within the area of IORT administration, but recurrences developed surrounding the radiation field. This was considered to represent a significant step toward designing a new treatment strategy for pancreatic cancer. The IORT portal was expanded from the 6- to 8-cm circular applicator used initially to a much larger radiation field encompassing the area from the diaphragm to the level of the inferior mesenteric artery. A special variable applicator was made to irradiate the extended area according to individual body size [3].

As a surgical development, extended radical resection was then taken up with almost complete resection of the lymph nodes and lymphatic chains around the celiac axis, mesenteric vessels, and aorta from the diaphragm to the level of the inferior mesenteric artery. Such an approach on its own, however, was also found not to improve survival, again because of local cancer recurrence around the aorta [9].

Of 33 patients who underwent extended resection with IORT, 4 survived more than 5 years after treatment, and 1 of the 4 was a noncuratively resected case. The 5-year cumulative survival rate of all the cases including operative deaths and noncuratively resected cases was 19.4%, and that of 21 patients with macroscopic tumor clearance was 26.6%; moreover, that of 22 patients with stage IVa tumor stage was 20.3%. These results are not superior to results reported by other authors [8–13], but extended radical surgery and expansion of the IORT portal seemed to result in improvement of local disease. This combined therapy will not be beneficial for patients with advanced tumor. In fact, these patients died of distant metastases (mainly hepatic metastases).

Sindelar observed that pancreatectomy plus IORT was superior to pancreatectomy alone with respect to patient survival in a randomized trial of IORT with a dose of 20 Gy with 8–14 MeV in resected carcinoma of the pancreas [14]. Moreover, Sindelar tried combination treatment of IORT in 11 of 20 patients with regional pancreatectomy for far-advanced cancer. In this trial, however, he reported that a significant improvement in the IORT group was not obtained compared to patients with external radiation therapy in terms of long-term survival, but the local recurrence rate at 1 year postoperatively was lower in the IORT group [15].

This extended combined therapy for far-advanced cancer may not be beneficial. Manabe et al. reported that a modest improvement has been obtained in survival rate and local recurrence rate using the combination of IORT at a dose of 25–30 Gy with 6–10 MeV and extended resection, but this was not significant [16]. Hanyu et al. did not find any benefit from IORT with a dose of 25 Gy with 9–15 MeV in resected pancreatic cancer [17].

Results of combined therapy using resection and radiation must be affected by differences in parameters of IORT, the stage of the tumor, and the degree and extent of dissection of lymph nodes in resection. In particular, suitable matching in combination between parameters of IORT and degree and extent of dissection is very important to obtain a better local effect. The tumor must be reduced as little as possible to get a better effect with radiation therapy on the tumor. Therefore, the combination of extended surgery with extended IORT may be the best approach in combination therapy of resection with radiation for advanced cancer. A further study with large numbers will be required to clarify the clinical significance of such combined therapy.

Judging from the autopsy and cause of death in patients with extended operation combined with IORT, we think that even if resection and radiation therapy were extended and combined, local recurrence of the tumor could not be completely controlled; however, the incidence of local recurrence is decreased by introducing the extended combined therapy. Two patients who had incomplete tumor clearance showed no local recurrence. Moreover, at autopsy of two patients with local recurrence of those who underwent this combined therapy, local microscopic recurrence was only found enclosed by thick, firm connective tissues. Such findings will not directly cause death. In this series of patients with combined therapy, the cause of death of patients with tumor recurrence was almost always metastasis via vessels.

We have often found local recurrence and hepatic metastases after the standard operation, but could not evaluate which factor is more important in the prognosis for patients with resection for pancreatic cancer. Now we can clearly recognize the gravity of liver metastases in treatment for pancreatic cancer by introducing extended resection combined with IORT. We think that extended pancreatectomy combined with IORT is best used as a treatment for local disease control at present. Enhanced local control induced by this combined therapy, however, has only a limited impact on overall survival because of systemic disease progression, especially hepatic metastases. Therefore, as a next step, anticancer treatment toward metastases of the liver will become very important for the cure of pancreatic cancer.

Anticancer treatment for hepatic metastases must be considered from two points of view: treatment for hepatic metastases after resection for pancreatic cancer and prophylactic treatment to prevent lodging of cancer cells in the blood vessels. If we can inhibit local recurrence after resection, some metastatic lesions may be resected. We performed partial resection of the liver on one patient who had not had local recurrence after resection for pancreatic cancer. This patient survived more than 8 years after the first operation and 4 years after hepatic resection for metastases [18]. Hereafter, the number of such successful cases will increase by continuing this combined therapy.

At present, it is important to perform an extended pancreatectomy with extended IORT on carefully selected patients. This extended approach may not be needed for patients with tumor at a very early stage. We think that this extended approach should be indicated for patients with cancer that is not far advanced according to tumor staging. This combined approach, however, is only significant as treatment for local control of cancer. Therefore, anticancer treatment for metastases of the liver must be established for the cure of pancreatic cancer as soon as possible.

References

1. Hiraoka T, Watanabe E, Mochinaga M, Tashiro S, Miyauchi Y, Nakamura I, Yokoyama I (1984) Intraoperative irradiation combined with radical resection for cancer of the head of the pancreas. World J Surg 8:766–771
2. Japan Pancreas Society (1996) Classification of pancreatic cancer. Kanehara, Tokyo, pp 5–14
3. Hiraoka T, Nakamura I, Tashiro S, Miyauchi Y (1989) Intraoperative radiation therapy for pancreatic cancer in Japan. In: Dobelbower RR Jr, Abe M (eds) Intraoperative radiation therapy. CRC Press, Boca Raton, FL, pp 181–193
4. Fortner JG (1984) Regional pancretectomy for cancer of the pancreas, ampulla, and other related sites, tumor staging and results. Ann Surg 199:418–425
5. Longmire WP Jr (1984) Cancer of the pancreas: palliative operation, Whipple procedure, or total pancreatectomy. World J Surg 8:872–879
6. Moosa AR, Scott MH, Lavell-Jones M (1984) The place of total and extended total pancreatectomy in pancreatic cancer. World J Surg 8:895–899
7. Van Heerden JA (1984) Pancreatic resection for carcinoma of the pancreas: Whipple versus total pancreatectomy—an institutional perspective. World J Surg 8:880–888
8. Brooks JR, Brooks DC, Levine JD (1989) Total pancreatectomy for ductal cell carcinoma of the pancreas. An update. Ann Surg 209:405–410
9. Hiraoka T (1990) Extended radical resection of cancer of the pancreas with intraoperative radiotherapy. Bailliéres Clin Gastroenterol 4:985–993
10. Michelassi F, Erroi F, Dawson PJ, Pietrabissa A, Noda S, Handcock M, Block GE (1989) Experience with 647 consecutive tumors of the duodenum, ampulla, head of the pancreas, and distal common bile duct. Ann Surg 210:544–556
11. Ishikawa O, Ohigashi H, Sasaki Y, Kabuto T, Fukuda I, Furukawa H, Imaoka S, Iwanaga T (1988) Practical usefulness of lymphatic and connective tissue clearance for the carcinoma of the pancreas head. Ann Surg 208:215–220
12. Trede M, Schwall G, Saeger HD (1990) Survival after pancreatoduodenectomy: 118 consecutive resections without an operative mortality. Ann Surg 211:447–458
13. Cameron JL, Crist DW, Sitzmann JV, Hruban RH, Boitnott JK, Seidler AJ, Coleman J (1991) Factors influencing survival after pancreatoduodenectomy for pancreatic cancer. Ann J Surg 161:120–125
14. Sindelar WF (1988) Intraoperative radiotherapy in carcinoma of the stomach and pancreas. Recent Results Cancer Res 110:226–243
15. Sindelar WF (1989) Clinical experience with regional pancreatectomy for adenocarcinoma of the pancreas. Arch Surg 24:127–132
16. Manabe T, Sibamoto Y, Ono K, Sasai K, Baba N, Takahashi M, Abe M, Tobe T (1991) Combined modality treatment for cancer of the pancreas. In: Abe M, Takahashi M (eds) Intraoperative radiation therapy. Pergamon, New York, pp 242–243
17. Hanyu F, Hatori T, Imaizumi T, Suzuki M, Nakasako T, Ookawa T, Kita M (1991) Intraoperative radiation therapy for patients with carainoma of the head of the pancreas. In: Abe M, Takahashi M (eds) Intraoperative radiation therapy. Pergamon, New York, pp 242–243
18. Takamori H, Hiraoka T, Kanemitsu K, Tsuji T, Saito N, Nishida H, Sakaguchi H, Miyauchi Y (1994) Treatment strategies for hepatic metastases from pancreatic cancer in patients previously treated with radical resection combined with intraoperative radiation therapy. J Hep Bil Pancr Surg 8:107–110

Extended Pancreatoduodenectomy for Adenocarcinoma of the Pancreatic Head

Osamu Ishikawa, Hiroaki Ohigashi, Takushi Yasuda,
Hiroshi Nakano, Shoji Nakamori, Masahiro Hiratsuka,
Masao Kameyama, Yo Sasaki, Hiroshi Furukawa,
Toshiyuki Kabuto, Shingi Imaoka, and Takeshi Iwanaga

Summary. This chapter reviews the role of extended pancreatectomy in resection of adenocarcinoma of the pancreatic head. Because cancer cells are likely to spread into the lymph nodes and neighboring connective tissues, locoregional recurrence had been common in traditional or conventional pancreatectomy. Differing from the techniques in the conventional Whipple's procedure, our extended pancreatectomy is characterized by skeletonizing the major vessels to clear a wide range of lymphatic and connective tissues. By this procedure, a significant improvement has been obtained in the long-term survival rates and the locoregional control. However, such a beneficial effect is limited to the less advanced tumors: these are less than 4 cm in diameter, nodal involvement is absent or limited in the n1 group, and cancer invasion to the portal vein is either absent or less than 2 cm in length and hemilateral. For more advanced cancers, this procedure seems to be of no use at present. In the future, however, we can expect to increase the long-term survival rate after an extended pancreatectomy and thereby widen its indication, when we combine more effective adjuvant therapy that can reduce both locoregional recurrence and liver metastasis.

Key words. Extended pancreatectomy—Pancreatic cancer—Indication—Adjuvant therapy

Why Is an Extended Pancreatectomy Needed for Pancreatic Cancer?

Surgical resection is the only curative treatment of pancreatic adenocarcinoma, and recent advances in surgical techniques and postoperative care have succeeded in decreasing postoperative mortality and morbidity rates [1–3]. However, the long-term outcome after pancreaticoduodenectomy for this cancer has been very poor. In 1976, Tepper et al. [4] reported that more than 50% of patients developed locoregional recurrence after curative pancreatectomy. Thereafter, many surgeons and oncologists

Department of Surgery, Osaka Medical Center for Cancer and Cardiovascular Diseases (The Center for Adult Diseases, Osaka), Higashinari-ku, Osaka 537, Japan.

paid special attention to the causes of locoregional recurrence and concentrated on trying to prevent it when surgically resecting a pancreatic cancer.

At one time, intrapancreatic cancer residuals, the result of multifocal lesions [5,6] or continuous extension along the main pancreatic duct [7] from the main tumor, were proposed as the causes of locoregional recurrence. However, no obvious recurrence was seen in the remnant pancreas when the cut end of the pancreas had been proven to be negative for cancer cells by intraoperative histology [8]. Likewise, van Heerden et al. [9] and Sarr et al. [10] showed that total pancreatectomy was not superior to the Whipple procedure in improving the long-term survival rate. Because pancreatic fistula currently remains the most common cause of postoperative complication, it is generally considered that the only benefit of total pancreatectomy is the obviation of the pancreatic anastomosis.

On the other hand, the cause of locoregional recurrence was attributed to extrapancreatic cancer extension: nodal involvement and invasion (microinvasion, MI) into the lymphatic channels, vascular vessels, soft tissues, and perineural spaces. Among the patients who received pancreatectomy, the incidence of nodal involvement was reported to be 90% by Cubilla et al. [11], 80% by Ishikawa et al. [12], and 77% by Nakao et al. [13]. Tsuchiya et al. [14] collected small pancreatic cancers measuring 2 cm or less in diameter from the Japanese registry and reported that the nodal involvement was about 40%. In cases of cancer of the pancreatic head, it is well known that nodal involvement is common in the anterior and posterior pancreaticoduodenal regions and the region along the superior mesenteric vessels [12,13].

Although the positive nodes in these three regions are removable even by conventional pancreaticoduodenectomy, Cohen et al. [15] reported that no 5-year survivors existed among the patients who had positive nodes and underwent a conventional pancreatectomy. Thus, it is possible that incomplete eradication of MI is the more possible cause of locoregional recurrence in the conventional pancreatectomy. Cubilla et al. [16] reported that 90% of patients had cancer invasion in the perineural spaces. In addition, Nagai et al. [17] and Nagakawa et al. [18] showed that this type of

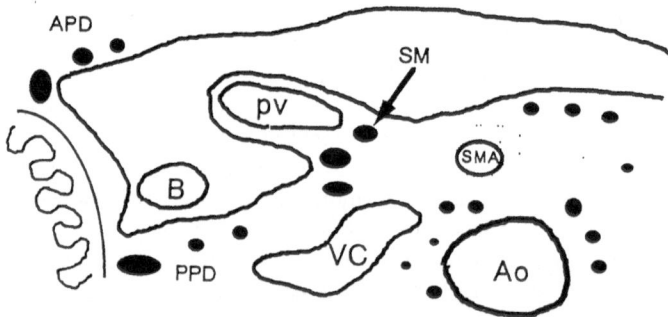

FIG. 1. Anatomical schema of the pancreatic head and neighboring vessels. The superior mesenteric artery (SMA) is encircled by a dense connective tissue that is rich in nerve fibers. The lymph nodes at the anterior (APD) and posterior pancreaticoduodenal (PPD) region and around the superior mesenteric vessels (SM) offer the common site of cancer metastasis. Ao, Aorta; VC, inferior vena cava; pv, portal vein; B, bile duct

cancer invasion was not rare, even though the tumor was as small as 2 cm or less in diameter.

To eradicate not only positive nodes but also MI, it is necessary to clear the connective tissues around the aorta, celiac artery, and superior mesenteric artery (Fig. 1). Thus, beginning in 1981, we [12] have performed an extended pancreatectomy— a wide range of lymphatic and connective tissue clearance—when resecting cancer of the pancreatic head. Our previous report [12] showed that the 3-year survival rate was improved from 13% in the group having undergone conventional pancreatectomy to 38% in the group having undergone extended pancreatectomy. Likewise, the 5-year survival rate was improved from 9% to 28%, with a significant decrease in locoregional recurrence. Long-term survival could be expected even if the regional lymph node or portal vein/superior mesenteric vein (PV/SMV) were involved by cancer [19].

Although these reports were not based on a prospective randomized study, the group of conventional pancreatectomy (historical control group, before 1981) included higher incidence of less advanced cancers because the resection of the portal vein had been abandoned when it was involved with cancer. In addition, when at least one positive node was detected at any site, no long-term (3- or 5-year) survivor existed in the control group, although there were long-term survivors in the extended pancreatectomy group. Additionally, Henne-Bruns et al. [20] performed a prospective randomized study and recognized the superiority of extended pancreatectomy to conventional pancreatectomy in the locoregional control.

Yeo et al. [21] and Cameron et al. [22] have presented an argument against our extended pancreatectomy, citing the fact that the 5-year survival rate was more than 20% in their experience of performing conventional pancreatectomies. However, we should note that their 3-year survival rate was as low as less than 10% when positive nodes were detected. Thus, the traditional or conventional pancreatectomy should be replaced by our extended pancreatectomy, and its appropriate indication is limited to the following tumors: 4 cm or less in diameter; negative in n2 group (according to the

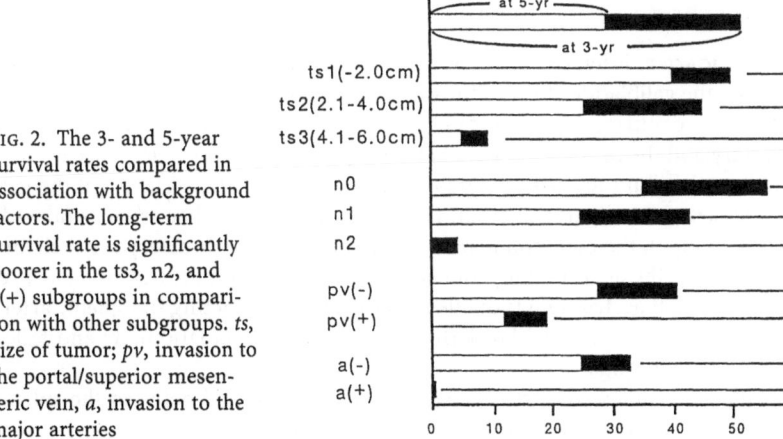

FIG. 2. The 3- and 5-year survival rates compared in association with background factors. The long-term survival rate is significantly poorer in the ts3, n2, and a(+) subgroups in comparison with other subgroups. *ts*, Size of tumor; *pv*, invasion to the portal/superior mesenteric vein, *a*, invasion to the major arteries

classification proposed by the Japan Pancreas Society [23]); and the PV/SMV-invasion is either negative or less than 2 cm in length and hemilateral (Fig. 2).

Surgical Techniques of Extended Pancreatectomy

Mobilization of the Pancreaticoduodenal Region (Extended Kocher's Maneuver)

After laparotomy, it should be confirmed that there is no hepatic metastasis, perito-neal seeding, or nodal involvement that spreads beyond the line of resection. When a curative pancreatectomy is intended, an incision of the retroperitoneum is made to remove the underlying connective tissues for the following ranges: the upper margin is 2 cm on the upper side of the root of the celiac truncus (the inferior subphrenic artery is usually cut together with the muscular tissue of the aortic crus); the lower margin should cover the root of the inferior mesenteric artery; the right margin should be 2–3 cm outside the right margin of the inferior vena cava; and the left margin is at 3 cm outside the left margin of the aorta. By this procedure, the aorta, the inferior vena cava, and the renal veins are clearly revealed, and the roots of the superior mesenteric artery and the celiac truncus can be hung by catch tape (Fig. 3). The third and fourth portions of the duodenum (including the duodenum at the ligament of Treitz) are freed from the retroperitoneal spaces (Fig. 4). The right half of the greater omentum is separated from the transverse colon. The stomach is transected by automatic suture, on the line of the distal one-fifth.

At the same time as this procedure, the mesocolon, which is attached to the inferior pancreatic head, is resected. Likewise, by preserving the bundles including the supe-rior mesenteric vessels alone, this incision is extended to the point between the body and tail of the pancreas. During this procedure, the inferior mesenteric vein is divided where it joins into the splenic vein at the point that is more cranial (right side) to the borderline between the pancreatic body and tail. Around this point, the pancreatic body is elevated and freed from the retroperitoneal cavity exposing the underlying left renal vein. We do not perform the traditional type of dissection between the anterior surface of the PV/SMV and the confines of the pancreatic neck (tunneling).

Dissection of the Hepatoduodenal Ligament and Mobilization of the Pancreatic Body

After the cystic artery is ligated and divided, the gallbladder is detached from the liver. By retracting the gallbladder toward the duodenum, the common hepatic duct is cut. The cut end is confirmed histologically to be negative in cancer cells. Along the hepatic artery and the portal vein, lymphatic and connective tissue clearance is made from the hepatic hilum toward the duodenum. The right gastric artery and the gas-troduodenal artery are ligated and cut. From the root of the celiac truncus (already hung by catch tape), the common hepatic artery and the splenic artery are skeleton-ized by removing the surrounding connective tissues. The left gastric artery is pre-served while the left gastric vein is divided after ligation. Retracting the splenic artery upward, the splenic vein at the borderline between the pancreatic body and tail is exposed and cut after ligation.

If the spleen becomes congestive, anastomosis is performed between the splenic vein and the inferior mesenteric vein after resection of the pancreatic head. Because

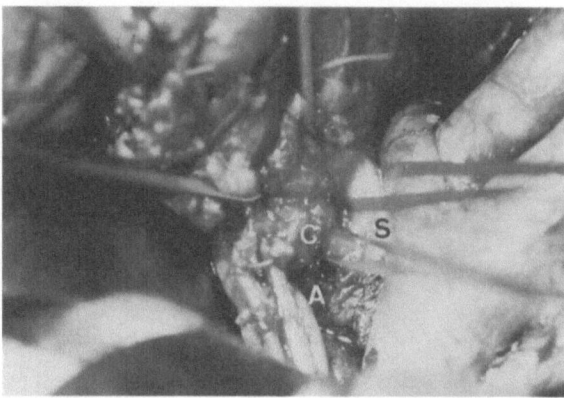

FIG. 3. Extended Kocher's maneuver. The pancreatic head and its neighboring connective tissues are elevated from the retroperitoneal space. The right half of the aortic crus is divided (*A*). A catch tape is hung aroung the root of the superior mesenteric artery (*S*) and another around the root of the celiac truncus (*C*)

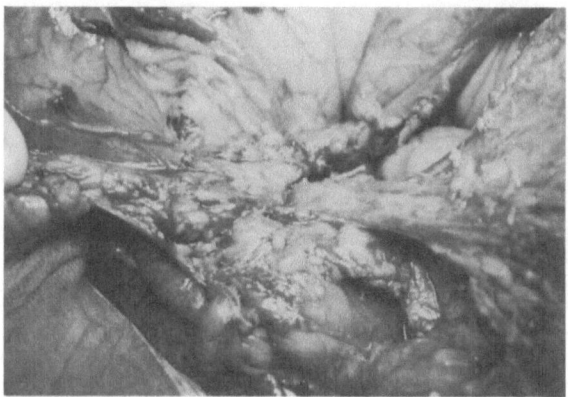

FIG. 4. Mobilization of the inferior pancreatic head. During Kocher's maneuver, the inferior pancreatic head area is freed from the retroperitoneum, mesocolon, and greater omentum. Although the bundle that includes the superior mesenteric vessels is revealed at this point, no further dissection is made between the anterior surface of PV/SMV and the posterior surface of the pancreatic neck ("tunneling" procedure)

the pancreas has been freed from the retroperitoneal space at this area, it is divided at a right angle to the main pancreatic duct using a pair of noncrushing clamps (Fig. 5). The cut end is used for the frozen section of intraoperative histology. A pancreatic catheter with a node (S.B. Medical, Tokyo, Japan) is placed in the main pancreatic duct of the caudal segment and is fixed by the pursestring suture that is made around the main pancreatic duct. Hemostasis is established for the cut surface by electric coagulation; the cut surface is oversewn with a continuous suture in a fishmouth fashion when pancreaticogastrostomy is intended.

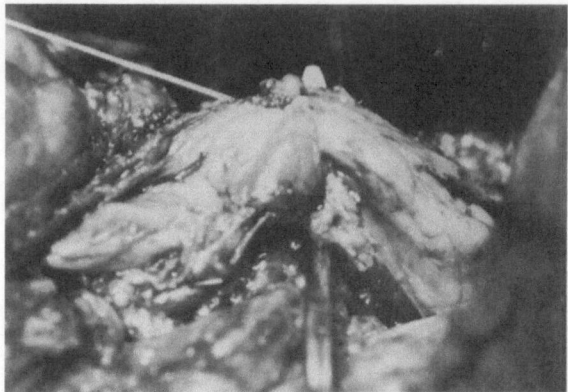

FIG. 5. Mobilization of the pancreatic body. After the splenic artery and vein are disclosed, the pancreatic body is elevated from the retroperitoneal space and transected at a right angle with the main pancreatic duct. After this procedure, we expose the superior mesenteric artery

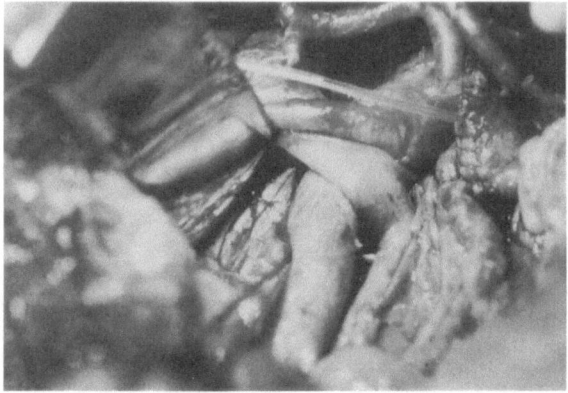

FIG. 6. Exposure of the superior mesenteric artery. When the pancreatic head is retracted to the right side, the superior mesenteric artery is disclosed clearly. The surrounding connective tissues are removed, and some branching arteries are ligated and cut. After this procedure, the PV/SMV is separated from the pancreatic head or cut together with it

Exposure of the Superior Mesenteric Vessels

With the guide of a catch tape, the anterior surface of the superior mesenteric artery is disclosed by cutting the hard connective tissue between the branching point from the aorta and the branching point to the second jejunal artery. In removing the connective tissues all around this artery, some branching arteries (the first jejunal artery, anterior and posterior inferior pancreaticoduodenal arteries, communicating arteries with dorsal pancreatic artery, and the middle colic artery) are ligated and divided. When the second jejunal artery is preserved, the mesojejunum is divided along this artery. The jejunum is transected by an automatic suture, and the oral end is pulled out under the superior mesenteric vessels (Fig. 6). At this time, the pancreatic head is attached to the PV/SMV alone. As the pancreatic head is retracted toward the right, it can be confirmed whether the cancer has infiltrated the PV/SMV. Even though no obvious invasion is detected macroscopically, we take a touch-smear for cytological examination to determine the indication for PV/SMV resection.

We Should Be More Careful in Determining the Indication of Extended Pancreatectomy

The importance of case selection should be emphasized in the indication for extended pancreatectomy. As shown in Fig. 2, for advanced tumors (more than 4 cm in diameter, positive for nodal involvement in the n2 group [23], and direct invasion to the surrounding major arteries), we can scarcely expect that an extended pancreatectomy will be effective. In reviewing the causes of cancer death after extended pancreatectomy, hepatic metastasis was more frequent than the locoregional recurrence [12], suggesting the limited effectiveness of surgical resection alone. We must remember that Fortner [24] failed to produce long-term survivors even by his aggressive regional pancreatectomy, possibly because most of his patients might have cancer of far-advanced stages (more than 5 cm in diameter). With regard to the postoperative quality of life after an extended pancreatectomy, it generally requires 1 postoperative year for the disease-free patients to recover the 0–2 levels of performance according to the criteria proposed by Zubord [25]. We can easily speculate that, in the patients who die of cancer recurrence within 1 postoperative year, their remaining life had been full of pain. Also, from the standpoint of cost–performance analysis, Gudjonsson [26] doubted the role of pancreatectomy itself in the treatment of pancreatic cancer.

Future Problems

In the future, further advances in imaging techniques will increase the number of candidates for extended pancreatectomy by detecting smaller and earlier cancer of the pancreas. Likewise, we can expect that adjuvant therapy may improve postoperative survival rates, because the Gastrointestinal Tumor Study Group [27] showed that the 2-year survival rate was 43%–46% in the patients who had received postoperative chemoradiation in combination with conventional pancreatectomy but 18% in the control group. Furthermore, neoadjuvant therapy seems to be more promising, because we can expect both down-staging of the tumor and more strict patient selection during the period of preoperative irradiation. For instance, nonvisible metastatic foci in the peritoneal cavity and liver may grow to be visible foci before laparotomy. Pilepich and Miller [28] showed that of 17 patients who had been once judged as unsuitable for surgical resection, 6 were judged as suitable candidates after irradiation, and 2 patients survived 5 years after pancreatectomy. Our histopathological study indicated that the peripheral areas of the tumor were more sensitive to preoperative irradiation [29], which was clinically useful in preventing locoregional recurrence after pancreatectomy [30].

A high incidence of hepatic metastasis was the bottleneck in our preoperative irradiation therapy. Yeung et al. [31] and Evans et al. [32] showed that a preoperative combination of chemotherapy and radiation improved the long-term survival rates. More recently, we [33] developed a new method of postoperative liver perfusion chemotherapy via the portal vein and hepatic artery that has proven to be effective in preventing the postoperative development of liver metastasis. Thus, with the aid of adjuvant therapies that are effective not only for locoregional control but also for preventing distant (hepatic) metastasis, the role of extended pancreatectomy will be more appreciated in the near future.

References

1. Grace PA, Pitt HA, Tompkins RK, DenBeston L, Longmire WP Jr (1986) Decreased morbidity and mortality after pancreaticoduodenectomy. Am J Surg 15:141–147
2. Crist DW, Sitzman JV, Cameron JL (1987) Improved hospital morbidity, mortality and survival after the Whipple procedure. Ann Surg 206:358–365
3. Spencer MP, Sarr MG, Nagorney DM (1990) Radical pancreatectomy for pancreatic cancer in the elderly. Is it safe and justified? Ann Surg 212:140–143
4. Tepper TG, Nardi G, Suit H (1976) Carcinoma of the pancreas—review of MGH experience from 1963 to 1973. Analysis of surgical failure and implications for radiation therapy. Cancer (Phila) 37:1519–1524
5. Tryka AF, Brooks JR (1979) Histopathology in the evaluation of total pancreatectomy for ductal carcinoma. Ann Surg 190:373–381
6. Collins JJ, Craighead JE, Brooks JR (1966) Rationale for total pancreatectomy for carcinoma of the pancreatic head. N Engl J Med 274:599–602
7. Matsui Y, Aoki Y, Ishikawa O, et al (1979) Ductal carcinoma of the pancreas. Arch Surg 114:722–726
8. Ishikawa O, Ohigashi H, Imaoka S, et al (1984) Clinicopathological study on the appropriate range of pancreatic resection to obtain operative curability of the pancreatic head cancer (in Japanese; abstract in English). Jpn J Surg 195:274–281
9. van Heerden JA, ReMine WH, Weiland LH, McIlrath DC, Ilstrup DM (1981) Total pancreatectomy for ductal adenocarcinoma of the pancreas: Mayo Clinic experience. Am J Surg 142:308–311
10. Sarr MG, Behrns KE, van Heerden JA (1993) Total pancreatectomy—an objective analysis of its use in pancreatic cancer. Hepato-Gastroenterology 40:418–421
11. Cubilla AL, Fortner PJ, Fitzgerald PJ (1978) Lymph node involvement in carcinoma of the head of the pancreas area. Cancer (Phila) 41:880–887
12. Ishikawa O, Ohigashi H, Sasaki Y, et al (1988) Practical usefulness of lymphatic and connective tissue clearance for the carcinoma of the pancreas head. Ann Surg 208:215–220
13. Nakao A, Harada A, Nonami T, et al (1995) Lymph node metastases in carcinoma of the head of the pancreas region. Br J Surg 82:399–402
14. Tsuchiya R, Noda Y, Harada H, et al (1986) Collective review of small carcinoma of the pancreas. Ann Surg 203:77–81
15. Cohen JR, Akuchta N, Geller N, et al (1982) Pancreaticoduodenectomy: a 40-year experience. Ann Surg 195:608–617
16. Cubilla AL, Fitzgerald PJ (1980) Surgical pathology of tumors of the exocrine pancreas. In: Moossa AR (ed) Tumors of the pancreas. Williams and Willkins, Baltimore, pp 159–193
17. Nagai H, Kuroda A, Morioka Y (1986) Lymphatic and local spread of T1 and T2 pancreatic cancers. A study of autopsy material. Ann Surg 204:65–71
18. Nagakawa T, Kayahara M, Ueno K, et al (1992) A clinicopathologic study on neural invasion in cancer of the pancreatic head. Cancer (Phila) 69:930–935
19. Ishikawa O, Ohigashi H, Imaoka S, et al (1992) Preoperative indications for extended pancreatectomy for locally advanced pancreas cancer involving the portal vein. Ann Surg 215:231–236
20. Henne-Bruns D, Kremer B, Meyer-Pannwitt U, Vogel I, Schroder S (1993) Partial duodenopancreatectomy with radical lymphadenectomy in patients with pancreatic and periampullary carcinomas: initial results. Hepato-Gastroenterology 40:145–149

21. Yeo CJ, Cameron JL (1994) Arguments against radical (extended) resection for adenocarcinoma of the pancreas. Adv Surg 127:273–284
22. Cameron JL, Crist DW, Sitzmann JV, et al (1991) Factors influencing survival after pancreaticoduodenectomy for pancreatic cancer. Am J Surg 161:120–125
23. Japan Pancreas Society (1993) General rules for the study of pancreatic cancer, 4th edn. Kanehara, Tokyo, pp 14–15
24. Fortner JG (1981) Surgical principles for pancreatic cancer. Regional total and subtotal pancreatectomy. Cancer (Phila) 47:1712–1718
25. Ishikawa O, Ohigashi H, Imaoka S, et al (1992) Extended lymphadenectomy for pancreas cancer—an evaluation of the curability and postoperative quality of life (in Japanese; abstract in English). Jpn J Gastroenterol Surg 25:2661–2665
26. Gudjonsson B (1995) Carcinoma of the pancreas—critical analysis of costs, results of resections and the need for standardized reporting. J Am Coll Surg 181:483–503
27. Gastointestinal Tumor Study Group (1987) Further evidence of effective adjuvant combined radiation and chemotherapy following curative resection of pancreatic cancer. Cancer (Phila) 59:2006–2010
28. Pilepich MV, Miller HH (1980) Preoperative irradiation in carcinoma of the pancreas. Cancer (Phila) 46:1945–1949
29. Ishikawa O, Ohigashi H, Teshima T, et al (1989) Clinical and histopathological appraisal of preoperative irradiation for adenocarcinoma of the pancreatoduodenal region. J Surg Oncol 40:143–151
30. Ishikawa O, Ohigashi H, Imaoka S, et al (1994) Is the long-term survival rate improved by preoperative irradiation prior to Whipple's procedure for adenocarcinoma of the pancreatic head? Arch Surg 129:1075–1080
31. Yeung RS, Weese JL, Hoffman JP, et al (1993) Neoadjuvant chemoradiation in pancreatic and duodenal carcinoma. Cancer (Phila) 72:2124–2133
32. Evans DB, Rich TA, Byrd DR, et al (1992) Preoperative chemoradiation and pancreaticoduodenectomy for adenocarcinoma of the pancreas. Arch Surg 127:1335–1339
33. Ishikawa O, Ohigashi H, Sasaki Y, et al (1994) Liver perfusion chemotherapy via both hepatic artery and portal vein to prevent hepatic metastasis after extended pancreatectomy for adenocarcinoma of the pancreas. Am J Surg 168:361–364

The Long-Term Survival of Patients with Ductal Carcinoma of the Pancreatic Head and Body

Hisashi Mimura[1], Masanobu Mori[2], Takuji Mimura[3],
Keisuke Hamazaki[2], and Hiromu Tsuge[2]

Summary. Seventy-six patients with ductal carcinoma of the pancreatic head and body who underwent resection during the past 20 years were studied. Included were 1 patient in stage I, 5 patients in stage II, 27 patients in stage III, 24 patients in stage IVa, and 19 patients in stage IVb. Curative resection was achieved in 100% of the patients with stage I and II, 81.5% of stage III, 41.7% of stage IVa, and 10.5% of stage IVb. The surgical procedure involved pancreatoduodenectomy or total pancreatectomy with extensive skeletonization. Intraoperative radiotherapy and perioperative chemotherapy were seldom performed. Surgical mortality (deaths within 3 months after surgery) decreased from 19.4% before 1986 to 2.5% after 1987. There were 11 (18.6%) long-term survivors of more than 3 years among 59 patients and 7 (15.2%) survivors of more than 5 years among 46 patients. These long-term survivors were all found in the group that underwent pathologically curative resection, and there were no long-term survivors among patients with pathologically noncurative resection. In the group receiving curative resection, 28.9% (11/38) of patients survived more than 3 years and 24.1% (7/29) of patients survived more than 5 years. The 3-year-survival rates were 60% in stages I and II, 26.9% in stage III, 4.2% in stage IVa, and none in stage IVb; the 5-year-survival rates were 40% in stages I and II, 19.2% in stage III, and none in stage IV. Curative resection should be applied to patients with stages I, II, III, and IVa tumors, and excessive surgery should be avoided for patients with stage IVb.

Key words. Pancreatic cancer—Pancreatectomy—Survival rate—Long-term survivors—Surgical mortality

[1] School of Health Sciences, Okayama University, Okayama 700, Japan.
[2] First Department of Surgery, Okayama University Medical School, Okayama 700, Japan.
[3] Department of First Surgery, Kagawaken Saiseikai Hospital, Takamatsu, Kagawa 760, Japan.

143

Introduction

Application of extended resection for advanced ductal carcinoma of the pancreas remains controversial because of the poor survival rates reported [1–9]. However, long-term survivors have recently been reported [10–16]. We observed 76 patients who underwent pancreatectomy for ductal carcinoma of the pancreas; 11 patients survived more than 3 years and 7 patients survived more than 5 years. Pathological and surgical factors that might influence long-term survival were evaluated.

Patients and Methods

A total of 76 patients with ductal carcinoma of the pancreatic head and body underwent resection between 1976 and 1995. Their pathological findings were analyzed, and pathological staging was determined on the basis of the "General Rules for the Study of Pancreatic Cancer" [17]. Surgical procedures, surgical mortality, pathological findings, and survival rates were compared between long-term survivors and other patients.

Our Surgical Method

Our routine surgical procedure for ductal carcinoma of the pancreas is "isolated pancreatectomy", which is defined as no-touch isolation resection of the pancreas. This method was devised by the authors in 1987 and first presented in 1991 [18]; the survival curves by this method were reported in 1994 [16].

In this method, the feeding and draining vessels of the pancreatic tumor are ligated and divided before pancreatectomy so that intraoperative migration of carcinoma

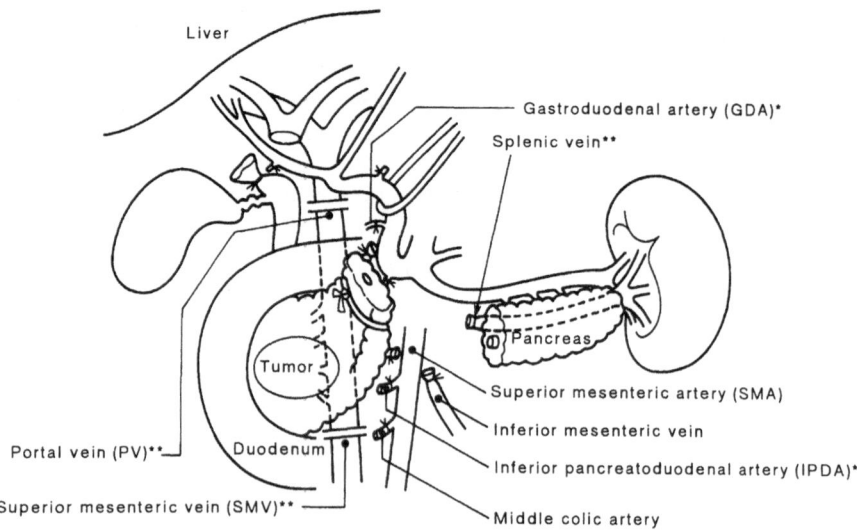

FIG. 1. Schematic of isolated pancreatectomy. *, Inflow vessels into the tumor in pancreatic head; **, outflow vessels from the tumor in pancreatic head. Both inflow vessels (*GDA, IPDA*) and outflow vessels (*PV, SMV, SpV*) for the pancreatic head are cut in advance before pancreatectomy

cells into the portal vein can be avoided. The feeding vessels supplying the pancreatic head are the gastroduodenal artery (GDA) and the inferior pancreatoduodenal artery (IPDA); the draining vessels are the portal vein (PV), the inferior mesenteric vein (SMV), and the splenic vein (SPV).

Figure 1 shows a diagram of isolated pancreatoduodenectomy. The confluence of the portal vein, the superior mesenteric vein, and the splenic vein was resected, providing a wide surgical field, which facilitates extended retroperitoneal skeletonization. Before 1987, the portal vein was not routinely removed. After 1987, the portal vein was removed almost routinely by isolated pancreatectomy. Intraoperative radiotherapy was not applied. Postoperative chemotherapy using 5-fluorouracil (5-FU) was begun 3 months after surgery and continued for 2 years.

Results

Stages, Surgical Procedures, and Curability

Pathological stages of all 76 patients who underwent pancreatectomy are shown in Table 1. The patients included 1 case in stage I, 5 cases in stage II, 27 cases in stage III, 24 cases in stage IVa, and 19 cases in stage IVb, respectively. Curative resection was achieved in 100% of the patients with stage I and II, 81.5% of stage III, 41.7% of stage IVa, and 10.5% of stage IVb.

Table 2 shows the surgical procedures applied in 76 patients. Pancreatoduodenectomy (PD) was performed in 47 patients and total

TABLE 1. Stage and curability

Stage[a]	Number of patients	Curative resection[a]	Noncurative resection[a]
I	1	1	
II	5	5	
III	27	22 (81.5%)	5
IVa	24	10 (41.7%)	14
IVb	19	2 (10.5%)	17
Total	76	40 (52.6%)	36

[a] Determined pathologically.

TABLE 2. Surgical procedures

Method	Curative resection[a] (n = 40)	Noncurative resection[a] (n = 36)	Total (n = 76)
Pancreatectomy (PD)	47		
Standard	4	10	14
Extended	21	12	33
Total pancreatectomy (TP)	29		
Standard	1	2	3
Extended	14	12	26
Total:			76
Standard	5	12	17
Extended	35	24	59

[a] Determined pathologically.

pancreatectomy (TP) in 29 patients. Standard resection, which indicates simple pancreatectomy without extended skeletonization, was performed in 17 cases, while extended resection including extensive retroperitoneal skeletonization was done in 59 patients.

Surgical Mortality

Surgical mortality (deaths within 3 months after surgery) was high at 19.4% before 1986. However, as a result of the renovation of surgical techniques and perioperative management, surgical mortality decreased to 2.5% after 1987 despite the more aggressive surgery being performed (Table 3).

Survival Curves After Surgery

Survival curves at each stage are shown in Fig. 2. Three-year survival rates were 60% in stages I and II, 26.9% in stage III, 4.2% in stage IVa, and none in stage IVb.

TABLE 3. Surgical mortality: deaths within
3 months after pancreatectomy

Chronological change and mortality:
   Before 1986, 7/36 (19.4%)
   After 1987, 1/40 (2.5%)
   Total: 8/76 (10.5%)
Operative methods and mortality:
   PD
      Extended pancreatectomy, 1/33 (3.0%)
      Standard pancreatectomy, 1/14 (7.1%)
   TP
      Extended pancreatectomy, 5/26 (19.2%)
      Standard pancreatectomy, 1/3 (33.3%)
   Total
      Extended pancreatectomy, 6/59 (10.2%)
      Standard pancreatectomy, 2/17 (11.8%)

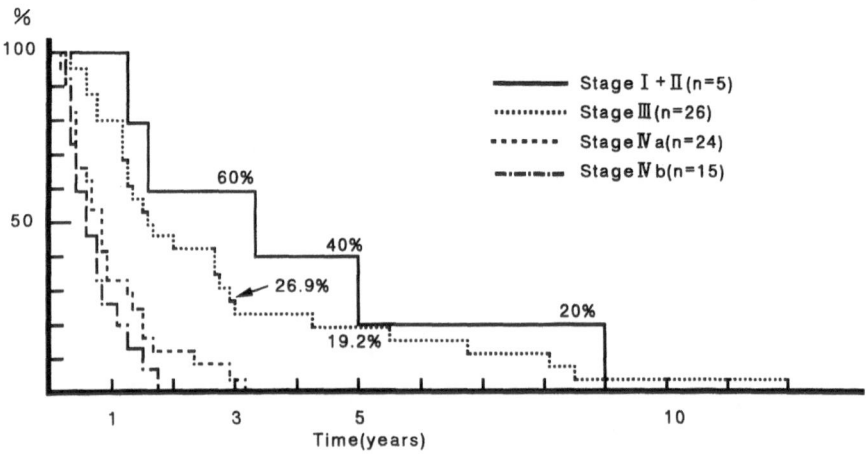

FIG. 2. Cumulative survival rate for stages I, II, III, IVa, and IVb. Deaths within 3 months after pancreatectomy are excluded

Five-year survival rates were 40% in stages I and II, 19.2% in stage III, and none in stage IV.

Long-Term Survivors

Eleven patients (18.6%) of 59 patients who had undergone pancreatectomy more than 3 years earlier survived longer than 3 years, while 7 (15.2%) of 46 patients who had undergone pancreatectomy more than 5 years earlier survived longer than 5 years (Table 4). Pathologically curative resection had been performed in all long-term survivors, and there were no long-term survivors in the group with noncurative

TABLE 4. Long-term survivors

Years after pancreatectomy	3	5
Background:		
Curative resection	38	29
Noncurative resection	21	17
Survivors:		
Stage I[a]	1	0
Stage II[a]	2	2
Stage III[a]	7	5
Stage IVa[a]	1	0
Total	11 (18.6%)[b]	7 (15.2%)[b]
Operative method:		
PD	7	4
TP	4	3
Curative resection[a]	11	7
Noncurative resection[b]	0	0
Vessel resection:		
Portal vein	6	3
Hepatic artery	0	1

[a] Determined pathologically.
[b] Survivors/patients having undergone resection in each time × 100.

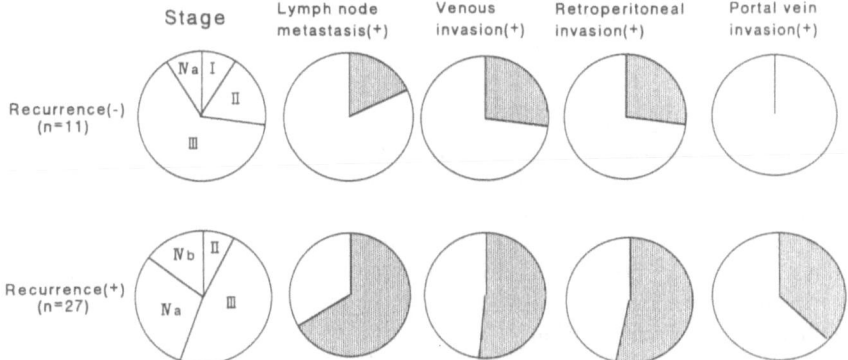

FIG. 3. Pathological cancer involvement and recurrence within 3 years after pathologically curative resection. The *shaded areas* show the percentage of patients with cancer invasion

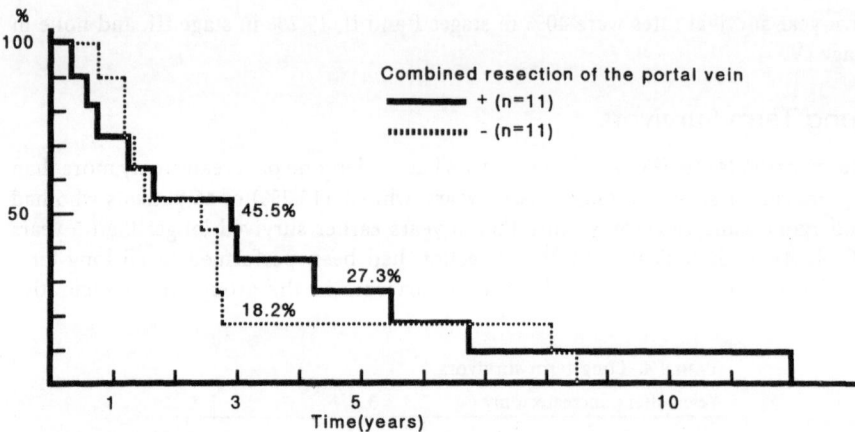

FIG. 4. Effect of combined resection of the portal vein on survival rates in stage III. An advantage from portal vein resection is suggested. Deaths within 3 months after pancreatectomy are excluded

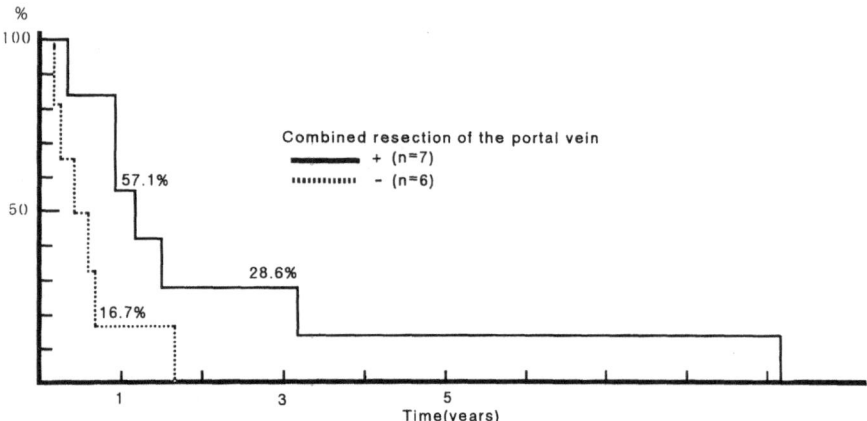

FIG. 5. Effect of combined resection of the portal vein on survival rates in stage IVa. An advantage from portal vein resection is suggested. Deaths within 3 months after pancreatectomy are excluded

resection. Of the patients who underwent curative resection, 28.9% (11/38) survived longer than 3 years and 24.1% (7/29) survived longer than 5 years.

Figure 3 shows the pathological cancer involvement and recurrence within 3 years after surgery among patients who underwent curative resection. None of the patients in stage IVb survived longer than 3 years. Some patients with lymph node metastasis, venous invasion, or retroperitoneal invasion survived more than 3 years, although their incidence was lower than that of patients without recurrence. Three-year survivors had no portal vein invasion.

Figures 4 and 5 show the effect of combined resection of the portal vein on survival rates in stages III and IVa. Advantages from portal vein resection were suggested for both stages.

Discussion

Recently improved survival rates after resection of invasive ductal carcinoma of the pancreas were obtained by curative resection for patients with early disease. In the most recent Japanese survey [19] covering 11671 patients with pancreatic cancer treated between 1981 and 1993, postoperative survival curves during 11 years of ductal carcinoma were reported by histological cell differentiation. The 3-year survival rates among 2447 patients were 20.1% in well-differentiated carcinoma ($n = 856$), 13.7% in moderately differentiated carcinoma ($n = 1268$), and 12.8% in poorly differentiated carcinoma ($n = 323$). The 5-year survival rates were 11.8% in well-differentiated carcinoma and 9.3% each in moderately and poorly differentiated carcinoma.

Compared with this very large report covering all Japan, our local report appeared to show compatible or better results, especially for stages I, II, and III. Regarding the pathological stages, the 3-year survival rates were 40% in stages I and II, 26.9% in stage III, and 4.2% in stage IVa, while the 5-year survival rates were 20% in stages I and II and 19.2% in stage III. Pathological factors affecting patient prognosis after surgery were not specified. Patients showing a minimal degree of lymph node metastasis, and minimal invasion of the small vein or portal vein and retroperitoneum, achieved better results.

In addition to the pathological stage, the surgical procedure is thought to play an important role, because all long-term survivors without exception had undergone histologically curative resection and none of the patients with noncurative resection survived more than 3 years. As a result, extensive curative resection is recommended for patients in stage I, II, or III. For patients in stage IVb, resection is not indicated, although some patients with stage IVa survive longer than 3 years after curative resection. The role of postoperative chemotherapy remains uncertain.

References

1. Marks S, Stahlgren LH (1987) Is resection appropriate for adenocarcinoma of the pancreas? Am J Surg 15:651–654
2. Gudjonsson B (1987) Cancer of the pancreas. 50 years of surgery. Cancer (Phila) 60:2284–2303
3. Sindelar WF (1989) Clinical experience with regional pancreatectomy for adenocarcinoma of the pancreas. Arch Surg 124:127–132
4. Tred M (1987) Treatment of pancreatic carcinoma: the surgeon's dilemma. Br J Surg 74:79–80
5. Crile G (1970) The advantages of bypass operations over radical pancreatoduodenectomy in the treatment of pancreatic carcinoma. Surg Gynecol Obstet 130:1049–1053
6. Warshaw AL, Swanson RS (1988) Pancreatic cancer in 1988, possibilities and probabilities. Ann Surg 208:541–553
7. Sunada S, Miyata M, Okumura K, Nakamura M, Kitagawa T, Shirakura R, Kawashima Y (1992) Aggressive resection for advanced pancreatic carcinoma. Surg Today 22:74–77
8. Sperti C, Bonadimani B, Pasquali C, Piccoli A, Cappellazzo F, Rugge M, Pedrazzoli S (1993) Ductal adenocarcinoma of the pancreas: clinicopathologic features and survival. Tumori 79:325–330
9. Farthman EH, Ruf G (1994) Chirurgishe Therapie des Pankreackarzinoms—Indikation und Resultate. Sweiz Rundsh Med Prax 83:870–872

10. Fortner JG (1973) Regional resection of cancer of the pancreas: a new surgical approach. Surgery 73:307–320
11. Fortner JG (1987) The rationale, technique and results of treating pancreatic and peripancreatic cancer by regional pancreatectomy. Acta Gastro-Enterol Belg 50:121–127
12. Lygidakis NJ, van der Heyde MN, Houthoff HJ, Schipper MEI, Huibregtse K, Tytgat NJ, Lubber MJ, Reeders JWAJ, Bosey M MEM, Oosting J (1989) Resectional surgical procedures for carcinoma of the head of the pancreas. Surg Gynecol Obstet 168:157–165
13. Ishikawa O (1993) What constitutes curative pancreatectomy for adenocarcinoma of the pancreas? Hepato-Gastroenterology 40:414–417
14. Ishikawa O, Ohigashi H, Imaoka S, Furukawa H, Sasaki Y, Fujita M, Kuroda C, Iwanaga T (1992) Preoperative indications for extended pancreatectomy for locally advanced pancreas cancer involving the portal vein. Ann Surg 215:231–236
15. Baumel H, Huguir M, Manderscheid JC, Fabre JM, Houry S, Fagot H (1994) Results of resection for cancer of the exocrine pancreas: a study from the French Association of Surgery. Br J Surg 81:102–107
16. Mimura H, Mori M, Hamazaki K, Tsuge H (1994) Isolated pancreatectomy for ductal carcinoma of the head of the pancreas. Hepato-Gastroenterology 41:483–488
17. Japan Pancreatic Society (1993) General rules for the study of pancreatic cancer, 4th ed. Kanehara Shuppan, Tokyo
18. Mimura H, Mori M, Hamazaki K, Kashino H, Tsuge H, Takakura N, Sakata T (1991) Isolated pancreatectomy for ductal carcinoma of the head of the pancreas. J Biliary Tract Pancreas (Japan) 12:293–298
19. Saito Y (1994) A survey on pancreatic cancer in Japan (in Japanese). J Jpn Pancreas Soc 9:499–527

Extended Radical Pancreatoduodenectomy for Carcinoma of the Head of the Pancreas

Takukazu Nagakawa, Tetsuo Ohta, and Masato Kayahara

Summary. Since 1973, we have utilized a unique method of extended radical pancreatectomy, using the translateral retroperitoneal approach (TRA) to facilitate combined portal resection. The advantages of this operation for patients with carcinoma of the head of the pancreas are described here. In addition, the problems associated with this operation are discussed. Survival was calculated on the basis of the type of resection, degree of invasion of the retroperitoneal tissues, degree of lymph node involvement, and cancer stage. Extensive surgery has been performed for pancreatic carcinoma in 229 patients. Of these, 155 had carcinoma of the head of the pancreas. Of 63 patients who underwent macroscopically curative resections, only 44 were microscopically curative; 10 patients who underwent microscopically curative resections survived for 5 years (25.1%). There were no statistically significant differences in survival based on tumor size. However, there was a significant difference in survival based on extent of invasion of the anterior capsule of the pancreas, extent of invasion of the retroperitoneal tissue, extent of lymph node involvement, cancer stage, and extent of invasion at the surgical margin of resection. The results suggest that extended radical pancreatectomy may be indicated for the treatment of cancer of the head of the pancreas.

Key words. Extended radical pancreatoduodenectomy—Carcinoma of the head of the pancreas—Retroperitoneal dissection—Translateral retroperitoneal approach—Postoperative prognosis

Introduction

Total pancreatectomy and lymph node dissection have been reported for the radical cure of carcinoma of the head of the pancreas [1-4 Extended radical pancreatectomy including en bloc resection of the portal vein and superior mesenteric artery has not been routinely employed, although Fortner [5] has described the feasibility of resection and reanastomosis of the portal vein and hepatic or superior mesenteric arteries

Second Department of Surgery (Department of Health Science), School of Medicine, Kanazawa University, Kanazawa, Ishikawa 920, Japan.

during regional pancreatectomy. Since 1973, we have utilized a unique method of extended radical pancreatectomy, using the translateral retroperitoneal approach (TRA) to facilitate combined portal resection [6,7]. The technique and the advantages of this operation are described here for patients with carcinoma of the head of the pancreas. In addition, the problems associated with this operation are discussed. Survival was calculated on the basis of the type of resection, degree of invasion of the retroperitoneal tissues, degree of lymph node involvement, and cancer stage.

Patients and Methods

The elements of extended radical pancreatectomy by the translateral retroperitoneal approach (TRA) include complete excision of the lymph nodes and nerve plexes of the trunks of both celiac axis and superior mesenteric artery. Adequate lymphadenectomy requires wide retroperitoneal dissection of the nodes from the adrenal glands to the iliac bifurcation. The extent of the pancreatectomy depends on the site of the cancer. For cancers localized to the head, the pancreas is transected to the left of the celiac artery (Fig. 1). This is performed in combination with resection of the portal vein and the retropancreatic tissues, including the nerve plexes of the trunks of the celiac axis and the superior mesenteric artery. For cancers not localized to the head, a total pancreatectomy together with resection of the portal vein and the retropancreatic tissues is performed. In all except 7 of our cases, the TRA facilitated an adequate lymphadenectomy.

Since 1973, 229 patients with pancreatic cancer underwent surgical exploration, of whom 155 had cancer of the head of the pancreas. Patients with cystoadenocarcinoma, islet carcinoma, and carcinoma of the inferior bile duct and papilla of Vater were not included in this study. There were 106 men and 49 women, with ages at the time of

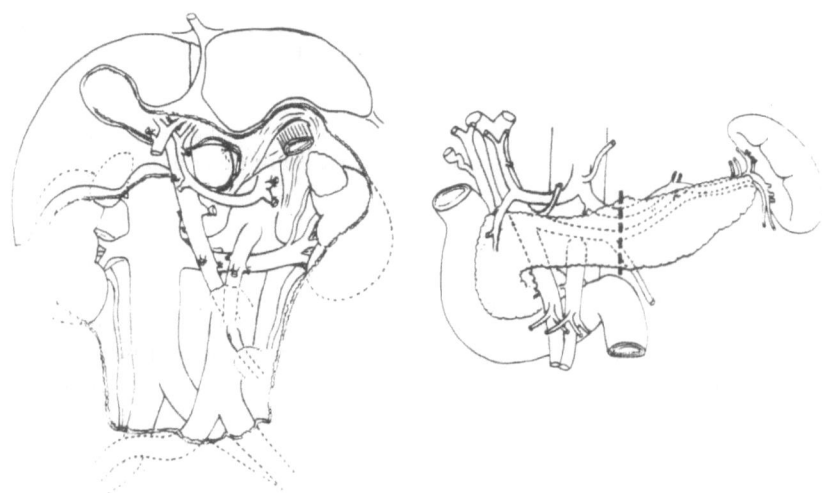

a   b

Fig. 1a,b. Resection of pancreatic cancer. a Area of retroperitoneal dissection. b Incisional line on the pancreas

operation ranging from 31 to 82 years (mean, 61.2 years). Resection was performed in 78 patients (50.3%), including 63 patients (40.6%) undergoing curative resection based on macroscopic criteria and 44 patients (28.4%) whose resection was based on microscopic criteria. In this chapter, we describe the results of carcinoma of the head of the pancreas according to type of resection and evaluate histopathologically the local extent of the tumor, the staging of the cancer, and the presence of cancer at the surgical margin.

Tumor size was classified as follows: t_1, less than 2.0 cm in diameter; t_2a, 2.1–3.0 cm in diameter; t_2b, 3.1–4.0 cm in diameter; t_3, 4.1–6.0 cm in diameter; and t_4, more than 6.1 cm in diameter. The local extent of disease was also evaluated as s_0, anterior capsule of the pancreas not invaded; s_1, slightly invaded; or s_2, invasion of the capsule; and rp_0, rp_1, or rp_2, depending on whether the retroperitoneal tissue had been invaded. Further, invasion of the portal vein was evaluated as pv_0, negative invasion; pv_1, positive invasion to the adventitia or media of the portal vein; or pv_2, positive invasion to the intima or the internal lumen of the portal vein, in correlation with retroperitoneal invasion. Invasion to the surgical margin of resection was classified as ew_0, negative invasion; ew_1, positive invasion within 5 mm from the surgical margin; and ew_2, positive invasion. Lymph node metastases and the stages were classified into n_0 to n_2 and stage I to stage IV, respectively, according to the General Rules published by the Japan Pancreas Society [8].

The generalized Wilcoxon test was used for statistical analysis, and differences were considered significant if the probability was less than .05.

Technique of Retroperitoneal Dissection Followed by Translateral Retroperitoneal Approach

The abdomen is opened through a chevron incision in the epigastric region.

Retroperitoneal Dissection

Using an electric scalpel, the retroperitoneum is entered by incising the peritoneum at the lower margin of the liver, carrying the incision inferiorly about 3 cm laterally along the right side of the duodenum. The incision is extended further along the right margin of the ascending colon to the cecum, and the duodenocolic ligament is divided. The duodenum is mobilized and elevated along with the pancreas, the ascending colon, and the transverse colon, thus allowing full access to the retroperitoneum (Fig. 2).

The right kidney is first exposed at the lateral aspect of the duodenum, and the fatty tissue attached to it is removed. The right renal artery and vein are now visible. The dissection then proceeds leftward, exposing the inferior vena cava. Care should then be taken not to damage the suprarenal vein. Once the inferior vena cava is fully exposed, the dissection is directed inferiorly to remove the soft tissue and lymph nodes along the vena cava. During this maneuver, the testicular or ovarian vein is ligated and dissected. Care should be taken not to injure the right ureter.

Dissection of the retroperitoneum is carried as far as the bifurcation of the commom iliac artery. At this point, dissection proceeds superiorly, exposing the abdominal aorta. Small-caliber vessels to the inferior vena cava and from the abdomi-

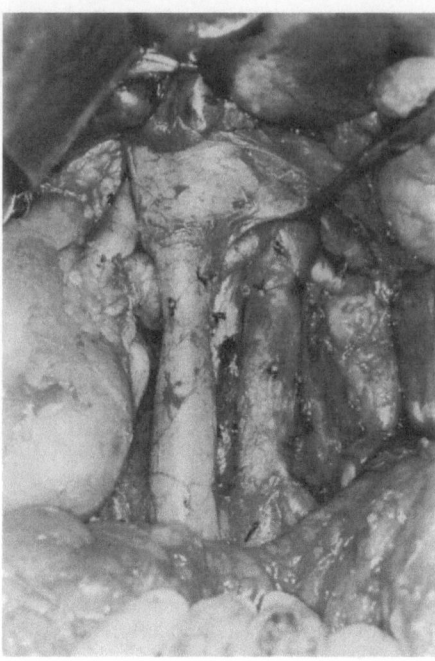

FIG. 2. Appearance of the retroperitoneum following completion of the dissection. Abdominal aorta and inferior vena cava have been completely skeletonized. Both renal arteries and veins are exposed

nal aorta are ligated and divided. The lymph nodes around both renal arteries, particularly the right renal artery, are dissected carefully, retracting these vessels with vascular tapes. Particular attention should be paid to the dissection around the root of the inferior mesenteric artery and the left ureter. The exposure of the abdominal aorta is carried as far as the root of the superior mesenteric artery. The field of dissection is shifted to the retroperitoneum in the vicinity of the foramen of Winslow, exposing the inferior vena cava and left renal vein. Next, as much fatty tissue and as many lymphatics around the left side of the abdominal aorta as possible are ligated to prevent excessive postoperative lymphorrhea.

Treatment of the Transverse Mesocolon, Dissection of the Hepatoduodenal Ligament, Cholecystectomy, and Gastrectomy

The greater omentum is divided at its attachment to the transverse colon, and the transverse mesocolon is divided by an electric scalpel 3 cm distal to its attachment to the pancreas. The middle colic artery and vein are ligated and divided. It is advisable in the subsequent procedure to keep several centimeters of the superior mesenteric vein free distally.

Attention now shifts to the hepatoduodenal ligament. The gastroduodenal artery is ligated and divided at its root, the lesser omentum is divided along the lower margin of the liver, and the stomach is resected. Total gastrectomy is performed in conjunction with total pancreatectomy, and subtotal gastrectomy is done when a proximal pancreatoduodenectomy is performed.

Dissection Around the Celiac Artery and Left-Upper Quadrant of the Retroperitoneum, and Division of the Pancreas

Keeping the stomach elevated toward the right, the lymph nodes around the root of celiac artery are removed en bloc with the ganglion and nerve plexus. The pancreas is divided along the line of the celiac axis, and the splenic vein is ligated and divided as in a standard pancreatoduodenectomy. The dissection is directed toward the left border of the abdominal aorta. In particular, lymph nodes around the left renal artery are dissected at this time. This establishes a connection with the site of the initial dissection, inferiorly. The splenic artery is ligated and divided in a total pancreatectomy; this maneuver exposes the common hepatic artery.

Dissection Around the Superior Mesenteric Artery

The jejunum is transected 10–20 cm from the ligament of Treitz. The jejunal crus, which had been divided, is lifted upward from the opening of the previously mentioned incision. The jejunal crus and pancreas are pulled downward and to the right, and the superior mesenteric vein is pulled to the left with a hook. This maneuver exposes the superior mesenteric artery along with its nerve plexus. The nerve plexus can be separated from the vessels easily using Kelly hemostats. However, the surgeon must take care not to avulse any small vessels arising from the superior mesenteric artery. The dissection is continued to the root of the superior mesenteric artery (Fig. 3). The nerve plexus is dissected using scissors, and the superior mesenteric artery is divided between ligatures. At this point all retroperitoneal soft tissue and ganglia can be removed en bloc together with the pancreas. In the quasi-dissection, a thin layer of

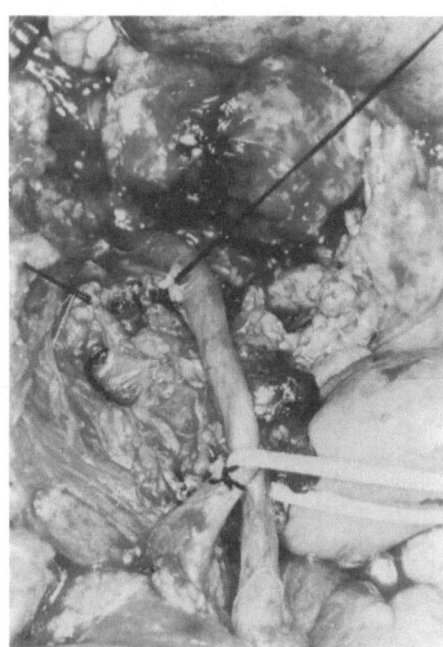

FIG. 3. Dissection around the superior mesenteric artery. The inferior pancreatoduodenal artery is ligated and divided. The superior mesenteric artery is exposed

nerve plexus around the superior mesenteric artery and the left ganglion at the root of the celic artery are preserved.

Combined Resection of the Portal Vein

When a combined resection of the portal vein is required, the procedures for handling the portal vein just described above can be eliminated. Once the retroperitoneum has been dissected, the portal vein can be divided at the upper and lower margins of the pancreas and removed with the pancreas. An end-to-end anastomosis of the portal vein can be performed easily using 5-0 proline sutures (Fig. 4).

The technique of the reconstruction method is not described here.

Abdominal Drainage

In an attempt to prevent the fatal complications of pancreatic leakage, we developed a new method of intraabdominal drainge that involves continuous suction.

First, an 18-Fr double-lumen sump tube is positioned beside the pancreaticoenterostomy with Penrose drains and a duple drain, ensuring that the sump drain tube is not kinked (Fig. 5). Immediately after the operation, continuous suction drainage is commenced at a pressure of about $-20\,cmH_2O$. We usually use the common thoracic pump as the suction machine. If the sump tube does not work effectively, it should be changed in the ward and the position immediately checked by a plain abdominal roentgenogram.

The amylase level and bacterial cultures of the sump tube fluid should be examined regularly to monitor for the early detection of dehiscence of the pancreaticoenterostomy. The sump tube should be removed when it is draining less than 50 ml and the amylase level has normalized.

Two Penrose and one duple or φ con tubes are inserted toward the pancreaticoenterostomy, following which fluid from the abdominal cavity is allowed to exude passively. The other abdominal drainage methods are the same as those used for the continuous intraabdominal suction drainage (CISD) method.

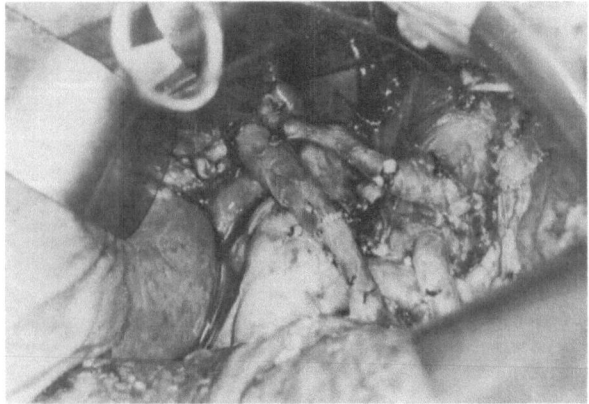

FIG. 4. Anastomosis after combined resection of the portal vein. The roots of the dissected celiac axis and superior mesenteric artery are visible

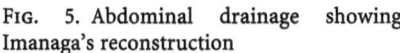

Fig. 5. Abdominal drainage showing Imanaga's reconstruction

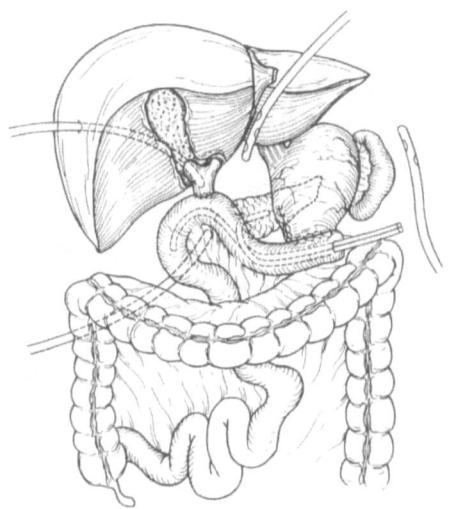

Results

Of the 63 patients who underwent macroscopically curative resections, there were 5 (7.9%) perioperative deaths from peritonitis or intraperitoneal hemorrhage. Another 2 patients died within 60 days of sepsis or hepatorenal failure. Major postoperative complications included wound infection, postoperative hemorrhage, pneumonia, and hepatic and renal insufficiency. The overall incidence of complications in this group was 37.2%. Survival was calculated for the 63 patients who underwent a macroscopically curative resection (Fig. 6); there were 14 three-year survivors and 10 five-year survivors in this group. The 5-year survival rate was 21.3% in macroscopically curative resection and 25.1% in microscopically curative resection. The overall median survival period was 13 months in macroscopically curative resection and 16 months in microscopically curative resection. Late postoperative complications including diarrhea and nutritional disturbances were observed in most of the patients.

Prognoses were compared according to cancer spread in 38 patients who underwent microscopically curative resection and survived the operation. There was no correlation between tumor size and prognosis. There was no 5-year survivor among the patients with s_2 disease ($n = 3$), while the 5-year survival rate in patients with s_0 disease ($n = 32$) was 43.8% ($P < .05$).

There were 5-year survivors in all three groups (rp_0, rp_1, and rp_2) (Fig. 7). The survival was significantly better in the rp_0 group than in the rp_1 or rp_2 group ($P < .05$). Four of the patients with retroperitoneal invasion survived more than 3 years. There was no 5-year survivor among the patients with positive invasion to the intima or the internal lumen of the portal vein, but there was no statistically significant difference in survival between these groups.

The lymph nodes were positive in 24 patients. All patients with n_2 disease were dead within 3 years (Fig. 8). Patients with n_0 disease had a 5-year survival of 60.0%. There was a significant difference between survival in the patients with n_0 and n_1 disease ($P < .05$). In all patients with metastases to the periaortic lymph nodes, the nodes around the superior mesenteric artery were involved. Five patients with metastasis to

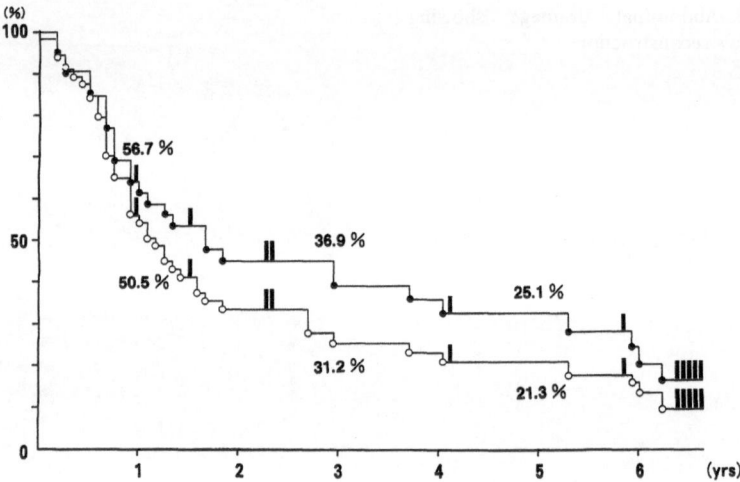

FIG. 6. Survival rate according to the type of curative resection for carcinoma of the head of the pancreas (Kaplan–Meier method). Percentages are given for the 5-year survival rate. Median survival period was 16 months for microscopically curative resection (n = 44) and 13 months for microscopically curative resection (n = 63)

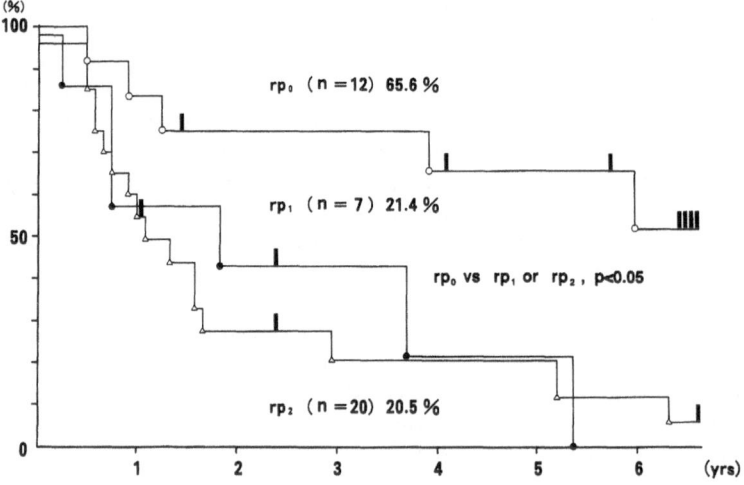

FIG. 7. Survival rate according to invasion of the retroperitoneal tissue behind the pancreas (rp)

the periaortic lymph nodes lived for more than 1 year. Metastases to the lymph nodes were present in 46 of the 63 patients (73.0%). The average number of involved lymph nodes in specimens examined from patients with metastatic disease was 6.1 (8.1%). The prevalence of metastases of area no. 13 was highest, followed by areas no. 17 and 14. There were 10 patients (18.9%) with metastases to the paraaortic area no. 16 (Fig. 9).

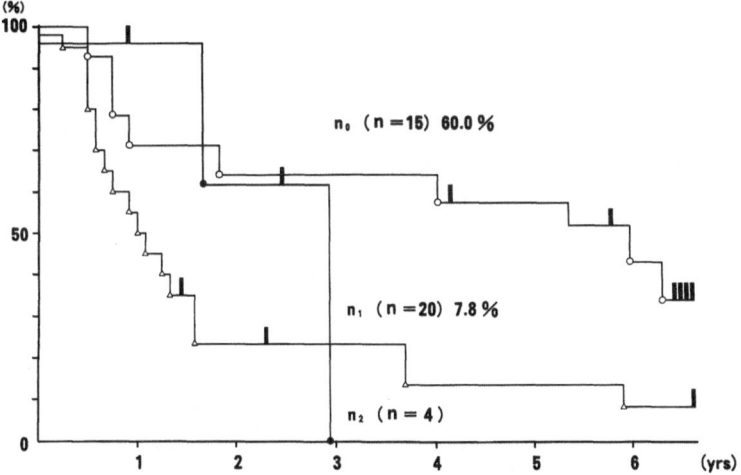

FIG. 8. Survival rate according to lymph node metastasis (n)

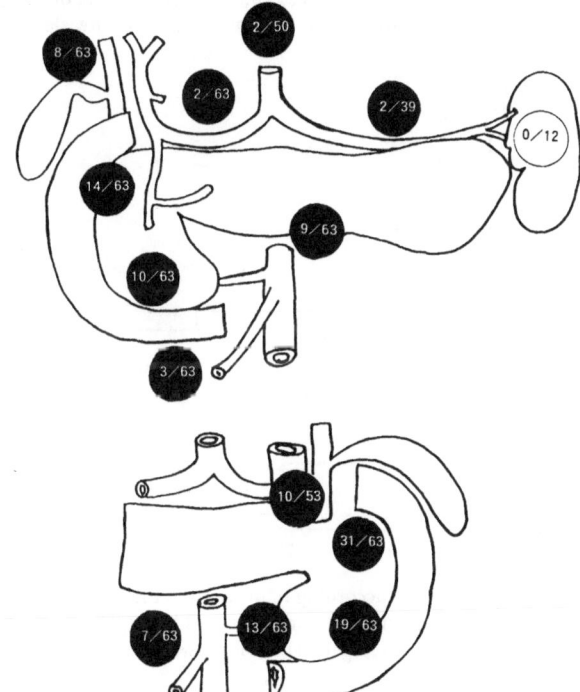

FIG. 9. Distribution of lymph node involvement in carcinoma of the head of the pancreas. Positive metastatic cases, 46/63 (73.0%); average number of positive lymph nodes; 6.1 (8.1%). Numbers of metastatic cases in each area are shown

All the patients with stage IVb disease died within 3 years (Fig. 10), but three patients with stage IVa disease survived more than 5 years. Survival was significantly better in patients with stage I or II disease compared to those with stage IVb disease.

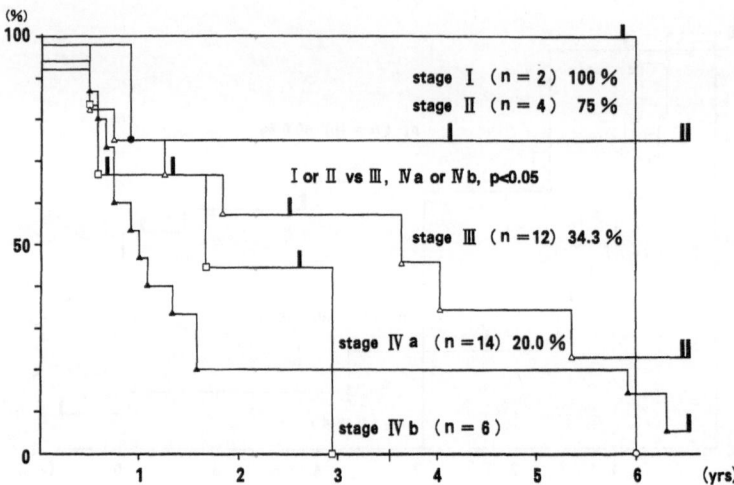

FIG. 10. Survival rate according to cancer stage. Survival was significantly better in patients with stage I or II disease compared to those with stage IVb disease ($P < .005$). Percentages are given for the 5-year survival rate. Stage I, t_1, s_0, rp_0, pv_0, and n_0; stage II, s_0, rp_0, pv_0, and n_1; stage III, s_1, rp_1, pv_1, or n_2; stage IVa, n_2 and s_2, rp_2, or pv_2, stage IVb, others. t, Tumor size; s, local extent of disease; rp, retroperitoneal invasion; pv, portal vein invasion; n, lymph node metastases

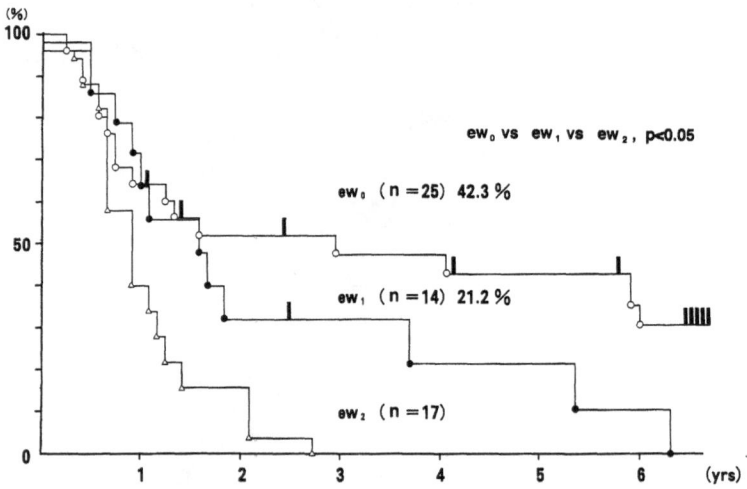

FIG. 11. Survival rate according to invasion to the excisional margin (ew). Survival was significantly better in patients with ew_0 compared to ew_2 ($P < .05$). Percentages are given for the 5-year survival rate. ew_0, Negative invasion; ew_1, invasion within 5 mm from surgical margin; ew_2, positive invasion

All patients with microscopic evidence of cancer at the resection margin were dead within 3 years. Of those with a negative margin, a 5-year survival rate of 42.3% was noted. Cancer at the resection margin was statistically correlated with survival ($P < .05$) (Fig. 11). Among the 63 patients who underwent macroscopically curative resection, only 44 (69.8%) were microscopically cured. Figure 12 shows the correla-

FIG. 12. Correlation between retropancreatic invasion (rp) and cancer cells on the excisional margin (ew)

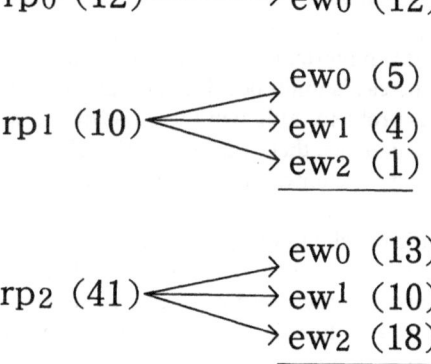

tion between rp and ew (retroperitoneal invasion and invasion to the surgical margin, respectively).

Discussion

The resection rate for pancreatic carcinoma is increased when advanced techniques such as en bloc removal of the portal vein are used. At the same time, the mortality of extensive operations for pancreatic cancer can be reduced by utilizing ancillary techniques such as percutaneous transhepatic biliary drainage, and perioperative nutritional support [3,9,10]. Despite these approaches, however, the 5-year survival rate is still disappointing, ranging from 2.3% to 14.3% for cancer of the head of the pancreas [10–21]. Because of disappointing long-term survival rates following radical surgery for pancreatic cancer, some authors have suggested that bypass should be used as the procedure of choice [22–24].

Our extended radical pancreatectomy involves complete resection of the local extent of cancer cells and wide dissection of the metastatic lymph nodes. Combined resection of the portal vein and the nerve plexes around the trunks of the celiac axis and the superior mesenteric artery are performed to dissect the local extent. Such procedures may be associated with a high postoperative mortality rate [3,9,10]. Although we lost seven patients within 60 days of the operation, five died in the early days of this study. The recent postoperative mortality rate was less than 5%.

The safety of en bloc resection of the portal vein is reasonably well established [25], although the necessity of routine removal of the portal vein is not clear. The observed invasion of the portal vein in our patients suggests that a resection that does not include the periportal tissues would leave cancer cells in the operative field. However, patients with invasion into the intima or the internal lumen of the portal vein did not live very long despite combined resection [26,27].

Invasion of the extrapancreatic nerve plexes was correlated with invasion of the surgical margin of resection, which shows that an extensive dissection of the extrapancreatic nerve plexes is necessary to perform a microscopically curative resection for cancer of the head of the pancreas [27]. Although our procedures are similar to those reported by Fortner [5], our 5-year survival rate was higher. There is also a difference between the two procedures with respect to the completeness of retroperitoneal dissection, in particular in the dissection of the nerve plexus around the superior mesenteric artery.

It is important to consider the argument of those who maintain that cancer of the pancreas is multifocal [28] and that total pancreatectomy is the only way to handle this problem. Although there was direct invasion of the neck of the pancreas in 2 of our patients, there was no multifocal disease in the 12 patients who underwent total pancreatectomy. Moreover, we have previously evaluated autopsy specimens from 68 patients and were unable to confirm a high rate of multifocal disease [29]. Of the 12 patients who underwent total pancreatectomy, only 1 patient survived more than 5 years. Consequently, we now depend on histological examination of the tissues at the margin of the resection specimen to determine the need for total pancreatectomy. However, the role of total pancreatectomy for carcinoma of the head of the pancreas may be limited.

The most serious nutritional disturbance that resulted was postoperative diarrhea. This is related to the excision of the sympathetic nerves to the small intestine and can be affected by the method of reconstruction. We have previously investigated this problem clinically and experimentally and found that the degree of disturbance is related to the extent of nerve dissection [30]. Furthermore, reconstruction by the Imanaga method [31], in which the stomach, pancreas, and bile duct are reconstructed in order, was associated with a more favorable outcome compared to the Child reconstruction [32]. Because this disorder is caused by the complete excision of lymph vessels and nerve plexes, dissection that leaves a thin layer of the nerve plexus around the superior mesenteric artery is recommended in patients with stage I or stage II disease [33].

Our method of extensive surgery for carcinoma of the head of the pancreas resolves the problems of local extension of disease, particularly retropancreatic invasion, but not the problems of lymphatic metastasis, particularly around the superior mesenteric artery and the abdominal aorta. Thus, combined resection of the superior mesenteric artery or the abdominal aorta may be necessary to improve the surgical results in patients with lymphatic metastases around these arteries.

References

1. Pliam MB, ReMine WH (1975) Further evaluation of total pancreatectomy. Arch Surg 110:506–512
2. Brooks JR, Culebras JM (1979) Carcinoma of the pancreas: palliative operation, Whipple procedure, or total pancreatectomy? Am J Surg 131:516–530
3. Connoly MM, Dawson PJ, Michelassi F, Moosa AR, Lowenstein F (1987) Survival in 1001 patients with carcinoma of the pancreas. Ann Surg 206:366–373
4. Moosa AR, Scott M, Lavelle-Jones M (1984) The place of total and extended pancreatectomy in pancreatic cancer. World J Surg 8:895–899
5. Fortner JG (1973) Regional resection of cancer of the pancreas: a new surgical approach. Surgery 73:307–320
6. Nagakawa T, Konishi K, Kurachi M, Miyazaki I (1979) Retroperitoneal dissection for pancreatic carcinoma—translateral retroperitoneal approach (in Japanese). Igaku No Ayumi 111:339–341
7. Nagakawa T, Kurachi M, Konishi K, Miyazaki I (1982) Translateral retroperitoneal approach in radical surgery for pancreatic carcinoma. Jpn J Surg 12:229–233
8. The Japan Pancreas Society (1993) The general rules for surgical and pathological studies on cancer of the pancreas (in Japanese). Kanehara Shuppan, Tokyo

9. Manabe T, Ohshio G, Baba N, Miyashita T, Asano N, Tamura K, Yamaki K, Nonaka A, Tobe T (1989) Radical pancreatectomy for ductal cell carcinoma of the head of the pancreas. Cancer (Phila) 64:1132–1137
10. Crist DW, Sitzmann JV, Cameron JC (1987) Improved hospital morbidity, mortality, and survival after the Whipple procedure. Am J Surg 206:358–365
11. Sato T, Saito Y, Noto T, Matsuno S (1977) Follow-up studies of radical resection for pancreaticoduodenal cancer. Ann Surg 186:581–588
12. Tsuchiya R, Tomioka T, Izawa K, Noda T, Yamamoto K, Tsunoda T, Harada N, Yamaguchi T, Yoshino R, Miyamoto T, Eto T (1986) Collective review of small carcinomas of the pancreas. Ann Surg 283:77–80
13. Nakase A, Matsumoto Y, Uchida K, Honjo I (1977) Surgical treatment of cancer of the pancreas and the periampullary region: cumulative results in 57 institutions in Japan. Ann Surg 185:52–57
14. Fortner JG (1981) Surgical principles for pancreatic cancer. Regional total and subtotal pancreatectomy. Cancer (Phila) 47:1712–1718
15. Nix GA, Schmitz PIM, Wilson JHP, van Blankenstein M, Groeneveld CFM, Hofuijk R (1984) Carcinoma of the head of the pancreas. Gastroenterology 87:37–43
16. Bjorck S, Svensson JO, Macpherson S, Edlund Y (1981) Cancer of the head of the pancreas and choledochoduodenal junction: a clinical study of 88 Whipple resections. Acta Chir Scand 148:353–359
17. van Heerden JA (1984) Pancreatic resection for carcinoma of the pancreas: Whipple versus total pancreatectomy—An institutional perspective. World J Surg 8:880–888
18. Kummerle F, Ruckert K (1984) Surgical treatment of pancreatic cancer. World J Surg 8:889–894
19. Longmire WP Jr (1984) Cancer of the pancreas: palliative operation, Whipple procedure, or total pancreatectomy? World J Surg 8:872–879
20. Grace PA, Pitt HA, Longmire WP (1986) Pancreatoduodenectomy with pylorus preservation for adenocarcinoma of the head of the pancreas. Br J Surg 73:647–650
21. Lygidakis NJ, Hyde MN, Houtoff HJ, Schipper MEI, Huibregste K, Tytgat GNJ, Lubber MJ, Reeders JWA, Bosey MMEM, Oosting J (1989) Resectional surgical procedures for carcinoma of the head of the pancreas. Surg Gynecol Obstet 168:157–165
22. Lea MS, Stahlgren LH (1987) Is resection appropriate for adenocarcinoma of the pancreas—a cost-benfit analysis. Am J Surg 154:651–654
23. Crile G Jr (1970) The advantages of by-pass operation over radical pancreatoduodenectomy in the treatment of pancreatic carcinoma. Surg Gynecol Obstet 130:1049–1053
24. Hertzberg J (1974) Pancreatoduodenal resection and by-pass operation in patients, ampulla, and distal end of the common duct. Acta Chir Scand 140:523–527
25. Nakao A, Horisawa M, Kondo T, Ando H, Kishimoto W, Ichihara T, Sakamuki T, Tanimoto H, Ito N (1983) Total pancreatectomy combined with resection of the portal vein employing portal perfusion method (in Japanese). Shujutsu 7:1–6
26. Nagakawa T, Konishi I, Ueno K, Ohta T, Akiyama T, Kayahara M, Miyazaki I (1991) Surgical treatment of pancreatic cancer. Int J Pancreatol 9:135–143
27. Nagakawa T, Konishi I, Ueno K, Ohta T, Akiyama T, Kanno M, Kayahara M, Miyazaki I (1991) The results and problems of extensive radical surgery for carcinoma of the head of the pancreas. Jpn J Surg 21:262–267
28. Tryka AF, Brooks JR (1979) Histopathology in the evaluation of total pancreatectomy for ductal carcinoma. Ann Surg 190:373–381
29. Nagakawa T, Asano E, Konishi K, Kurachi M, Kinami Y, Miyazaki I (1987) Significance of the extended radical operation for pancreatic cancer. New Trends Gastroenterol 205–214
30. Nagakawa T, Yoshimitsu Y, Suzaki Y, Takeda T, Sanada H, Kayahara M, Ohta T, Ueno K, Konishi I, Miyazaki I (1993) Postoperative digestive function and nutritional management after pancreaticoduodenectomy. Jpn J Biliary-Pancreatic Physiol 9:96–103
31. Imanaga H (1960) A new method of pancreaticoduodenectomy designed to preserve life and pancreatic function. Surgery 47:577–586

32. Child CG III (1944) Pancreaticojejunostomy and other problems associated with the surgical management of carcinoma involving the head of the pancreas. Ann Surg 119:845–855
33. Nagakawa T, Mori K, Kayahara M, Ohta T, Ueno K, Sanada H, Miyazaki I (1994) Three-dimensional studies on the structure of the tissue surrounding the superior mesenteric artery. Int J Pancreatol 15:129–138

Pylorus-Preserving Pancreatoduodenectomy by the Imanaga Procedure for Pancreatic and Periampullary Cancer

YOSHIRO OGATA[1], SHOICHI HISHINUMA[1], JUNICHI MATSUI[1], IWAO OZAWA[1], and SHIN TAKAHASHI[2]

Summary. Ninety-three patients with diseases of the periampullary region underwent pylorus-preserving pancreatoduodenectomy (PPPD) between March 1983 and March 1996. For 106 patients with cancer of the pancreatic head, the survival rate of 36 patients who underwent PPPD was compared with that of 50 patients who underwent standard pancreatoduodenectomy (PD) and 12 patients who underwent total pancreatectomy during the same period. There were no significant differences among the three procedures. The PPPD by the Imanaga procedure has shown advantages of (1) better recovery of body weight after surgery and (2) high possibility of observation of the pancreatic and bile duct orifice. We found local recurrence in 2 patients, 1 with malignant lymphoma and another with cancer of the bile duct, before elevation of tumor markers or detection by computed tomography or ultrasonography.

Key words. Pylorus-preserving pancreatoduodenectomy—Imanaga procedure—Pancreatic cancer—Periampullary cancer—Standard pancreatoduodenectomy

Introduction

The standard approach to pancreatic head resection has been the Whipple procedure, originally described for ampullary carcinoma in 1935. This type of procedure has a number of disadvantages, particularly related to the arrangement in gastrointestinal reconstruction and the partial gastrectomy. Postoperatively, patients have suffered from cholangitis because of retention of bile in the blind loop of the intestine and retained poor nutritional status.

Since 1981, we have adopted the Imanaga procedure [1] for gastrointestinal reconstruction after pancreatoduodenectomy in the hope of dissolving these problems. Moreover, we started using the operation of pylorus-preserving pancreatoduodenectomy (PPPD) reported by Traverso in 1983 and modified it to

[1] Department of Surgery, Tochigi Cancer Center, Tochigi 320, Japan.
[2] Department of Surgery, Keio University, School of Medicine, Shinjuku-ku, Tokyo 160, Japan.

PPPD by the Imanaga procedure for patients with cancer of the head of the pancreas in 1987 [2]. This chapter analyzes the indication, technique, and results of this procedure for patients with cancer of the head of the pancreas.

Patients and Methods

Patients

Ninety-three patients with diseases of the periampullary region underwent PPPD between March 1983 and March 1996 at Tochigi Cancer Center and the Keio University Hospital (Table 1). Of 39 patients with cancer of the pancreatic head undergoing PPPD, 36 patients with invasive ductal carcinoma were admitted to this study and the remaining 3 patients with cystadenocarcinoma were excluded. Other pancreatic resection for patients with cancer of the pancreatic head was by pancreatoduodenectomy (PD) in 58 patients and by total pancreatectomy (TP) in 12 patients.

All resected patients were classified into three categories of "Curability": Curability A and B resections were performed in 12.0% and 79% of 58 PDs, respectively, and 25.0% and 61.1% of 36 PPPDs; Curability B resection was done in all patients of 12 TPs (Table 2). Statistical analysis was performed using the t-test and log rank test.

TABLE 1. Pylorus-preserving pancreatoduodenectonc (PPPD) for diseases of the periampullary region, March 1983–March 1996

| | | Gastrointestinal reconstruction procedure | |
	Number of patients	Traverso (March 1983– June 1988)	Imanaga (July 1988-)
Malignant disease ($n = 86$)			
Cancer of the head of the pancreas	39 (19)[a]	5 (2)	34 (17)
Cancer of the bile duct	17 (1)	7 (1)	10
Cancer of the ampulla of Vater	19	7	12
Cancer of the duodenum	2	2	5
Cancer of the gallbladder	5	1	
Cancer of the duodenum	1		1
Malignant lymphoma of the duodenum	1		1
Cancer of the transverse colon	1		
Cancer of the right kidney	1	1	
Benign disease ($n = 7$)			
Chronic pancreatitis	3	1	2
Adenoma of the head of the pancreas	1		1
Adenoma of the ampulla of Vater	1		1
Arteriovenous malformation of the head of the pancreas	1		1
Benign stricture of the common bile duct	1		1
	93 (20)	24 (3)	69 (17)

Numbers in parentheses indicate numbers of patients undergoing combined resection of vessels.
[a] Includes three cases of cystadenocarcinoma.

TABLE 2. Characteristics of resections for 106 patients with cancer of the pancreatic head

Operative procedure		Number of resections	Curability	Number of patient
PD (*n* = 58)	With PV resection	27	A	1
			B	24
			C	2
	Without PV resection	31	A	6
			B	22
			C	3
TP (*n* = 12)	With PV resection	11	B	11
	Without PV resection	1	B	1
PPPD (*n* = 36)	With PV resection	20	A	4
			B	14
			C	2
	Without PV resection	16	A	5
			B	8
			C	3

PD, Pancreatoduodenectomy; TP, total pancreatectomy; PPPD, pylorus-preserving pancreatoduodenectomy; PV, portal vein.

Definition of Curability

Judging from operative findings as to the extent of tumor invasion to the adjacent organs or tissues, surgical margins, and lymph node and distant metastases, "Curability" is classified into the three categories according to the General Rules for Study of Pancreatic Cancer (Japan Pancreas Society) [3]. Curability A is defined as "no residual tumor and a high probability of cure", Curability B as "curability other than "A or C", and Curability C as "definite residual tumor". If "Curability" is based on histological findings, "Curability" should be recorded using small letters such as "curability A, B, or C".

Indication for PPPD

PPPD was indicated for patients who had no metastases to the perigastric lymph nodes and no tumor involvement of the first portion of the duodenum. Patients for whom PPPD was not indicated underwent PD or TP. In patients with portal vein or adjacent artery (the hepatic or superior mesenteric artery) involvement and no distant metastases, we performed combined resection of these vessels [4,5].

PPPD Procedure

It is our consistent policy that the cancer should be extirpated with en bloc clearance of both lymph nodes and peripancreatic soft tissue, along with excision of the nerve plexus in the retroperitoneum. Lymph nodes were extensively dissected in the primary and secondary lymph node groups regulated by the General Rules for the Study of Pancreatic Cancer (Japanese Pancreas Society) [3]. Thus, the dissection skeletonized the aorta from the level of the superior mesenteric artery and celiac axis. This dissection is termed D_2 dissection of lymph nodes.

We carefully dissected the suprapyloric lymph nodes in patients with cancer of the bile duct and also the infrapyloric lymph nodes in patients with cancer of the pancre-

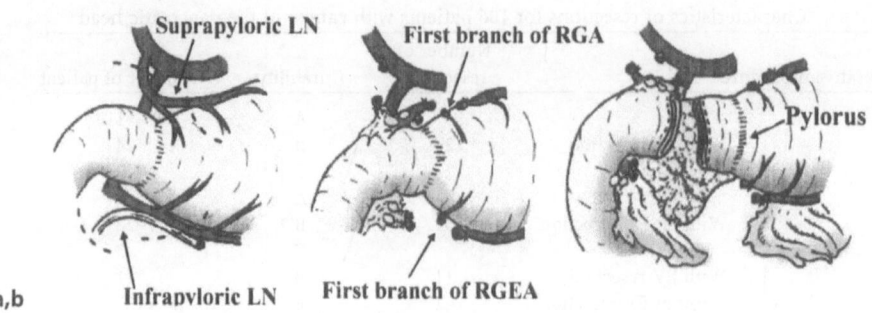

FIG. 1a–c. Dissection of the supra- and infrapyloric lymph nodes (*LN*). **a, b** The peripheries of the right gastric (*RGA*) and right gastroepiploic arteries (*RGEA*) and veins with their first branches to the stomach are divided along the gastric wall to completely remove both the supra- and infrapyloric lymph nodes. **c** The blood supply to the first portion of the duodenum is thus reduced, and the length of duodenum that can be preserved is limited to less than 2 cm

TABLE 3. Incidence of lymph node metastasis in periampullary cancer

Lymph node site	Pancreatic head, % (n = 73)	Distal bile duct, % (n = 64)	Ampulla of Vater, % (n = 28)
Along the lesser curvature of the stomach	0 (0/26)	0 (0/27)	0 (0/5)
Along the greater curvature of the stomach	2.0 (1/43)	0 (0/32)	0 (0/11)
Suprapyloric	1.5 (1/67)	7.1 (1/14)	0 (0/9)
Infrapyloric	7.5 (5/67)	0 (0/44)	0 (0/14)
Along the left gastric artery	6.0 (3/32)	0 (0/11)	20.0 (1/5)
Along the common hepatic artery	11.0 (4/37)	7.3 (4/55)	6.0 (1/17)
Around the celiac axis	11.0 (4/37)	0 (0/25)	0 (0/9)

Numbers in parentheses indicate numbers of patients with positive lymph nodes/total number of resected patients.

atic head (Fig. 1) because a relatively high incidence of metastasis to these regions was observed in each disease (Table 3). If nodal metastases were found in those lymph nodes, we abandoned PPPD and performed PD.

After dissection of lymph nodes in these region, the blood supply to the first portion of the duodenum was reduced and the length of the duodenum that could be reserved was limited to less than 2 cm. When the portal vein, hepatic, and superior mesenteric arteries could not be separated from the tumor during the operation after skeletonization of these blood vessels, they were judged to be invaded by the cancer and were resected if there were no distant metastases. Reconstruction of the portal vein was done by a direct end-to-end anastomosis, but for patients undergoing resection of a long segment more than 4 cm in length reconstruction was by grafting the external iliac vein [4] or the left renal vein [6]. The hepatic and superior mesenteric arteries were reconstructed by grafting the saphenous vein. Of 36 patients with invasive ductal carcinoma undergoing PPPD, 19 (52.7%) underwent combined resection of the portal vein, and 1 patient with cancer of the uncinate process also underwent resection of the superior mesenteric artery. Of 58 patients of PD and 12 patients

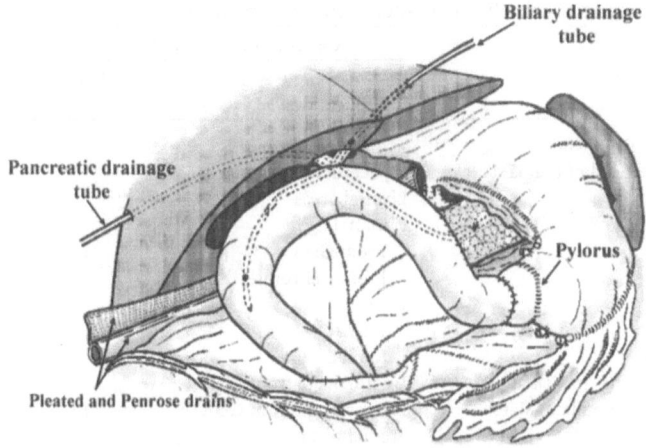

FIG. 2. Gastrointestinal continuity is restored by the Imanaga procedure. Two transhepatic catheters are used to stent and decompress the anastomotic portion of the pancreatic and biliary ducts

of TP, 27 (46.6%) and 11 (91.7%) underwent resection of the portal vein. In our series portal vein resection was adopted to 58 (54.7%) of 106 resected patients.

Intraoperative Radiation Therapy

Following resection, patients with pancreatic cancer received intraoperative radiation therapy (IORT) 16–20 Gy with 6–12 MeV electron beams. The radiation field included the tumor bed, with adequate margins covering the roots of celiac axis and superior mesenteric artery, the porta hepatis, and the 2-cm cut stump of the remnant pancreas.

Gastrointestinal Reconstruction by the Imanaga Procedure

We used the Imanaga procedure for restoring gastrointestinal continuity. The proximal jejunum, which was brought through the transverse mesocolon, was anastomosed end-to-end to the distal end of the duodenum with a layer-to-layer anastomosis, an end-to-side to the pancreas with the jejunal mucosa to the pancreatic duct anastomosis method 2–3 cm distal to the duodenojejunostomy, and an end-to-side to the bile duct with a single-layer anastomosis, in that order (Fig. 2). As a result of this type of gastrointestinal reconstruction, we can easily insert an endoscope to observe the stoma of the pancreatic and bile duct postoperatively.

Results

Postoperative Complications

The 30-day operative mortality rate was 1.1% (1 of 93). One patient with cancer of the bile duct died of intraperitoneal hemorrhage because of a pancreatic fistula. The hospital mortality rate was 5.4% (5 of 93). Three patients with cancer of the pancreatic head died of a myocardial infarction on postoperative day 107, a liver abscess on

TABLE 4. Postoperative complications after PPPD in 93 patients

Disease	Complieation	Traverso (n = 24)	Imanaga (n = 69)
		Gastromtestmal reconstruction procedure	
Malignant disease (n = 86)			
Cancer of the head of the pancreas	Myocardial infarction		1 (1)
(n = 39)	Liver abscess		1 (1)
	Hemorrhage		
	From GDA	1	
	From gastrointestinal tract		2 (1)
	Ulcer		
	Gastric	1	
	Stomal		1
Cancer of the bile duct (n = 17)	Hemorrhage from CHA		1[a]
Cancer of the ampulla of Vater	Hemorrhage from GDA	1 (1)	
(n = 19)	Stomal ulcer		1
Benign disease (n = 7)	Stomal ulcer		2
		3 (1)	9 (3)

GDA, Gastroduodenal artery; CHA, common hepatic artery.
Numbers in paren theses are hospital deaths;
[a] Operative death (<30 days). Operative mortality rate, 1.1% (1/93); hospital mortality rate, 5.4% (5/93).

TABLE 5. Incidence of delayed gastric emptying[a]

Traverso	41.7%	(10/24)
Imanaga	33.3%	(23/69)
Total	35.5%	(33/93)

[a] Gastric drainage for more than 14 days.

postoperative day 140, and gastrointestinal hemorrhage on postoperative day 113, respectively, 1 patient with cancer of the ampulla died of arterial hemorrhage from the stump of the gastroduodenal artery on postoperative day 91, and 5 patients (1 in Traverso, 4 in Imanaga) developed a gastric or stomal ulcer, which was treated conservatively (Table 4).

Delayed Gastric Emptying

Delayed gastric emptying, defined as a requirement of gastric drainage for more than 14 days after operation, was observed with a high incidence of 41.7% by the Traverso procedure and 33.3% by the Imanaga procedure. However, this complication was transient and resolved on postoperative course in all patients (Table 5).

Survival

The survival rates for 106 patients with cancer of the pancreatic head were calculated by the Kaplan–Meier method for the three different procedures (PD, PPPD, and TP). The 1-, 3-, and 5-year survival rates were 52.8%, 18.6%, and 14.5% in PD; 65.9%, 27.6%, and 18.4% in PPPD; and 18.1%, 9.1%, and 9.1% in TP, respectively. There were

Survival Rate

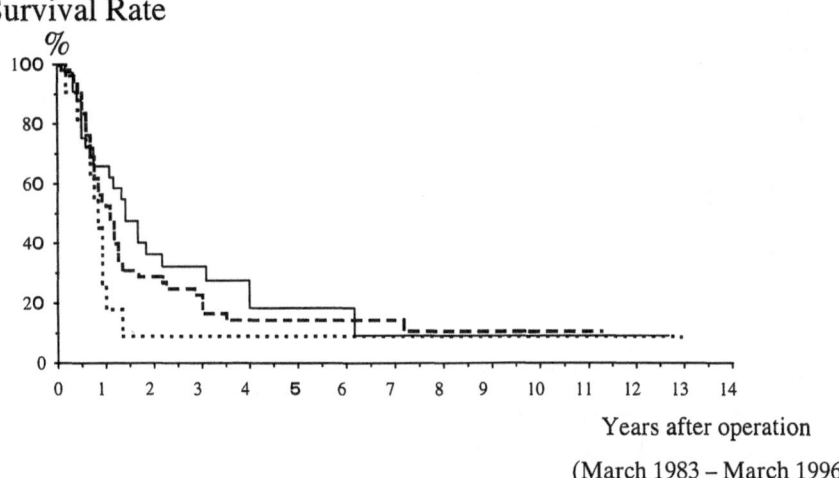

Years after operation

(March 1983 – March 1996)

FIG. 3. Survival curves after pylorus-preserving pancreatoduodenectomy (PPPD; *continuous line*, n = 36), standard pancreatoduodenectomy (PD; *dashed line*, n = 58), or total pancreatectomy (TP; *dotted line*, n = 12). There were no statistically significant differences among the three procedures

Survival Rate

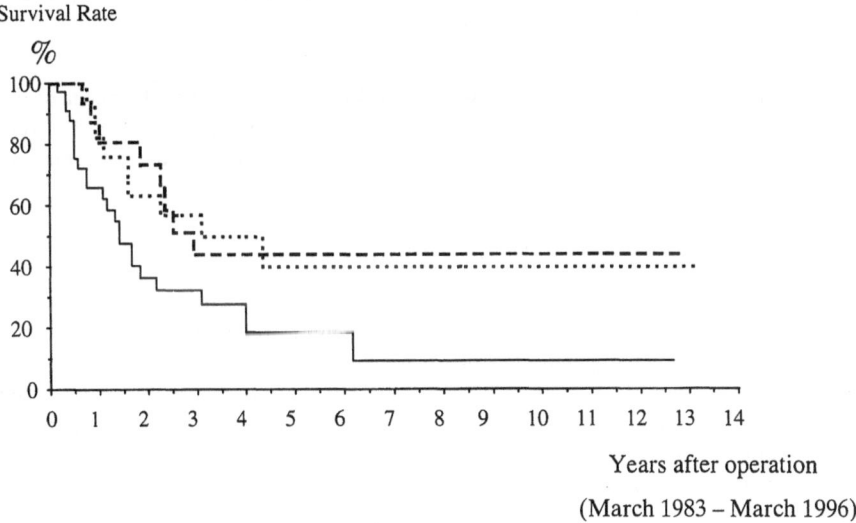

Years after operation

(March 1983 – March 1996)

FIG. 4. Survival curves after PPPD for patients with cancer of the pancreatic head (*continuous line*; n = 36), cancer of the ampulla of Vater (*dotted line*; n = 19), or cancer of the bile duct (*dashed line*; n = 17)

no significant differences among the three procedures (Fig. 3). For 36 patients with cancer of the pancreatic head, 17 patients with cancer of the bile duct, and 19 patients with cancer of the ampulla who underwent PPPD, the 5- and 10-year survival rates were 18.4% and 9.2%, 44.0% and 44.0%, and 39.9% and 39.9%, respectively (Fig. 4).

Survival Rate

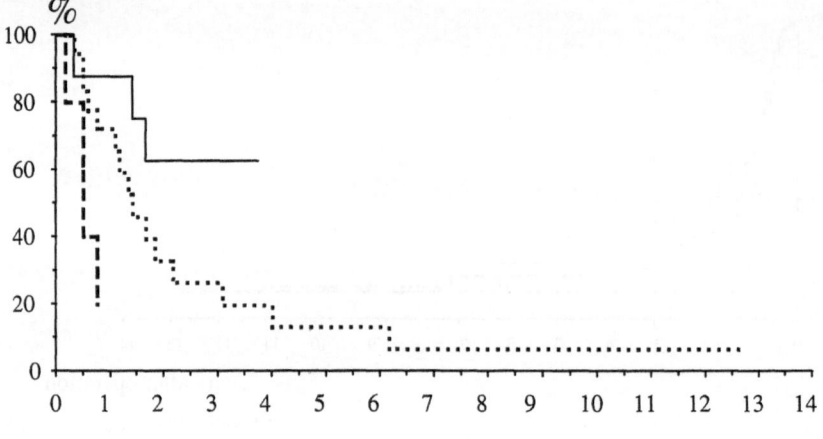

FIG. 5. Survival curves for patients with cancer of the pancreatic head after "Curability A" resection (*continuous line*; *n* = 9), "Curability B" resection (*dotted line*; *n* = 21), and "Curability C" resection (*dashed line*; *n* = 5). There were statistical differences between "Curability A" and "C", and between "Curability B" and "C", at *P* < .05

The survival rates by the classification of curability for patients with cancer of the pancreatic head who underwent PPPD indicated that "Curability A" and "B" were significantly higher than "Curability C", but there was no significant difference between "Curability A" and "B" (Fig. 5).

Postoperative Change in Body Weight

Chemotherapy and radiotherapy were scheduled for patients with pancreatic cancer, but good nutritional status was required. Thus, gastrointestinal reconstruction should be the mode to preserve digestive and absorptive functions as much as possible and to maintain good performance status. Postoperative change in body weight was analyzed as an aspect of evaluation for nutritional status. Each group showed that the patients had a tendency to recover in body weight from 3 months after surgery. Body weight was recovered better in the PPPD group than in the PD group. There was a significant difference between PPPD-Imanaga and PD-Imanaga groups (*P* < .05) in body recovery ratio at 18 months after surgery (Fig. 6).

Postoperative Findings of Gastrointestinal Series and Endoscopy

The gastrointestinal reconstruction by the Imanaga procedure has some advantages because food passes physiologically through the upper part of the jejunum (Fig. 7) and thus we can insert an endoscope postoperatively to observe the anastomotic stoma of the pancreatic and bile ducts and to perform cholangiopancreatography (Fig. 8). Radioisotope studies have showed better mixing of food with bile and no reflux of bile into the stomach.

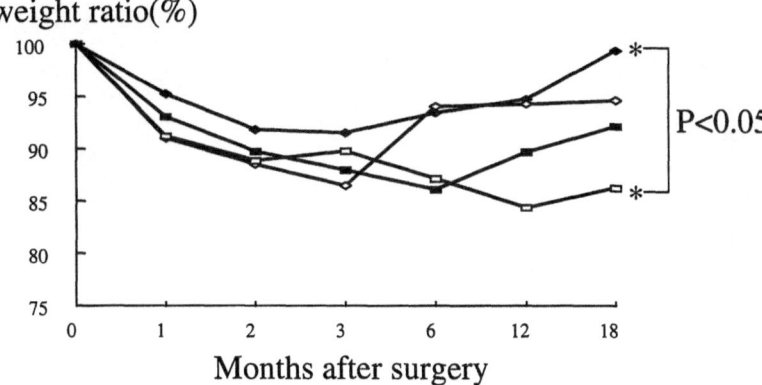

FIG. 6. Postoperative change in body weight. The difference in body weight ratio between PPPD-Imanaga (*solid diamonds*) and PD-Imanaga (*open rectangles*) was significant at 18 months after surgery

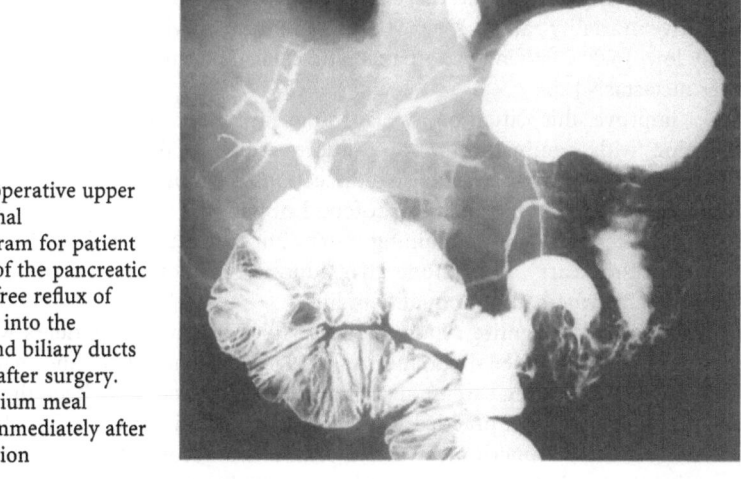

FIG. 7. Postoperative upper gastrointestinal roentogenogram for patient with cancer of the pancreatic head shows free reflux of barium meal into the pancreatic and biliary ducts at 8 months after surgery. Reflux of barium meal disappears immediately after the examination

We succeeded in postoperative observation of the pancreatic and bile duct by endoscopy with 88.9% (24/27) and found local recurrence in 2 patients: 1 with malignant lymphoma was diagnosed as recurrence in the pancreatic duct at 1 year 3 months and another with cancer of the bile duct at the choledochojejunostomy at 2 years 1 month postoperatively.

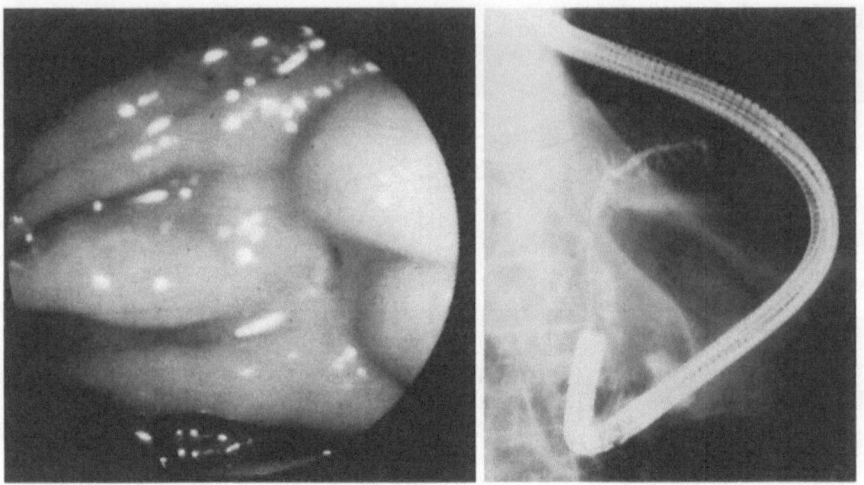

a   b

FIG. 8. Observation of the pancreatic orifice (a) and the pancreatogram (b) taken by postoperative endoscope for the patient shown in Fig. 7

Discussion

The resectability rate for patients with cancer of the pancreatic head undergoing conventional pancreatoduodenectomy was about 20%–30%. We began to perform combined resection of the pancreas, the portal vein, and adjacent arteries in 1976 [4]. The resectability rate was increased to 61.9% (151/244) with 2.6% (4/151) of the 30-day operative mortality rate in 1995. The overall 5-year survival rate was still unsatisfactorily low, 16.0%. Patients with pancreatic cancer succumbed to local recurrence or liver metastasis [7].

To improve this situation, we introduced IORT and postoperative external radiation with administration of 5-fluorouracil. As the Whipple type of pancreatoduodenectomy with extensive dissection of lymph nodes and excision of the retroperitoneal nerve plexus has profound nutritional sequelae, many patients not only found difficulty in maintaining weight but suffered from fatty liver. It became very difficult to carry out postoperative adjuvant chemotherapy or radiotherapy for these patients who had poor quality of life.

Traverso and Longmire reported successful PPPD in two patients with chronic pancreatitis and duodenal carcinoma in 1978 [8]. Since that time, periampullary malignancies, including carcinoma of the pancreatic head, have been the list of indications for PPPD. In our practice, PPPD with extensive dissection of lymph nodes, and excision of the retroperitoneal nerve plexus has become the standard means of resecting the head of the pancreas and since 1983 PD has been reserved for those few patients with metastasis to perigastric lymph nodes or with direct invasion to the bulb of the duodenum.

Our study showed that patients treated by PPPD had gained postoperative weight better than patients with PD. PPPD by the Imanaga procedure has another advantage in allowing insertion of an endoscope and observation of the stoma of the pancreatic and bile duct postoperatively. We could check the patency of these ducts, evaluate function of the residual pancreas and the liver correctly, and find recurrence around the anastomotic site earlier than detection by elevation of tumor markers and computed tomography or ultrasonography. As a result, we were able to start early chemotherapy or radiation therapy for recurrences.

The applicability of PPPD to malignant diseases of the periampullary region is still debatable. Moossa [9] has stated that PPPD should be used cautiously until further data become available, and a controlled trial with the standard Whipple procedure is needed.

Adequate conclusions on the suitability of PPPD for cancer resection depend on the analysis of survival rates according to stage. Roder et al. [10] reported that PPPD was associated with a significantly worse survival rate than the Whipple resection for stage III pancreatic carcinoma but that there was no difference among patients with carcinoma of the pancreas, ampulla of Vater, or distal common bile duct. We need further information on this report, because Roder et al. calculated the survival rate of stage III including curative and noncurative patients, and their operative procedure was not known. Patel et al. [11] noted that the analysis of operative mortality rates, operative times, delayed gastric emptying, hospitalization, and cost provided no evidence of any advantage for PPPD in patients with malignant periampullary tumors.

Several authors have found no difference between the two procedures in survival for periampullary malignancy, including adenocarcinoma of the pancreatic head. Braasch et al. [12] applied PPPD to patients with periampullary malignancy if the nodes in the resectable field were positive but no spread outside this field was observed. They have shown a 5-year survival rate of 17% for 14 patients with cancer of the pancreatic head with good quality of gastrointestinal function, and this result is comparable with results after the standard Whipple procedure.

Cameron et al. [13] found that the factors influencing survival after pancreatoduodenectomy for pancreatic cancer were blood vessel invasion and lymph node involvement. Their 5-year survival rate following PPPD was 22% for 27 patients with cancer of the pancreatic head. This figure is compatible with survival rates after Whipple resection. PPPD allows patients a better quality of life and provides a chance to accomplish adjuvant chemotherapy or radiotherapy, which will improve the results of pancreatic surgery.

References

1. Imanaga H (1960) A new method of pancreaticoduodenectomy designed to preserve liver and pancreatic function. Surgery (St. Louis) 47:577–586
2. Ogata Y, Hishinuma S, Matsui J, Ozawa I, Takahashi S (1994) Pylorus-preserving pancreaticoduodenectomy with combined resection of the portal vein and gastrointestinal reconstruction by Imanaga procedure for ductal cancer of the head of the pancreas. J Hep Bil Pancr Surg 4:372–378
3. Japanese Pancreas Society (1993) General rules for the study of pancreatic cancer. Kanehara, Tokyo
4. Ogata Y, Ohyama R, Kobayashi K, Kojima M, Marugami Y, Amemiya T, Takami H, Tsuzuki T, Abe O (1981) Pancreatectomy with combined resection of the portal vein (in Japanese). Gekashinryo (Surg Diagn Treat) 23:418–428
5. Takahashi S, Ogata Y, Tsuzuki T (1994) Combined resection of the pancreas and portal vein for pancreatic cancer. Br J Surg 81:1190–1193
6. Miyazaki M, Itoh H, Kaiho T, Ambiru S, Togawa A, Sasada K, Shiobara M, Shimizu Y, Yoshioka S, Yoshitome H, Nakajima N (1995) Portal vein reconstruction at the hepatic hilus using a left renal vein. J Am Coll Surg 180:497–498

7. Ogata Y, Takahashi S, Hishinuma S, Matui J, Ozawa I (1994) Surgical treatment for pancreatic cancer (in Japanese). Gan no Rinsho (Jpn J Cancer Clin) 40:1566–1576
8. Traverso LM, Longmire WP (1978) Preservasion of the pylorus in pancreatectomy. Surg Gynecol Obstet 146:959–962
9. Moossa AR, Veeragandham RS (1994) Preservation of the pylorus in resection of the head of the pancreas. J Hepatic Biliary Pancr Surg 4:349–354
10. Roder JD, Stein HJ, Huttl W, Siewert JR (1992) Pylorus-preserving versus standard pancreaticoduodenectomy: an analysis of 110 pancreatic and periampullary carcinomas. Br J Surg 79:152–155
11. Patel AG, Toyama MT, Kusske AM, Alexander P, Ashley SW, Reber HA (1995) Pylorus-preserving Whipple resection for pancreatic cancer. Is it any better? Arch Surg 130:838–843
12. Braasch JW, Rossi R, Watkins E JR, Deziel DJ, Winter PF (1980) Pyloric and gastric preserving pancreatic resection. Experience with 87 patients. Ann Surg 204:411–418
13. Cameron JL, Crist DW, Sitzmann JV, Hruban RH, Boitnott JK, Seidler AJ, Coleman J (1991) Factors influencing survival after pancreaticoduodenectomy for pancreatic cancer. Am J Surg 161:120–125

Hepatopancreatoduodenectomy for Biliary Cancer

Yuji Nimura

Summary. Hepatopancreatoduodenectomy (HPD), that is, en bloc hepatic resection with pancreatoduodenectomy (PD), has been used as a radical operation for advanced carcinoma of the biliary tract. From September 1979 to December 1994, HPD was performed on 37 patients with advanced biliary cancer. Several kinds of hepatic segmentectomies with caudate lobe resection were applied in 17 cases of bile duct cancer, and four types of liver resections with PD were carried out in 20 patients with gallbladder cancer. Combined HPD and portal vein resection were performed in 7 cases of bile duct cancer and 9 cases of gallbladder cancer. Postoperative morbidity was high, both in bile duct cancer patients (76%) and in gallbladder cancer patients (45%). The 30-day operative mortality rate for patients undergoing HPD was 14% and hospital mortality was 22%. However, no fatal complication has been encountered after employing preoperative portal vein embolization for 4 patients undergoing major hepatectomy with PD. The 1- and 2-year survival rates for 15 patients with bile duct cancer undergoing curative HPD were 30% and 20%, respectively, and 15 patients died within 3 years. The 1-, 3-, and 5-year survival rates for 18 patients undergoing curative PD and hepatectomy of more than 4a,5,6 segmentectomy for gallbladder cancer were 50%, 6%, and 6%, and those for 12 patients undergoing curative PD and extended right lobectomy were 50%, 8%, and 8%, respectively. It should be considered that HPD was associated not only with an unexpectedly long survival period but also with high morbidity and mortality.

Key words. Hepatectomy—Bile   duct   cancer—Pancreatectomy—Pancreato-duodenectomy—Gallbladder cancer

Introduction

Recent advances in techniques for diagnosing hepatobiliary and pancreatic diseases have allowed a gradually increasing number of cancers to be detected early; however, most carcinoma of the biliary tract is still first encountered at an advanced stage.

First Department of Surgery, Nagoya University School of Medicine, Showa-ku, Nagoya, Aichi 466, Japan.

Aggressive surgical approaches to carcinoma of the biliary tract using liver resection have been applied by many surgeons with varying degrees of success [1–6]. On the other hand, several Japanese surgeons have attempted to remove advanced carcinoma of the biliary tract, often in combination with hepatectomy and pancreatectomy [7–14]. In this chapter, the author describes a procedure of hepatopancreatoduodenectomy (HPD), that is, en bloc hepatic resection with pancreatoduodenectomy (PD) for advanced carcinoma of the bile duct or the gallbladder.

Materials and Method

From September 1979 to December 1994, HPD was performed on 37 patients with advanced carcinoma of the bile duct or gallbladder. The 37 patients included 17 (16.0%) of 106 hepatectomized cases of bile duct carcinoma and 20 (29.0%) of 69 cases of liver resection for gallbladder carcinoma. HPD included en bloc hepatic segmentectomy or lobectomy with PD. Combined liver bed resection and PD for gallbladder carcinoma was excluded from HPD. The smallest hepatectomies were a segment 4a (anterior subsegment of S4),5,6 resection for gallbladder carcinoma and an independent caudate lobectomy for bile duct carcinoma. HPD was indicated for diffuse carcinoma of the bile duct and for advanced carcinoma of the gallbladder that showed macroscopic invasion of the liver, distal bile duct, duodenum, or pancreas.

Selective cholangiography through percutaneous transhepatic biliary drainage (PTBD) or percutaneous transhepatic cholangioscopy (PTCS) [15–19] was performed for precise diagnosis of the extent of cancer in the bile duct. Ultrasonography, dynamic computed tomography, selective arteriography, percutaneous transhepatic portography (PTP), and selective hepatic venography were carried out to investigate the involvement of the liver, duodenum, colon, hepatic artery, portal vein, and regional lymph nodes. An operative procedure was designed according to these assessments. Special attention was paid to the pathophysiological effects of jaundice, to cholangitis, and to the anticipated functional capacity of preserved liver segments. Since 1989, percutaneous transhepatic portal vein embolization (PTPE) has been performed before major hepatectomy: right lobectomy, extended right lobectomy, right trisegmentectomy, or left trisegmentectomy [20–22] to reduce functional capacity of the resected liver and to increase the safety of major hepatectomy.

Seven kinds of hepatic lobectomies or segmentectomies with PD (10 cases) or pylorus-preserving pancreatoduodenectomy (PPPD) (7 cases) were carried out in 17 patients with bile duct carcinoma. The caudate lobe was also resected in all cases. Independent total caudate lobectomy with PD was indicated for diffuse carcinoma of the proximal bile duct as a minimum hepatectomy. Portal vein resection and reconstruction was concomitantly performed in 7 cases of HPD (Table 1).

Four kinds of liver resections with PD (19 cases) or PPPD (1 case) were carried out for 20 patients with gallbladder carcinoma. S4a,5,6 resection with PD or PPPD was indicated for gallbladder carcinoma with limited direct invasion of the liver bed. As a maximum hepatectomy, right hepatic trisegmentectomy with caudate lobectomy and PD were performed together with combined resection of the portal vein for advanced carcinoma of the gallbladder involving both the hepatic hilus and adjacent organs (Table 2).

TABLE 1. Hepatopancreatoduodenectomy (HPD) for bile duct cancer

	Pancreatectomy		Combined resection	
Hepatectomy	PD	PPPD	PV	IVC
Right trisegmentectomy + S_1 ($n = 1$)	1		1	
Extended right lobectomy + S_1 ($n = 7$)	4	3	4	1
Right lobectomy + S_1 ($n = 3$)	2	1	2	
Right anterior segmentectomy + S_1 ($n = 2$)		2		
Left trisegmentectomy + S_1 ($n = 1$)	1			
Extended left lobectomy + S_1 ($n = 1$)	1			
S_1 ($n = 2$)	1	1		
Totals ($n = 17$)	10	7	7	1

S_1, caudate lobectomy; PD, pancreatoduodenectomy; PPPD, pylorus-preserving pancreatoduodenectomy; PV, portal vein; IVC, inferior vena cava.

TABLE 2. Hepatopancreatoduodenectomy (HPD) for gallbladder cancer

	Pancreatectomy		Combined resection		
Hepatectomy	PD	PPPD	PV	IVC	Colon
Right trisegmentectomy (+S_1) ($n = 4$)	4	0	2	0	0
Exterior right lobectomy (+S_1) ($n = 8$)	8	0	7	1	2
Right anterior segmentectomy (+S_1) ($n = 2$)	2	0	0	0	0
$S_{4a,5,6}$ ($n = 6$)	5	1	0	0	3
Totals ($n = 20$)	19	1	9	1	5

Results

Several postoperative complications such as hyperbilirubinemia, hepatic failure, anastomotic insufficiencies, and intraperitoneal bleeding occurred in 13 (76%) of the 17 patients with bile duct cancer and 9 (45%) of the 20 patients with gallbladder cancer.

Five patients (2 bile duct cancer and 3 gallbladder cancer) died of acute hepatic failure within 30 days after HPD. Three other patients (2 bile duct cancer and 1 gallbladder cancer) developed persistent postoperative hepatic failure complicated by intraperitoneal abscess caused by anastomotic leakage or low-output syndrome caused by myocardiac infarction progressed to a fatal complication within 3 months after HPD. The overall 30-day operative mortality rate for patients undergoing HPD was 14% (5/37), and hospital mortality was 22% (8/37). However, no fatal complication has been encountered after employing PTPE for 4 patients undergoing major hepatectomy with PD. There was a close relation between the rate of hospital mortality and the extent of liver resection. All 4 patients with bile duct cancer who died underwent major hepatectomy of more than a right lobectomy with PD, and all 5 patients undergoing three kinds of liver resections of less than a right lobectomy survived the HPD. No fatal complication occurred in 6 patients with gallbladder cancer undergoing a S4a,5,6 hepatectomy with PD. One of 8 patients with advanced gallbladder cancer undergoing PD with hepatectomy of less than a right lobectomy developed fatal liver damage. Three of 12 patients undergoing PD with an extended right lobectomy or a right trisegmentectomy died of acute or chronic hepatic failure (Table 3).

The 1- and 2-year survival rates for 15 patients with bile duct cancer were 30% and 20%, respectively, and all 15 patients died within 3 years after curative HPD, while the 1-, 3-, 5-, and 10-year survival rates for 89 patients with hilar bile duct cancer undergoing hepatectomy without PD were 83%, 45%, 29%, and 23%, respectively. The 1-year survival rate for 29 patients with unresectable advanced bile duct cancer was 23%, and almost all patients died within 2 years after PTBD. There was, however, no statistically significant difference in survival between patients with HPD and those with unresectable tumor (Fig. 1).

The 1-, 3-, and 5-year survival rates for 18 patients undergoing curative PD and hepatectomy of more than 4a,5,6 segmentectomy for gallbladder cancer were 50%,

TABLE 3. Extent of liver resection and mortality in HPD

Liver resection	Hospital mortality (%)
Bile duct cancer	4/17 (24)
<Right lobectomy	0/5 (0)
≧Right lobectomy[a]	4/12 (33)
Gallbladder cancer	4/20 (20)
<Right lobectomy	1/8 (13)
≧Right lobectomy	3/12 (25)

[a] Includes a left trisegmentectomy.

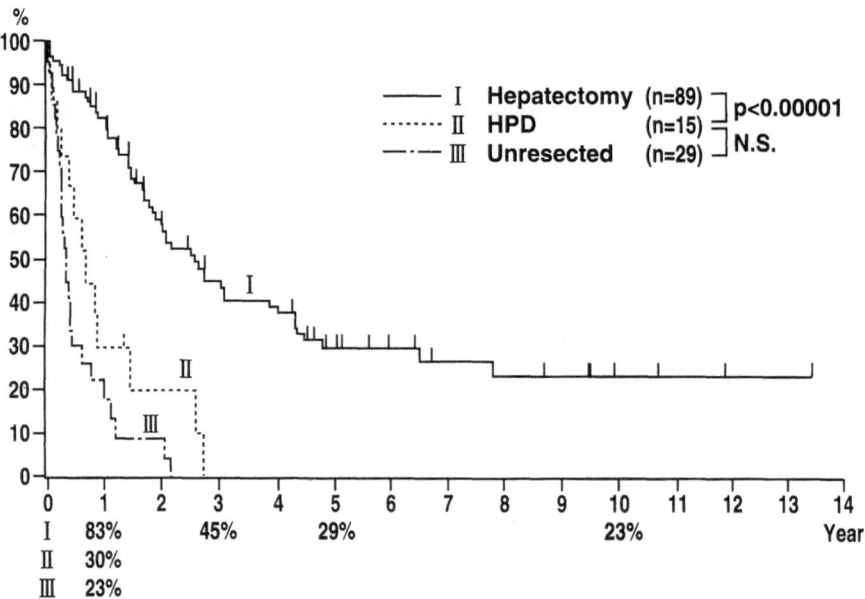

FIG. 1. Postoperative life table survival curves according to type of treatment in patients with hilar bile duct carcinoma, comparing hepatectomy with hepatopancreatoduodenectomy (HPD). Statistically significant differences were found between groups I and II ($P < .00001$); group II versus III was not significant

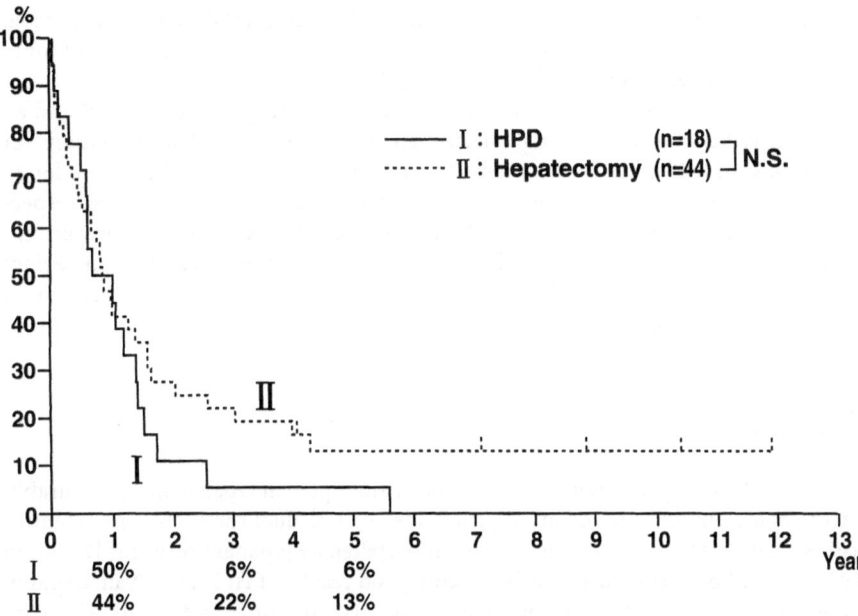

FIG. 2. Postoperaive life table survival curves according to type of surgery in patients with gallbladder cancer undergoing curative liver resection of more than a S4a,5,6 segmentectomy. There was no statistically significant difference between the two groups

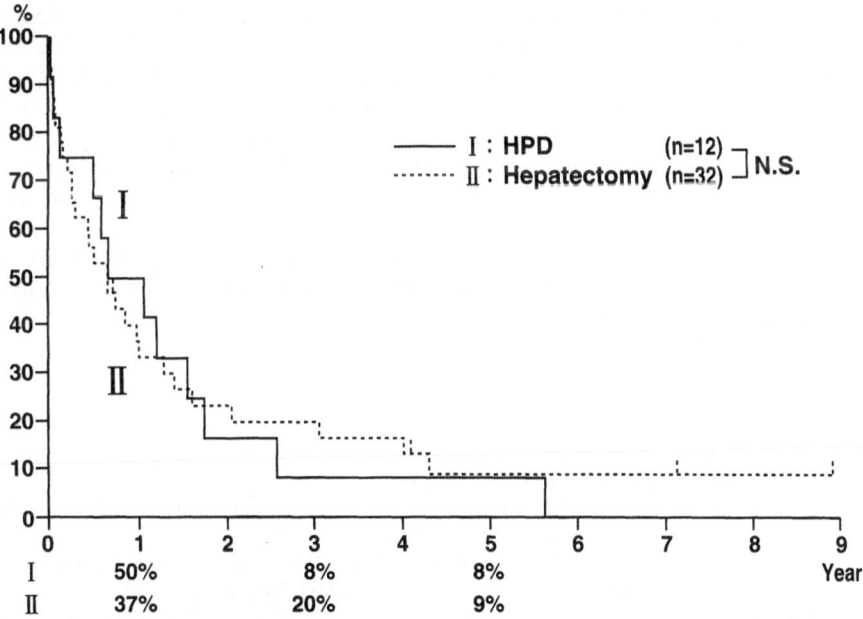

FIG. 3. Postoperative life table survival curves according to type of surgery in patients with advanced gallbladder cancer undergoing curative major hepatectomy of more than an extended right hepatic lobectomy. No statistically significant difference was found between the two groups

6%, and 6%, respectively. There was no statistically significant difference in survival between these 18 patients and 44 patients undergoing curative hepatectomy of more than S4a,5,6 segmentectomy without PD (Fig. 2).

The 1-, 3-, and 5-year survival rates for 12 patients undergoing curative PD and an extended right lobectomy or right trisegmentectomy with caudate lobectomy for advanced gallbladder cancer were 50%, 8%, and 8%, respectively, while those for 32 patients undergoing the same curative hepatectomy were 37%, 20%, and 9%, respectively. No statistically significant difference was observed between the two groups (Fig. 3). The longest survivor with advanced gallbladder carcinoma undergoing a right hepatic trisegmentectomy with total caudate lobectomy and PD died of recurrent carcinoma on the right fonsilla at 5 years and 7 months without any recurrent tumor in the peritoneal cavity.

Discussion

Although clinical application of HPD had been attempted in Japan to increase curability of radical surgery for advanced gallbladder or bile duct carcinoma, no scientific assessments of this procedure have been undertaken by Japanese surgeons [7–14]. In 1991, the author [23] reported unexpectedly good results of HPD for advanced carcinoma of the biliary tract involving adjacent vascular structures and intestinal organs, and showed 39.7% of 1-year, 20.4% of 2-year, and 6.8% of 5-year survival rates, and 11.0 months of median survival for all 21 patients surviving HPD, with an acceptable mortality rate of 12.5%.

However, 44 postoperative complications occurred in 19 (79.2%) of the 24 patients undergoing HPD. Some patients with highly advanced carcinoma developed early postoperative hepatic failure attributable to preoperative cholangitis or intraoperative manipulation and died of the disease [24,25]. Recently, fairly good surgical results have also been reported by several Japanese surgeons who applied limited liver resections or extended right hepatic lobectomy in HPD with varying degrees of morbidity and succeeded in reducing mortality by selecting the surgical patients and providing several perioperative managements [26–28]. Therefore, operative indications should be carefully reexamined, taking into consideration the fact that HPD was associated not only with an unexpectedly long and good quality of survival period, but also with unexpected postoperative hepatic failure or early cancer recurrence in some cases.

References

1. Longmire WP Jr, McArthur MS, Bastounis EA, Hiatt J (1973) Carcinoma of the extra-hepatic biliary tract. Ann Surg 178:333–345
2. Fortner JG, Kallum BO, Kim DK (1976) Surgical management of carcinoma of the junction of the main hepatic ducts. Ann Surg 184:68–73.
3. Launois B, Campion JP, Brissot P, Gosselin M (1983) Carcinoma of the hepatic hilus. Surgical management and the case for resection. Arch Surg 190:151–157
4. Evander A, Fredlung P, Hoevels J, Ihse I, Bengmark S (1980) Evaluation of aggressive surgery for carcinoma of the extrahepatic bile ducts. Ann Surg 191:23–29
5. Tsuzuki T, Ogata Y, Iida S, Nakanishi I, Takenaka Y, Yoshii H (1983) Carcinoma of the bifurcation of the hepatic ducts. Arch Surg 118:1147–1151

6. Bengmark S, Ekberg H, Evander A, Klofver-Stahl B, Tranberg KG (1988) Major liver resection for hilar cholangiocarcinoma. Arch Surg 207:120-125

7. Takasaki K, Kobayashi S, Mutoh H, Akimoto S, Tada K, Asado S, Fukushima Y, Yoshikawa E, Imaizumi T, Sato Y, Takada T, Nakamura M, Hanyu F (1980) Our experience (5 cases) of extended right lobectomy combined with pancreatoduodenectomy for carcinoma of the gallbladder (in Japanese). Tan to Sui (Biliary Tract Pancreas) 1:923-932

8. Sugiura Y, Shima S, Yonekawa H, Ogata T (1983) Post-surgical management of hepatopancreatoduodenectomy (in Japanese). Nippon Shokaki Gekagakkai Zasshi (Jpn J Gastroenterol Surg) 15:1631-1635

9. Nakamura S, Hishiki S, Sakaguchi S (1983) Extended radical resection of advanced gallbladder cancer (in Japanese). Nippon Shokaki Gekagakkai Zasshi (Jpn J Gastroenterol Surg) 16:601-606

10. Nimura Y, Hayakawa N, Hasegawa H, Asai M, Kamiya J, Shionoya S (1985) Right hepatic trisegmentectomy with total caudate lobectomy and pancreatoduodenectomy for diffuse carcinoma of the bile duct (in Japanese). Shujutsu (Operation) 39:297-304

11. Nimura Y, Hayakawa N, Kamiya J, Kondo S, Kohno S, Shionoya S (1987) Clinical significance of extended operation for advanced carcinoma of the gallbladder (in Japanese with English abstract). Nippon Geka Gakkai Zasshi (J Jpn Surg Soc) 88:1343-1346

12. Nimura Y, Hayakawa N, Kamiya J, Maeda S, Okamoto K, Shionoya S (1989) Present status and surgical results of operative procedures employing pancreatoduodenectomy (in Japanese). Nippon Shokaki Gekagakkai Zasshi (Jpn J Gastroenterol Surg) 22:2521-2524

13. Sugiura Y, Shima S, Yonekawa H, Yoshizumi Y, Ohtsuka H, Tsuchiya C, Ogata T (1987) Hepatopancreatoduodenectomy for carcinoma of the gallbladder invasive to both the liver and the hepatoduodenal ligament (in Japanese with English abstract). Nippon Geka Gakkai Zasshi (J Jpn Surg Soc) 88:1332-1335

14. Hanyu F, Nakamura M, Yoshikawa T (1988) Hepato-ligamento-pancreatoduodenectomy (in Japanese). Geka Chiryo (Surg Ther) 59:12-21

15. Nagino M, Hayakawa N, Nimura Y, Dohke M, Kitagawa S (1992) Percutaneous transhepatic biliary drainage in patients with malignant biliary obstruction of the hepatic hilus. Hepato-Gastroenterology 39:296-300

16. Nimura Y, Kamiya J, Kondo S, Nagino M, Kanai M (1995) Technique of inserting multiple biliary drains and management. Hepato-Gastroenterology 42:323-331

17. Nimura Y, Shionoya S, Hayakawa N, Kamiya J, Kondo S, Yasui A (1988) Value of percutaneous transhepatic cholangioscopy (PTCS). Surg Endosc 2:213-219

18. Nimura Y, Kamiya J, Hayakawa N, Shionoya S (1989) Cholangioscopic differentiation of biliary strictures and polyps. Endoscopy 21:351-356

19. Nimura Y (1993) Staging of biliary carcinoma: cholangiography and cholangioscopy. Endoscopy 25:76-80

20. Nagino M, Nimura Y, Hayakawa N (1993) Percutaneous transhepatic portal embolization using newly devised catheters: preliminary report. World J Surg 17:250-255

21. Nagino M, Nimura Y, Kamiya J, Kondo S, Uesaka K, Kin Y, Kutsuna Y, Hayakawa N, Yamamoto H (1995) Right or left trisegment portal vein embolization before hepatic trisegmentectomy for hilar bile duct carcinoma. Surgery (St Louis) 117:677-681

22. Nagino M, Nimura Y, Kamiya J, Kondo S, Kanai M (1996) Selective percutaneous transhepatic embolization of the portal vein in preparation for extensive liver resection: the ipsilateral approach. Radiology 200:559-563

23. Nimura Y, Hayakawa N, Kamiya J, Maeda S, Kondo S, Yasui A, Shionoya S (1991) Hepatopancreatoduodenectomy for advanced carcinoma of the biliary tract. Hepato-Gastroenterology 38:170-175

24. Nagino M, Nimura Y, Hayakawa N, Kamiya J, Kondo S, Sasaki R, Hamajima N (1993) Logistic regression and discriminant analyses of hepatic failure after liver resection for carcinoma of the biliary tract. World J Surg 17:250-255

184   Y. Nimura

25. Kanai M, Nimura Y, Kamiya J, Kondo S, Nagino M, Miyachi M, Goto Y (1996) Preoperative intrahepatic segmental cholangitis in patients with advanced carcinoma involving the hepatic hilus. Surgery (St Louis) 119:498–504
26. Tsukada K, Yoshida K, Aono T, Koyama S, Shirai Y, Uchida K, Muto T (1994) Major hepatectomy and pancreatoduodenectomy for advanced carcinoma of the biliary tract. Br J Surg 81:108–110
27. Nakamura S, Nishiyama R, Yokoi Y, Serizawa A, Nishiwaki Y, Konno H, Baba S, Muro H (1994) Hepatopancreatoduodenectomy for advanced gallbladder carcinoma. Arch Surg 129:625–629
28. Miyagawa S, Makuuchi M, Kawasaki S, Hayashi K, Harada H, Kitamura H, Seki H (1996) Outcome of major hepatectomy with pancreatoduodenectomy in advanced biliary malignancies. World J Surg 20:77–80

Hepatoligamentopancreatoduodenectomy in Patients with Advanced Gallbladder Carcinoma

Tatsuya Yoshikawa, Tatsuo Araida, Mitsuji Nakamura,
Tsukasa Azuma, Takehiro Oota, Ken Takasaki, and Fujio Hanyu

Summary. Advanced carcinomas of the gallbladder often involve the hepatoduodenal ligament and have a poor prognosis. Dissection of the hepatoduodenal ligament with preservation of the portal vein and hepatic artery has a high risk of residual tumor and early death. Curative resection in patients with invasion of the hepatoduodenal ligament ideally requires en bloc resection of the entire ligament. F. Hanyu of our department has developed an extended procedure, referred to as hepatoligamentopancreatoduodenectomy (HLPD), for en bloc resection of the right lobe of the liver and head of the pancreas with the hepatoduodenal ligament. This chapter describes the surgical technique of HLPD and outlines the background of its development as well as its indications, long-term outcome, and problems. Curative resection could be performed in all patients using HLPD; however, long-term survival could not be determined and operative mortality was extremely high, thus the clinical significance of HLPD was not established. We concluded that the clinical significance of HLPD for patients with advanced gallbladder carcinoma with hepatoduodenal ligament invasion should be evaluated after the safety of the procedure has been established and the cumulative results of a number of cases have been obtained.

Key words. Advanced gallbladder carcinoma—Hepatoligamentopancreato-duodenectomy—Invasion of the hepatoduodenal ligament—Portal active bypass

Introduction

Advanced carcinomas of the gallbladder often involve the hepatoduodenal ligament and have a very poor prognosis [1,2]. The tumor typically spreads laterally from the neck of the gallbladder to the hepatoduodenal ligament and encompasses the entire ligament. Gallbladder cancer may also spread horizontally toward the hilum of the liver or the head of the pancreas [3]. Dissection of the hepatoduodenal ligament with

Department of Surgery, Institute of Gastroenterology, Tokyo Women's Medical College, Shinjuku-ku, Tokyo 162, Japan.

preservation of the portal vein and hepatic artery therefore has a high risk of residual tumor and early death.

Curative resection in patients with invasion of the hepatoduodenal ligament ideally requires en bloc resection of the entire ligament. In 1986 Hanyu of our department developes an extended procedure, referred to as hepatoligamentopancreatoduodenectomy (HLPD), for en bloc resection of the right lobe of the liver and head of the pancreas with the hepatoduodenal ligament, and successfully performed this procedure for the first time ever in the medical world [4,5]. This chapter describes the surgical technique of HLPD and outlines the background of its development as well as its indications, long-term outcome, and problems.

Background of Development

Invasion of the hepatoduodenal ligament is chiefly responsible for the poor prognosis of patients with gallbladder cancer [1–3]. In the past, ligament invasion was treated by skeletonization with preservation of the major blood vessels, which were resected only in patients with vascular involvement. Thus, in many patients residual cancer cells were evident on histological examination. Patients with hepatoduodenal ligament invasion experienced very poor long-term survival, estimated at only 2.4% at 5 years.

Invasion of the hepatoduodenal ligament in gallbladder carcinoma proceeds from the serosa and envelops the entire ligament. Dissection of the ligament with ablation of involved blood vessels alone carries an extremely high risk of local recurrence from residual cancer cells as well as from intraoperative abdominal seeding of cancer cells. Theoretically, therefore, the hepatoduodenal ligament must be resected en bloc. In patients with evidence of hepatoduodenal ligament invasion, the tumor often spreads deeply on the hepatic side and infiltrates along the intrahepatic portion of Glisson's capsule. On the pancreatic side, the tumor usually spreads below the pancreatic capsule or along the connective tissue surrounding the intrapancreatic bile duct. These characteristics of gallbladder carcinomas require resection of the right lobe of the liver and the head of the pancreas concurrent with en bloc resection of the hepatoduodenal ligament. HLPD, an extended procedure combining extended right lobectomy with resection of the hepatoduodenal ligament and pancreatoduodenectomy, was therefore developed and first performed in 1986 [4,5]. This procedure is also indicated even in extensive carcinomas of the bile duct with remarkable lateral spread.

Indications for HLPD

Based on the characteristics of tumor spread, HLPD is indicated primarily for gallbladder cancer with distinct involvement of the hepatoduodenal ligament. HLPD is indicated for some extensive carcinomas of the bile duct with remarkable lateral extension within the ligament. The possibility of vascular anastomosis and no invasion to the transverse part of the left branch of the portal vein or to the origin of the common hepatic artery are prerequisite to HLPD. However, as is mentioned later, the extremely great extent of surgical invasion and the high rate of operative mortality with HLPD require strict screening of patients. The procedure is contraindicated in patients with persistent jaundice, in those likely to have an inadequate reserve capacity of the residual liver, in elderly patients, and in patients with seriously compromised cardiac, pulmonary, or renal function or serious metabolic diseases such as diabetes mellitus.

Practical Aspects of Surgical Technique

Preoperative Imaging Findings

A 40-year-old woman underwent bilateral percutaneous transhepatic cholangiodramage (PTCD) for obstructive jaundice. Imaging of the bile duct revealed separation of the left and right hepatic ducts by the tumor (Fig. 1). Cholangiography

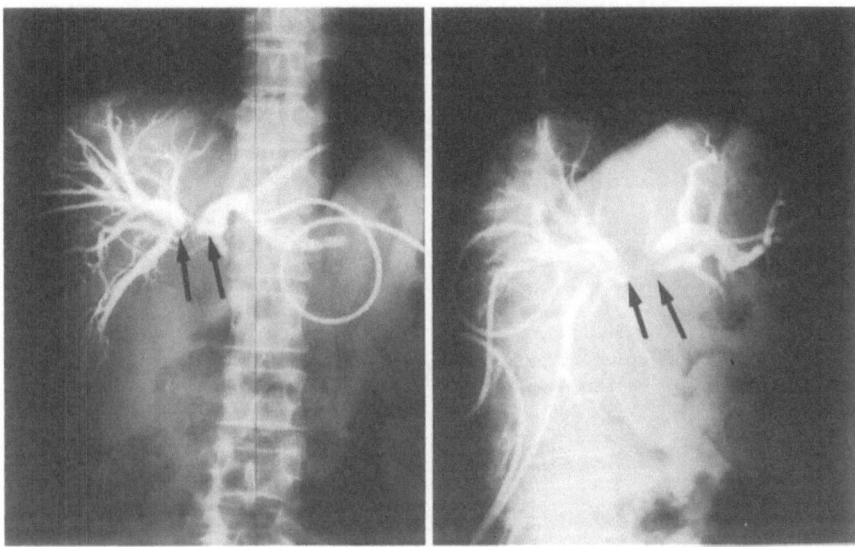

FIG. 1. A 40-year-old woman underwent bilateral percutaneous transhepatic cholangiodrainage (PTCD) for obstructive jaundice. Imaging of the bile duct (cholangiography, *right* and *left*) revealed separation of the left and right hepatic ducts by tumor (*arrows*)

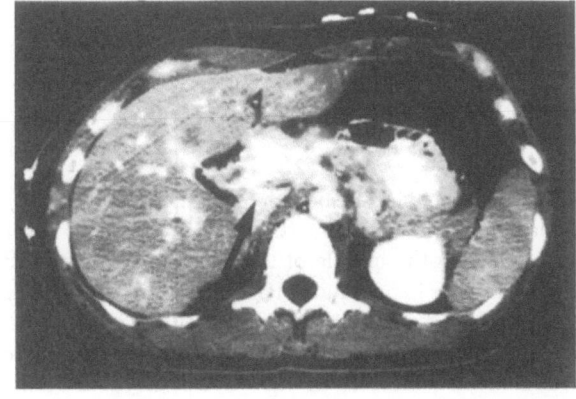

FIG. 2. A computed tomographic scan of this patient showed invasion of the hepatoduodenal ligament from the hilum of the liver to the superior margin of the pancreas

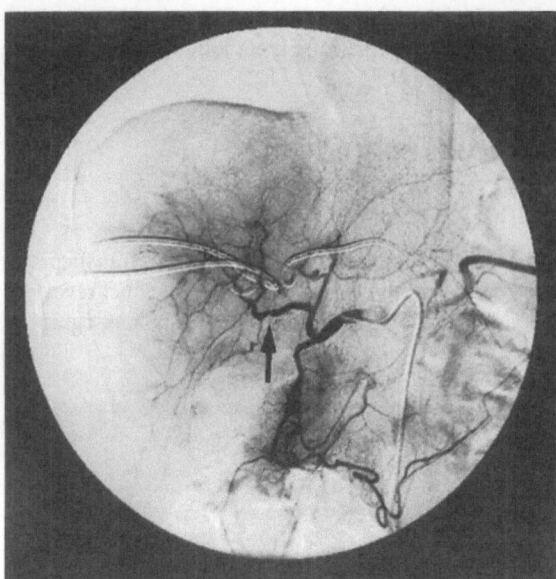

FIG. 3. Encasement of right and left hepatic arteries was seen on selective celiac angiography of the common hepatic artery

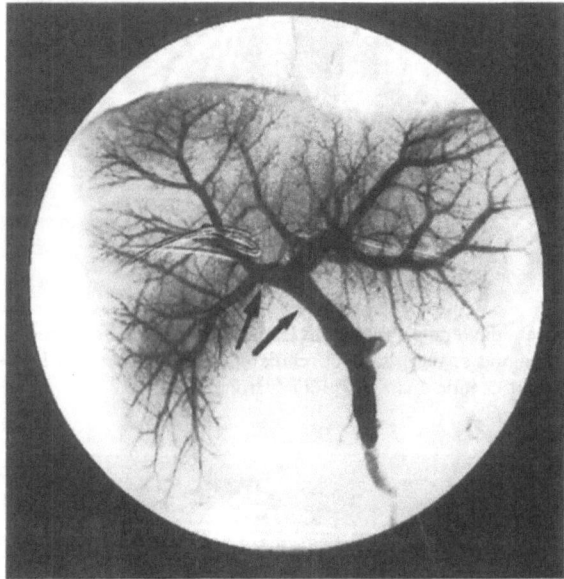

FIG. 4. Percutaneous transhepatic portography revealed encasement from the right side of the main trunk to the anterior and posterior branches of the portal vein

with percutaneous transhepatic cholangiography (PTC) and endoscopic retrograde cholangiopancreatography (ERCP) demonstrated severe stenosis from the hilum of the liver to the middle of the bile duct. A computed tomographic scan showed invasion of the hepatoduodenal ligament from the hilum of the liver to the superior margin of the pancreas (Fig. 2). Encasement of the right and left hepatic arteries was seen on selective angiography (Fig. 3). Percutaneous transhepatic portography revealed encasement from the right side of the main trunk to the anterior and posterior branches of the portal vein (Fig. 4).

Findings at Laparotomy

Laparotomy revealed severe invasion of the hepatoduodenal ligament, which had shrunk. The left branch of the portal vein and the origin of the common hepatic artery showed no signs of invasion. HLPD was therefore indicated.

Kocher's Mobilization and Separation of the Duodenum

First, Kocher's mobilization was performed. The descending aorta was exposed, and mobilization was performed to expose the anterior surface of the abdominal aorta. The metastatic status of periaortic lymph nodes was confirmed. In this patient, there was no evidence of direct invasion to the stomach or duodenal bulb or of perigastric lymph node metastasis. A pancreatoduodenectomy with preservation of the entire stomach and pyloric sphincter (PpPD) was therefore performed to minimize loss of gastrointestinal function. First, the right gastric artery and the right gastroepiploic artery were ligated and divided, and the lymph nodes superior and inferior of the pylorus were dissected prophylactically. Next, the duodenum was divided at 4–5 cm distal portion from the pyloric sphincter (Fig. 5).

Pancreatectomy

The common hepatic artery was exposed at the superior margin of the pancreas, and the lymph nodes were dissected from the common hepatic artery to the trunk of the celiac artery. The gastroduodenal artery was exposed, ligated, and divided. The common hepatic artery was taped and raised, exposing the portal vein. Next, to perform Kocher's mobilization, the superior lobe of the transverse mesocolon was divided, exposing the superior mesenteric vein. This vein was abraded and exposed to the superior margin of the pancreas (Fig. 6). Next, a tunnel was made between the posterior surface of the pancreas and the anterior surface of the portal vein, appearing at the superior and inferior margins of the pancreas, and the side toward the head of the pancreas was ligated with silk suture. The superior and inferior margins on the side toward the body of the pancreas were anchored with stay sutures, and the pancreas was sharply divided immediately superior to the portal vein (Fig. 7). The main pancreatic ducts were confirmed, and a pancreatic duct tube was inserted 2–

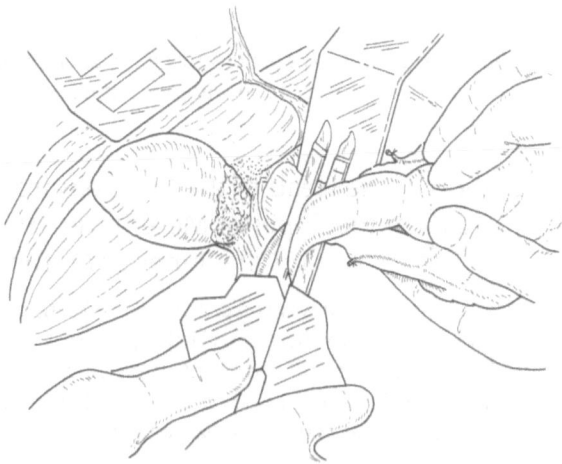

FIG. 5. Division of the duodenum

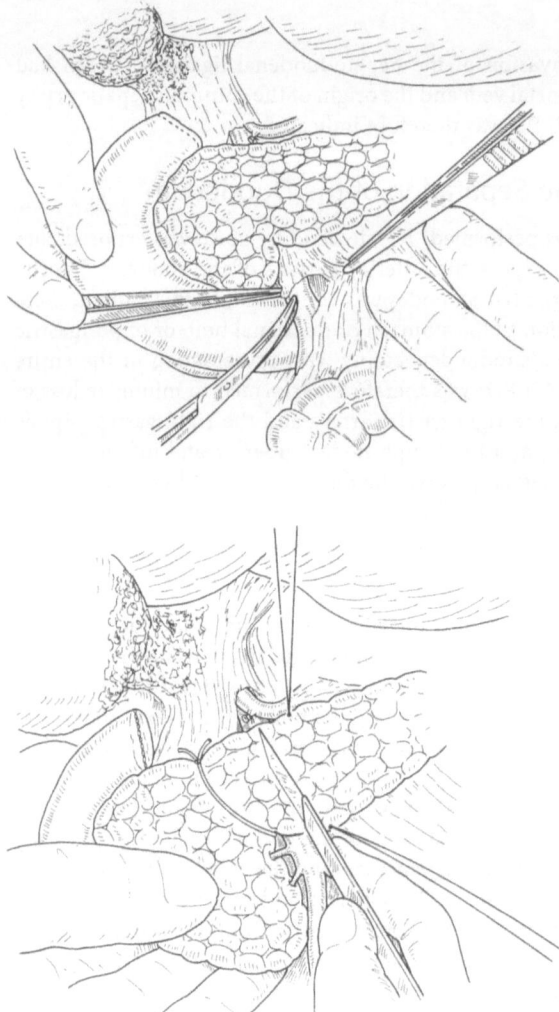

FIG. 6. Exposure of the superior mesenteric vein and the portal vein

FIG. 7. Division of the pancreas at the front surface of the portal vein

3 cm. The smooth outflow of pancreatic juice was confirmed, and the tube and the wall of the pancreatic duct were fixed with one suture with the use of 5–0 polydioxanone suture (PDS®).

Separation of the Head of the Pancreas from the Portal Vein and from the Superior Mesenteric Artery and Vein, and Dissection Around the Superior Mesenteric Artery

The origin of the jejunum was freed from Treitz' ligament, and the duodenum and jejunum were pulled to the right via the posterior part of the superior mesenteric artery. The jejunum was divided about 10 cm from its origin. The superior mesenteric vein and portal vein were each taped and extended anteriorly to the left. Several veins running from the head of the pancreas to the portal vein and superior mesenteric vein were ligated and divided. The portal vein and superior mesenteric vein were then freed from the head of the pancreas. Next, an incision was made in the anterior aspect of the superior mesenteric artery along its long axis to its origin. The first branch of the jejunal arteries and the inferior pancreaticoduodenal artery were successively ligated and divided, as dissection proceeded toward the origin of the superior mesenteric artery (Fig. 8).

Preparation of a Portal Active Bypass

When the head of the pancreas had been freed from its main blood vessels, and before hepatectomy, an active bypass was created between the umbilical part of the portal

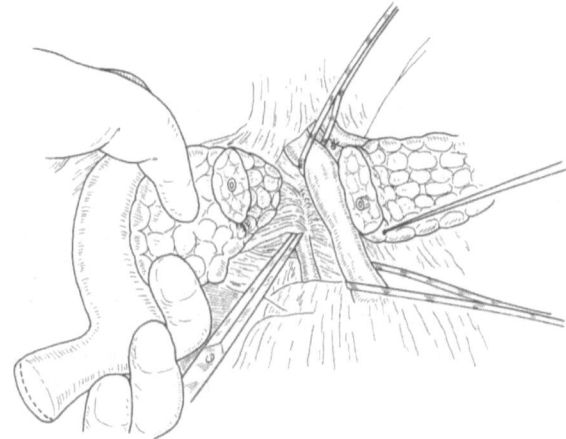

FIG. 8. Dissection of the lymph node along the superior mesenteric artery and division of the pancreas head

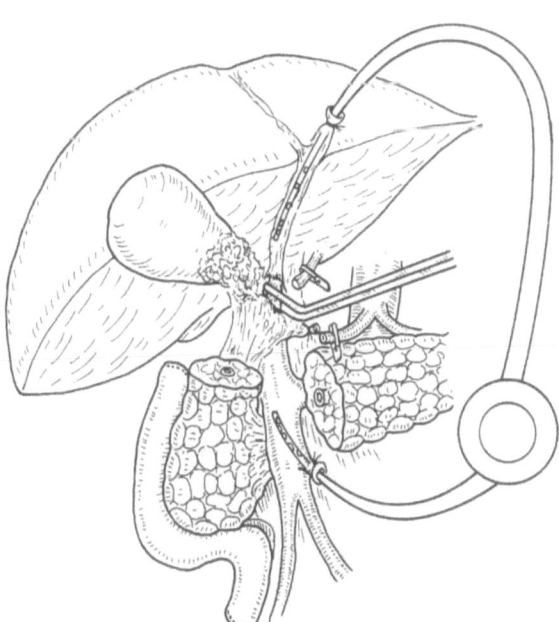

FIG. 9. Interposition of the bypass between the superior mesenteric vein and the umbilical vein

vein and the superior mesenteric vein to prevent hepatic ischemia and reperfusion injury. First, the umbilical part of the portal vein was reopened and cannulated with one end of an Anthron catheter (Toray Industries, Tokyo, Japan). The opposite end of the catheter was inserted into a branch of the superior mesenteric vein (Fig. 9). The main trunk and the left branch of the portal vein were clamped, and the Bio-pump (Medtronic Bio-Medicus, Eden Prairie, MN, USA) was confirmed to operate with no problem. The common hepatic artery and left hepatic artery were clipped with a microclip just before the point of entry into the liver parenchyma and were divided. The main trunk and the left branch of the portal vein were then clamped and divided.

The blood flow rate during bypass was 500 ml/min on average (maximum, 800 ml/min). Respiration was controlled at FiO_2, 80%. The PVO_2 of the portal blood at that time was 80 mm Hg.

Division of the Liver Parenchyma

To divide the liver parenchyma, we use an anterior approach whenever possible to avoid blood flow disturbances caused by turning over the liver. We do not divide the falciform ligament or triangular ligament or turn over the right lobe from the bare area until the liver parenchyma has been completely divided. The short hepatic veins are also manipulated from below the liver.

First, the inferior surface of the liver was pulled caudally. The short hepatic vein arising directly from the inferior vena cava was successively ligated and divided in a caudal direction. This procedure was performed with care to avoid damaging the short hepatic veins (Fig. 10). The Spiegel's region of the caudate lobe was then freed from the inferior vena cava by dividing the inferior vena cava ligament. Before division of the liver parenchyma, the liver was separated as much as possible from the inferior vena cava. Segment 4b was preserved to maintain the reserve capacity of the liver. Glisson's branches were successively ligated and divided in the direction of the medioinferior part of the liver.

Discoloration was seen at the region corresponding to segment 4a. The liver was divided along this discolored area, leaving segment 4b. The liver was divided in a

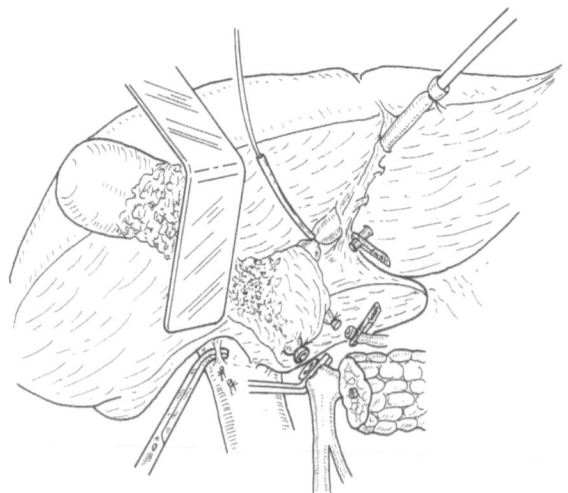

Fig. 10. Ligation of the short hepatic vein

Fig. 11. Resection of the liver
by anterior approach and
resection of the right hepatic
vein

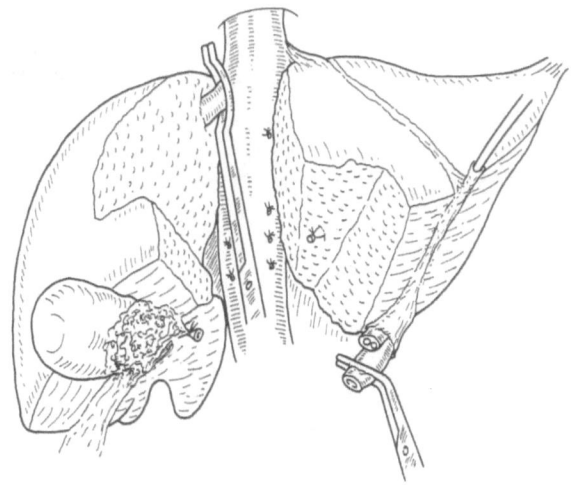

right, transverse direction, starting from the right side of the falciform ligament. Branches of the middle hepatic veins appearing on the cut surface of the liver were ligated and divided. When the middle hepatic veins were reached, the parenchyma on the dorsal side of the middle hepatic veins was freed in the direction of Arantius' duct, while pulling Spiegel's region to the right. The inferior vena cava region of the caudate lobe and Spiegel's region were resected en bloc with the right lobe.

Finally, when the origin of the right hepatic vein was reached, a Glover's forceps was applied and the vein was divided (Fig. 11). The inferior vena cava side was closed with a continuous suture with 4-0 Prolin. After the right lobe was completely separated from the inferior vena cava, the right triangular ligament and the right coronary ligament were divided, and the right lobe was lifted from the retroperitoneum to complete en bloc resection of the right lobe and caudate lobe.

Vascular Reconstruction

The posterior wall of the portal vein was anchored with an introverted suture and the anterior wall with an extroverted suture. The sutures consisted of 4-0 Prolin, placed while washing the lumen with heparinized physiological saline. Adequate intake of growth factors and the avoidance of stenosis are essential in preventing the formation of thrombi (Fig. 12).

The hepatic artery is most often reconstructed with an autologous graft taken from the great saphenous vein. Occasionally, the gastroduodenal artery is inverted and used. In this patient, the lumen was damaged when prostaglanding E_1 was injected into the left hepatic artery. Because the artery could not be reconstructed, the ileocolic artery and the ileocolic vein were anastomosed to achieve partial arterialization of the portal vein.

Periaortic Lymph Node Dissection

After vascular reconstruction was completed, the periaortic lymph nodes were dissected. Periaortic lymph node dissection extended from the left anterior aspect of the

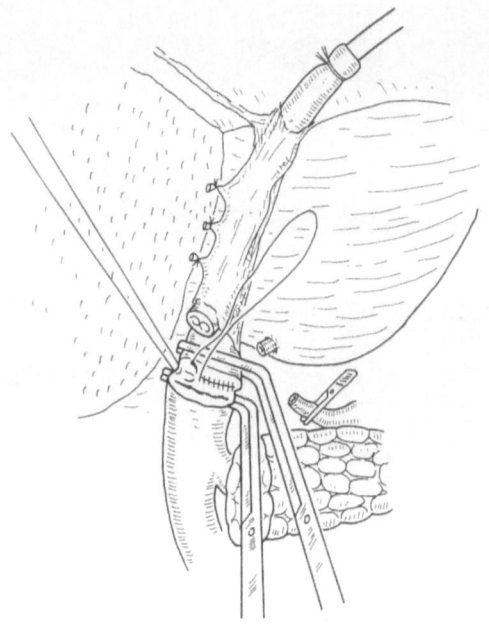

FIG. 12. Reconstruction of the portal vein (end-to-end anastomosis between the main portal vein and the left branch of the portal vein)

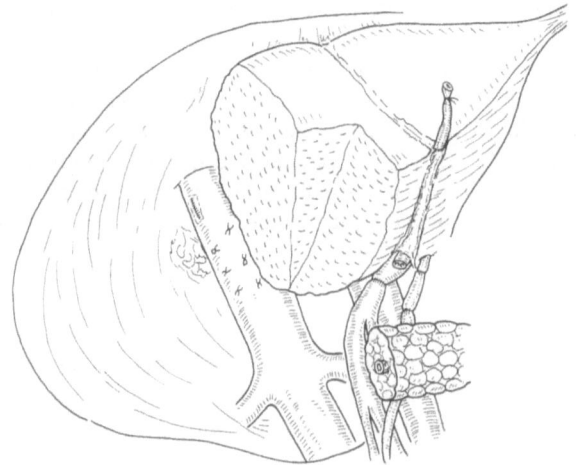

FIG. 13. Dissection of the lymph node along the aorta

aorta superior to the left renal vein and to the left and right anterior aspects of the aorta inferior to the left renal vein (Fig. 13).

Reconstruction

Reconstruction was performed by a modification of Child's method (Fig. 14). For the pancreatojejunostomy, the pancreatic duct and jejunal wall were anastomosed with six sutures with the use of 5-0 PDS. The choledochojejunostomy was made with knotted single-layer suture using 4-0 Opepollix.

FIG. 14. Reconstruction of the
digestive tract with
pancreaticobiliogastro
arrangement

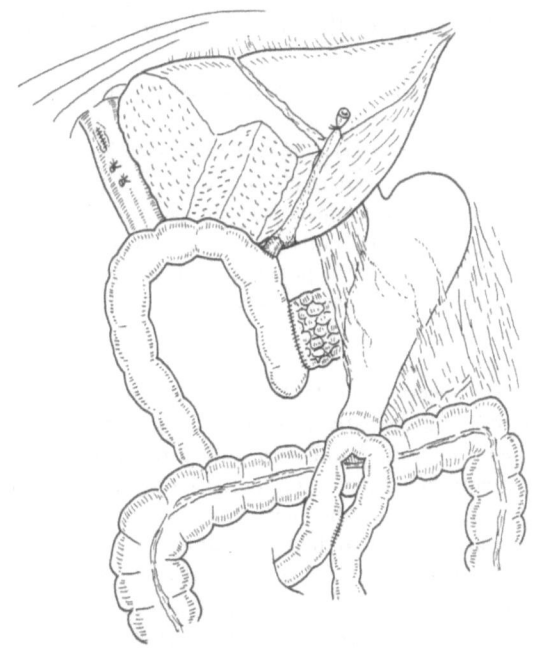

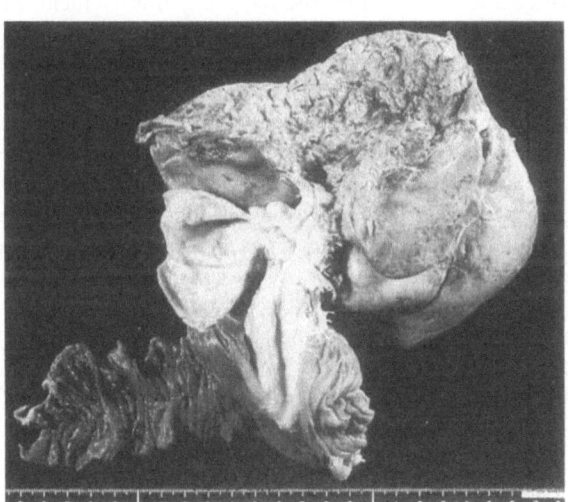

FIG. 15. Resected specimen

Resected Specimen

The main lesion was located in the neck of the gallbladder. There was evidence of
invasion to the liver and severe invasion of the hepatoduodenal ligament (Fig. 15).
Lymph node metastasis was evident around the bile duct, head of the pancreas, and
posterior surface of the common bile duct. The patient died of retroperitoneal recurrence after 1 year.

Results, Problems, and Future Outlook for HLPD

We have performed HLPD in a total of 15 patients, 9 with carcinoma of the gallbladder and 6 with carcinoma of the bile duct. The portal vein was reconstructed by end-to-end anastomosis in 11 patients; an artificial blood vessel was used in 2 patients; and an autologous vein graft was used in 2 patients. Arterial reconstruction was performed by anastomosis with the gastroduodenal artery in 1 patient; an autologous vein graft was used in 3 patients (great saphenous vein); an end-to-end anastomosis was performed in 2 patients; and no reconstruction was performed in 9 patients (accessory hepatic artery, 3 patients; preoperative transcatheter arterial embolization, 2 patients).

Curative resection was possible in all patients. There were seven operative deaths for an operative mortality rate of 47%; all operative deaths were from hepatic failure. In five of these patients, hepatic failure was triggered by postoperative bleeding from the liver stump, portal vein, and gastroduodenal artery, respectively. In the other two patients, hepatic failure was caused by bleeding from the hepatic artery. As for long-term outcome in the eight survivors, six died of cancer within 13 months after the operation, and two died of another cause after 10 months.

The major problem with HLPD is the extremely high rate of operative mortality; improvement of the safety of this procedure is urgently required. The management of hepatic insufficiency and factors that may trigger hepatic insufficiency, such as infection and intraperitoneal bleeding, is essential to improving the prognosis of HLPD. There is a long list of factors requiring improvement, which include the preoperative reduction of jaundice, elimination of biliary tract infections, metabolic hypertrophy of the residual liver by preoperative portal infarction of the lobe scheduled to undergo resection [6], measures to minimize intraoperative bleeding and liver ischemia (for example, by creation of a vascular bypass before resection of blood vessels), improved competence in vascular surgery techniques, reliable intraoperative hemostasis of the liver stump, the appropriate placement of drains to prevent intraperitoneal infection postoperatively, and improved perioperative management.

Whether HLPD will remain as an ultraextended radical procedure depends on the establishment of its safety. At present, however, with no other effective means available for treatment except surgery, it is hoped that HLPD will contribute to improved survival in carcinoma of the gallbladder with invasion of the hepatoduodenal ligament. After establishing its safety, the clinical significance of HLPD should be evaluated on the basis of long-term survival and quality of life.

References

1. Hanyu F, Yoshikawa T, Ryo H (1987) Procedures following to the modes of spread of gallbladder cancer (in Japanese). J Biliary Pancr 8:123–131
2. Yoshikawa T, Hanyu F, Nakamura M, Araida T, Azuma T, Ota T, Toda H (1992) The radical resection for the gallbladder cancer with tumor exposed serosa or more severe infiltration according to its mode of spread (in Japanese). J Biliary Pancr 13:165–172
3. Yoshikawa T (1988) Clinicopathological study on spreading modes of gallbladder cancer (in Japanese). J Jpn Biliary Assoc 2:34–43
4. Hanyu F, Nakamura M, Yoshikawa T (1988) Radical operation for carcinoma of the biliary tract—hepatoligamentopancreatoduodenectomy (in Japanese). Surg Ther 59:12–21

5. Hanyu F, Nakamura M, Yoshikawa T, Azuma T (1989) Extended lobectomy of the liver, total resection of the hepatoduodenal ligament and pancreatoduodenectomy (in Japanese). J Biliary Pancr 10:143–149
6. Hanyu F, Araida T, Yoshikawa T, Nakamura M (1992) Hepato-ligamento-pancreatoduodenectomy (HLPD) for advanced gallbladder carcinoma. In: New frontiers in hepato-biliary-pancreatic surgery. Bangkok, pp 317–321

Pancreatoduodenectomy for Cancer: Technique, Complications, and Results

M. TREDE, B. RUMSTADT, M. SCHWAB, G. SCHWALL, and M. SCHMID

Summary. Between 1972 and 1995, 519 duodenopancreatectomies—459 Whipple procedures and 60 total resections—were performed at the Mannheim Surgical Clinic. The standard resection was the Whipple pancreatoduodenectomy. Overall there were 116 complications, i.e., 22%; 53 of them required relaparotomy and 10 ended fatally. Following 459 Whipple operations, we saw 40 complications at or around the pancreatic anastomosis. This complication carried a mortality of 17%. The overall operative and hospital mortality was 2.5%. The actual 5-year survival rate of 97 patients whose adenocarcinoma of the head of the pancreas was resected by pancreatoduodenectomy more than 5 years ago is 27%. These results were obtained by surgery alone.

Key words. Pancreatic cancer—Pancreatoduodenectomy—Complications—Pylorus-preserving—Survival rate

Introduction

Although the rate of successful surgery has increased steadily and operative mortality has declined all over the world, the overall results of the therapy of pancreatic carcinoma are unsatisfactory as concerns 5-year survival. The diagnosis of early cancer is still left to lucky chance, and the results of adjuvant radio- and chemotherapies are disappointing [1,2]. So far, only surgery offers a realistic chance for definitive cure.

Diagnosis

Today, the diagnosis and staging of pancreatic carcinoma are dominated by the trend toward simplification, as exemplified by the slogan "Less is better" [3]. In 1972, diagnosis of pancreatic carcinoma relied on two steps only: a history and clinical examination of the patient (possibly a barium meal and scintigraphy) and then an exploratory laparotomy. Preoperative staging, as we know it, just did not exist.

Department of General Surgery, University Hospital Mannheim, Klinikum Mannheim, Theodor-Kutzer-Ufer, 68135 Mannheim, Germany.

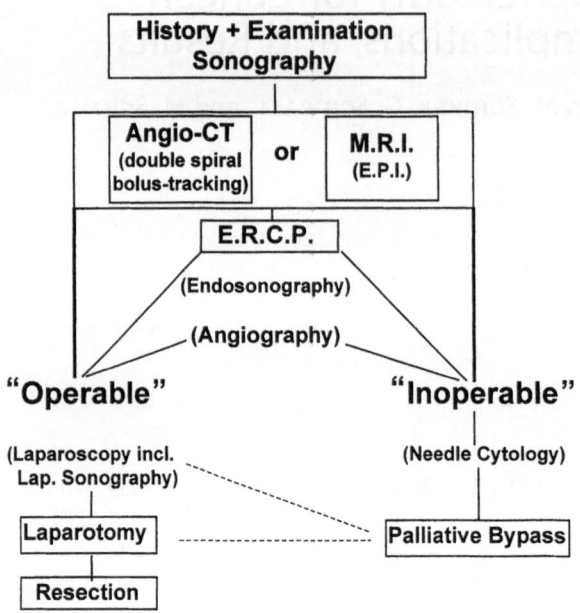

Fig. 1. Diagnosis and staging of pancreatic cancer. *Angio-CT*, angiography–computed tomography; *M.R.I.*, magnetic resonance imaging; *E.P.I.*, echoplanar imaging; *E.R.C.P.*, endoscopic retrograde cholangio pancreato graphy

Today, in the early 1990s, we have a huge armamentarium of more or less invasive endoscopic and imaging modalities at our disposal (Fig. 1), and the temptation is great, particularly in an academic environment, to use them all just because they are there.

Tomorrow, at the end of this century, we may be back to just two steps again: a history and physical examination (which today includes sonography) and echoplanar imaging (EPI). This single noninvasive procedure will probably replace endoscopic retrograde cholangiopancreatography (ERCP), computed tomography (CT) scans, and angiography and pave the way for the final step of laparotomy.

Technique

Confronted with the diagnosis of a resectable pancreatic carcinoma in an operable patient, the surgeon has three basic options: the nihilist, the activist, and the realistic approaches (Fig. 2). The nihilist avoids any resection for pancreatic cancer as being too dangerous and essentially ineffective [4]. The activist is one who would favor regional pancreatectomy on principle, for all patients. The realistic approach attempts resection of every operable pancreatic tumor, tailoring the procedure individually to the site and size of the tumor. Thus, our spectrum reaches from a (rare) local excision (for a papillary adenoma with malignant change in an elderly and frail patient, for instance) to total duodenopancreatectomy with portal vein resection, if that turns out to be necessary [5].

The standard resection is the Whipple pancreatoduodenectomy, which was first successfully performed by Professor Kausch of Berlin in 1909 [6]. From among the numerous technical questions that are worth discussing, four were selected and are presented here:

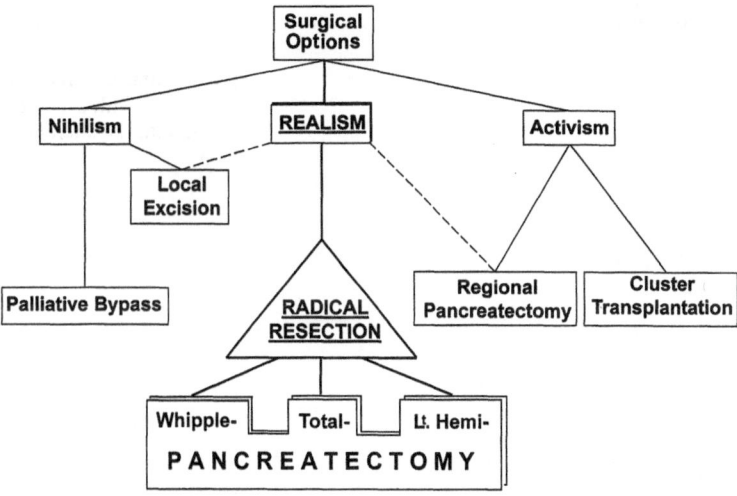

FIG. 2. Surgical options for periampullary and pancreatic carcinoma

TABLE 1. Pancreatoduodenectomy for cancer: pylorus-preserving (PPPD) versus Standard Whipple (SW) procedure

Criterion	Klinken bijl et al. [7]		Zerbi et al. [8]		Patel et al. [9]	
	PPPD	SW	PPPD	SW	PPPD	SW
Operation time (mm)	10	255	370	410	506	508
Blood loss (ml)	1800	2500	590	725	701	799
Body weight (% of preoperative weight at 6 months postoperative)	—	—	92%	89%	96%	92%

1. Standard resection versus pyloric preservation?
2. Anastomosis of the pancreatic remnant with jejunum or stomach?
3. Does extensive lymphadenectomy improve long-term survival?
4. Should the pancreatic or the bile duct be drained or not?

Pylorus-preserving pancreatoduodenectomy (PPPD) has two advantages (one practical, one theoretical) and some drawbacks. The practical advantage consists of some reduction in operating time (because antrectomy is avoided) and possible reduction of blood loss (Table 1) [7,8]. The alleged physiological advantage of preserving the stomach appears theoretical, and in fact the originators of the method at the University of California at Los Angeles (UCLA) admit that "the long-term benefits remain unproven" [9].

As for the disadvantages of PPPD, it is not realistic to overemphasize the possible reduction in radicality, because of course long-term survival is not very good with the standard Whipple either [10]. However, delay in gastric emptying, requiring the nasogastric tube to be left in place for a mean of 14 days (we remove it on the morning following our standard resection), and the high rate of jejunal ulceration (13% has been reported by the Mayo Clinic [11] while in our experience, following more than 450 standard Whipples, it is as low as 2.3%), are two drawbacks that convince us that PPPD is not worthwhile in resections for pancreatic cancer.

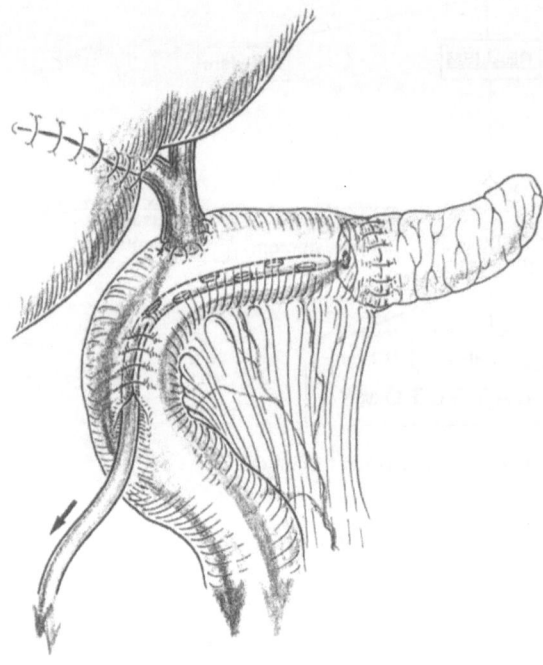

Fig. 3. After pancreatoduodenectomy with a Völker tube
placed into the afferent jejunal
loop

The Johns Hopkins group has demonstrated by a randomized trial [12] that it does not matter whether the pancreatic remnant is anastomosed to the jejunum or to the stomach, provided the anastomosis is performed with meticulous care. Thus, we continue to implement the end-to-end or end-to-side telescopic anastomosis.

The value of extended as compared to standard lymphadenectomy, as suggested by some Japanese studies [13,14], has so far not been confirmed by many Western surgeons. However, extended lymphadenectomy provides for more accurate staging and may be of benefit in cases with small (T1) tumors.

Intraductal drainage seems unnecessary for the bile duct unless this is very narrow. Similarly, we never drain the pancreatic duct because it is either too narrow to accommodate a stent without obstruction or too widely dilated to require one. We do, however, put a Völker tube into the draining jejunal loop (Fig. 3), which helps to decompress it and also serves as a port for the radiological control of both anastomoses in case a leak is suspected.

Complications

Table 2 lists all the surgical complications we have encountered in more than 500 pancreatoduodenectomies (partial and total) during the past 22 years. There were 116 in all, i.e., 22%, of which 53 required relaparotomy and 10 ended fatally. Another 3 deaths were added by purely medical complications, such as myocardial infarction. The most common and most serious complication is leakage from the pancreatic anastomosis. Following 459 Whipple operations, we saw 40 complications at or around the pancreatic anastomosis, i.e., 9% (Table 3); this complication carried a mortality of 17%.

TABLE 2. Surgical complications, relaparotomy, and mortality rates after 519 pancreatectomies[a]

Complication	n	Relaparotomy	Mortality
Pancreatic leak	40	21	7
Abdominal pain	7	4	—
Bleeding			
Gastrointestinal	24	8	2
Operating field	9	9	—
Bile fistula	16	5	—
Mesenteric ischemia	1	—	1
Abscess			
Hepatic	6	2	—
Abdominal	3	2	—
Chylous ascites	8	—	—
Gastric perforation	1	1	—
Jejunal torsion	1	1	—
Totals	116	53	10

[a] Surgical University Clinic, Mannheim, January 10, 1972–January 1, 1995.

TABLE 3. Complications occuring at or around 459 pancreatojejunostomies[a]

Complication	n	Deaths (n)
Anastomotic leak	17	6
Acute pancreatitis	16	1
Pancreatic fistula	7	—
Totals	40	7

[a] Surgical University Clinic, Mannheim, January 10, 1972–January 1, 1995.

TABLE 4. Treatment of 40 postoperative pancreatic complications[a]

Complications	n	Treatment			Deaths (n)
		Conservative	Drainage	Total pancreatectomy	
Anastomotic leak	17	2	6 (2)	9 (4)	6
Acute pancreatitis	16	10 (1)	—	6	1
Pancreatic fistula	7	7	—	—	—
Totals	40	19 (1)	6 (2)	15 (4)	7

The numbers in parentheses are the number of deaths.
[a] Surgical University Clinic, Mannheim, January 10, 1972–January 1, 1995.

Table 4 summarizes the treatment of these 40 complications over the past 22 years. Seven clinically bland pancreatic fistulae dried up spontaneously within 2–3 weeks, and probably there were many more that were never recognized. We saw 16 cases of acute postoperative pancreatitis, with unusual pain and raised amylase levels. Of these, 10 were treated conservatively and only 1 patient died (the first death in our series), because we underestimated the severity of her pancreatitis; she should have undergone relaparotomy with completion pancreatectomy as did the remaining 6 cases.

TABLE 5. The prevention of pancreatic anastomotic leaks

1. Total pancreatectomy
2. Esophagus–stomach pancreatojejunostomy with jejunoplication
3. Pancreatogastrostomy
4. Anastomoses with three separate jejunal loops
5. Ductal drainage
6. Closure of pancreatic remnant
    Ductal ligature
    Ductal occlusion (Ethibloc)
    Oversewing
7. Open drainage of pancreas

TABLE 6. Consecutive pancreatoduodenectomies without an operative mortality

Author	Year	Institution	Resections (n)
Howard [16]	1968	Philadelphia	41
Warren [17]	1973	Lahey Clinic	56
Trede [18]	1991	Mannheim	144
Cameron [19]	1993	Johns Hopkins	145
Warshaw [20]	1995	Massachusetts General Hospital	160

TABLE 7. Early results of pancreatoduodenectomy[a]

Procedure	Patients (n)	Diagnosis		Operative and hospital mortality
		Neoplasm	Pancreatitis	
Whipple operation	459	329 (8)	130 (1)	9
Total pancreatectomy	60	43 (3)	17 (1)	4
Totals	519	372 (11)	147 (2)	13 (2.5%)

[a] Surgical University Clinic, Mannheim, January 10, 1972–January 1, 1995.

The problem with clinically overt pancreatic leaks is to recognize them early enough and then to do a relaparotomy before the patient has become septic. In 6 patients, closure of the jejunal loop, blockage of the pancreatic duct, and placement of an additional irrigation-suction drain was all that could be done; 2 patients died. Completion pancreatectomy performed 9 times as a last resort was successful 5 times; actually, we did a total of 15 completion pancreatectomies, 11 of which were successful [15]. Of course, they key to dealing with these complications is their prevention (Table 5). It does not seem to matter how one handles the pancreatic remnant, whether with jejunoplication, pancreatogastrostomy, three separate loops, drainage, closure, or even leaving the pancreatic duct open, provided one does it with meticulous technique.

Results

Operative mortality has declined all over the world, and indeed there are series of consecutive pancreatoduodenectomies without any mortality at all (Table 6). At the Mannheim Surgical Clinic, we have performed 519 duodenopancreatectomies in the past 22 years, 459 Whipples and 60 total resections (Table 7). Thirteen patients died

Table 8. Long-term survival after Whipple operation for cancer

Author	Institution	Patients (n)	5-year survival rate (%)
Cooperman [21] 1981	Columbia, NY	70	7.1
Lerut [22] 1984	Insel Spital Bern	25	6.0
Jones [23] 1985	Toronto	28	7.0
Grace [24] 1986	UCLA	37	3.0
Tsuchiya [25] 1986	Collected Japanese series (<2 cm)	103	30.3
Conolly [26] 1987	Chicago University	89	3.4
Sarr [27] 1993	Mayo Clinic	104	10.0
Baumel [28] 1994	Collected French series	555	15.0
Fong [29] 1995	Sloan Kettering (>70)	138	21.0
Klempnauer [30] 1995	M.H. Hannover	107	13.8
Yeo [12] 1995	Johns Hopkins	201	21.0
Trede 1996	Mannheim (R_o)	134	27.0

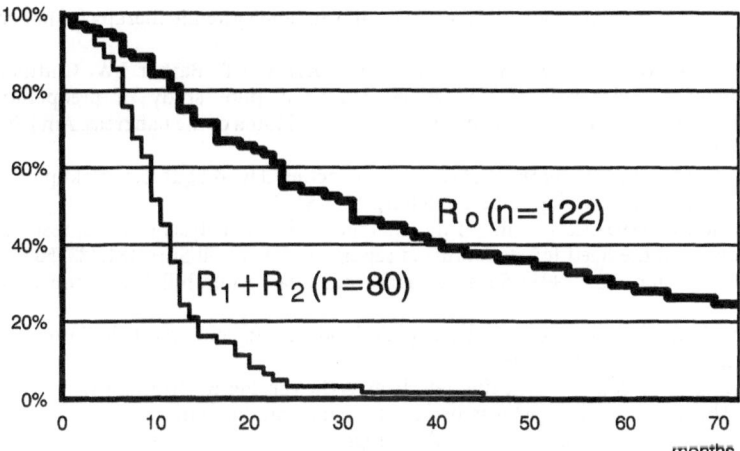

Fig. 4. Actuarial survival rate after pancreatectomy for adenocarcinoma of the pancreas (n = 202), Surgical University Clinic, Mannheim, 1972–1995

Table 9. Actual survival after R_o pancreatectomy for cancer[a]

Operative site	Number of patients operated on before January 1990	Number of 5-year survivors as of January 1995
Head of pancreas	97	26 (27%) (−18)[b]
Papilla	62	36 (58%) (−14)[b]
Choledochus and duodenum	33	7 (21%) (−5)[b]
Totals	192	69 (36%) (−37)[b]

[a] Surgical University Clinic, Mannheim, January 10, 1972–January 1, 1995.
[b] Number who died more than 5 years after surgery.

before being discharged from the hospital, which adds up to an operative and hospital mortality of 2.5%. With the 329 Whipple resections performed for cancer, with 8 deaths the mortality rate is the same, 2.4%. Partly as a result of this lower operative mortality, reports of improved 5-year survival rates are now coming from many countries (Table 8).

The actuarial survival curve of 122 patients whose adenocarcinoma of the pancreas was resectable in an R_0 fashion crosses the 5-year survival line at 26% (Fig. 4). However, actual survival is more important. Table 9 shows that of 97 patients whose adenocarcinoma of the head of the pancreas was resected by pancreatoduodenectomy more than 5 years ago, i.e., before January 1990, 26 were actually still alive 5 years later. This includes all patients of all stages, provided an R_0 resection was possible, and these results were achieved by surgery alone.

References

1. Clark JW, Glicksman A, Wanebo HJ (1995) Adjuvant and systemic therapy for pancreatic cancer. Semin Surg Oncol 11:149–153
2. Hoffmann JP, Weese JL, Solin LJ, Engstrom P, Agarwal P, Barber LW, Guttmann MC, Litwin S, Salazar H, Eisenberg BL (1995) A pilot study of preoperative chemoradiation for patients with localized adenocarcinoma of the pancreas. Am J Surg 169:71–78
3. Olen R, Pickleman J, Freeark RJ (1989) Less is better. The diagnostic workup of the patient with obstructive jaundice. Arch Surg 124:791–795
4. Gudjonsson B (1995) Carcinoma of the pancreas: critical analysis of costs, results of resections, and the need for standardized reporting. J Am Coll Surg 181:483–503
5. Trede M, Carter DC (1993) Surgery of the pancreas. Churchill Livingstone, New York
6. Kausch W (1912) Das Carcinom der Papilla duodeni und seine radikale Entfernung. Beitr Klinisch Chir 78:439–486
7. Klinkenbijl JHG, van der Schelling GP, Hop WCJ, van Pel R, Bruining HA, Jeekel J (1992) The advantages of pylorus-preserving pancreatoduodenectomy in malignant disease of the pancreas and periampullary region. Ann Surg 216:142–145
8. Zerbi A, Balzano G, Patuzzo R, Calori G, Braga M, Di Carlo V (1995) Comparison between pylorus-preserving and Whipple pancreatoduodenectomy. Br J Surg 82:975–979
9. Patel AG, Toyama MT, Kusske AM, Alexander P, Ashley SW, Reber HA (1995) Pylorus-preserving Whipple resection for pancreatic cancer. Is it any better? Arch Surg 130:838–842
10. Carter DC, Trede M, Beger HG, Roder JD, Siewert JR (1994) Hat die Pyloruserhaltung bei der Pankreatoduodenektomie wegen periampullären Karzinoms einen Stellenwert? Langenbecks Arch Chir 379:58–63
11. McAfee MK, van Heerden JA, Adson MA (1989) Is proximal pancreatoduodenectomy with pyloric preservation superior to total pancreatectomy? Surgery (St Louis) 105:347–351
12. Yeo CJ, Cameron JL, Maher MM, Sauter PK, Zahurak ML, Talamini MA, Lillemoe KD, Pitt HA (1995) A prospective randomized trial of pancreaticogastrostomy versus pancreaticojejunostomy after pancreaticoduodenectomy. Ann Surg 222:580–592
13. Ishikawa O, Ohhigashi H, Sasaki Y, Kabuto F, Fukuda I, Furukawa H, Imaoka S, Iwanaga T (1988) Practical usefulness of lymphatic and connective tissue clearance for the carcinoma of the pancreatic head. Ann Surg 208:215–220
14. Satake K, Nishiwaki H, Yokomatsu H, Kawazoe Y, Kim K, Haku A, Umeyama K, Miyazaki I (1992) Surgical curability and prognosis for standard versus extended resection for T1 carcinoma of the pancreas. Surg Gynecol Obstet 175:259–265

15. Farley DR, Schwall G, Trede M (1996) Completion pancreatectomy for surgical complications after pancreaticoduodenectomy: experience of the Mannheim Surgical Clinic 1972–1994. Br J Surg 83:176–179
16. Howard JM (1968) Pancreatico-duodenectomy: forty-one consecutive Whipple resections without an operative mortality. Ann Surg 168:629–640
17. Warren KW (1973) Current concepts in management of periampullary carcinoma. Am Surg 39:667–672
18. Trede M, Schwall G, Saeger HD (1990) Survival after pancreatoduodenectomy. 118 consecutive resections without an operative mortality. Ann Surg 211:447–458
19. Cameron JL, Pitt HA, Yeo CJ, Lillemoe KD, Kaufman HS, Coleman J (1993) One hundred and forty-five consecutive pancreaticoduodenectomies without mortality. Ann Surg 217:430–438
20. Fernandez-del Castillo C, Rattner DW, Warshaw AL (1995) Standards for pancreatic resection in the 1990s. Arch Surg 130:295–300
21. Cooperman AM (1981) Cancer of the pancreas: a dilemma in treatment. Surg Clin North Am 61:107–115
22. Lerut JP, Gianello PR, Otte JB, Kestens PJ (1984) Pancreaticoduodenal resection. Surgical experience and evaluation of risk factors in 103 patients. Ann Surg 199:432–437
23. Jones BA, Langer B, Taylor BR, Girotti M (1985) Periampullary tumors: which ones should be resected? Am J Surg 149:46–52
24. Grace PA, Pitt HA, Tompkins RK, DenBesten L, Longmire Jr WP (1986) Decreased morbidity and mortality after pancreatoduodenectomy. Am J Surg 151:141–149
25. Tsuchiya R, Tomioka T, Izawa K, Noda T, Yamamoto K, Tsunoda T (1986) Collective review of small carcinomas of the pancreas. Ann Surg 203:77–81
26. Conolly MM, Dawson PJ, Michelassi F, Moossa AR, Lowenstein F (1987) Survival in 1001 patients with carcinoma of the pancreas. Ann Surg 206:366–371
27. Sarr MG, Behrns KE, van Heerden JA (1993) Total pancreatectomy. An objective analysis of ist use in pancreatic cancer. Hepatogastroenterology 40:418–421
28. Baumel H, Huguier M, Manderscheid JC, Fabre JM, Houry S, Fagot H (1994) Results of resection for cancer of the exocrine pancreas: a study from the French Association of Surgery. Br J Surg 81:102–107
29. Fong Y, Blumgart LH, Fortner J, Brennan MF (1995) Pancreatic or liver resection for malignancy is safe and effective for the elderly. Ann Surg 222:426–437
30. Klempnauer J, Ridder GJ, Bektas H, Pichlmayr R (1996) Extended resections of ductal pancreatic cancer—impact on operative risk and prognosis. Oncology 53:47–53

Studies of Surgical Resection and Intraoperative Radiotherapy in Carcinoma of the Pancreas

WILLIAM F. SINDELAR

Introduction

Carcinoma of the pancreas occurs with a relatively low incidence of 9 per 100 000 in the United States; however, it is the fourth leading cause overall of cancer mortality [1]. Gudjonsson [2] found that of 22 319 patients collected from 85 published series from 1949 to 1986, only 0.4% were resected and lived at least 5 years following diagnosis. The current relative 5-year survival rate for the disease is less than 5% [2].

The dismal overall prospects for survival in patients with pancreatic cancer result from three major factors. First, the natural history of pancreatic cancer often involves the early dissemination of malignant cells, frequently during the preclinical phase of the disease. The second factor associated with poor prognosis in pancreatic cancer relates to the lack of sufficiently sensitive screening and diagnostic techniques to identify truly localized disease at the early stages, which are the most likely to be cured. The third factor related to poor survival is the paucity of effective therapeutic agents for advanced-stage disease, which accounts for the extent of malignancy in at least 70%–80% of all patients at the time of presentation [1,3].

Treatment Methods and Results

Surgical resection currently is the only therapeutic modality capable of curing pancreatic cancer, although long-term survival is observed only in small numbers of patients. In a literature review of 2398 resected patients, Gudjonsson [2] found only 92 individuals (3.8%) who survived 5 years or longer. In certain series of highly selected patients undergoing pancreatic resection, 5-year survival rates at high as 18%–25% have been recently reported [4–6]. In part, the increments in long-term survival have been attributed to declining morbidity and mortality following pancreatic resection in the last decade [7–9].

Department of Surgery, Good Samaritan Hospital, Baltimore, MD 21239-2995, U.S.A.

When potentially complete resections are performed in patients with carcinoma of the pancreas, local recurrences are common, observed in at least 50% of resected patients [10]. The observation of local recurrence as the initial site of disease relapse in many resected patients suggests that improvements in the treatment of local disease could provide therapeutic benefit. Extended resections have been described and are currently utilized at some centers [11,12], but local failures still occur following the most aggressive surgical extirpations [13]. Radiation therapy, widely used to promote the local control of a variety of malignancies, is frequently utilized in the treatment of advanced cancers of the pancreas [14]. Radiation therapy has been used as an adjunct to surgical resection, and combined with 5-fluorouracil chemotherapy has been demonstrated to improve the survival of resected patients compared to surgery alone [15]. However, the toxicity of external beam radiotherapy to the upper abdomen is considerable, and the high dosage of radiation necessary to control residual disease following resection is often poorly tolerated.

Intraoperative Radiotherapy

Intraoperative radiotherapy (IORT) involves the administration of large single doses of radiation during operative procedures directly to surgically exposed tissues. IORT offers the opportunity to deliver high doses of radiation to areas of neoplastic involvement while simultaneously minimizing the risk of radiation toxicity by limiting the dose to surrounding radiosensitive normal tissues, which may be physically shielded or displaced from the radiation treatment volume. IORT was explored in various malignancies during the 1970s in Japan, with reports of benefit in both disease control and survival in selected patients with various types of malignancies [14,16,17].

Several early clinical trials investigated IORT as a potential treatment modality in pancreatic cancer. An early pilot series was reported by Goldson [18] in which 19 patients demonstrated the feasibility of defining IORT in pancreatic cancer. A larger Japanese experience of 108 patients with pancreatic cancer demonstrated a median survival of 6 months in patients with advanced disease [19]. The Massachusetts General Hospital (MGH) accumulated a series of 16 patients with unresectable pancreatic cancer treated with IORT in combination with external beam radiotherapy (EBRT). These patients had an encouraging median survival of 18 months [20]. Further experience in treating selected patients with IORT at the MGH suggested a median survival of 17 months, considerably longer than that expected from conventional therapies for pancreatic carcinoma [21]. Large early experiences with IORT in unresectable pancreatic cancer were also accumulated at the Mayo Clinic, where the median survival was 11 months for 44 patients who had unresectable pancreatic cancers without distant metastases [22]. Disease progression was clinically documented in 71% of treated patients, although only 7% were considered to have progressed within the IORT field. The Radiation Therapy Oncology Group (RTOG) conducted a multi-institutional phase I–II trial of IORT in locally advanced pancreatic carcinoma [23]. Patients received IORT at the time of palliative biliary and gastric surgical bypass. Postoperative EBRT was delivered concomitantly with 5-fluorouracil chemotherapy. The median survival of 51 patients who received IORT according to protocol was 9 months. The RTOG study suggested little impact of IORT upon survival, although local tumor progression appeared to be controllable with little overall radiation-related toxicity.

Intraoperative Radiotherapy
Combined with Pancreatic Resection

The feasibility of the use of IORT in combination with pancreatic resection for cancer was demonstrated by 1983 at the National Cancer Institute (NCI) [24], where a patient with advanced cancer was reported to be disease–free for more than 19 months following extended pancreatectomy with portal vein resection and intraoperative radiotherapy delivered to the resection bed and regional nodal basins. Because of the technical complexity of delivering IORT in combination with extensive pancreatic surgery, relatively few institutions accumulated a significant experience with IORT as a adjunct to pancreatectomy.

The use of IORT with pancreatic resection was explored early at Kyoto University [25,26]. Twenty-three patients underwent potentially curative resection of pancreatic cancers, with IORT (25–30 Gy) delivered to the resection bed. Additionally, conventional EBRT was given pre- or postoperatively to most patients (total EBRT dose, 60–70 Gy). The 5-year survival was 19% for patients receiving IORT. Eighteen patients who had resections that were considered noncurative because of disease extension or nodal involvement received IORT and EBRT. The noncuratively resected patients receiving IORT had a median survival of 14 months, significantly greater than the 4-month median survival of a comparative series of noncuratively resected patients who received no radiotherapy.

Hiraoka and colleagues [27] at Kumamoto University resected 12 pancreatic cancer patients and administered adjunctive IORT (30 Gy), comparing the clinical results with 12 patients undergoing similar resections without radiotherapy. Although there were 4 treatment-related deaths in the series, no deaths occurred among patients receiving IORT. At 12 months, 50% of IORT and 25% of resection-alone patients were alive. In a subsequent report, Hiraoka [28] treated 16 patients with extended pancreatectomy, including wide nodal dissection and portal vein resection, and delivered IORT (30 Gy) to the resection bed. Nine patients underwent extended pancreatectomy alone. At 5 years, 29% of IORT patients were alive, compared to none of the non-IORT patients.

A comparative study of IORT in patients with resectable pancreatic cancer was reported from the University of Milan by Zerbi et al. [29]. Ninety patients underwent pancreaticoduodenectomy between 1985 and 1993. IORT (13–20 Gy) was delivered to the tumor bed in 43 patients, and no IORT was given to 47 patients. No postoperative adjunctive radiotherapy or chemotherapy was administered. Tumor size, adequacy of resection, morbidity, and mortality were similar between IORT and non-IORT patients. IORT significantly improved the median time to relapse (13 months for IORT patients, 8 months for surgery-alone patients) and the local control rate (27% local recurrence for IORT patients, 57% for surgery-alone patients). At 1 year, the overall survival was higher in IORT patients (71%) compared to surgery alone (49%). Similarly, higher survivals at 2 years were observed in IORT patients (24%) compared to non-IORT patients (16%). The observed survival differences were not statistically significant because of the small patient numbers.

A prospectively randomized controlled clinical trial of IORT in resectable pancreatic cancer was performed at NCI. Twenty-four patients with completely resected adenocarcinoma of the pancreatic head were randomized to receive IORT (20 Gy) to the resection bed or to receive standard treatment (standard control therapy was defined as 45–55 Gy postoperative EBRT for patients with extrapancreatic extension or nodal disease; control patients with disease confined within the pancreatic capsule received surgery alone, without postoperative EBRT). Nineteen patients had locally advanced disease, which would be considered unresectable by conventional criteria, and underwent extensive extirpative surgery. The overall perioperative mortality was 27% and overall morbidity was 71%. Mortality and morbidity did not differ statistically between IORT and control groups. Median survival of IORT patients was 18 months, compared to 12 months for control patients. Local recurrences occurred in all of 12 control patients (100%) but only in 4 of 12 IORT patients (33%). One IORT patient remains alive without evidence of disease more than 10 years following therapy at the NCI. Because of small patient numbers, statistically significant survival differences were not reached between IORT and control groups.

Conclusions

Available studies indicate that the combination of IORT with pancreatic resection is feasible and does not lead to substantially increased morbidity and mortality compared to surgical resection alone. At present, IORT must be considered an experimental treatment. IORT permits higher doses of radiation to be delivered, at least in intraabdominal sites, than conventional fractionated radiotherapeutic techniques, with acceptable toxicity to most normal tissues. The higher total dose seems to enhance local control rates in pancreatic carcinoma after resection with IORT, as compared to conventional surgical treatment alone. Although major improvements in survival have not been seen in most reports of IORT used adjunctively to pancreatic resection, it seems reasonable to speculate that the enhanced local control provided by IORT may have an important potential survival benefit. It is likely that the enhancement of survival provided by improved local control may become more apparent when effective systemic therapeutic adjuncts are discovered that reduce the incidence of widespread metastases, the usual clinical finding of pancreatic cancer late in its course.

In institutions with the capability to deliver IORT, intraoperative irradiation should be considered routinely in patients with locally advanced pancreatic carcinomas that appear technically possible to resect. Alternatively in centers without the capability to deliver IORT, referral of patients to centers with IORT facilities should be contemplated. The application of IORT in such patients should be performed in the context of approved trials designed to evaluate the efficacy and toxicity of IORT in specific clinical situations. The referral and inclusion of patients with pancreatic malignancies will be important in the final assessment of IORT in cancer treatment.

References

1. Warshaw AL, Fernandez-Del Castellio C (1992) Pancreatic carcinoma. N Engl J Med 326:455–465
2. Gudjonsson B (1987) Cancer of the pancreas: 50 years of surgery. Cancer (Phila) 60:2284–2303
3. Warshaw AL, Swanson RS (1988) Pancreatic cancer in 1988: possibilities and probabilities. Ann Surg 208:541–553
4. Crist DW, Sitzmann JV, Cameron JL (1987) Improved hospital morbidity, mortality, and survival after the Whipple procedure. Ann Surg 206:358–368

5. Trede M, Schwall G, Saefer H-D (1990) Survival after pancreatoduodenectomy. Ann Surg 211:447–458
6. Cameron JL, Crist DW, Sitzmann JV, et al (1991) Factors influencing survival after pancreaticoduodenectomy for pancreatic cancer. Am J Surg 161:120–125
7. Grace PA, Pitt HA, Tompkins RK (1986) Decreased morbidity and mortality after pancreatoduodenectomy. Am J Surg 151:141–149
8. Pellegrini CA, Heck CF, Raper S, et al (1989) An analysis of the reduced morbidity and mortality rates for pancreaticoduodenectomy. Arch Surg 124:778–781
9. Cameron JL, Pitt HA, Yeo CJ, et al (1993) One hundred and forty-five consecutive pancreaticoduodenectomies without mortality. Ann Surg 217:430–438
10. Tepper J, Nardi G, Suit HD (1978) Carcinoma of the pancreas: review of the MGH experience from 1963 to 1973. Analysis of surgical failure and implications for radiation therapy. Cancer (Phila) 37:1519–1524
11. Fortner JG (1973) Regional resection of the pancreas: a new surgical approach. Surgery (St Louis) 73:307–320
12. Fortner JG (1984) Regional pancreatectomy for cancer of the pancreas, ampulla, and other related sites. Tumor staging and results. Ann Surg 199:418–425
13. Sindelar WF (1989) Clinical experience with regional pancreatectomy for adenocarcinoma of the pancreas. Arch Surg 124:127–132
14. Johnstone PAS, Sindelar WF, Kinsella TJ (1994) Experimental and clinical studies of intraoperative radiation therapy. Curr Probl Cancer 18:249–292
15. Kalser MH, Ellenberg SS (1985) Pancreatic cancer: adjuvant combined radiation and chemotherapy following curative resection. Arch Surg 120:899–903
16. Abe M, Yabumoto E, Takahashi M, et al (1974) Intraoperative radiotherapy of gastric cancer. Cancer (Phila) 34:2034–2041
17. Abe M, Takahashi M, Yabumoto E, et al (1980) Clinical experiences with intraoperative radiotherapy of locally advanced cancers. Cancer (Phila) 45:40–48
18. Goldson AL (1978) Preliminary clinical experience with intraoperative radiotherapy. J Natl Med Assoc 70:493–495
19. Abe M, Takahashi M, Yabumoto E, et al (1975) Techniques, indications and results of intraoperative radiotherapy of advanced cancers. Radiology 116:693–702
20. Wood W, Shipley WU, Gunderson LL, et al (1982) Intraoperative irradiation for unresectable pancreatic carcinoma. Cancer (Phila) 49:1272–1275
21. Shipley WU, Wood WC, Tepper JC, et al (1984) Intraoperative electron beam irradiation for patients with unresectable pancreatic carcinoma. Ann Surg 200:289–296
22. Gunderson LL, Martin JK, Kvols LK, et al (1987) Intraoperative and external beam irradiation ± 5-FU for locally advanced pancreatic cancer. Int J Radiat Oncol Biol Phys 13:319–329
23. Tepper JE, Noyes D, Krall JM, et al (1991) Intraoperative radiation therapy of pancreatic carcinoma. A report of RTOG-8505. In: Abe M, Takahashi M (eds) Intraoperative radiation therapy. Proceedings of the third international symposium on intraoperative radiation therapy. Pergamon, New York, pp 231–233
24. Sindelar WF, Kinsella T, Tepper J, et al (1983) Experimental and clinical studies with intraoperative radiotherapy. Surg Gynecol Obstet 157:205–219
25. Manabe T, Shibamoto Y, Ono K, et al (1991) Combined modality treatment for cancer of the pancreas: intraoperative and external radiotherapies. In: Abe M, Takahashi M (eds) Intraoperative radiation therapy. Proceedings of the third international symposium on intraoperative radiation therapy. Pergamon, New York, pp 246–248
26. Manabe T, Baba N, Ono K, et al (1991) Radical pancreatectomy with intraoperative radiation therapy for pancreatic head cancer. In: Abe M, Takahashi M (eds) Intraoperative radiation therapy. Proceedings of the third international symposium on intraoperative radiation therapy. Pergamon, New York, pp 249–250
27. Hiraoka T, Watanabe E, Mochinaga M, et al (1984) Intraoperative irradiation combined with radical resection for cancer of the head of the pancreas. World J Surg 8:766–769

28. Hiraoka T (1990) Extended radical resection of cancer of the pancreas with intraoperative radiotherapy. Ballière's Clin Gastroenterol 4:985–993
29. Zerbi A, Fossati V, Parolini D (1994) Intraoperative radiation therapy adjuvant to resection in the treatment of pancreatic cancer. Cancer (Phila) 73:2930–2935

Resection of the Superior Mesenteric–Portal Vein Confluence During Pancreaticoduodenectomy

Douglas B. Evans, Jeffrey E. Lee, and Peter W.T. Pisters

Summary. The current management of patients with pancreatic cancer at our institution involves: (1) a selective approach to the use of laparotomy based on accurate preoperative radiographic imaging techniques and the availability of reliable minimally invasive techniques for biliary decompression, (2) the use of multimodality therapy in all patients with localized, potentially resectable disease, and (3) a standardized approach to surgery and perioperative patient management. The goals of this approach are to maximize length and quality of patient survival while minimizing treatment-related toxicity and limiting the social and economic impact of complicated, multimodality therapy. This chapter focuses on our technique for resection and reconstruction of the superior mesenteric–portal vein (SMPV) confluence at the time of pancreaticoduodenectomy. Our data suggest that tumors invading the SMPV confluence are not associated with histologic parameters suggesting a poor prognosis, and patients who undergo venous resection have a survival similar to patients who undergo standard pancreaticoduodenectomy. Tumor invasion of the SMPV confluence is a function of tumor location rather than an indicator of aggressive tumor biology.

Key words. Pancreatic cancer—Pancreaticoduodenectomy—Superior mesenteric vein

Introduction

The first resection and anastomosis of the superior mesenteric vein (SMV) as part of pancreaticoduodenectomy was reported by Moore et al. from the University of Minnesota in 1951 [1]. The resection was prompted by their finding of tumor involvement of the SMV after gastric and pancreatic transection:

"An exploratory laparotomy May 25, 1950, was done . . . the superior mesenteric vessels and the portal veins were not thought to be involved . . . the pancreas was cut across . . . further dissection revealed the tumor to be firmly attached to the lateral wall of the superior mesenteric vein

Department of Surgical Oncology, The University of Texas M.D. Anderson Cancer Center, Houston, TX 77030, U.S.A.

for a distance of 2 cm. At this point it was decided to remove the vein wall involved with tumor . . . ."

As illustrated in this case, tumor involvement of the SMV or superior mesenteric-portal vein (SMPV) confluence may not be apparent to the surgeon until after gastric and pancreatic transection, a point in the operation when nonresectional procedures are no longer an option. Tumor invasion of the lateral wall of the SMV is the most frequent unexpected finding at the time of pancreaticoduodenectomy [2]. In contrast to tumor involvement of the superior mesenteric artery (SMA), tumor invasion of the SMV can occur in the absence of extensive retroperitoneal invasion and therefore may represent the only barrier to the performance of a negative-margin pancreaticoduodenectomy [3].

The Need for Accurate Preoperative Radiographic Imaging

At the time of surgical exploration for pancreatic head cancer, a Kocher maneuver is the first procedure performed to assess the relationship of the tumor to the SMA by palpation (Fig. 1). This maneuver has proved to be an insensitive method of evaluating this vital tumor-vessel relationship as demonstrated by the high incidence of positive-margin resections recently reported [4]. The close proximity of adenocarcinomas of the pancreatic head to the SMA makes assessment of this vital tumor–vessel relationship (by palpation) an unrealistic expectation; the performance of this maneuver as an assessment of resectability is a vestige of our surgical past and is of only historical value. Direct intraoperative assessment of the extent of retroperitoneal tumor growth in relation to the SMA origin is not possible until the final step in tumor resection, after gastric and pancreatic transection, when the surgeon is committed to resection even if all the tumor cannot be safely removed. Tumor in-

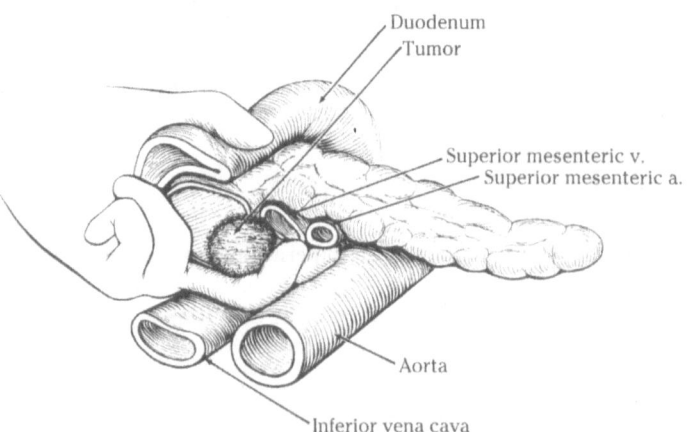

FIG. 1. Illustration of intraoperative palpation (surgeon's left hand) of the relationship of the tumor to the mesenteric vessels at the time of the Kocher maneuver. The surgeon attempts to palpate the relationship of the tumor to the superior mesenteric artery. This technique does not provide the accuracy necessary to assess this vital tumor–vessel relationship. (From [2], with permission)

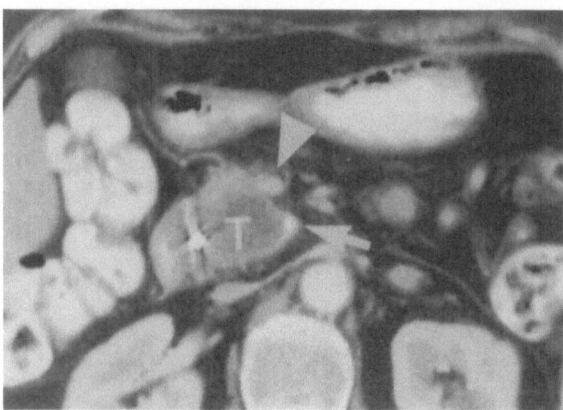

FIG. 2. Computed tomographic scan performed at 3-mm section thickness demonstrating a locally advanced tumor (*T*) of the pancreatic head involving both the superior mesenteric artery (*arrow*) and the superior mesenteric vein (*arrowhead*). A biliary stent is in the intrapancreatic portion of the common bile duct

volvement of the proximal SMA or celiac axis usually includes extensive involvement of the mesenteric neural plexus, rendering radical resections not only technically difficult but oncologically unsound because of the frequent finding of margin positivity. Patients who undergo pancreaticoduodenectomy and are found to have a positive resection margin have a median survival of less than 12 months, no different than patients with locally advanced disease treated with palliative chemoradiation without surgery [4–7].

Work from our institution has demonstrated the value of thin-section, contrast-enhanced computed tomography (CT) in increasing resectability rates, largely by defining the anatomy of the tumor in relation to the proximal SMA [8]. A tumor is deemed unresectable when there is clear evidence on CT scans of encasement of the SMA or celiac axis or occlusion of the SMPV confluence (Fig. 2). The accuracy of CT in predicting unresectability is well established [9–10]. Therefore, the majority of patients with locally advanced, unresectable disease can be spared needless laparotomy; biliary decompression, when necessary, can be performed using endoscopic, percutaneous, or laparoscopic methods.

The second intraoperative maneuver performed to assess local tumor resectability is to develop a plane of dissection between the anterior surface of the SMPV confluence and the posterior surface of the neck of the pancreas (Fig. 3); tumor encasement of this region, in the opinion of most surgeons, precludes resection. However, the rationale for this maneuver early in the operation is also unclear as tumors of the pancreatic head or uncinate process are prone to invade the lateral or posterior wall of the SMPV confluence; the anterior wall is rarely involved in the absence of encasement of the celiac axis or SMA orgin (as seen in locally advanced tumors of the pancreatic neck or body). The relationship of a pancreatic head tumor to the lateral and posterior walls of the SMPV confluence (and the SMA) can be directly inspected only after gastric and pancreatic transection. The loss of the normal fat plane between the tumor and the SMV (Fig. 4) should alert the surgeon preoperatively to the potential for direct tumor invasion of the vessel wall. If the

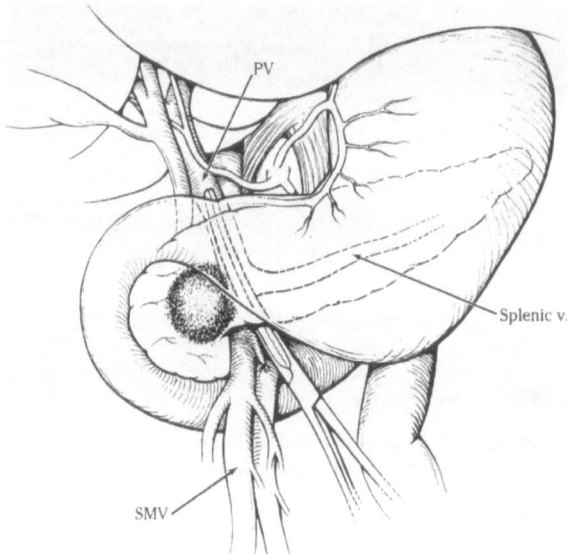

FIG. 3. Illustration of a tumor-free plane between the anterior surface of the superior mesenteric–portal vein confluence and the posterior surface of the pancreas. This plane can often be developed despite fixation of the tumor to the lateral wall of the superior mesenteric vein (*SMV*). We therefore do not perform this maneuver early in the operation because tumor invasion of the lateral wall of the SMV or portal vein (*PV*) is apparent only after pancreatic transection. (From [12], with permission)

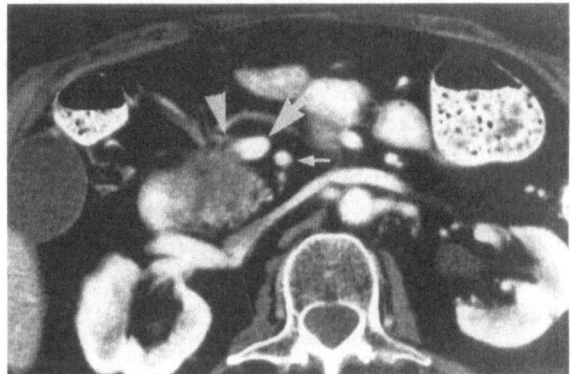

FIG. 4. Computed tomographic scan performed at 1.5-mm section thickness demonstrating no separation of the tumor (*arrowhead*) from the lateral wall of the superior mesenteric vein (*large arrow*). At surgery, the tumor was densely adhered to the vein in this region, and successful resection required segmental resection of the superior mesenteric–portal venous confluence. Note the normal fat plane between the tumor and the superior mesenteric artery (*small arrow*)

tumor is inseparable from the lateral wall of the SMV on preoperative CT scan, surgery should not be undertaken unless the surgeon has developed a technical strategy for the intraoperative management of this condition.

Extended Pancreaticoduodenectomy

Extended pancreaticoduodenectomy is the term used to described the operation performed at our institution for adenocarcinoma of the pancreatic head. It incorporates selected aspects of both the traditional Whipple procedure and regional pancreatectomy [11,12]. It differs from standard pancreaticoduodenectomy in three major areas:

1. A wide Kocher maneuver is performed, thereby removing all lymphatic tissue over the medial aspect of the right kidney, inferior vena cava, and left renal vein. The rationale for an extended Kocher maneuver is the high incidence of lymph node positivity in the posterior pancreaticoduodenal region, as initially reported by Cubilla et al. [13] and confirmed in recent studies [14,15]. This maneuver adds little time to the operation, incures no additional blood loss, is technically not difficult, and may decrease the risk of local tumor recurrence. Although it is unlikely that therapeutic maneuvers directed at the primary tumor and regional nodal basins will have any impact on the incidence of distant metastatic disease, improved tumor control in the bed of the resected pancreas and regional nodal basins may improve the quality and length of patient survival [16].

2. A wide retroperitoneal dissection is performed with complete exposure of the SMA. The high incidence of local recurrence following standard pancreaticoduodenectomy mandates that greater attention be paid to the retroperitoneal margin [8]. Perineural invasion involving the mesenteric plexus at the SMA origin, and tumor cell infiltration of lymphatic vessels and connective tissue, may extend beyond the confines of the palpable tumor. This more extensive retroperitoneal dissection with full mobilization of the SMPV confluence and dissection of the proximal SMA is necessary to obtain a negative retroperitoneal margin. As is true for other solid tumors, adequate local-regional control of pancreatic cancer requires a negative margin of excision (along the proximal SMA). In addition, clear identification of the SMA avoids the potential for iatrogenic injury.

3. Segmental resection of the SMPV confluence is performed when the tumor is inseparable from the lateral wall of the SMV or portal vein. Although an occasional patient may have such a small area of venous involvement that saphenous vein-patch angioplasty is an obvious choice, the majority of patients with involvement of the SMPV confluence require segmental venous resection. Primary closure of the vein without a patch or segmental resection has not been a feasible option in our experience. The technical feasibility of portal vein resection was first reported by Fortner in his large series of type I regional pancreatectomies that included routine portal vein resection [17]. More recently, Ishikawa and co-workers reported the safety of pancreatectomy with resection of the SMPV confluence in 35 patients; the perioperative mortality rate was 5.7% [18].

Extended pancreaticoduodenectomy, as defined here, clearly differs from regional pancreatectomy in the extend of retroperitoneal dissection and lymphadenectomy performed. Regional pancreatectomy for adenocarcinoma of the pancreatic head involves removal of lymphatic tissue to the left of the celiac axis and SMA with circumferential skeletonization of these vessels. Regional pancreatectomy as performed in the United States and Japan assumes that a wider lymphadenectomy will increase rates of long-term patient survival [19,20]. However, evidence for this is lacking.

There are three principal concerns over the use of regional pancreatectomy for adenocarcinoma of the pancreatic head: (1) the high morbidity and mortality of the procedure; (2) the long-term complications related to poor gastrointestinal function, leading to weight loss and chronic debilitation; and (3) the application of such an extensive local-regional therapy, with its associated sequelae, to a disease with such a dominant site of distant organ metastasis (liver). The high morbidity and mortality historically associated with regional pancreatectomy may have been the result of poor patient selection (i.e., the inappropriate application of a more extensive operation to patients with advanced disease), as recent reports of regional pancreatectomy demonstrate its safety in the hands of experienced surgeons [18]. However, in patients who survive the operation, skeletonization of both sides of the celiac axis and SMA deinnervates the proximal gastrointestinal tract, resulting in rapid gastrointestinal transit and chronic nutritional depletion. Therefore, dissection to the left of the SMA and celiac axis with the intent of removing possible micrometastatic disease within lymph nodes in patients with adenocarcinoma of the pancreatic head has little justification.

In contrast, extended pancreaticoduodenectomy as performed at our institution applies basic principles of oncologic surgery to the removal of the pancreatic head, with no additional perioperative morbidity or blood loss. In our published experience, median operative blood loss was 1300 ml and median hospital stay was 17 days, this despite the fact that many of our patients had undergone palliative surgical procedures before definitive resection at our institution [16]. The extended lymphadenectomy and retroperitoneal dissection described in extended pancreaticoduodenectomy are done to improve local-regional control by achieving negative retroperitoneal excision margins and adequate regional lymphadenectomy. Prospective data from our institution have demonstrated improved local-regional control when extended pancreaticoduodenectomy is performed as part of a multimodality treatment program. This has resulted in a shift in patterns of disease recurrence from a predominance of local recurrence to a predominance of liver metastases [16].

Local-regional anticancer therapy in the form of surgery, irradiation, or biochemotherapy must be based on knowledge of the natural history and patterns of disease recurrence for the specific solid tumor. Therefore, while being critical of regional pancreatectomy, there is an equal lack of justification for performing an inadequate retroperitoneal dissection at the time of pancreaticoduodenectomy by not removing all tissue to the right of the SMA or by leaving tumor on the posterior or lateral aspect of the SMV. Leaving a grossly positive margin at the time of pancreaticoduodenectomy confers no survival advantage over palliative chemotherapy and irradiation without surgery [3].

Resection of the SMPV Confluence

Before segmental resection of the SMPV confluence and tumor removal, the right colon is returned to its normal anatomical position, removing the clockwise twist in the mesentery that often occurs during the retroperitoneal dissection. Tumor adherence to the lateral wall of the SMPV confluence prevents dissection of the confluence off the pancreatic head and uncinate process, thereby inhibiting medial rotation of the confluence and lateral retraction of the specimen. Transection of the splenic vein allows identification of the SMA, located medial to the SMV, while also providing adequate length for a primary venous anastomosis following segmental vein resection (Fig. 5). The retroperitoneal dissection is completed by sharply dividing the soft tissues anterior to the aorta and to the right of the exposed SMA; the specimen is then attached only by the SMPV confluence. Vascular clamps are placed 2–3 cm proximal and distal to the involved venous segment, and the vein is transected, allowing tumor removal. The free ends of the vein are reapproximated using 6-0 Prolene (Ethicon,

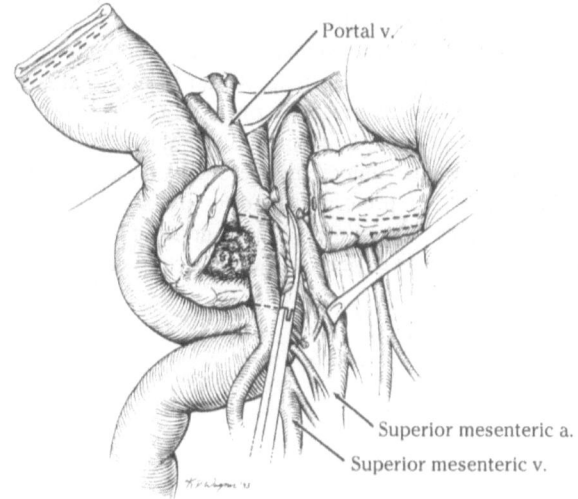

FIG. 5. Illustration of the final step in pancreaticoduodenectomy when segmental venous resection is required. In preparation for segmental resection of the superior mesenteric vein, the splenic vein has been divided and the superior mesenteric artery identified. The retroperitoneal dissection is completed by dissecting the specimen free from the lateral wall of the artery. The tumor is then attached only by the superior mesenteric–portal venous confluence. (From [2], with permission)

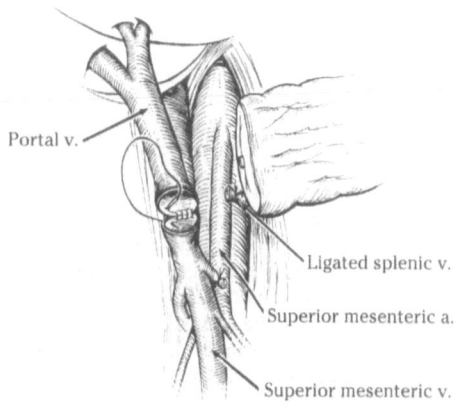

FIG. 6. Illustration of end-to-end anastomosis of the portal vein and the superior mesenteric vein with a 6-0 Prolene (Ethicon, Someville, NJ, USA) suture. (From [2], with permission)

Somerville, NJ, USA) interrupted sutures or a running suture incorporating a growth factor (Fig. 6).

Contrary to previously published reports, we have seen upper gastrointestinal hemorrhage caused by sinistral portal hypertension following splenic vein ligation. Therefore, in contrast to the technique just described, we currently preserve the splenic vein–portal vein junction whenever possible (Fig. 7). However, preservation of this confluence increases the complexity of the proximal SMA dissection. Tumor adherence to the SMPV confluence prevents medial retraction of this confluence, which is necessary for direct dissection of the tumor specimen from the lateral wall of the proximal SMA. Similarly, the SMA cannot be exposed medial to the SMV (as discussed previously) if the splenic vein–portal vein junction is left intact. Therefore, venous resection (and interposition grafting) is usually performed with the specimen still attached to the lateral aspect of the proximal SMA.

The need to perform venous reconstruction before complete specimen removal results in the requirement for an interposition graft in most patients who undergo SMV resection with splenic vein preservation. Additionally, preservation of the splenic vein–portal vein junction significantly limits the mobilization of the portal vein and prevents primary anastomosis of the SMV unless segmental resection is limited to less than 2 cm. Our preferred conduit for interposition grafting is the internal jugular vein (Fig. 8). When interposition grafting is performed, the SMA is temporarily cross-clamped so as to prevent vascular congestion of the small bowel.

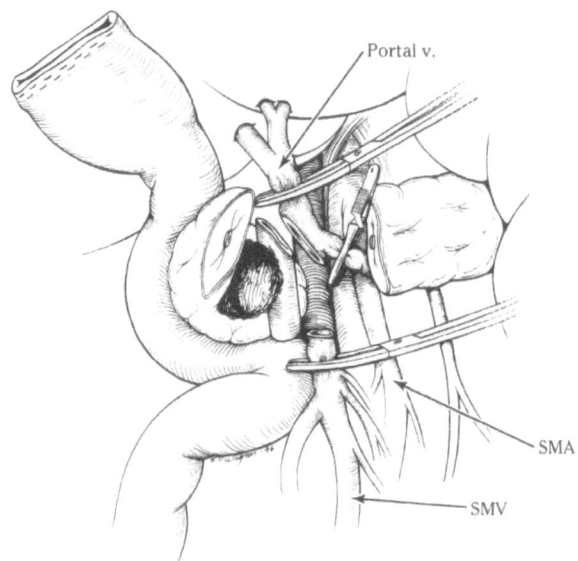

FIG. 7. Illustration of segmental resection of the superior mesenteric–portal vein confluence with splenic vein preservation. With the splenic vein intact, exposure is often inadequate to separate the specimen from the lateral aspect of the proximal superior mesenteric artery (*SMA*). Therefore, the graft is usually placed before completing the retroperitoneal dissection. The reconstructed superior mesenteric–portal vein confluence can then be retracted medially allowing the specimen to be removed from the proximal SMA under direct vision. When interposition grafting is performed, the SMA is temporarily cross-clamped (not shown) to prevent vascular congestion of the small bowel. *SMV*, superior mesenteric vein

Fig. 8. Illustration of our preferred method of reconstruction of the superior mesenteric vein (*SMV*) using an internal jugular vein interposition graft. *SMA*, superior mesenteric artery. (From [2], with permission)

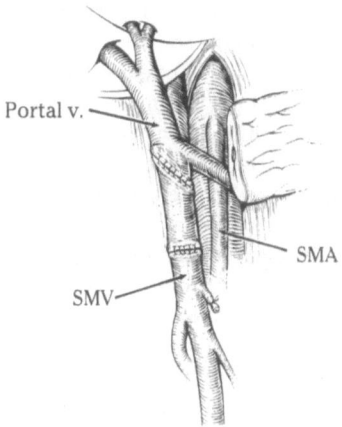

Portal v.

SMA

SMV

Table 1. Pathologic findings for 59 consecutive patients who underwent pancreaticoduodenectomy (P) or pancreaticoduodenectomy with en bloc segmental venous resection (VR)

Surgery	No. of patients	Median tumor size (cm)	No. with positive retroperitoneal margin	No. with positive nodes	No. with perineural invasion
P	36	3.0	5 (14%)[a]	22 (61%)	19 (53%)
VR	23	3.7	4 (17%)[b]	9 (39%)	19 (83%)
P value[c]		NS	NS[d]	NS[e]	<.05[e]

[a] One specimen classified as margin-negative had acellular mucin within perineural tissue.
[b] In one specimen (classified as margin-positive), tumor cells were seen in perineural tissue at the retroperitoneal margin in the absence of direct extension from the primary tumor.
[c] Differences were assessed by unpaired Student's *t*-test, Fisher's exact test,[d] or chi-squared analysis[e]; NS, not significant.
From [3], with permission.

We recently reported on 23 patients who underwent en bloc segmental resection of the SMPV confluence during pancreaticoduodenectomy for periampullary adenocarcinoma (pancreatic head, 21; duodenum, 1; bile duct, 1) [3]. CT correctly predicted the need for SMPV resection in 19 (83%) of these patients. Reconstruction was performed using either an end-to-end anastomosis or an interposition graft. The only perioperative death (in hospital or within 30 days of surgery) occurred in a patient who had undergone two previous operations, radiation therapy (including intraoperative radiation therapy), and chemotherapy for a localized duodenal carcinoma before definitive resection, which required en bloc resection of the SMV. Pathologic findings in these 23 patients were compared with those of 36 consecutive patients who underwent pancreaticoduodenectomy without venous resection (Table 1). There was a higher incidence of perineural invasion in patients who required venous resection; however, no differences in retroperitoneal margin positivity, or nodal positivity were observed between patients who required venous resection and those who did not.

SMPV patency and survival in our updated series were presented at the 1996 meeting of the Society of Surgical Oncology [21]. Patency of the SMPV confluence was 100% for jugular vein interposition graft, 82% for primary end-to-end anastomosis, 0% for Gore-Tex interposition graft, and 100% for vein-patch angioplasty. Our experience with jugular vein interposition grafting is increasing, and this technique appears to be the superior method for restoring portal–mesenteric flow while preserving splenic vein patency. In contrast to previous reports, patients with pancreatic head adenocarcinoma requiring resection of the SMPV confluence had a survival rate equivalent to patients who underwent pancreaticoduodenectomy without venous resection. These data suggest that tumor adherence to the SMPV confluence is a function of tumor location rather than an indicator of biologic aggressiveness and should not represent a contraindication to pancreaticoduodenectomy.

The goal of vascular resection as part of a multimodality treatment program involving pancreaticoduodenectomy is improved local-regional tumor control; only through this mechanism does surgical resection have potential to increase quality and length of patient survival. In the absence of more uniformly effective treatments for pancreatic cancer, the surgeon will best serve patients by observing the following guidelines:

1. Avoid surgery in patients with locally advanced or metastatic disease by thorough preoperative assessment with high-quality imaging studies. The relationship of the tumor to the SMA and celiac axis should be clearly delineated on preoperative CT. If the low-density tumor involves the lateral wall of either of these two arterial structures, resection should not be attempted. Palliative biliary decompression, if necessary, can be performed with minimally invasive techniques.

2. If preoperative CT suggests tumor invasion of the lateral or posterior wall of the SMPV confluence, proceed to laparotomy only if one has a technical strategy for the management of this condition.

3. Encourage patient participation in protocols examining the efficacy of innovative multimodality treatment programs [22].

References

1. Moore GE, Sako Y, Thomas LB (1951) Radical pancreaticoduodenectomy with resection and reanastomosis of the superior mesenteric vein. Surgery (St Louis) 30:550–553
2. Cusack JC, Fuhrman GM, Lee JE, Evans DB (1994) Management of unsuspected tumor invasion of the superior mesenteric-portal venous confluence at the time of pancreaticoduodenectomy. Am J Surg 168:352–354
3. Fuhrman GM, Leach SD, Staley CA, Cusack JC, Charnsangavej C, Cleary KR, El-Naggar AK, Fenoglio CJ, Lee JE, Evans DB (1996) Rational for en-bloc vein resection in the treatment of pancreatic adenocarcinoma adherent to the superior mesenteric-portal vein confluence. Ann Surg 223:154–162
4. Willet CG, Lewandrowski K, Warshaw AL, Efird J, Compton CC (1993) Resection margins in carcinoma of the head of the pancreas: implications for radiation therapy. Ann Surg 217:144–148
5. Nitecki SS, Sarr MG, Colby TV, vanHeerden JA (1995) Long-term survival after resection for ductal adenocarcinoma of the pancreas. Is it really improving? Ann Surg 221:59–66
6. Trede M, Schwall G, Saeger HD (1990) Survival after pancreaticoduodenectomy: 118 consecutive resections without an operative mortality. Ann Surg 211:447–458

7. Yeo CJ, Cameron JL, Lillemore KD, Sitzmann JV, Hruban RH, Goodman SN, Dooley WC, Coleman J, Pitt HA (1995) Pancreaticoduodenectomy for cancer of the head of the pancreas: 201 patients. Ann Surg 221:721–733

8. Fuhrman GM, Charnsangavej C, Abbruzzese JL, Clearly KR, Martin RG, Fenoglio CJ, Evans DB (1994) Thin-section contrast-enhanced computed tomography accurately predicts the resectability of malignant pancreatic neoplasms. Am J Surg 167:104–113

9. Freeny PC, Traverso LW, Ryan JA (1993) Diagnosis and staging of pancreatic adenocarcinoma with dynamic computed tomography. Am J Surg 165:600–606

10. Warshaw AL, Gu Z, Wittenberg J, Waltman AC (1990) Preoperative staging and asessment of resectability of pancreatic cancer. Arch Surg 125:230–233

11. Evans DB, Lee JE, Leach SD, Fuhrman GM, Cusack JC, Rich TA (1995) Vascualr resection and intraoperative radiation therapy during pancreaticoduodenectomy: rationale and technique. Adv Surg 29:235–262

12. Evans DB, Lee JE, Pisters PWT (1997) Pancreaticoduodenectomy (Whipple operation) and total pancreatectomy for cancer. In: Nyhus LM, Baker RJ, Fishcer JF (eds) Mastery of surgery, 3rd edn. Little, Brown, Boston, pp 1233–1249

13. Cubilla AL, Fortner J, Fitzgerald PJ (1978) Lymph node involvement in carcinoma of the head of the pancreas area. Cancer (Phila) 41:880–887

14. Kayahara M, Nagakawa T, Kobayashi H, Mori K, Nakano T, Kadoya N, Ohta T, Ueno K, Miyazaki I (1992) Lymphatic flow in carcinoma of the head of the pancreas. Cancer (Phila) 70:2061–2066

15. Nagakawa T, Kobayashi H, Ueno K, Ohta T, Kayahara M, Miyazaki I (1994) Clinical study of lymphatic flow to the paraaortic lymph nodes in carcinoma of the head of the pancreas. Cancer (Phila) 73:1155–1162

16. Staley CA, Lee JE, Cleary KA, Abbruzzese JL, Fenoglio CJ, Rich TA, Evans DB (1996) Preoperative chemoradiation, pancreaticoduodenectomy, and intraoperative radiation therapy for adenocarcinoma of the pancreatic head. Am J Surg 171:118–125

17. Fortner J (1985) Technique of regional subtotal and total pancreatectomy. Am J Surg 150:593–600

18. Ishikawa O, Ohigashi H, Imaoka S, Furukawa H, Sasaki Y, Fujita M, Kuroda C, Iwanaga T (1992) Preoperative indications for extended pancreatectomy for locally advanced pancreas cancer involving the portal vein. Ann Surg 215:231–236

19. Ishikawa O, Ohigashi H, Sasaki Y, Kabuto T, Fukuda I, Furukawa H, Imaoka S, Iwanaga T (1988) Practical usefulness of lymphatic and connective tissue clearance for the carcinoma of the pancreas head. Ann Surg 208:215–220

20. Fortner JG (1989) "Radical" abdominal cancer surgery: current state and future course. Jpn J Surg 19:503–509

21. Leach SD, Lowy AM, Fuhrman GM, Lee JE, Pisters PWT, Evans DB (1996) Pancreatic malignancy involving the superior mesenteric-portal vein confluence (SMPV) is not a contraindication to pancreaticoduodenectomy. In: Program of the 49th Annual Cancer Symposium of the Society of Surgical Oncology 10(18)

22. Evans DB, Abbruzzese JL, Rich TA (1997) Cancer of the Pancreas. In: Devita VT, Hellman S, Rosenberg SA (eds) Cancer, Principles and Practice of Oncology, Fifth Edition. J.B. Lippincott Co., Philadelphia, pp 1054–1087

Extended Duodenopancreatectomy: Is More Better? Commentary

WALDEMAR KOZUSCHEK[1] and HANS-BERND REITH[2]

Summary. The Whipple procedure with its modifications has become a safe operation with a low mortality rate. Long-term results have not improved despite the introduction of imaging techniques in early diagnosis. The only chance for cure remains radical surgical resection; however, only a few patients benefit from this.

Key words. Pancreatoduodenectomy—Extension of resection

The extension of the Whipple procedure, including total pancreatectomy with removal of the spleen and more extensive regional lymph nodes, was advocated by the van Heerden group in the Mayo Clinic, Rochester, MN (USA) [1] and by Andren-Sandberg and Ihse from Lund, Sweden, in the early 1980s [2].

The overall poor long-term survival after the standard Whipple operation was the impetus for the concept of extending the resection to a total pancreatectomy. Advocates of total pancreatectomy cite eliminating multicentric disease and eradicating the spread of disease to the distal pancreas by either direct extension, intraductal seeding, or lymphatic permeation. In addition, total pancreatectomy is believed by some surgeons to be a better cancer operation, including a wider en bloc resection of the pancreas and the lymph nodes [3]. Another advantage is the elimination of the pancreaticojejunal anastomosis, which is the major cause of morbidity and mortality [4]. However, in our experience there is no reduction in morbidity and mortality for those patients because of the length of operation.

The major disadvantage of the total pancreatectomy is the inevitable loss of pancreatic endocrine function, often resulting in a brittle diabetes. Therefore, total pancreatectomy should be reserved for those patients with histological evidence of tumor at the margin or multicentric disease [5,6].

[1] Department of Surgery, Ruhr-University Bochum, Knappschaftskrankenhaus, In der Schornau 23, D-44892 Bochum, Germany.
[2] Department of Surgery, University Würzburg, Josef-Schneider Str. 2, D-97080 Würzburg, Germany.

The study from Lund, Sweden (1991), is very important for our understanding as to why the Whipple procedure fails for pancreatic adenocarcinoma of the head of the pancreas, whether using the radical or standard procedure and regardless of pylorus preservation or hemigastrectomy. From 1958 through 1985, Andren-Sandberg et al. performed an extended radical standard Whipple procedure with total pancreatectomy. More recently, during 1985–1989, they performed the same operation excepting the tail of the pancreas to avoid diabetes. The 3-year survival rate was 2% and 6% in the first and second period and 25% in the latest period. Thus, their survival rate increased with a slightly less radical procedure and better patient selection. Despite radical resection, local recurrence was seen in approximately 90% of the patients in each of these three time periods [7].

The concept of supraradical pancreatectomy also has been suggested. These procedures include total resection of the portal vein with reanastomosis or graft and also an extensive lymph node dissection. Reports from Japanese centers, such as by, Hanyu et al. in Tokyo, have suggested very satisfactory results and also an improvement in long-term survival [8]. However, these results are nearly all retrospective and uncontrolled. A prospective, controlled study is necessary to demonstrate significant better results. In my experience, major vascular resection is associated with increased perioperative morbidity and mortality.

The Boston study group, led by Warshaw [9], investigated the surgical margins after the Whipple procedure. It was not surprising that there were no 5-year survivors with positive surgical margins and a 22% 5-year survival rate with negative margins. Half the patients had positive margins, and the most common area was the retropancreatic soft tissue just posterior to the pancreatic head. This is the weak area for any Whipple procedure for clearance of tumor, not the area of the pylorus. It makes little sense to have a millimeter margin posteriorly and centimeter-long margins on the stomach.

We conclude, from our experience, that a radical local resection of the head of the pancreas with extensive lymph node dissection has satisfactory results with pylorus preservation.

References

1. Reber HA (1993) The Whipple pancreaticoduodenectomy. In: Beger HG, Büchler M, Malfertheimer P (eds) Standards in pancreatic surgery. Springer, Berlin Heidelberg New York, pp 637–640
2. Ihse I, Andren-Sandberg A, Permerth J, Larsson J (1993) Early results of subtotal pancreatectomy for cancer. In: Beger HG, Büchler M, Malfertheimer P (eds) Standards in pancreatic surgery. Springer, Berlin Heidelberg New York, pp 641–645
3. Fortner JG (1984) Regional pancreatectomy for cancer of the pancreas, ampulla and other related sites. Ann Surg 199:418–425
4. Brooks JR, Culebras JM (1976) Cancer of the pancreas: palliative operation, Whipple procedure of total pancreatectomy? Am J Surg 131:516–520
5. Kozuschek W, Reith HB, Waleczek H, Haarmann W, Edelmann M, Sonntag D (1994) A comparision of long-term results of the standard Whipple procedure and the pylorus-preserving pancreatoduodenectomy. J Am Coll Surg 178:443–458
6. Traverso LW, Longmire WP (1980) Preservation of the pylorus in pancreatico-duodenectomy. A follow-up evaluation. Ann Surg 192:306–310
7. Andren-Sandberg A, Ahren B, Tranberg KG, Bengmark S (1991) Surgical treatment of pancreatic cancer. Int J Pancreatol 9:145–151

8. Hanyu F, Suzuki M, Imaizumi T (1993) Whipple operation for pancreatic carcinoma: Japanese experience. In: Beger HG, Büchler M, Malfertheimer P (eds) Standards in pancreatic surgery. Springer, Berlin Heidelberg New York, pp 646–653
9. Willett CG, Lewandrowski K, Warshaw AL, Efird J, Compton CC (1993) Resection margins in carcinoma of the head of the pancreas: implication for radiation therapy. Ann Surg 217:144–148

Duodenum-Preserving
Pancreatoduodenectomy

Duodenum-Preserving Total Pancreatic Head Resection with Preservation of the Vascular Arcades for Benign Lesions or Low-Grade Malignancies

Shuichi Miyakawa, Akihiko Horiguchi, Makoto Hayakawa, Shin Ishihara, Naotatu Niwamoto, and Kaoru Miura

Summary. Beger's procedure for pancreatic resection has been performed in patients with benign lesions or low-grade malignancies, such as mucin-producing tumors. When this procedure is applied in the treatment of tumors, it is modified to include a total resection of the head of the pancreas with the preservation of the blood supply to the bile duct and duodenum. A duodenum-preserving total resection of the head of the pancreas with preservation of the arterial arcades and their branches to the duodenum and the bile duct was performed in two patients with benign or low-grade malignant tumors without chronic pancreatitis. The blood flow in the duodenum and bile duct was based on both arterial arcades, and the color of the second portion of the duodenum was good. The postoperative results were satisfactory. The new technique for total resection of the head of the pancreas with preservation of the arterial arcades can be performed in patients with a normal pancreatic gland. This results in good blood flow to the duodenum and the bile duct.

Key words. Beger's procedure—Bile duct—Duodenum—Total pancreatic head resection—Arterial arcades

Introduction

It is now generally recognized that a duodenum-preserving resection of the head of the pancreas is one of the best procedures currently available for the treatment of chronic pancreatitis [1,2]. Recently, this procedure has been performed in patients with benign lesions or low-grade malignancies. These include mucin-producing tumors, which exhibit a very slight tendency to invade and a good prognosis [3–6]. However, there are some problems with the application of this procedure to mucin-producing tumors because the paraduodenal pancreatic remnant may contain residual disease resulting from intraductal spread to the pancreatic duct. On the other hand, during total resection of the head of the pancreas, it is absolutely essential to preserve the blood supply to the bile duct and the duodenum to prevent early postop-

Second Department of Gastroenterological Surgery, Fujita Health University School of Medicine, Toyoake, Aichi 470-11, Japan.

erative complications [7–9]. Therefore, a duodenum-preserving procedure for benign and low-grade malignant tumors is essentially a total resection of the head of the pancreas with the preservation of the blood supply to the bile duct and duodenum [6]. We report a duodenum-preserving total resection of the head of the pancreas with preservation of the arterial arcades and their branches to the duodenum and the bile duct for patients with normal glands and benign or low-grade malignant tumors.

Surgical Technique

The aim of our procedure is the complete resection of the head of the pancreas with preservation of the blood supply to the duodenum and the bile duct (Fig. 1). After laparotomy, both gastro- and duodenocolic ligaments are dissected without performing Kocher's maneuver. Then, the right gastroepiploic vein is ligated and divided on the anterior surface of the pancreas. The superior mesenteric vein is exposed from the inferior border of the pancreas to the anterior of the third portion of the duodenum. Next, the common hepatic artery is dissected on the superior border of the pancreas. After these maneuvers, the pancreas is dissected from the portal and mesenteric vein.

The resection itself begins with the division of the pancreas over the portal vein. Careful hemostasis is then obtained at the divided edge of the left side of the pancreas with ligation and coagulation of the vessels. A polyvinyl tube is inserted into the main pancreatic duct and fixed with 5-0 Prolene sutures. The superior and inferior pancreatoduodenal veins from the portomesenteric vein are preserved. The total

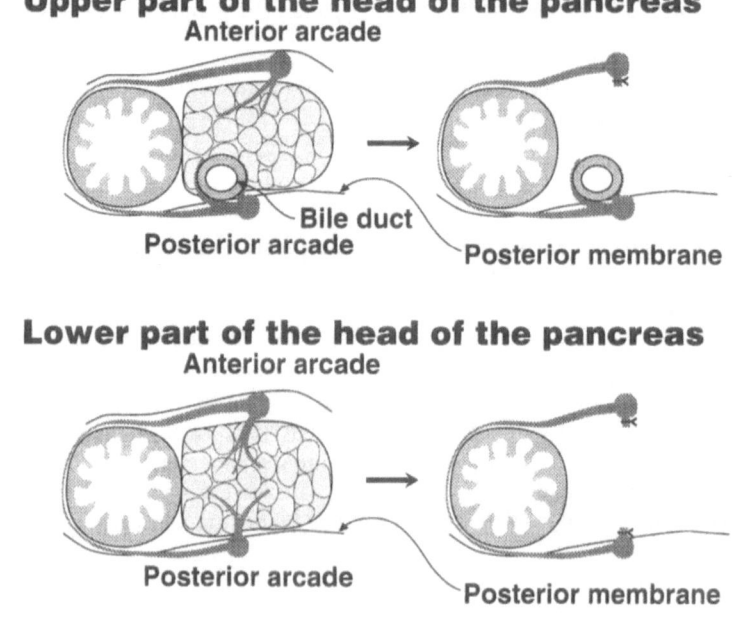

FIG. 1. Duodenum-preserving total resection of the head of the pancreas with preservation of both arterial arcades

resection of the head of the pancreas is carried out from the divided edge at the portal vein toward the prepapillary common bile duct. During resection of the uncinate lobe, the inferior pancreaticoduodenal artery (IPDA) is taped, and the pancreatic branches of the anterior inferior pancreaticoduodenal artery (AIPDA) are ligated and divided one by one toward the papilla of Vater, preserving the branches of the AIPDA to the duodenum (Fig. 2). As a matter of course, the mesoduodenal vessels are preserved.

During resection of the dorsal side of the head of the pancreas, the pancreatic branches of the posterior inferior pancreaticoduodenal artery (PIPDA) and the inferior pancreaticoduodenal vein (IPDV) are ligated and divided, with preservation of the PIPDA, the IPDV, and the pancreatic posterior membrane. It is important for the blood supply and venous drainage of the duodenum to preserve the AIPDA, PIPDA, IPDV, and the membrane because the PIPDA and the IPDV run under the posterior membrane. While ligating and dividing the pancreatic branches of the gastroduodenal artery (GDA) and the anterior superior pancreaticoduodenal artery (ASPDA) toward the papilla of Vater, the duodenal branches are preserved. Several traction sutures are placed at the divided edge of the pancreas, after which the head of the pancreas is dissected from the duodenum and the bile duct.

When dissecting between the pancreatic tissue and the bile duct, it is important for the preservation of the blood supply to the bile duct from the posterior superior pancreaticoduodenal artery (PSPDA) to dissect the pancreatic tissue at the anterior wall of the bile duct because the PSPDA and its bile duct branches run from the cranial side to the dorsal side of the bile duct (Fig. 3). It is also important to preserve the superior pancreaticoduodenal vein for the venous drainage from the first and second portions of the duodenum, the papilla of Vater, and the bile duct. These vessels also run under the posterior membrane. As the pancreas is dissected from the bile duct,

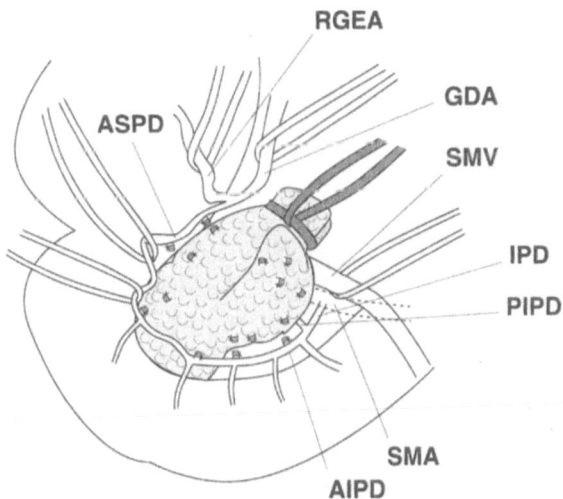

FIG. 2. The pancreatic branches of the anterior inferior pancreaticoduodenal artery (*AIPD*) and the anterior superior pancreaticoduodenal artery (*ASPD*) are ligated and divided one by one toward the papilla of Vater, preserving the branches to the duodenum. *SMV*, Superior mesenteric vein; *SMA*, superior mesenteric artery; *RGEA*, gastroepiploic artery; *IPD*, inferior pancreaticoduodenal artery; *PIPD*, posterior inferior pancreaticoduodenal artery; *GDA*, gastroduodenal artery

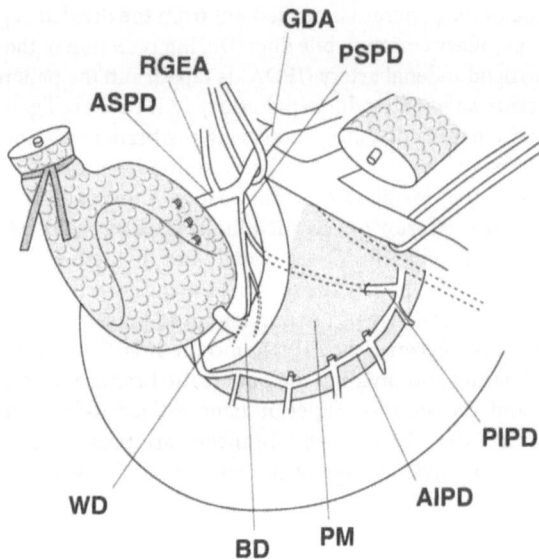

FIG. 3. The preservation of the bile duct and its blood supply from the posterior superior pancreaticoduodenal artery (PSPD) requires dissection of the pancreatic tissue along the anterior wall of the bile duct. The posterior pancreatic membrane (PM) is also preserved. GDA, Gastroduodenal artery; IPD, inferior pancreaticoduodenal artery; RGEA, gastroepiploic artery; ASPD, anterior superior pancreaticoduodenal artery; AIPD, anterior inferior pancreaticoduodenal artery; PIPD, posterior inferior pancreaticoduodenal artery; BD, bile duct; WD, wirsung duct

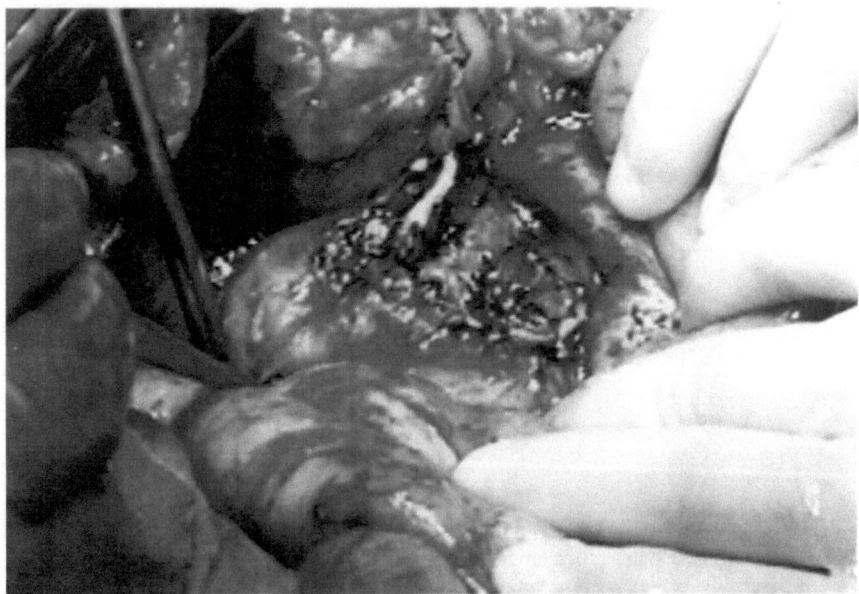

FIG. 4. After total resection of the head of the pancreas, the anterior arterial arcades and the posterior membrane were preserved, and the color of the duodenum in reconstruction was good

the confluence of the pancreatic duct is noted. The pancreatic duct is ligated and divided at the confluence. The pancreas is dissected from the duodenum while preserving the accessory papilla and the papilla of Vater. The head of the pancreas is removed after dividing the accessory pancreatic duct. Reconstruction is accomplished by an end-to-side pancreaticojejunostomy using a Roux-en-Y jejunal loop.

Intraoperative and Postoperative Course

This surgical procedure was performed in two patients with mucinous cystic tumors of the pancreatic duct in the uncinate portion of the pancreas. The mean operative time was 429 min, and the mean blood loss was 810 ml. Immediately after resection of the head of the pancreas, the second portion of the duodenum remained pink in both patients (Fig. 4). The mean postoperative hospitalization was 20 days. Neither of the patients had early or late postoperative complications. These patients have been well without recurrence for 18 months.

Discussion

The duodenum-preserving resection of the head of the pancreas (Beger's procedure) is an organ-saving procedure in the treatment of severe chronic pancreatitis [1]. However, there are some problems when Beger's procedure is utilized in treatment of patients with benign lesions or low-grade malignancies, such as mucin-producing tumors. First, tumor may remain in the paraduodenal pancreatic remnant because mucin-producing tumors can spread along the lumen of the pancreatic duct. Second, a pancreatic fistula from the paraduodenal pancreatic remnant may result because of congenital obstruction of the accessory papilla. Third, it is difficult to preserve the blood supply and the venous drainage of the duodenum and the bile duct because collaterals from the hepatoduodenal ligament and the retropancreatic space are not developed in patients with a normal gland compared to those with chronic pancreatitis [10]. This may cause ischemia of the bile duct and the duodenum following resection of the head of the pancreas, resulting in early postoperative complications such as perforation. Therefore, Beger's procedure should not be used in patients with a normal gland and benign lesions or low-grade malignancies. For these patients, a new operative procedure is needed.

The aims of the new operative procedure are total resection of the head of the pancreas with preservation of the blood supply and the venous drainage of the bile duct and the duodenum. Total resection of the head of the pancreas might be incompatible with preservation of the blood supply and the venous drainage. Kimura and Nagai [11] have reported that the preservation of the blood supply and the venous drainage of the bile duct and the duodenum is possible topographically during resection of the head of the pancreas. Takada et al. [7] have reported that the blood flow in the duodenum is based on an intact duodenal blood supply from the mesoduodenum and the retroperitoneum. This can be preserved by avoiding the disruption caused by Kocher's maneuver and by saving the posterior superior pancreaticoduodenal artery. In their report, however, the blood supply to the second portion of the duodenum is limited because it is provided only by the duodenal branches of the posterior superior pancreaticoduodenal artery and the arteries from the retroperitoneum, which may not be developed in the normal gland.

To avoid ischemia of the second portion of the duodenum and the intrapancreatic bile duct, one must preserve the superior pancreaticoduodenal vein (SPDV) and the inferior pancreaticoduodenal vein (IPDV) during exploration of the mesentericoportal vein, the duodenal branches of the AIPDA and the ASPDA (the vasa rectus to the duodenum), and the posterior pancreatic membrane. In our patients who were treated using these methods, the blood flow was based on both arterial arcades. The color of the second portion of the duodenum was good, and the postoperative results were satisfactory. The new techniques for the preservation of the arterial arcades can be performed in patients with a normal pancreatic gland.

References

1. Beger HG, Krautzberger W, Bittner R, Buchler M, Limmer J (1985) Duodenum-preserving resection of the head of the pancreas in patients with severe chronic pancreatitis. Surgery (St Louis) 97:467–473
2. Izbicki JR, Bloechle C, Knoefel WT, Kuechler T, Binmoeller KF, Broelsch CE (1995) Duodenum-preserving resection of the head of the pancreas in chronic pancreatitis. A prospective, randomized trial. Ann Surg 221:350–358
3. Ryo H, Hanyu F, Seiyo K, Toda H, Imaizumi T (1990) New operative technique of the head of the duodenum-preserving pancreatic head resection (in Japanese). Shujutu (Operation) 44:447–451
4. Yasuda H, Takada T, Uchiyama K, Hasegawa H, Tuchiya S, Iwagaki T, Narazaki Y, Sikata J (1990) Resection of the head of the pancreas with preservation of biliary tract and duodenum (in Japanese). Tan to Sui (J Biliary Tract Pancreas) 11:967–973
5. Imaizumi T, Hanyu H, Suzuki M, Nakasako T, Harada N, Komatsu E, Kimura T, Hatori T (1991) Duodenum-preserving total resection of the head of the pancreas (in Japanese). Shoukaigeka (Gastroenterol Surg) 14:475–488
6. Takada T, Yasuda H, Uchiyama K, Hasegawa H (1993) Duodenum-preserving pancreaticoduodenostomy. A new technique for complete excision of the head of the pancreas with preservation of biliary and alimentary integrity. Hepato-Gastroentrology 40:356–359
7. Takada T, Yasuda H, Uchiyama K, Iwagaki T, Yamakawa Y (1995) Complete duodenum-preserving resection of the head of the pancreas with preservation of the biliary tract. J Hep Bil Pancr Surg 2:38–44
8. Frey CF, Child CG, Frey W (1978) Pancreatectomy for chronic pancreatitis. Ann Surg 184:403–414
9. Warren WD, Milikan WJ, Henderson JM, Hersh T (1984) A denervated pancreatic flap for control of chronic pain in pancreatitis. Surg Gynecol Obstet 159:581–583
10. Lambert MA, Linehan IP, Russel RCG (1987) Duodenum-preserving total pancreatectomy for end-stage chronic pancreatitis. Br J Surg 74:35–39
11. Kimura W, Nagai H (1995) Study of surgical anatomy for duodenum-preserving resection of the head of the pancreas. Ann Surg 221:359–363

Surgical Procedure of Complete Duodenum-Preserving Pancreatoduodenostomy with Preservation of the Biliary Tract

Hideki Yasuda, Tadahiro Takada, Hodaka Amano, Masahiro Yoshida, and Katsuhiro Uchiyama

Summary. Duodenum-preserving pancreatic head resection began with the report by H. Beger in 1980. However, the procedure of Beger was subtotal resection of the pancreatic head, and its indication was limited to chronic pancreatitis. We therefore developed total pancreatic head resection with preservation of not only the duodenum but also the biliary tract in 1990 and have since applied the procedure clinically. To perform duodenum-preserving total pancreatic head resection safely, preservation of the mesoduodenal vessel as well as the posterior superior pancreatoduodenal artery is important, and Kocher's maneuver should be avoided for this purpose.

Key words. Duodenum-preserving pancreatic resection—Pancreatoduodenectomy—Duodenal blood supply—Mesoduodenal blood vessels—Preservation of the biliary tract

Introduction

The Whipple procedure has been a standard resectional operation for pancreatic head lesions for years. However, the procedure has been associated with problems such as postoperative dumping syndrome and postgastrectomy syndrome.

In 1978, Traverso and Longmire reported pylorus-preserving pancreatoduodenectomy (PPPD), and the procedure has been widely accepted because of its superiority to the Whipple procedure with regard to postoperative quality of life [1–4]. In PPPD, however, only about 4 cm of the duodenum from the pyloric ring is preserved, while the entire stomach and the pyloric ring are left intact. In 1980, Beger reported duodenum-preserving pancreatic head resection (DPPHR) for patients with chronic pancreatitis [5]. In the Beger operation, however, pancreatic tissue attached to the duodenal wall must be left unresected to preserve duodenal blood flow. This reduced the procedure to partial resection of the pancreatic head and limited its indication to chronic pancreatitis.

First Department of Surgery, Teikyo University School of Medicine, Itabashi-ku, Tokyo 173, Japan.

Since 1988, we have developed pancreatic segmentectomy in consideration of anatomical segments of the pancreas [6]. We succeeded in total resection of the pancreatic head by preserving the biliary tract and the alimentary tract [7] and have applied the procedure to clinical cases [8,9]. This total pancreatic head resection has enlarged the indication of DPPHR beyond chronic pancreatitis to conditions such as mucin-producing tumor of the pancreas.

In this chapter, we describe the procedure and characteristics of complete duodenum-preserving pancreatic head resection.

Characteristics of the Operative Procedure

Characteristics of this surgical procedure are (1) avoidance of Kocher's maneuver, (2) division of the anterosuperior pancreatoduodenal artery but preservation of the posterosuperior pancreatoduodenal artery, (3) preservation of the duodenal papilla and the biliary tract, (4) preservation of the duodenum, and (5) complete resection of the pancreatic parenchyma of the pancreatic head from the upper margin of the portal vein to the attachment to the duodenum (Fig. 1).

Concerning preservation of the duodenal blood supply, which is the greatest problem in this procedure: (1) the mesoduodenal vessel as well as the retroperitoneal vessels are preserved by not performing Kocher's maneuver, and these play an important role in maintaining the blood supply to the duodenum; (2) the blood flow of the gastroduodenal artery, which is the primary vessel supplying the duodenum, is maintained by separating only the anterosuperior pancreatoduodenal artery but preserving the posterosuperior pancreatoduodenal artery.

Another characteristic of our procedure is end-to-side pancreatoduodenostomy, which has become possible because of the absence of residual pancreatic tissue around the duodenum. This procedure, which allows the flow of not only bile but also pancreatic juice into the duodenum, is considered to be more physiological than foregoing procedures.

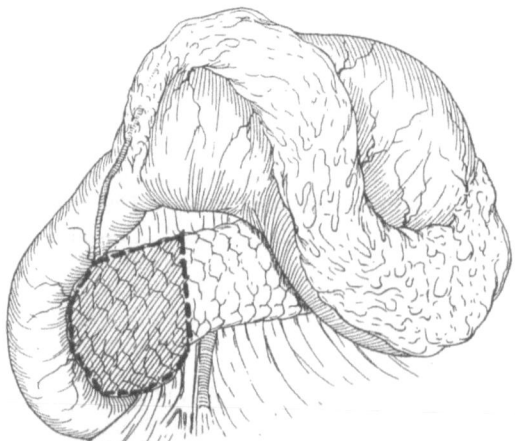

FIG. 1. Area of resection: pancreatic tissue is resected from its duodenal attachment to the upper margin of the portal vein. *Dashed line enclosing shaded area* is head of pancreas

Operative Procedure

Laparotomy

Laparotomy is performed by a median incision in the upper abdominal region. The gastrocolic membrane and duodenocolic membrane are separated, and the pancreatic head is exposed (Fig. 2). It is important here not to perform Kocher's maneuver so as to preserve the duodenal blood flow.

Separation of the Gastroepiploic Artery and Vein

The right gastroepiploic artery and vein are ligated and cut anteriorly to the pancreas (Fig. 3).

Portal Vein Tunneling

The superior mesenteric vein is exposed, and its anterior aspect is dissected toward the lower margin of the pancreatic body. The anterior aspect of the superior mesenteric vein and the posterior aspect of the pancreatic body are gradually detached. This method makes portal vein tunneling possible.

Separation of the Pancreatic Body and Intubation of the Pancreatic Duct

After portal vein tunneling, the pancreas is separated at the right-upper margin of the portal vein. After hemostasis of the pancreatic stump, a Fr. 4 or Fr. 6 polyvinyl tube is

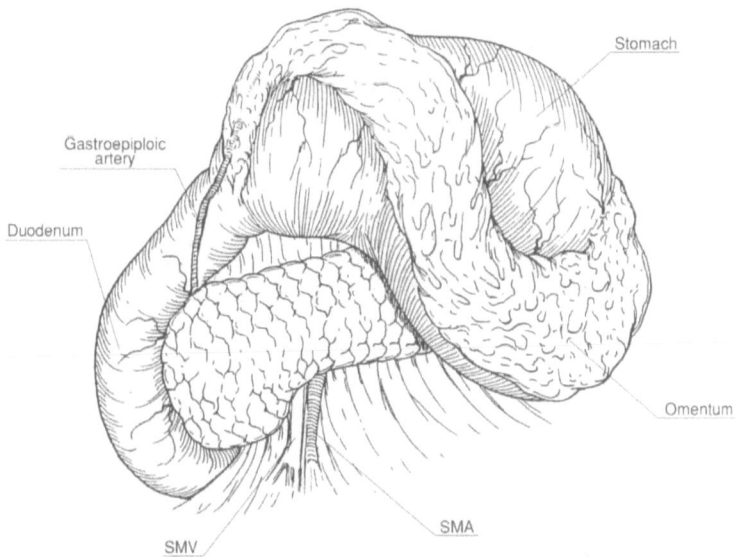

FIG. 2. Exposure of the pancreatic head. *SMV*, superior mesenteric vein; *SMA*, superior mesenteric artery

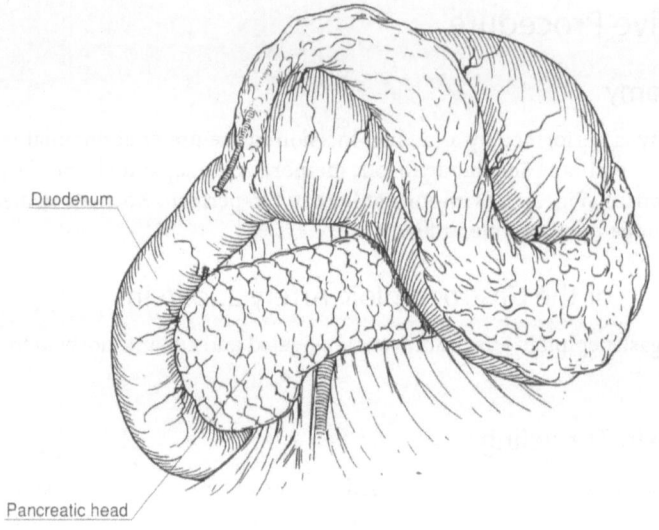

FIG. 3. Treatment of the gastroepiploic artery and vein

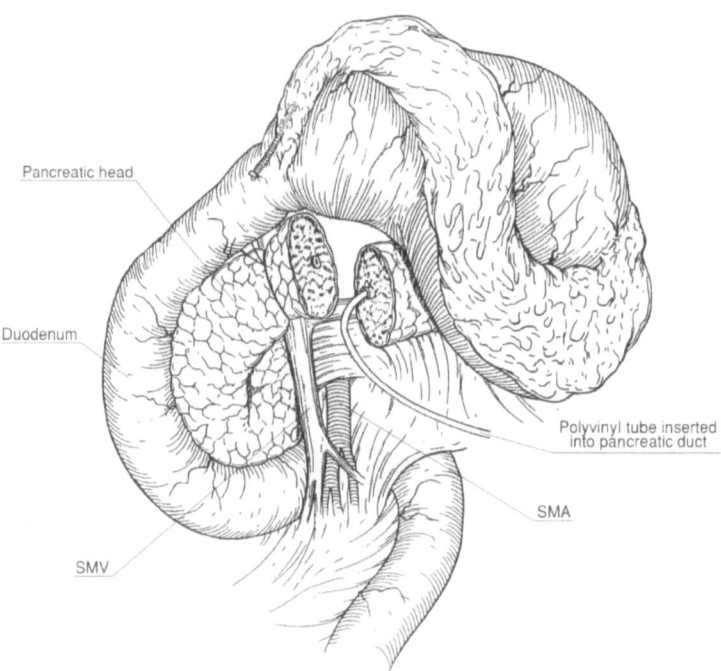

FIG. 4. Separation of the pancreas and intubation of the pancreatic duct

inserted into the caudal pancreatic duct and immobilized there by fixing suture using a 5-0 nylon thread (Fig. 4).

Separation of the Anterosuperior Pancreatoduodenal Artery

The anterosuperior pancreatoduodenal artery alone is exposed at the duodenal margin and is cut after ligation (Fig. 5). At this time, caution is needed not to separate or damage the gastroduodenal artery or the posterosuperior pancreatoduodenal artery.

Dissection of the Pancreatic Head

The pancreatic parenchyma is slowly and bluntly detached from the duodenal wall while retracting the pancreatic parenchyma of the pancreatic head. The anterior aspect of the bile duct is exposed by further advancing the detachment of the pancreatic tissue from the duodenum and retracting the pancreatic head below. Dissection is continued until the bile duct is completely detached from the pancreatic parenchyma.

When the pancreas is detached from the third portion of the duodenum, mesoduodenal vessels can be clearly observed. The pancreatic head is detached from the duodenum with sufficient caution not to damage these vessels. Then, the uncinatus process is detached from the superior mesenteric artery and vein. The inferior pancreatoduodenal artery is exposed during this detachment process. This artery is preserved as much as possible, but branches of the anteroinferior pancreatoduodenal artery that flow into the pancreatic tissue may be separated. As

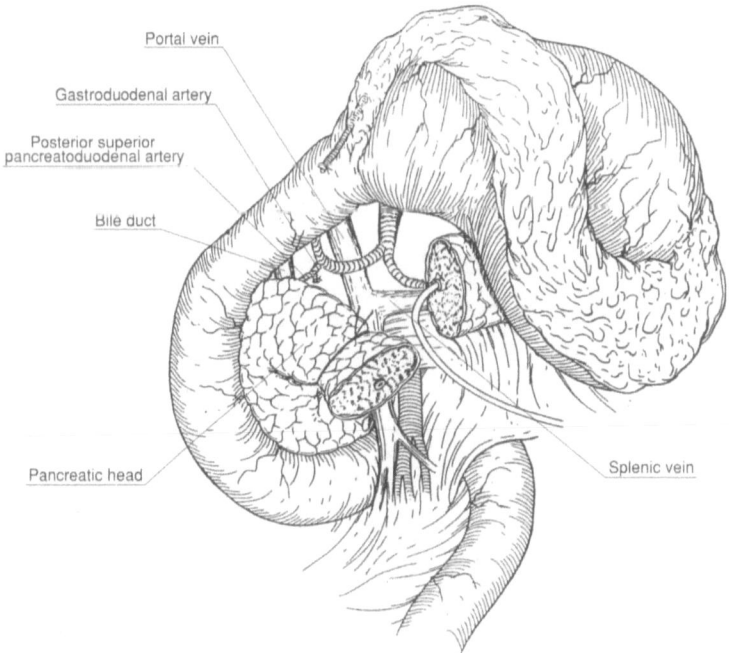

Fig. 5. Treatment of the anterosuperior pancreatoduodenal artery

the posteroinferior pancreatoduodenal artery is detached downward from the pancreatic parenchyma, it is seen to communicate with the posterosuperior pancreatodudenal artery. However, its branches may be ligated and cut at their entry into the resected portion of the pancreas if the mesoduodenal vessels are confirmed to be preserved.

Resection of the Pancreatic Head

When detachment of the bile duct is advanced toward the papilla while lifting the pancreatic head, the pancreatic duct is seen to join the bile duct. The pancreatic duct is ligated and separated at this site. As the pancreas is detached from the duodenum by lifting the pancreatic head eventually to the duodenal papilla, the pancreatic head is resected by carefully preserving the papilla (Fig. 6).

Reconstruction of the Digestive Tract

After confirmation of preservation of the duodenal blood flow (note the absence of color changes in the duodenal wall), the remaining pancreas is anastomosed end-to-side with the duodenum 1–2 cm above the duodenal papilla (Fig. 7).

First, the posterior wall of the pancreas is fixed to the duodenal serosa by intermittent suture using a 3-0 nylon thread. Then, a small hole is made in the duodenal wall opposite the caudal pancreatic duct. A small hole is opened in the anterior wall of the stomach; dissection forceps are inserted, and their tips are brought slightly out of the duodenum through the hole made in the duodenal wall. The end of the pancreatic

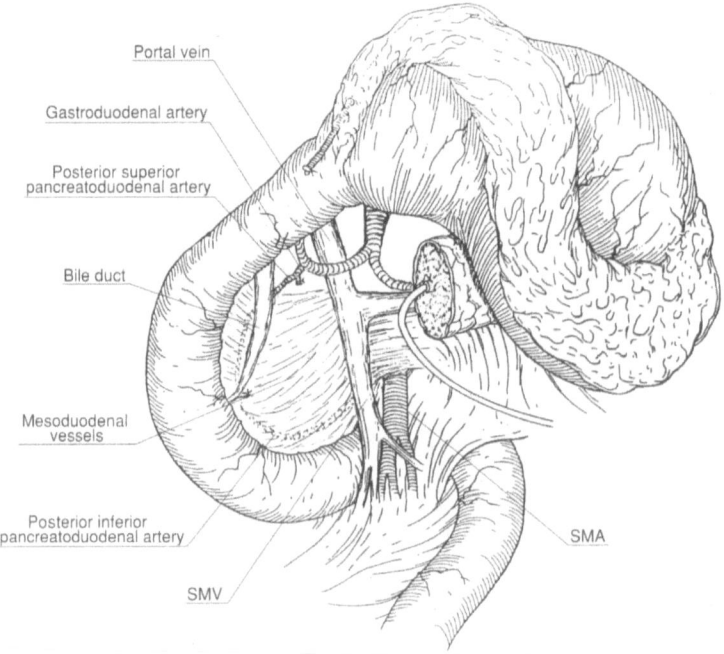

FIG. 6. Resection of the pancreatic head

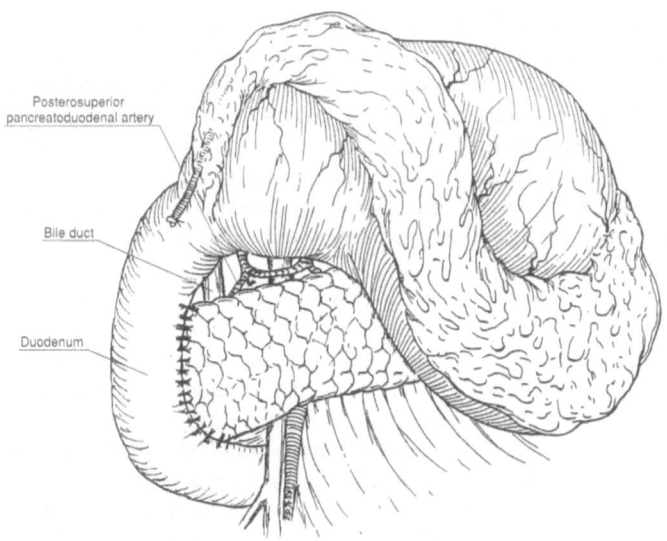

FIG. 7. Pancreatoduodenostomy

tube is held with the tips of the dissection forceps, and it is pulled out transgastrically. Next, the pancreatic duct and the duodenal mucosa are sutured by five or six stitches of intermittent suture using vicryl 5-0. The anterior aspect of the pancreatic stump and the duodenal serosa are then sutured by intermittent suture using a nylon 3-0 thread. The pancreatic duct tube is fixed in the anterior wall of the stomach by Witzel's method.

Installation of Peritoneal Drains

A Penrose drain is inserted into the upper margin of the site of the pancreatoduodenostomy and the posterior aspect of the spleen, and the abdomen is closed.

Discussion

How to maintain the duodenal blood flow is an important point in complete duodenum-preserving pancreatic head resection. The importance of this problem is understood from the fact that various methods have been developed to maintain the duodenal blood flow. Historically, in 1980 Beger et al. [5] reported duodenum-preserving pancreatic head resection. They preserved the duodenal blood flow by leaving 5–10mm of pancreatic parenchyma on the duodenal side. In 1984, Warren et al. [10] reported duodenum-preserving pancreatic head resection with a denervated pancreatic flap. In their procedure, also, pancreatic parenchyma was left on the duodenal wall for complete preservation of the gastroduodenal artery system to maintain the duodenal blood flow. In 1987, Frey et al. [11] described a procedure to cut out part of the pancreatic parenchyma in the pancreatic head. However, pancreatic tissue was also left 3–4mm from the duodenal wall to preserve the duodenal blood flow.

On the other hand, Lambert et al. [12] in 1987 performed duodenum-preserving total pancreatectomy by extending the pancreatic resection line from the duodenal margin. They reported that the color of the duodenum became dusky blue during the operation, suggesting impairment of the blood flow, but that intraoperative responses to stimulation were maintained well and that there were no clinical problems except for duodenal edema observed during the postoperative period. In this procedure, no pancreatic parenchyma was left medially to the duodenum so that the duodenum is considered to have been supplied entirely by the blood flow through the duodenal wall.

In 1993, Takada et al. [8] reported that the color of the second portion of the duodenum changed intraoperatively, so that the procedure had to be changed to PPPD, in the 3 early cases that received Kocher's maneuver simultaneously with separation of the gastroduodenal artery of the 11 cases undergoing duodenum-preserving pancreatic head resection. However, they succeeded in complete duodenum-preserving pancreatic head resection without impairment of the duodenal blood flow in the following 8 consecutive cases by preserving the anterosuperior pancreatoduodenal artery and not performing Kocher's maneuver. On the basis of our clinical experience, we would like to emphasize the importance of (1) preservation of the posterosuperior pancreatoduodenal artery and (2) preservation of retroperitoneal vessels and mesoduodenal vessels by avoiding Kocher's maneuver.

Complete duodenum-preserving pancreatic head resection, as described here, has enlarged the indication of Beger's operation from chronic pancreatitis further to benign pancreatic head tumor and mucin-producing tumor of the pancreatic head. Also, in Beger's operation, bile juice flows into the duodenum but pancreatic juice flows into the jejunum as a result of Roux-en-Y pancreatojejunostomy. Our procedure, however, which allows influx of not only bile juice but also pancreatic juice into the duodenum as a consequence of the pancreatoduodenostomy, is considered to be more physiological than Beger's operation with regard to mixing of the digestive juices with food.

References

1. Takada T (1993) Pylorus-preserving pancreatoduodenectomy: technique and indications. Hepato-Gastroenterology 40:422–425
2. Yasuda H, Takada T, Uchiyama K, Hasegawa H (1993) Social function following pylorus-preserving pancreaticoduodenectomy for cancer of the head of the pancreas. Asian J Surg 16:228–231
3. Traverso LW, Longmire WP Jr (1978) Preservation of the pylorus in pancreatoduodenectomy. Surg Gynecol Obstet 146:959–962
4. Takada T, Yasuda H, Uchiyama K, et al (1989) Postprandial plasma gastrin and secretin concentrations after a pancreatoduodenectomy: a comparison between a pylorus-preserving pancreatoduodenectomy and the Whipple procedure. Ann Surg 210:47–51
5. Beger HG, Witte CH, Krautzbeger W, et al (1980) Erfahrung mit einer das Duodenum erhaltenden Pankreaskopfresection bei chronischer Pankreatitis. Chirurg 51:303–307
6. Takada T, Yasuda H, Uchiyama K, Hasegawa H, Iwagaki T, Yamakawa Y (1994) A proposed new pancreatic classification system according to segments: operative procedure for a medial pancreatic segmentectomy. J Hep Bil Pancr Surg 1:322–325
7. Yasuda H, Takada T, Uchiyama K, Hasegawa H, Tuchiya S, Iwagaki T, Narasaki Y, Shikata J (1990) Resection of the head of the pancreas with preservation of biliary tract and duodenum (in Japanese). Tan to Sui (J Biliary Tract Pancreas) 11:967–973

8. Takada T, Yasuda H, Uchiyama K, Hasegawa H (1993) Duodenum-preserving pancreatoduodenostomy: a new technique for complete excision of the head of the pancreas with preservation of biliary and alimentary integrity. Hepato-Gastroenterology 40:356–359
9. Takada T, Yasuda H, Uchiyama K, Hasegawa H, Iwagaki T, Yamakawa Y (1995) Complete duodenum-preserving resection of the head of the pancreas with preservation of the biliary tract. J Hepato Biliary Pancr Surg 2:32–37
10. Warren WD, Millikan WJ Jr, Henderson JM, et al (1984) A denervated pancreatic flap for control of chronic pain in pancreatitis. Surg Gynecol Obstet 159:581–583
11. Frey CF, Smith GJ (1987) Description and rationale of a new operation for chronic pancreatitis. Pancreas 2:701–707
12. Lambert MA, Linehan IP, Russell RCG (1987) Duodenum-preserving total pancreatectomy for end-stage chronic pancreatitis. Br J Surg 74:35–39

Duodenum-Preserving Total Resection of the Head of the Pancreas with Pancreaticocholedochoduodenostomy

N. Harada, T. Imaizumi, M. Suzuki, T. Nakasako, T. Hatori, and F. Hanyu

Summary. A duodenum-preserving total resection of the head of the pancreas (DpTRHP) with pancreaticocholedochoduodenostomy was carried out in 20 patients with periampullary benign disease. The postoperative results of DpTRHP were assessed in comparison with the results in a control group of 20 patients with periampullary benign disease who underwent pylorus-preserving pancreatoduodenectomy (PpPD) with gastropancreaticobiliary reconstruction. In the patients with DpTRHP, complications developed in 5 patients, including duodenal leakage ($n = 4$) that was thought to be associated with duodenal ischemia, but was managed conservatively, and distal bile duct necrosis ($n = 1$), which required reoperation. There was no mortality during hospital stay. The mean postoperative hospitalization period was 41.5 days, and postoperative weight gain at 6 months in comparison with preoperative weight (100%) averaged 99.4%; 90% of the patients were professionally rehabilitated. These early postoperative results were acceptable compared with that of PpPD. The secretin secretion test in response to a test meal and the pancreatic function diagnostant (PFD) test were carried out postoperatively in comparison with those of the patients who had undergone PpPD. The integrated secretion of secretin in response to a test meal 2h after ingestion was 9.0 ng-min./ml in patients with DpTRHP, higher than that in patients with PpPD (7.5 ng-min./ml). The PFD value at 1 year after the operation decreased to 64% of the preoperative value in patients with PpPD but was preserved in patients with DpTRHP (88%). These data suggest that preservation of the duodenum contributes in part to maintain the exocrine function of the pancreas in the late postoperative course, DpTRHP is feasible in some patients with benign disease that requires pancreatic head resection.

Key words. Duodenum-preserving pancreas head resection—Pylorus-preserving pancreatoduodenectomy—Gastrointestinal hormone—Exocrine pancreatic function

Department of Gastroenterological Surgery, Tokyo Women's Medical College, Shinjuku-ku, Tokyo 162, Japan.

Introduction

The one-stage pancreatoduodenectomy primarily described by Whipple [1] in 1945 has been used for the management of periampullary cancer or benign diseases that require pancreatic head resection. Although the consensus is that surgical resection is the only curative modality for malignant diseases [2,3], some surgeons are doubtful of applying the Whipple operation for patients with benign diseases because of the high morbidity and postoperative malnutrition. With advances in perioperative management, postoperative malnutrition has been improved, but some patients still suffer from postoperative digestive dysfunction. A pylorus-preserving pancreatoduodenectomy (PpPD) originally advocated by Traverso and Longmire [4] in 1978 is now widely employed for the management of periampullary disease with good results. More physiological, organ-preserving pancreatectomies have recently been reported by several authors [5–8]. Since 1989, we have performed a duodenum-preserving total resection of the head of the pancreas (DpTRHP) with pancreaticocholedochoduodenostomy [8]. This chapter concerns the operative procedure of DpTRHP and its postoperative results, including the assessment of gastrointestinal hormone secretion and exocrine pancreatic function in 20 patients.

Operative Procedure of DpTRHP

The remarkable feature of this procedure is to resect the whole part of the pancreatic head without resection of the duodenum. The blood supply to the duodenal bulb and the transverse portion of the duodenum is maintained by the supraduodenal artery and the duodenal branches from the inferior pancreatoduodenal artery, respectively. The blood supply to the descending portion of the duodenum depends on intramural blood flow. As Kocher's maneuver is not performed, venous blood from the duodenum is drained via the retroperitoneum to the portal vein.

After the right gastroepiploic artery and vein are dissected, the common hepatic artery is identified and the gastroduodenal artery is ligated and divided. Then the pancreas is divided on the right border of the portal vein. While lifting the cut edge of the pancreatic head forward, small vessels toward the portal vein are ligated and divided as close to the pancreas as possible, so as not to injure the mesoduodenal vessels. The common bile duct is divided from behind the pancreas head and the pancreas head is separated from the duodenum, taking care not to damage the duodenal wall. Neither pancreatic parenchyma nor the arterial arcade remain around the duodenum. At the ampulla of Vater and accessory papilla, the common duct and accessory pancreatic duct are exposed extramurally. Total resection of the head of the pancreas is completed by ligation and division of these ducts (Fig. 1).

The reconstruction is made by end-to-side pancreaticoduodenostomy (two-layer suture) and end-to-side choledochoduodenostomy (one-layer suture). The pancreaticoduodenostomy is normally positioned at the descending part of the duodenum, near the ampulla of Vater. In performing the innter-layer anastomosis or extraluminal pancreatic duct-to-duct anastomoses, or if the ampulla of Vater is excised, duodenal mucosa-to-duct anastomoses are available. The choledochoduodenostomy is placed on the duodenal bulb in the usual manner. Because no part of the gastrointestinal (GI) tract is resected or interrupted, gastrointestinal anastomoses are not necessary (Fig. 2).

FIG. 1. The whole pancreas head is excised, preserving the duodenum without Kocher's maneuver [9]

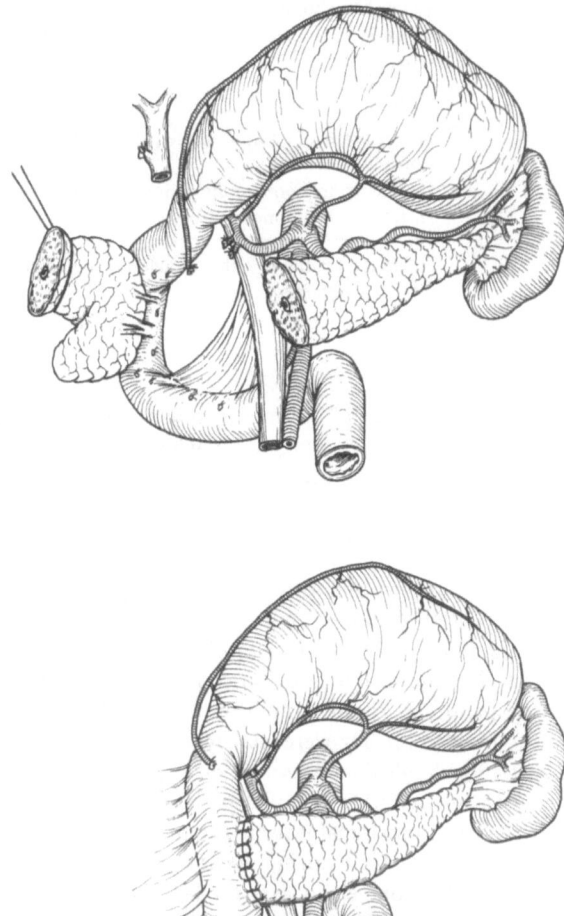

FIG. 2. End-to-side pancreaticoduodenostomy and end-to-side choledochoduodenostomy are accomplished [9]

Patients

During the period from 1989 to 1994, DpTRHP was performed in 20 patients with periampullary benign disease in the Department of Gastroenterological Surgery, Tokyo Women's Medical College. The male-to-female ratio of the patients was 1:1 and the mean age was 52.5 years (range, 26–70 years). The clinical diagnoses of this series of the patients were mucin-producing tumor (10), chronic pancreatitis (8), including 4 patients with an anomalous arrangement of the pancreatic and bile duct system, serous cystadenoma (1), and distal bile duct tumor (1) (Table 1). The postoperative results of DpTRHP in the 20 patients were assessed in comparison with the results in a control group of 20 patients with periampullary benign disease who underwent PpPD with gastropancreaticobiliary reconstruction. The difference be-

TABLE 1. Clinical diagnosis in 20 patients who received a duodenum-preserving total resection of the head of the pancreas (DpTRHP)

Diagnosis	Patients (n)
Mucin-producing tumor of the pancreas head	10
Chronic pancreatitis[a]	8
Serous cystadenoma of the pancreas head	1
Distal bile duct tumor	1

[a] Includes 4 patients with anomalous arrangement of pancreatic and bile duct system.

tween DpTRHP and PpPD is merely whether the descending and transverse portion of the duodenum exists and in which order the pancreaticoduodenostomy and choledochoduodenostomy are done.

Postoperative Assessment

Morbidity during a 2-month postoperative period was seen in 5 of 20 patients (25%) in the DpTRHP group as compared with 6 of 20 patients (30%) in the PpPD group. The most common early complication in the DpTRHP group was duodenal leakage, including leakage of the pancreaticoduodenostomy (2) and leakage at the duodenal suture point (2). These complications were thought to be associated with ischemia of the duodenum but were managed conservatively. One patient who underwent DpTRHP with bile duct preservation required reoperation because of distal bile duct necrosis. In the PpPD group, 3 patients developed anastomotic leakage, including pancreaticojejunostomal leakage (2) and choledochojejunostomal leakage (1). There was no operative death during the hospital stay in either group. The mean postoperative hospitalization period was 41.5 days for the DpTRHP group and 37.5 days for the PpPD group, the difference not being statistically significant. Postoperative weight gain at 6 months in comparison with preoperative weight (100%) averaged 99.4% for the DpTRHP group and 101% for the PpPD group. The proportion of patients who could return to their profession was 90% in both groups (Table 2).

A secretin secretion test in response to a test meal was carried out in five patients at 1 month after surgery. After 12h of fasting, each patient ingested a 580 kcal test meal, and serial blood samples were obtained at 15, 30, 60, 90, and 120 min after ingestion. The integrated secretion of secretin was compared with that of the patients who had undergone PpPD ($n = 4$). The integrated secretion of plasma secretin after taking the test meal was 9.0 ± 1.5 ng-min./ml in patients with DpTRHP, higher than that in patients with PpPD ($7.5 \pm .8$ ng-min./ml). No significant difference, however, was noted in this evaluation (Fig. 3).

Pancreatic function diagnostant (PFD) tests were carried out in six patients at 6 and 12 months postoperatively. The PFD test was carried out after 3 days' interruption of medication, and the ratio to the preoperative value was estimated in comparison with the PpPD group ($n = 4$). The PFD value at 1 year after the operation decreased to 64% of the preoperative value in patients with PpPD but was preserved in patients with DpTRHP (88%) (Fig. 4).

TABLE 2. Comparison of postoperative results between DpTRHP and PpPD

Result	DpTRHP ($n = 20$)	PpPD ($n = 20$)
Morbidity	25%	30%
Duodenal leakage	4	
Necrosis of distal bile duct	1	
Pa-Je anastomotic leakage		2
Ch-Je anastomotic leakage		1
Marginal ulceration		1
Gastric stasis		2
Mortality	0%	0%
Hospital stay (mean)	41.5 days	37.5 days
Body weight gain	99.4%	101%
Professional rehabilitation	90%	90%

PpPD, pylorus-preserving pancreatoduodenectomy; Pa-Je, pancreatojejuno; Ch-Je, choledochojejuno.

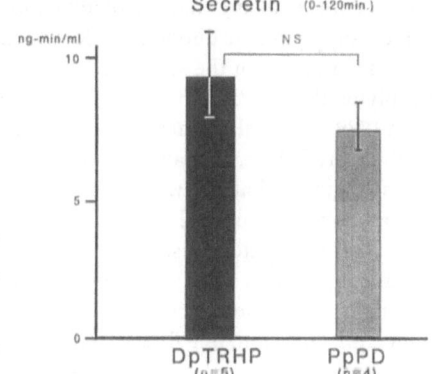

FIG. 3. Comparison of integrated secretion of secretin between duodenum-preserving total resection of the head of the pancreas (*DpTRHP*; *black bar*) and pylorus-preserving pancreato-duodenectomy (*PpPD*; *shaded bar*) in response to test meal [10]

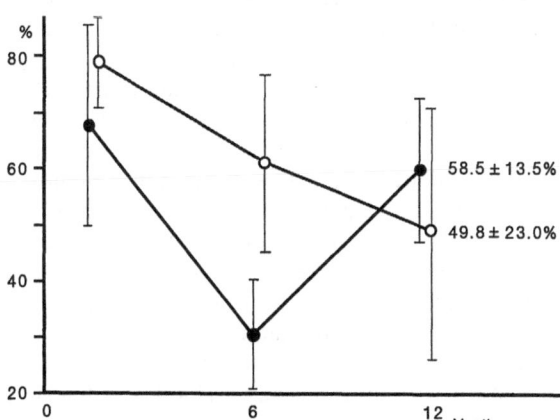

FIG. 4. Changes in pancreatic function diagnostant test before and after DpTRHP (*closed circles*; $n = 6$) and PpPD (*open circles*; $n = 4$) [10]

Discussion

Since Traverso and Longmire [4] reported the PpPD in 1978 with good results, this operation has been widely employed not only for the treatment of periampullary cancer but also for benign diseases [11,12] and has reduced the nutritional disability that follows pancreaticoduodenectomy [13]. Furthermore, some new surgical procedures attempting to preserve gastrointestinal and pancreatic function have been reported by several authors [5–8]. Beger et al. [6] reported a duodenum-preserving subtotal resection of the head of the pancreas for patients with severe chronic pancreatitis, leaving the common bile duct and a rim of pancreatic tissue between the wall of the duodenum and the common bile duct. Beger et al. stated that the mesoduodenal vessels should be preserved but that preservation of the gastroduodenal artery is not mandatory for duodenal blood flow. It has long been thought that separation of the pancreatic head from the duodenum was impossible, because they are closely related both anatomically and embryologically and their blood supply depends on the anterior and posterior arcade between gastroduodenal artery and inferior pancreatoduodenal artery. Lambert et al. [14] reported a two-stage duodenum-preserving total pancreatectomy for patients with end-stage chronic pancreatitis, showing that the blood supply to the duodenum was maintained by the vessels supplying the duodenal bulb, which receive their blood from the epiploic arch, and the branches of the superior mesenteric artery that course along the duodenum, supplying the fourth part of the duodenum.

In 1989, Ryo et al. [7] made a success of DpTRHP with a Roux-en-Y reconstruction. In their procedure, and also in our procedure, the gastroduodenal artery is divided at its origin so that the whole pancreatic head can be resected. The significance of complete excision of the head of the pancreas is that this procedure can be applied not only for inflammatory diseases but also for benign neoplastic tumors such as mucin-producing tumors, avoiding remnant lesion. Since 1989, we have performed DpTRHP and pancreaticocholedochoduodenostomy as previously described [8,9,15]. As both pancreatic juice and bile flow into the preserved duodenum, this reconstruction must be more physiological than Roux-en-Y reconstruction in terms of maintenance of chemical neutrality in the duodenum and secretion of the gastrointestinal hormones. Furthermore, continuity of the upper GI tract is not interrupted and innervation of the vagal nerve is preserved as much as possible, so that movement of the GI tract is maintained. In our series of patients, the postoperative barium meal examination showed normal contraction of the duodenum.

Concerning the role of the duodenum in postprandial release of gastrointestinal hormones, Malfertheiner et al. [16] reported that after duodenectomy cholecystokinin (CCK-8), gastric inhibitory polypeptide (GIP), and neurotensin (they did not measure secretin) exhibited a normal response to the test meal in duodenectomized dogs, and they suggested that the remaining proximal small bowel was sufficient to achieve normal levels. In this study, however, the postoperative assessment of secretin secretion in response to a test meal showed a tendency toward greater secretion in patients who had undergone DpTRHP than in those with PpPD. The PFD test 1 year after the operation indicated that pancreatic function decreased to 64% of the preoperative value in PpPD but was preserved at 88% in DpTRHP. It has been known that more than 80% of secretin-releasing cells localize in the duodenum, and some gastrointestinal hormones such as secretin and CCK have a trophic effect on the pancreas [17,18]. It seems reasonable to assume, therefore, that preservation of the duodenum contributes in part to maintain the exocrine function of the pancreas in the late postoperative course.

Conclusion

DpTRHP is feasible in some patients with benign disease that requires pancreatic head resection. We consider that it has advantages in terms of preservation of gastrointestinal hormone secretion and the exocrine function of the pancreas.

References

1. Whipple AO (1945) Pancreaticoduodenectomy for islet carcinoma: 5-year follow-up. Ann Surg 121:847–852
2. Hanyu F, Suzuki M, Imaizumi T (1993) Whipple operation for pancreatic carcinoma: Japanese experience. In: Beger HG, Büchler M, Malfertheiner P (eds) Standards in pancreatic surgery. Springer, Berlin Heidelberg New York, pp 646–653
3. Suzuki M, Hanyu F, Imaizumi T, Nakasako T, Harada N (1993) Indications for extended radical Whipple operation for ductal adenocarcinoma of the head of the pancreas. In: Takahashi T (ed) Recent advances in management of digestive cancers. Springer, Berlin Heidelberg New York Tokyo, pp 751–752
4. Traverso LW, Longmire WP Jr (1978) Preservation of the pylorus in pancreaticoduodenectomy. Surg Gynecol Obstet 146:959–962
5. Warren WD, Millikan WJ Jr, Henderson JM, Hersh T (1984) A denervated pancreatic flap for control of chronic pain in pancreatitis. Surg Gynecol Obstet 159:581–583
6. Beger HG, Witte C, Kraas E, Bittner R (1980) Erfahrung mit einer das Duodenum erhaltenden Pankreaskopfresektion bei chrinischer Pankreatitis (in German). Chirurg 51:303–307
7. Ryo H, Hanyu F, Watayo T, Toda H, Imaizumi T (1990) A new procedure for total resection of the head of the pancreas with duodenal preservation (in Japanese). Operation 44:447–451
8. Imaizumi T, Hanyu F, Suzuki M, Nakasako T, Matsuyama H, Ogata S, Yoshii K, Kimura T, Komatsu E, Harada N (1990) A new procedure duodenum-preserving total resection of the head of the pancreas with pancreatico- and choledochoduodenostomy (in Japanese). J Biliary Pancr 11:621–626
9. Imaizumi T, Hanyu F, Suzuki M, Nakasako T, Harada N, Hatori T (1995) Clinical experience with duodenum-preserving total resection of the head of the pancreas with pancreaticocholedochoduodenostomy. J Hepato Biliary Pancr Surg 2:38–44
10. Harada N (1994) Digestive functions and secretion of gastrointestinal hormones after duodenum-preserving pancreas head resection (in Japanese). Jpn J Gastroenterol Surg 27:781–788
11. Rossi RL, Rothschild J, Braasch JW (1987) Pancreatoduodenectomy in the management of chronic pancreatitis. Arch Surg 122:416–420
12. Hanyu F, Suzuki M, Imaizumi T (1990) Resection of the head of the pancreas in the treatment of chronic pancreatitis. In: Beger HG, Büchler M, Ditschineit H, Malfertheiner P (eds) Chronic pancreatitis. Springer, Berlin Heidelberg New York, pp 490–495
13. Braasch JW, Rossi RL, Watkins E Jr, Deziel DJ, Winter PF (1986) Pyloric and gastric preserving pancreatic resection. Ann Surg 204:411–418
14. Lambert MA, Linehan IP, Russell RCG (1987) Duodenum-preserving total pancreatectomy for end stage chronic pancreatitis. Br J Surg 74:35–39
15. Imaizumi T, Hanyu F, Suzuki M (1993) A new procedure for duodenum-preserving total resection of the head of the pancreas with pancreaticocholedochoduodenostomy. In: Beger HG, Büchler M, Malfertheiner P (eds) Standards in pancreatic surgery. Springer, Berlin Heidelberg New York, pp 464–470

16. Malfertheiner P, Sarr MG, Nelson DK, DiMagno EP (1994) Role of the duodenum in postprandial release of pancreatic and gastrointestinal hormones. Pancreas 9:13–19
17. Johnson LR (1976) The trophic action of gastrointestinal hormones. Gastroenterology 70:278–288
18. Dembinski AB, Johnson LR (1980) Stimulation of pancreatic growth by secretin, caerulein and pentagastrin. Endocrinology 16:323–328

Duodenum-Preserving Resection of the Head of the Pancreas in Patients with Chronic Pancreatitis or Low-Grade Malignancy

Toshiyuki Takahashi, Hiroyuki Katoh, Shunichi Okushiba, Mitsuru Dohke, Haruchika Ikenaga, and Toshiji Motohara

Summary. Duodenum-preserving resection of the head of the pancreas was performed in 41 patients with chronic pancreatitis and 23 with pancreatic neoplastic lesions. Denervation of the body and tail of the pancreas was added for the patients with chronic pancreatitis. The major advantage of this procedure is that only the small pancreas head is resected, leaving the endocrine and exocrine systems functioning normally. This procedure provides complete pain relief for the patients with chronic pancreatitis; 92% of patients experienced alleviation of pain and no recurrence. Postoperatively, 76% of patients could work well, and 87% maintained their preoperative body weight. Postoperative glucose tolerance test showed 21% of the patients with preoperative diabetic pattern improved to the nondiabetic pattern between 3 months and 3 years after surgery. In 23 patients with pancreatic neoplasms, 22 patients were alive during the follow-up period with no recurrence of the tumor, except 1 patient who died of acute myocardial infarction. We concluded that our procedure allows patients with chronic pancreatitis to be free from intractable pain and to maintain good endocrine function of the pancreas. Furthermore, this procedure can be applied to patients with low-grade malignant lesions of the pancreas.

Key words. Pancreas head resection—Chronic pancreatitis—Denervation—Endocrine function—Cystadenoma of the pancreas

Introduction

The clinical course of chronic pancreatitis is characterized by abdominal pain and often progresses to narcotic dependence. The major indication for surgical treatment is unrelenting pain. However, the progression to end-stage levels of functional impairment of the pancreas has never been arrested by any surgical procedure. We appreciated the usefulness of the duodenum-preserving resection of the head of the pancreas reported by Beger et al. [1] in 1980. However, we supposed that abdominal pain could be more effectively alleviated by a modification with complete dissection of the nerve plexus around the remnant pancreas. The primary advantage of our proce-

Second Department of Surgery, Hokkaido University School of Medicine, Sapporo, Hokkaido 060, Japan.

dure compared with others is that only a small portion of the pancreas is resected, allowing the drainage of pancreatic juice and preservation of the exocrine and endocrine function of the pancreas.

Moreover, we presumed that this procedure could be indicated for patients with low-grade malignancy in the head of the pancreas, such as mucinous cystadenoma, cystadenocarcinoma, and serous cystadenoma that was localized in the pancreas. In this study, we report the long-term results of our procedure in patients with severe chronic pancreatitis and low-grade malignancy in the pancreas head.

Patients and Methods

Surgical Methods

Our procedure of the duodenum-preserving resection of the head of the pancreas is begun through a bilateral subcostal incision. The pancreas is exposed by entering the lesser sac through the gastrocolic ligament. Before resection of the pancreas, we usually perform Kocher's maneuver to mobilize the pancreas head with the duodenum. This procedure is not disadvantageous for blood supply to the duodenum. Moreover, it is necessary for safe, complete resection of the head of the pancreas. We then dissect the hepatoduodenal ligament at the point on the head of the pancreas to find the common hepatic artery, the gastroduodenal artery (GD), and the portal vein. Consecutively, we dissect the superior mesenteric vein at the point under the pancreas. Vascular tapes are put on all these vessels. Preservation of the GD is required to maintain enough blood flow to the duodenum.

Resection is begun by dividing the pancreas at the right side of the portal vein in patients with chronic pancreatitis. If a neoplastic lesion is over the junction of the head and neck of the pancreas, we convert the dividing line so as to remove the tumor

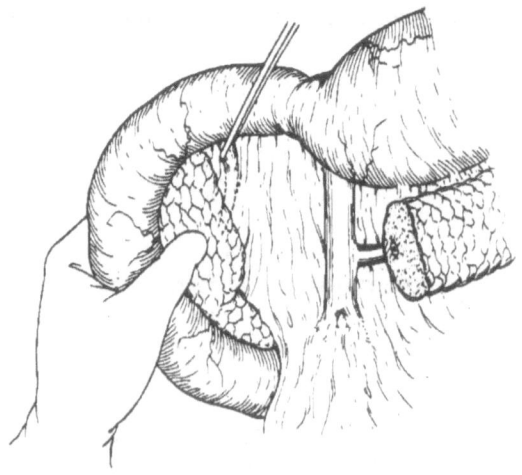

FIG. 1. Preservation of the common bile duct (CBD). The CBD should be carefully dissected and a vascular tape put around the CBD to preserve it. A small amount of pancreatic tissue behind the CBD is left to maintain the blood flow to CBD. The intrapancreatic bile duct is resected, and choledochoduodenostomy is performed in cases with jaundice or severe stenosis of the intrapancreatic bile duct

completely. Then, the pancreas surrounded by the duodenum is resected. The posterior superior pancreatoduodenal artery (PSPD) and the anterior superior pancreatoduodenal artery are taped, and their duodenal branches are preserved. The intrapancreatic common bile duct (CBD) is carefully dissected and taped (Fig. 1). A slight amount of pancreas tissue behind the CBD is left to preserve the blood supply to the CBD. In patients with stenosis of the intrapancreatic segment of the CBD, choledochoduodenostomy should be chosen. The inferior pancreatoduodenal artery, a branch of the superior mesenteric artery, is also preserved in removal of the uncinate lobe of the pancreas (Fig. 2).

Following removal of the pancreas head, the somatic nerve fibers around the splenic artery are dissected (Fig. 3). Reconstruction with drainage of pancreatic secretions from the remnant pancreas into the upper intestinal tract is performed by pancreatojejunostomy using a Roux-en-Y jejunal loop. In patients with dilatation of

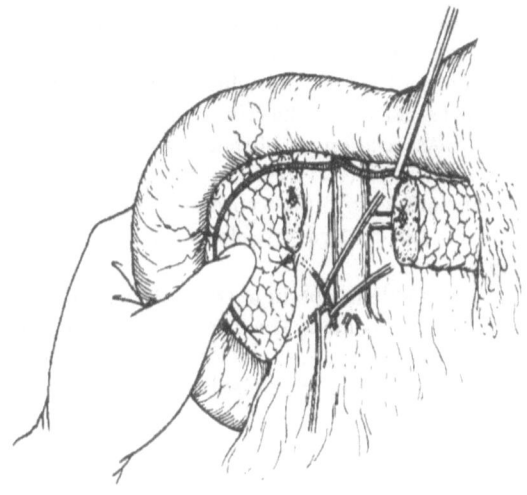

FIG. 2. Resection of the uncinate lobe. The inferior pancreatoduodenal artery is detected in the tissue behind the uncinate lobe, and a vascular tape is put on it to preserve it

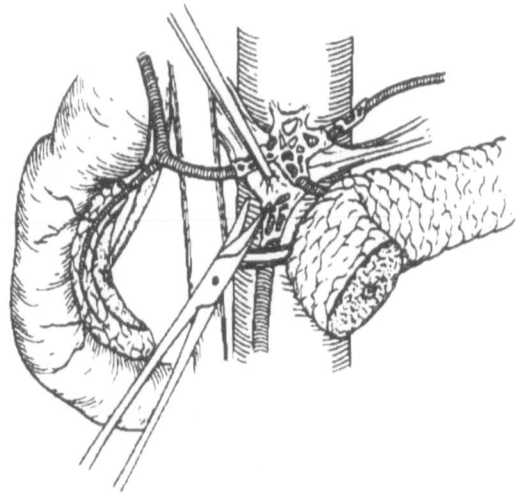

FIG. 3. Denervation of the remnant pancreas. Somatic nerve fibers around the splenic artery are dissected to denervate the remnant pancreas after pancreas head resection

the main duct and multiple pancreatic stones in the remnant pancreas, we perform the Partington modification to remove the stones; i.e., a longitudinal cut is made along the main duct, and side-to-side anastomosis of the duct and the jejunum is performed after removal of the stones (Fig. 4).

Patients with Chronic Pancreatitis

From March 1985 to April 1994, our procedure was performed in 41 patients with chronic pancreatitis, 34 men and 7 women aged from 19 to 74 years, with an average of 49 years. The period of time from the onset of abdominal pain until surgery ranged from 4 months to 26 years, with an average of 4.8 years. The etiology of the disease was alcohol related in 34 (82.9%) of the patients and idiopathic in 7. In all 41 patients, ultrasound (US), computerized tomography (CT), and endoscopic retrograde cholangiopancreatography (ERCP) were carried out for preoperative diagnosis. Celiac and superior mesenteric arteriography were performed in 34 patients. Surgical indication was intractable pain in 37 (90.2%) of the patients and suspected cancer in 4.

Preoperative and postoperative pancreatic endocrine function of all patients was evaluated by the 75-g oral glucose tolerance test (OGTT). Then the patients were classified according to the criteria specified by the Diagnosis Committee of the Japan Diabetes Association established in 1979 [2]; the categories are normal, glucose tolerance impairment (GTI), and diabetes mellitus (DM). Preoperatively, we classified the patients into two groups according to the preoperative OGTT findings. Those with a normal or GTI pattern were classified into group A and those with a DM pattern into group B.

We were able to obtain postoperative information from 39 (95.1%) of the 41 patients by direct contact. The median follow-up period was 36 months, the range being 3 months to 9 years. Postoperative conditions concerning abdominal pain, return to the workforce, and body weight were appraised in April 1994.

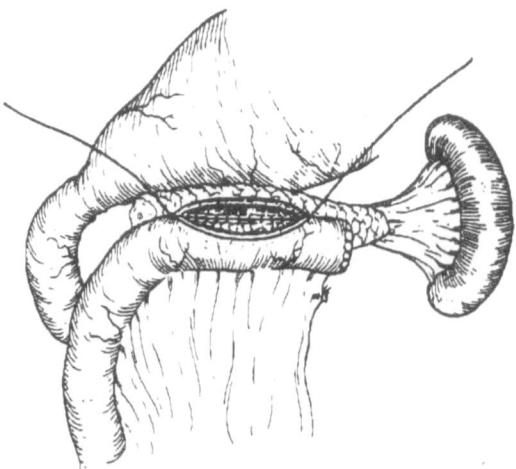

FIG. 4. Longitudinal pancreatojejunostomy in patients with dilatation and multiple stones of the main pancreatic duct. The Partington modification, i.e., a longitudinal cut along the main duct and side-to-side anastomosis of the duct and the jejunum, is performed in cases with dilatation of the main duct and multiple stones in the remnant pancreas

Patients with a Neoplastic Lesion of the Head of the Pancreas

We have applied duodenum-preserving pancreas head resection to a total of 23 patients, 14 men and 9 women, with pancreatic neoplasms. Patient age ranged from 15 to 72 years (average, 59.8 years). Preoperative imaging such as US, CT, and ERCP was performed in all these cases. Cytological examination of pancreatic juice was also carried out in several cases. The preoperative diagnoses of these patients were 17 mucinous cystadenomas, 3 serous cystadenomas, 2 solid and cystic tumors, and 1 nonfunctioning islet cell tumor. Thus, malignancy was not proved preoperatively in any case. During surgical treatment of these patients, we did not dissect the regional lymph nodes or the nerve plexus around the pancreas. The CBD was preserved in all patients.

Postoperatively, histopathological examination revealed that there was malignancy in 4 of 17 patients with mucinous cystadenomas. However, we did not perform additional resection because these cases were all carcinomas with no invasion into the surrounding tissue. The follow-up period ranged from 1 month to 80 months, an average of 30.0 months.

Results

Operative Results

In patients with chronic pancreatitis, secondary surgery was necessary for 1 patient because of bleeding from the cut edge of the pancreas 5 days after surgery. The period of hospitalization for the patients with pancreatitis was 22–129 days, with a median of 47 days. There was no hospital mortality in these 41 patients. On the other hand, there was 1 hospital death from acute myocardial infarction 1 month after surgery in the 23 patients with low-grade malignancy. Total mortality in this study was 1.6%.

Effectiveness in Regard to Pain Relief and Quality of Life in Patients with Chronic Pancreatitis

Thirty-seven patients required pain medication preoperatively. Symptoms of pain completely disappeared in 31 of the patients (84%) after surgery. In 3 of these 37 patients, there was improvement of pain. Another 3 patients required amelioration or occasional hospitalization because of recurrent abdominal pain or discomfort (Fig. 5a).

Twenty-eight patients (76%) were working well postoperatively, while 6 patients (16%) were unable to work well. Altogether, 92% of the patients returned to work. Only 3 patients have complained about social disability. Two of these 3 patients have occasionally been institutionalized with recurrent abdominal pain, and 1 became a habitual drinker (Fig. 5b). Thirty-four patients (87%) maintained more than ±10% of preoperative body weight (Fig. 5c). None of the patients had severe steatorrhea postoperatively.

Endocrine Function of Patients with Chronic Pancreatitis

As stated, we classified the patients into two groups according to the preoperative OGTT findings; group A, normal or GTI pattern of OGTT, consisted of 21 patients (4 normal and 17 GTI pattern). Twenty patients who had already shown a DM pattern

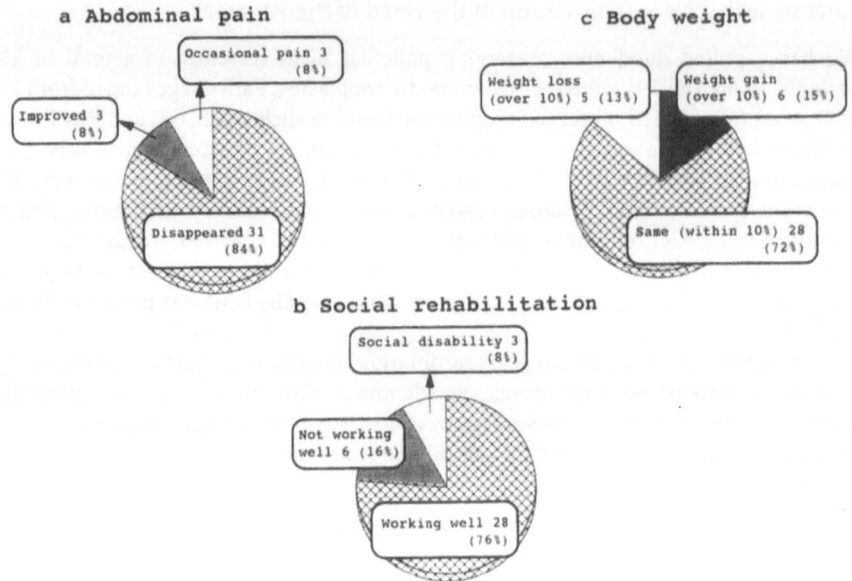

FIG. 5a–c. Postoperative effect of our procedure on relief of pain and quality of life in patients with chronic pancreatitis. **a** Relief of abdominal pain. **b** Social rehabilitation (return to the workforce). **c** Body weight change

before surgery were categorized as group B. The alterations of pancreatic endocrine function of the patients of group A are summarized in Table 1. Within 3 months after surgery, OGTT was examined in 16 patients of the 21 patients of group A. Patients with normal pattern increased from 4 preoperatively to 7 postoperatively. Two patients (12.6%) showed a DM pattern postoperatively, and 1 required insulin therapy. During the period from 3 months to 3 years after surgery, 18 patients were examined. Normal and GTI patterns were found in 7 patients (38.9%) and 5 patients (27.8%), respectively, while 6 patients (33.4%) had the DM pattern. Insulin therapy was necessary for 3 of these patients.

During the period beyond 3 years after surgery, OGTT was performed in 7 patients. Normal and GTI patterns were found in 1 (14.3%) and 3 (42.9%), respectively. There were 3 patients (42.9%) with DM pattern, 2 of whom were treated with insulin. In April 1994 (longest and mean follow-up periods, 9 years and 2 years, respectively), 15 of the 21 patients of group A had maintained endocrine function. The etiology of chronic pancreatitis in 15 of the 21 patients was alcohol related; 5 of the 15 patients had ceased drinking, and 10 had reduced their alcohol consumption compared to preoperative levels. Six patients of group A showed deterioration to DM pattern postoperatively; 3 of these 6 patients required insulin therapy.

The alterations of pancreatic endocrine function of the patients of group B are summarized in Table 2. Seventeen of the 20 patients of group B were examined within 3 months after surgery. One patient (5.9%) recovered to the normal pattern and 4 (23.5%) to the GTI pattern; 12 (70.6%) remained in the DM pattern. Seven of these 12 patients required insulin treatment. When OGTT was evaluated in 19 patients be-

TABLE 1. Alteration of endocrine function in patients of group A

		Postoperative period			
Patterns on OGTT[a]	Preoperative (%)	3 Months (%)	3 Months–3 years (%)	3–5 Years (%)	5 Years (%)
Normal	4/21	7/16	7/18	1/7	
	(19)	(43.8)	(38.9)	(14.3)	
GTI[b]	17/21	7/16	5/18	3/7	1/1
	(81)	(43.8)	(27.8)	(42.9)	(100)
DM[c] (NID[d])		1/16	3/18	1/7	
		(6.3)	(16.7)	(14.3)	
DM[c] (ID[e])		1/16	3/18	2/7	
		(6.3)	(16.7)	(28.6)	

[a] OGTT, Oral glucose tolerance test classified according to the criteria of the Japan Diabetic Society.
[b] GTI, Glucose tolerance impairment.
[c] DM, Diabetes mellitus.
[d] NID, Noninsulin-dependent.
[e] ID, Insulin-dependent.

TABLE 2. Alteration of endocrine function in patients of group B

		Postoperative period			
Patterns on OGTT	Preoperative (%)	3 Months (%)	3 Months–3 years (%)	3–5 Years (%)	5 Years (%)
Normal		1/17			1/3
		(5.9)			(33.3)
GTI		4/17	4/19	1/5	
		(23.5)	(21.1)	(20)	
DM (NID)	13/20	5/17	8/19	2/5	2/3
	(65)	(29.4)	(42.1)	(40)	(66.7)
DM (ID)	7/20	7/17	7/19	2/5	
	(35)	(41.2)	(36.8)	(40)	

tween 3 months and 3 years postoperatively, 4 patients (21.1%) showed amelioration to the GTI pattern. Fifteen (79.0%) remained in DM pattern and 7 required insulin therapy as they had done preoperatively. Five patients were followed postoperatively for more than 3 years after surgery, and 1 patient (20.0%) improved to the GTI pattern 5 years after surgery; 4 of the 5 patients (80.0%) remained in the DM pattern with 2 requiring insulin treatment.

In April 1994 (longest and mean follow-up period, 9 and 2 years, respectively), 4 patients with mild DM in the preoperative condition of group B showed recovery to normal or GTI pattern. Of these 4 patients, 3 had alcohol-related chronic pancreatitis and 1 was idiopathic. Two of the 3 alcohol-related patients could stop drinking, and 1 decreased his alcohol consumption. On the other hand, 7 of the remaining 20 patients of group B had severe DM preoperatively, requiring insulin treatment, and there was no evidence of deterioration in the condition of DM. All 16 patients who exhibited DM before and after surgery were alcoholic; 6 stopped drinking, 5 reduced their alcohol intake, and 5 continued drinking as previously.

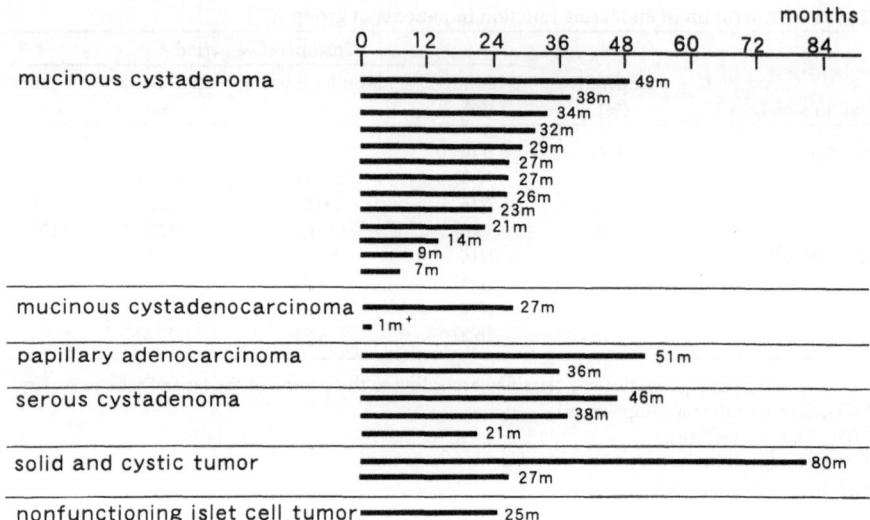

FIG. 6. Survival period of patients with low-grade malignancy. All patients are alive except one hospital death from acute myocardial infarction 1 month after surgery (+). No recurrence was found in any case

Long-Term Survival of Patients with Pancreatic Neoplasms

Twenty-two patients are alive with no recurrence except 1 hospital death from acute myocardial infarction. The survival period ranged from 7 to 80 months with a mean of 30 months (Fig. 6). No patients had complaints concerning abdominal conditions, jaundice, severe steatorrhea, body weight loss, or DM during the postoperative follow-up.

Discussion

The intractable pain of chronic pancreatitis remains a therapeutic problem. The ideal method would obtain reliable control of the pain while preserving endocrine or exocrine function of the pancreas. No definite surgical indications for chronic pancreatitis have been reported, and the selection of operative procedures depends on the surgeon. A major indication for surgical treatment of chronic pancreatitis is medically uncontrolled pain, and we decided operative indications according to this rule. Representative procedures that have been reported thus far are decompression of the pancreatic duct by longitudinal pancreaticojejunostomy and resection of the pancreas. Although pancreaticojejunostomy has had favorable results for the preservation of pancreatic function [3,4], there have been some problems, namely, difficulty in patients without dilatation of the pancreatic duct and incomplete relief of pain despite patent anastomosis [5–7].

In other institutes, subtotal distal pancreatectomy has been applied for patients with severe pancreatic fibrosis and nondilated pancreatic duct [8,9]. However, there are disadvantages such as incomplete long-term pain relief [8] or a high incidence of postoperative DM [9]. In addition to these two surgical procedures, near-total resection of the proximal pancreas by pancreatoduodenectomy has major disadvantages of a high incidence of postoperative DM and mortality from malnutrition, hypoglycemic episodes, or ketoacidosis [10]. We consider this procedure to be an exceedingly invasive treatment for patients with severe chronic pancreatitis.

In 1980, Beger et al. [1] reported duodenum-preserving resection of the head of the pancreas for chronic pancreatitis. This procedure includes resection of the head of the pancreas and pancreaticojejunostomy. They demonstrated excellent results of long-term follow-up in that 77% of patients were completely rehabilitated occupationally and 77% were completely free from abdominal pain. However, Beger et al. [11,12] have also reported that 12% of the patients postoperatively needed hospitalization because of recurrent abdominal pain. We appreciated the usefulness of their procedure and thought that the incidence of recurrent pain could be reduced by a slight modification.

The point of our modification is additional dissection of the nerve plexus around the remnant pancreas [13,14]. We believe this modification is valuable to prevent the abdominal pain of recurrent pancreatitis of the remnant pancreas. On the complete relief of pain, we consider that our results were satisfactory compared to those of Beger et al. [1,11,12]. Although three of our patients (8%) were subsequently hospitalized because of abdominal pain, this complaint was found to be postoperative ileus related. These three patients experienced no pain preoperatively. Therefore, we believe our procedure was effective for all patients. Social rehabilitation to occupational situation after our procedure was also satisfactory. This high incidence of complete return to the workforce probably resulted from the good pain control.

Our procedure preserves the stomach, the bile duct, the duodenum, and more pancreatic tissue compared with Whipple's operation. Therefore, functional defects are uncommon after our operation. It has been reported more than 50% of patients had steatorrhea after Whipple's procedure [15,16]. In contrast, none of our patients had severe diarrhea, and 87% maintained their preoperative body weight.

It is thought that endocrine dysfunction in patients with chronic pancreatitis is progressive. After Whipple's operation, it was stated that 3%–42% of the patients exhibited increased insulin dependence [15]. In our study, only 6 of 18 patients (33%) who showed a normal or GTI pattern on the preoperative OGTT deteriorated to DM after an average of 21 months follow-up. In 4 patients of 19 with preoperative DM (21%), there were improvements in glucose tolerance after an average of 18 months follow-up. Moreover, there was no increase in the number of insulin-dependent patients after our procedure, and no increase in the dose of insulin was required for the patients who had showed the DM pattern on preoperative OGTT. This result suggests that our procedure has no unfavorable effect on glucose tolerance even in patients with preoperative DM.

We consider that the indication of duodenum-preserving resection of the head of the pancreas for low-grade malignant neoplastic lesion is suitable. In these tumors, such as mucinous cystadenoma, serous cystadenoma, and solid and cystic tumor, the disease is usually localized. Therefore, adequate resection of small portion of he pancreas should be applied. We believe the Whipple operation, even if a pyloric ring-preserving pancreatoduodenectomy, is too invasive for these tumors.

Recent improvement of diagnostic methods has contributed to a high accuracy in determination of malignancy of pancreatic neoplasms and their extent to the surrounding tissues. Moreover, we have been able to obtain a histological or cytological diagnosis in almost all cases with malignant lesions that we have treated. We usually indicate an intraoperative histopathological examination for the cases in which no malignancy was proved preoperatively, and if the case is diagnosed as malignancy by this intraoperative pathological examination, we change the procedure to pancreatoduodenectomy. Although duodenum-preserving resection was indicated for four malignant lesions, two cystadenocarcinomas and two papillary adenocarcinomas, all these cases were diagnosed as cystadenoma or papillary adenoma intraoperatively, and carcinoma with no invasion was found postoperatively. Thus, we decided to perform no additional resection for these patients, and no recurrence has been detected during follow-up.

These results suggest the technique of duodenum-preserving resection can be indicated for low-grade malignancy in the pancreas head region. However, duodenum-preserving resection cannot be applied for the treatment of usual pancreatic malignant tumors because pancreatic ductal adenocarcinoma, even if a small tumor, can easily invade the surrounding tissues through the lymphatic canals or perineural routes [17,18]. An additional period of follow-up should be indicated for the precise decision of a suitable indication of this procedure for neoplastic lesions.

References

1. Beger HG, Witte CH, Krautzberger W, Bittner R (1980) Erfahrung mit einer das Duodenum erhaltenden Pankreaskopf resektion bei chronischer Pankreatitis. Chirurg 51:303–309
2. Kosaka K (1982) Report of the committee regarding diagnosis of diabetes mellitus (in Japanese). J Jpn Diabetes Soc 25:859–866
3. Drake DH, Fry WJ (1989) Ductal drainage for chronic pancreatitis. Surgery (St Louis) 105:131–140
4. Jalleh RP, Williamson RCN (1992) Pancreatic exocrine and endocrine function after operations for chronic pancreatitis. Ann Surg 216:656–662
5. Printz RA, Greenlee HB (1981) Pancreatic duct drainage in 100 patients with chronic pancreatitis. Ann Surg 194:313–320
6. Proctor HJ, Mendes OC, Thomas CG, Herbst CA (1979) Surgery for chronic pancreatitis. Ann Surg 189:664–671
7. Stone WM, Sarr MG, Nagorney DM, McIlrath DC (1988) Chronic pancreatitis; results of Whipple's resection and total pancreatectomy. Arch Surg 123:815–818
8. Keith RG, Saibil FG, Sheppard RH (1989) Treatment of chronic pancreatitis by pancreatic resection. Am J Surg 157:156–162
9. Frey CF, Child CG III, Fry W (1976) Pancreatectomy for chronic pancreatitis. Ann Surg 184:403–414
10. Longmire WP (1978) The surgical treatment of pancreatic disease. Jpn J Surg 8:249–260
11. Beger HG, Buchler M, Bittner R, Oettinger W, Roscher R (1988) Duodenum-preserving resection of the head of the pancreas in severe chronic pancreatitis. Early and late results. Ann Surg 209:273–278
12. Beger HG, Buchler M, Bittner R (1990) The duodenum-preserving resection of the head of the pancreas (DPPHR) in patients with chronic pancreatitis and an inflammatory mass in the head. An alternative surgical technique to the Whipple operation. Acta Chir Scand 156:309–315
13. Ikenaga H, Katoh H, Motohara T, Takahashi T, Dohke M, Okushiba S (1995) Duodenum-preserving resection of the head of the pancreas with denervation of the body and tail of the pancreas in patients with severe chronic pancreatitis. J Heptato Biliary Pancr Surg 2:19–24
14. Katoh H, Shimozawa E, Takahashi T, Nakajima K, Okushiba S, Tanabe T (1993) Duodenum-preserving resection of the head of the pancreas with complete denerva-

tion of the body and tail of the pancreas in severe chronic pancreatitis. In: Takada T, Vaniyapongs T, Nimsakul N, Shaipanich T (eds) New frontiers in hepato-biliary-pancreatic surgery. Bangkok Medical, Bangkok, pp 234–237

15. Frey CF, Suzuki M, Isaji S, Zhu Y (1989) Pancreatic resection for chronic pancreatitis. Surg Clin North Am 69:499–528
16. Howard JM, Zhang Z (1990) Pancreaticoduodenectomy (Whipple resection) in the treatment of chronic pancreatitis. World J Surg 14:77–82
17. Nagai H, Kuroda A, Morioka Y (1986) Lymphatic and local spread of T1 and T2 pancreatic cancer: a study of autopsy material. Ann Surg 204:65–71
18. Nagakawa T, Kayahara M, Ueno K, Ohta T, Konishi I, Ueda N, Miyazaki I (1992) A clinicopathologic study on neural invasion in cancer of the pancreatic head. Cancer (Phila) 69:930–935

Duodenum-Preserving Head Resection: A Standard Operation for Chronic Pancreatitis

H.G. Beger[1], T. Imaizumi[1,2], N. Harada[1,2], W. Schlosser[1], and R. Kunz[1]

Summary. Duodenum-preserving head resection of the pancreas has become a standard surgical procedure in benign lesions of the head of the pancreas. In patients with chronic pancreatitis and an inflammatory mass in the head of the pancreas, duodenum-preserving head resection offers major advantages in comparison to the Whipple resection: conservation of the stomach, duodenum, and biliary tree, and minimal restriction of endocrine pancreatic function. In 380 patients with chronic pancreatitis and an inflammatory mass, the duodenum-preserving head resection was carried out with a median postoperative hospitalization of 13.9 days, a frequency of reoperation of 5.3%, and a hospital mortality of 0.8%. The duodenum-preserving subtotal pancreatic head resection resulted in an improved glucose metabolism in 9% of the patients, preoperatively suffering latent or insulin-dependent diabetes. Only 2% of the patients showed deterioration with newly developed diabetes mellitus in the early postoperative phase. The late mortality after a median follow-up of more than 6 years is around 6%. In terms of the disease chronic pancreatitis, duodenum-preserving head resection leads to an interruption of the progression of the chronic inflammation of the pancreas.

Key words. Chronic pancreatitis—Pancreas divisum—Benign tumor—Duodenum-preserving head resection

Introduction

Chronic pancreatitis is a progressive inflammatory disease, in Western countries caused mainly by continuing alcohol abuse; irreversible morphological and functional damage to both the exocrine and endocrine pancreatic tissue compartments is typical. After a subclinical phase of variable duration, recurrent attacks of upper abdominal pain develop, frequently combined with back pain, and clinical signs of exocrine and endocrine insufficiency appear.

[1] Department of General Surgery, University of Ulm, 89075 Ulm, Germany.
[2] Department of Surgery, Institute of Gastroenterology, Tokyo Women's Medical College, Shinjuku-ku, Tokyo 162, Japan.

The hypersecretion from acinar cells forming protein plaques within interlobular and intralobular ducts early in the disease, leading to periductal inflammation and fibrosis, is thought to be its underlying cause [1–3]. A second hypothesis suggests that chronic pancreatitis results from relapsing acute pancreatitis that causes interstitial acinar and fat tissue necrosis, inducing perilobular fibrosis [4].

Anatomical, embryological, and pathomorphological data point to the head of the pancreas as the pacemaker of chronic pancreatitis. Some 15–30% of patients with chronic pancreatitis develop an inflammatory mass in the head of the pancreas, leading to head enlargement. Macroscopically, parenchymal calcifications, pancreatic duct calculi, small cystic cavities, and small areas of necrosis are found within the inflammatory mass in the pancreatic head [5]. Microscopically, atrophy of the exocrine pancreas as well as local increase of extracellular matrix proteins—collagen, fibronectin, laminin—are observed. The sensory nerves in the area of inflammation are enlarged in diameter, showing a loss of perineurium and infiltration of inflammatory cells under the electron microscope; the nerve network is rarefied per tissue area [6]. This pancreatitis-specific neuritis has been found to contribute to the clinical pain syndrome via local liberation of pain hormones, such as substance P and calcitonin gene-related protein (CGRP) [7]. A dominant inflammatory process in the head of the pancreas, including main duct changes, is observed in patients with pancreas divisum [8].

Chronic Pancreatitis with Inflammatory Mass in the Head of the Pancreas

Fifteen to 30% of patients with chronic pancreatitis develop an inflammatory mass in the head of the pancreas. In more than 80% of the patients of this subgroup the disease is alcohol induced; men are predominant and the mean age is less than 40 years at the time of diagnosis. Besides severe abdominal pain that may be persistent or episodic and which frequently does not respond to analgesic treatment, local complications occur, such as stenosis of the common bile duct, stenosis or thrombosis of the splenic vein or main trunk of the portal vein, and severe duodenum stenosis (Table 1).

Surgical treatment for chronic pancreatitis becomes mandatory after failure of medical and interventional management, e.g., analgesic medication, enzyme supplementation, or duct stenting. Surgical options in a big-duct disease are the Partington–

TABLE 1. Chronic pancreatitis with inflammatory mass in the head of the pancreas

About 30% of patients with chronic pancreatitis
More than 80% alcohol induced
Predominantly in men
Mean age: <40 years at time of diagnosis
Clinical features: Severe, medically intractable pain, 80%
                      Stenosis of the common bile duct, ≈50%
                      Severe duodenum stenosis, 5%–10%
                      Portal vein/superior mesenteric vein and hepatic artery/superior mesenteric
                      artery

From the Department of General Surgery, University of Ulm.

TABLE 2. Surgery of chronic pancreatitis: the Ulm experience with 841 patients[a]

		Head resection		
Duct drainage/pseudocyst drainage	Left resection	Whipple	PPPD	DPPHR
211[b] (25%)	197 (23%)	20 (2%)	40 (5%)	380 (45%)

PPPD, Pylorus-preserving pancreatoduodenectomy; DPPHR, duodenum-preserving pancreatic head resection.
[a] 11/1968–4/1982, Department of Surgey, FU Berlin Charlottenburg.
5/1982–9/1995, Department of General Surgery, University of Ulm.
[b] Data are number of patients.

Rochelle duct drainage procedure [9], left resection in segmental left-sided pancreatitis, and pancreatic head resection. In about 50% of the patients who had been referred to our clinic for operative treatment of chronic pancreatitis, a head resection was indicated (Table 2). Because neither the stomach nor the duodenum nor the common bile duct is involved in the inflammatory process in the pancreas, the use of the Whipple procedure goes far beyond the requirements for optimal surgical control of chronic pancreatitis.

After experimental investigations and studies of the blood supply to the duodenum, a duodenum-preserving subtotal resection of the head of the pancreas was introduced in 1972 and has since been regularly employed in patients with chronic pancreatitis and an inflammatory mass in the head of the pancreas [10]. The duodenum-preserving head resection aims at a subtotal resection of the pancreatic head with removal of the inflammatory mass while preserving the duodenum, the extrahepatic biliary tree, and the stomach as well as protecting the pancreatic parenchyma to a large extent.

Indications for Duodenum-Preserving Pancreatic Head Resection

Up to September 1995, 380 patients with chronic pancreatitis and an inflammatory mass in the head of the pancreas had been surgically treated using the duodenum-preserving head resection; 93% of all these patients suffered abdominal pain, and 78% had daily or daily severe pain. The preoperative pain period and time of medical treatment of chronic pancreatitis was 3.1 years on average (range, 1 month–21 years). Twenty-four percent of the patients were diabetic, dependent on insulin medication. The indications for surgery are listed in Table 3.

Techniques of Duodenum-Preserving Pancreatic Head Resection

There are three major steps in the resection: exposure of the head of the pancreas, subtotal resection of the head, and reconstruction using the upper jejunal loop for interposition. The head of the pancreas is exposed as described by Kocher, and the ligaments are divided. The resection starts with a transection of the pancreas ventrally to the portal vein at the level of the duodenal portal vein wall (Fig. 1). After transection of the pancreatic neck, the head of the pancreas is rotated to the ventral dorsal level

TABLE 3. Indication for surgical treatment in 380 patients[a] with chronic pancreatitis with inflammatory mass in the head of the pancreas (IMH)

Indication	Number of patients
Abdominal pain	354 (93%)
IMH (>4 cm)	302 (79%)
CBD stenosis	187 (49%)
Duodenum stenosis	23 (6%)
Vascular obstruction	65 (17%)

[a]11/1972–4/1982, Department of Surgery, FU Berlin.
5/1982–9/1995, Department of General Surgery, University of Ulm.

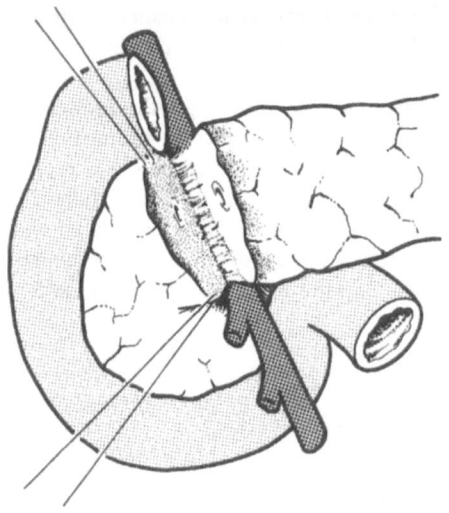

FIG. 1. Transection of the pancreas between the head and body along the duodenal border of the portal vein

(Fig. 2a). Subtotal resection of the pancreatic head is carried out from the dorsal surface of the pancreatic head toward the intrapancreatic common bile duct. In most patients it is not difficult to dissect the pancreatic tissue along the wall of the intrapancreatic common bile duct toward and up to the uncinate process. A 5- to 8-mm shell-like piece of the pancreatic head along the duodenal wall is preserved to maintain the blood supply of the third part of the duodenum (Fig. 2b). Preservation of the gastroduodenal artery is not necessary.

Restoration of the pancreatic secretory flow from the body and tail to the upper gastrointestinal tract is maintained by interposition of the first jejunal loop; two pancreatic anastomoses must be carried out (Fig. 3). In most patients, subtotal excision of the inflammatory mass in the head leads to a decompression of the pancreatic segment of the common bile duct. In patients in whom cholestasis is caused by narrowing of the prepapillary common bile duct segment because of intraductal wall inflammation, a biliary anastomosis with the jejunal loop is necessary (Fig. 4) [11]. In cases with multiple stenoses and dilatations of the pancreatic main duct, a Puestow

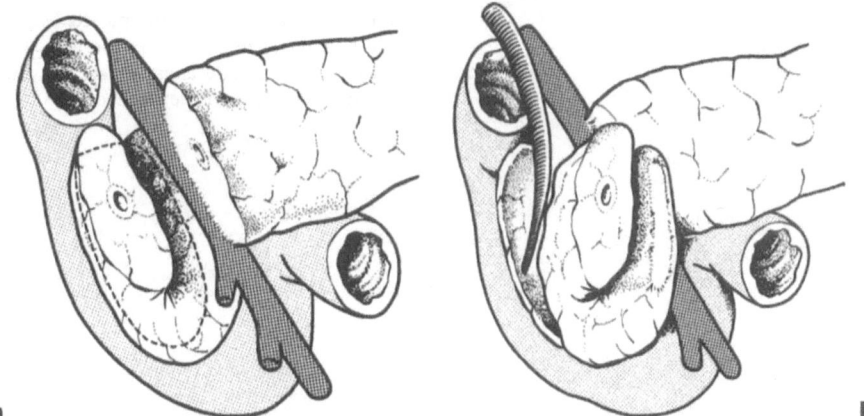

a   b

FIG. 2. **a** After transection of the pancreas, the pancreatic head is rotated to a ventrodorsal position. **b** A subtotal resection of the head of the pancreas results in a decompression of the intrapancreatic segment of the common bile duct

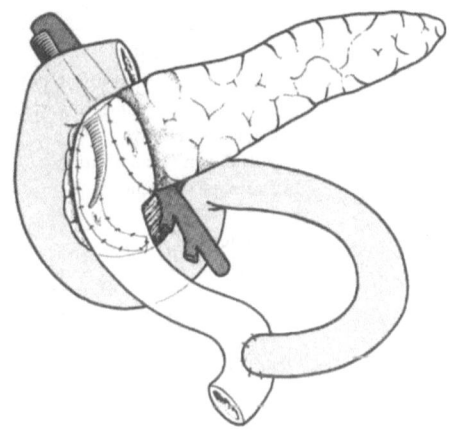

FIG. 3. Restitution of pancreatic secretory flow is accomplished by interposition of the upper jejunal loop between the left pancreas and the pancreatic shell along the duodenum. Two pancreatic anastomoses are carried out

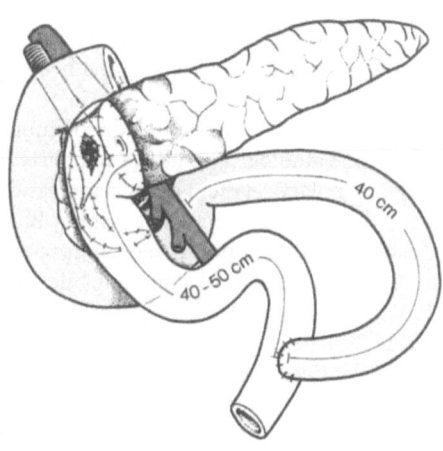

FIG. 4. In patients with chronic pancreatitis and an inflammatory mass, who suffer from a severe stricture of the common bile duct in the prepapillary intrapancreatic segment, an additional common bile duct anastomosis with the jejunal loop has to be carried out to restore the bile flow into the upper intestine

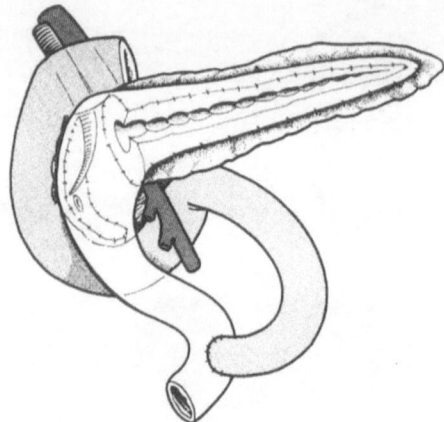

FIG. 5. In patients with multiple stenosis of the pancreatic main duct in the left pancreas, a side-to-side anastomosis like the Puestow procedure is performed

TABLE 4. Duodenum-preserving head resection in chronic pancreatitis: additional surgical procedures for 380 patients[a]

Procedure	Number of patients
CBD anastomosis	86 (23%)
Duct drainage (Puestow type)	26 (7%)
Decompression of ducodenum	16 (4%)
Cholecystectomy	102 (27%)
Portal vein recanalization	6 (2%)
Drainage of pseudocysts	4 (1%)
Left resection	2 (1%)
Splenectomy	3 (1%)
Other	15 (4%)

[a] 11/1972–4/1982, Department of Surgery, FU Berlin.
5/1982–9/1995, Department of General Surgery, University of Ulm.

modification using the side-to-side anastomosis must be performed (Fig. 5) [12]. To restore upper gastrointestinal tract continuity, a Roux-en-Y jejunal anastomosis must be carried out. The medium wet weight of dissected pancreatic tissue using the duodenum-preserving subtotal head resection in our series was 28 g (range, 18–52 g).

In 380 patients in whom the duodenum-preserving head resection was applied, the following pathological findings were listed: a single pancreatic main duct stenosis in the prepapillary segment of the pancreatic head in 39%, pseudocystic cavities in 51%, small focal necrosis in 9%, common bile duct stenosis in 48%, severe duodenum stenosis in 7%, and portal vein compression caused by pancreatic head enlargement in 13%. An additional common bile duct anastomosis had to be carried out in 23% and a Puestow drainage procedure of the left pancreas in 7%. Portal vein thrombosis necessitated an additional recanalization procedure in 6 patients, and an additional decompression procedure of the narrowed duodenum was performed in 4% (Table 4).

Early and Late Postoperative Course

Early results after duodenum-preserving head resection are displayed in Table 5. The median postoperative hospitalization time was 13.9 days; 5.3% of the patients had to be reoperated. The hospital mortality was 0.8%. Subtotal pancreatic head resection resulted in improved glucose metabolism (of preoperatively latent or insulin-dependent diabetes) in 9%; only 2% of the patients showed deterioration with newly developed diabetes mellitus in the early postoperative phase [13].

During the follow-up period (from 6 months to 23 years), it was demonstrated that late morbidity and mortality after duodenum-preserving head resection are surprisingly low. In 1983, 1987, and 1993, reevaluations of all patients after duodenum-preserving head resection were carried out; the follow-up response was 92%, 96%, and 88%, respectively [14] (M. Büchler, 1995, unpublished data). In terms of relief of abdominal complaints, 75%–82% of all patients were absolutely pain-free, and an additional 7%–11% did not need analgesic medication in spite of occasional upper abdominal pain sensations. Regarding pain recurrence, 8%–11% suffered further pain with a need for analgesic treatment at the reevaluation. As to work status, more than 60% of all patients were in professional employment. Body weight increase occurred in more than 80% in the first postoperative months. Late after surgical treatment, only one-third of the patients were still on a full dose of enzyme supplementation; 50% of the patients had only an occasional enzyme supplementation.

Late mortality after duodenum-preserving head resection was 4%, 4.7%, and 8.9%, respectively [12,13] (Büchler, unpublished). Only about 10% had to be hospitalized because of further attacks of pancreatitis. This low postoperative hospitalization rate in chronic pancreatitis deserves special mention, because on the basis of our knowledge of the natural course of chronic pancreatitis at least 50% of the patients should experience further severe attacks of pancreatitis. The low late morbidity in spite of progression of chronic pancreatitis provides evidence that the surgical excision of the inflammatory process in the head of the pancreas promotes the transformation of a clinically manifest chronic pancreatitis into a healing form of the disease (Table 6).

Endocrine Function After Duodenum-Preserving Head Resection

Subtotal resection of the head of the pancreas preserving the duodenum in chronic pancreatitis does not lead to a deterioration of glucose metabolism as an early consequence of surgical resection of pancreatic tissue. As compared to the preoperative

TABLE 5. Duodenum-preserving head resection in chronic pancreatitis: Early postoperative results in 380 patients[a]

Relaparotomy	20 patients (5.3%)
Postoperative newly developed diabetes mellitus	8 patients (2.0%)
Postoperative improved glucose metabolism	33 patients (9.0%)
Postoperative hospitalization	13.9 days (median)
Hospital mortality	3 patients (.8%)

[a] 11/1972–4/1982, Department of Surgery, FU Berlin.
5/1982–9/1995, Department of General Surgery, University of Ulm.

TABLE 6. Duodenum-preserving head resection in chronic pancreatitis: late outcome after DPPHR in 298 patients[a]

Early:	Hospital mortality	1.0%
	Relaparotomy	5.7%
	Postoperative newly developed diabetes mellitus	2%
	Postoperative hospitalization	13.9 days (median)
Late outcome after 6-year follow-up (median) in		
232 patients[b]:	Late mortality	8.9%
	Pain: none/rare	88%
	Professionally rehabilitated	63%
	Rehospitalization	10%

[a] 11/1972–12/1994, Department of General Surgery, University of Ulm.
[b] M. Büchler, unpublished data.

level of endocrine functions, glucose metabolism was unchanged in 82% of patients, improved in 9%, and deteriorated in only 2%. Glucose tolerance tests in a small group of patients early and late after duodenum-preserving head resection showed an improvement of glucose tolerance in the first 6–12 months after surgical treatment. The preoperative and late postoperative insulin secretion was almost identical. The basal levels of glucagon, pancreatic polypeptide, and somatostatin were postoperatively significantly reduced as compared to the preoperative levels, contributing to the postoperative improvement of glucose metabolism [15].

Advantages of the Duodenum-Preserving Head Resection as Compared to Traditional Resection Techniques

The rationale behind the use of the duodenum-preserving pancreatic head resection in patients with chronic pancreatitis and an inflammatory mass in the pancreatic head is based on our present knowledge of chronic pancreatitis. The inflammatory process as the pacemaker of the disease develops in a subgroup of patients in the head of the pancreas; pain is generated by the inflammatory process, which leads to a specific pancreatitis-associated neuritis and a liberation of pain hormones in the head of the pancreas. The preservation of the stomach, the duodenum, and the extrahepatic biliary tree offers the major advantage of retaining normal upper gastrointestinal physiology. The major advantage when using the duodenum-preserving head resection in chronic pancreatitis derives from the conservation of the endocrine capacity of the pancreas and duodenum in the early and late postoperative course. In contrast to the Whipple procedure, the duodenum-preserving pancreatic head resection means preservation of stomach, biliary tract, and duodenum. Early and late morbidity after Whipple's procedure are related to the reduction in insulin secretion, the occurrence of early and late dumping complaints, and attacks of cholangitis [16–23].

The results of two prospective clinical trials comparing the duodenum-preserving pancreatic head resection with the pylorus-preserving Whipple procedure in chronic pancreatitis have been published. After 6 months, patients who had undergone the duodenum-preserving resection had significantly less frequent pain, a greater weight gain, a significantly better glucose tolerance, and a higher insulin secretory capacity than patients after pylorus-preserving Whipple resection [4]. Duodenum-preserving head resection does not lead to a complete restoration of the reduced exocrine and endocrine function of the pancreas, because the impairment resulting from chronic pancreatitis cannot be compensated for by any surgical intervention. The coring-out technique of pancreatic head tissue advocated by Frey results in an operative tissue specimen of 5 g and is considered as a modification of the Partington–Rochelle duct drainage procedure [25].

Conclusion

Duodenum-preserving pancreas resection for chronic pancreatitis results in a subtotal resection of the pancreatic head, leading to a removal of 28 g of tissue on average. Of 380 patients suffering from chronic pancreatitis who did not respond to medical pain treatment, 79% had an inflammatory mass in the pancreatic head, 49% had a common bile duct stenosis, 6% a severe duodenum stenosis, and 13% a portal vein obstruction. Hospital mortality after duodenum-preserving head resection was 0.8%, late mortality after a follow-up of 6 years on average (range, 3 months–23 years) was 8.9%. In the late follow-up, 88% of patients were pain-free or had rare minor pain; 63% were professionally rehabilitated. The incidence of diabetes mellitus early postoperatively amounted to 2%, and in the late follow-up an additional 10% developed insulin-dependent diabetes mellitus; 9% of patients had a postoperative improvement of their glucose metabolism. In patients after duodenum-preserving head resection, early and late postoperative glucose metabolism and insulin secretion are significantly better than in patients after pylorus-preserving pancreatic head resection for chronic pancreatitis.

Duodenum-preserving head resection should be the standard surgical procedure in chronic pancreatitis because of the low early and late postoperative morbidity and mortality and a favorable maintenance of glucose metabolism and upper gastrointestinal tract physiology.

References

1. Pitchumoni CS (1990) Role of nutrition in chronic pancreatitis. In: Beger HG, Büchler M, Ditschuneit H, Malfertheiner P (eds) Chronic pancreatitis: research and clinical management. Springer, Berlin Heidelberg New York pp 15–25
2. Durbec JP, Sarles H (1978) Multicenter survey of the etiology of pancreatic diseases: relationship between the relative risk of developing chronic pancreatitis and alcohol, protein and lipid consumption. Digestion 18:337–350
3. Guy O, Robles-Diaz G, Adrich Z, Sahel J, Sarles H (1983) Protein contents of precipitates present in pancreatic juice of alcoholic subjects and patients with chronic calcifying pancreatitis. Gastroenterology 84:102–107
4. Singer MV, Gyr KE, Sarles H (1985) Revised classification of pancreatitis: report of the second international symposium on the classification of pancreatitis in Marseille, France, March 28–30, 1994. Gastroenterology 89:683–685
5. Beger HG, Bittner R, Büchler M, Block S, Senn T, Malfertheiner P (1988) Die chronische Pankreatitis mit entzündlicher Pankreaskopfvergrößerung. Früh- und Spätergebnisse nach duodenumerhaltender Pankreaskopfresektion. Med Klin 83:548–553
6. Bockman D, Büchler M, Malfertheiner P, Beger HG (1988) Analysis of nerves in chronic pancreatitis. Gastroenterology 94:1459–1469

7. Büchler M, Weihe E, Müller S, Malfertheiner P, Friess H, Beger HG (1989) Neurotransmitter in Pankreasnerven: Ein Beitrag zur Schmerzpathogenese bei chronischer Pankreatitis. Langenbecks Arch Chir (Suppl Chir Forum) 1989:375–379
8. Blair AJ III, Russell CG, Cotton PB (1984) Resection for pancreatitis in patients with pancreas divisum. Ann Surg 200:590–594
9. Partington PF, Rochelle REL (1960) Modified Puestow procedure for retrograde drainage of the pancreatic duct. Ann Surg 152:1037–1043
10. Beger HG, Witte C, Kraas E, Bittner R (1980) Erfahrung mit einer das Duodenum erhaltenden Pankreaskopfresektion bei chronischer Pankreatitis. Chirurg 51:303–307
11. Beger HG, Krautzberger W, Gögler H (1981) Résection de la tête du pancréas (pancréatectomie céphalique) avec conservation du duodénum dans les pancréatites chroniques, les tumeurs de la tête du pancréas et les compressions du canal cholédoque. Chirurgie 107:597–604
12. Beger HG, Krautzberger W, Bittner R, Büchler M, Limmer J (1985) Duodenum-preserving resection of the head of the pancreas in patients with severe chronic pancreatitis. Surgery (St Louis) 98:467–473
13. Beger HG, Büchler M, Bittner R, Oettinger W, Roscher R. Duodenum-preserving resection of the head of the pancreas in severe chronic pancreatitis. Early and late results. Ann Surg 209:273–278
14. Beger HG, Büchler M (1990) Duodenum-preserving resection of the head of the pancreas in chronic pancreatitis with inflammatory mass in the head. World J Surg 14:83–87
15. Bittner R, Butters M, Büchler M, Nägele S, Roscher R, Beger HG (1988) Glucose homeostasis and endocrine pancreatic secretion in patients with chronic pancreatitis before and after surgical therapy. Biomed Res 9:28
16. Doutre LP, Perissat J, Pernot F, Houdelette P (1977) Réflexions statistiques sur une série de 142 interventions pour pancréatite chronique primitive. Chirurgie 103:169–176
17. Gall FP, Mühe E, Gebhardt C (1981) Results of partial and total pancreaticoduodenectomy in 117 patients with chronic pancreatitis. World J Surg 5:269–275
18. Leger L, Lenriot JP, Lemaigre G (1980) L'hypertension et la stase portales ségmentaires dans les pancréatites chroniques. J Chir 95:599–608
19. Guillemin G, Cuilleret J, Michael A, Berard P, Foroldi J (1971) Chronic relapsing pancreatitis. Surgical management. Including 63 cases of pancreatico-duodenectomy. Am J Surg 122:802–807
20. Trede M (1987) Therapie der chronischen Pankreatitis—Schlußkommentar. Langenbecks Arch Chir 373:379–382
21. Warren KW, Hoffman G (1976) Changing patterns in surgery of the pancreas. Surg Clin North Am 56:615–629
22. Proctor HJ, Mendes OC (1979) Surgery for chronic pancreatitis. Ann Surg 189:664–671
23. Grant CSJ, van Heerden JA (1979) Anastomotic ulceration following subtotal and total pancreatectomy. Ann Surg 190:1–5
24. Büchler MW, Friess H, Müller MM, Beger HG (1995) Randomized trial of duodenum-preserving pancreatic head resection versus pylorus-preserving Whipple in chronic pancreatitis. Am J Surg 169:65–70
25. Frey CF, Smith GJ (1987) Description and rationale of a new operation for chronic pancreatitis. Pancreas 2:701–707

Duodenum-Preserving Total Pancreatectomy

R.C.G. Russell

Summary. Preservation of the duodenum in pancreatic surgery is a concept based on conservation of normal physiological function after surgery to ensure improved long-term results. Surgical procedures on infants in which all the pancreas was extirpated for hyperinsulinism showed that the duodenum could be separated from the pancreas and survive. Anatomical studies suggested that this was because there is a submucosal plexus of vessels similar to that found in the stomach. Selection of patients for duodenum-preserving procedures should be undertaken with care. The published results of total pancreatectomy show that the operation can be performed with low mortality. Long-term results, which are rarely reported, to date suggest that these patients have a high risk of death from disease-related problems. In my own series, 58 patients have undergone a total pancreatectomy, of which 32 have had a duodenum-preserving procedure. The operative mortality was 0 in the duodenum-preserving group but 3 in the standard group; the complication rates were similar. There have been 13 late deaths, 8 in the standard group and 5 in the duodenum-preserving group. Outcome in the two groups is similar, apart from weight gain, which is better with duodenum preservation. The conclusion from this study is that both procedures give adequate results, with a better nutritional status in the group with duodenum preservation.

Key words. Duodenum preservation—Total pancreatectomy—Chronic pancreatitis—Pancreatic surgery

Introduction

It was Whipple, in one of his original articles, who said that it was necessary to resect the duodenum because "complete removal of the pancreas so compromises the blood supply to the duodenum as to favor necrosis and fistula formation" [1]. Consequently, this ideal has been followed for many years without question. The first dissent from this classical teaching came from the paper by Traverso and Longmire [2], who thought that preservation of the pylorus was appropriate as this would aid gastric

The Middlesex Hospital, London, W1N 8AA, U.K.

emptying. At that time, proximal gastric vagotomy was considered to be the most suitable procedure for the treatment of duodenal ulcer as it was believed that a normal antropyloro-duodenal reflex ensured proper emptying of the stomach, with maximum utilization of the food and minimal chance of the old postvagotomy and postgastrectomy problems, which did much to distract from the success of surgery for ulcer disease.

The concept of preservation of some part of the duodenum was extended by Beger [3] to preservation of all the duodenum, leaving a rim of tissue around the duodenal loop to preserve the vascular arcade and so maintain the duodenal blood supply. Preserving the duodenum should preserve gastric emptying, normal duodenal and small intestinal motility, and bile mixing by preserving the normal hormonal release mechanisms from the antrum and duodenum and maintaining the antropyloric emptying mechanism as well as the duodenal pacemaker, which coordinates duodenal and jejunal contractions as a result of the undisturbed myenteric plexus. This normal physiology should ensure that the clinical outcome for the patient is better with an improved weight gain, better diabetic control as a result of more predictable absorption, and less diarrhea because there is more coordinated intestinal activity with less undigested food reaching the cecum.

Experience in the surgery of children who had nesidioblastosis showed that a 98% pancreatectomy can be performed in children under 5 years of age with preservation of the duodenum. Animal work performed during the early studies on pancreatic transplantation showed that the duodenum survived following meticulous dissection of the pancreas off the duodenum. This simplified the animal model, as it avoided the usual duodenal resection and the major reconstruction involved. Biochemical studies of the animals showed no detectable insulin or insulin activity, thereby indicating that the pancreatectomy was complete. Further, the duodenum appeared vascularized and functioned normally.

In 1971 Harken described a total pancreatectomy performed in infants with idiopathic hypoglycemia in whom a 50% pancreatectomy had failed to control the symptoms [4]. It was apparent that the duodenum in the neonate would survive after sacrifice of both superior and inferior pancreaticoduodenal arteries. A subsequent description of this procedure by Gough confirmed that this operation was safe and in fact was the only procedure that would satisfactorily relieve the symptoms of infantile hyperinsulinism [5]. My own experience in ten infants confirmed that the duodenum could be well separated from the pancreas in the infant and that a plane of cleavage could be developed along the pancreatic border of the duodenum by careful dissection [6]. In the infant, the color of the duodenum was completely normal at the end of the operation. Long-term follow-up of these children has shown no long-term sequelae; because of preservation of the duodenum, the pattern of growth is normal.

Terminology

As a result of development of the concept of preservation of the duodenum, the terminology has become confused. In the Beger procedure, a rim of pancreas is preserved to maintain the anterior and posterior vascular arcades that supply the duodenum. The amount of pancreas that is preserved appears variable, and in some instances the posterior capsule may be preserved. The Frey procedure can hardly be included in a discussion of duodenum-preserving pancreatectomy because most of the head of the pancreas is left behind and only a small amount of the head, namely, that in front of the main pancreatic duct, is removed. The usual amount of tissue that is removed at this operation is no more than 5 or 10 g. On the other hand, in true duodenum preservation procedures all the pancreas is removed such that the blood supply of the duodenum relies on its intramucosal anastomoses and the part of the anterior and posterior arcades that can be preserved.

Blood Supply of the Duodenum

Injection studies in the human suggest that there is an arcade of vessels within the mucosa of the duodenum similar to those of vessels in the stomach [7]. These injection studies suggested that contrast injected in the superior pancreaticoduodenal artery would perfuse through this submucosal plexus down to the fourth part of the duodenum [8]. Subsequent clinical experience in the adult has confirmed that the duodenum will survive devascularization extending from the first to the fourth part of the duodenum, and thus presumably the duodenum is preserved by this submucosal plexus.

Kimura and Nagai undertook a careful study of 40 autopsy cases to define the vascular anatomy of the pancreas [9]. They described an arcade formation between the anterosuperior pancreaticoduodenal artery and the anteroinferior pancreaticoduodenal artery. After leaving the gastroduodenal artery the anterosuperior pancreaticoduodenal artery runs toward a point 1.5 cm below the papilla of Vater, then turns to the posterior aspect of the pancreas to join the anteroinferior pancreaticoduodenal artery. In 88% of cases, an arcade was found between the posterosuperior pancreaticoduodenal artery and the posteroinferior pancreaticoduodenal artery. These vessels were not buried in the pancreatic parenchyma in any study. It was possible generally to dissect the pancreas from the duodenum, preserving some of the arterial arcade. Near the accessory papilla, however, the dissection of the vessels was difficult, and pancreatic parenchyma was found in the wall of the duodenum.

Dissection of the pancreas from the common bile duct and identification of the main pancreatic duct at the junction of the terminal portion of the bile duct was straightforward in all cases. The posterior arcade of arteries and veins runs on a connective tissue membrane situated on the posterior surface of the pancreas. It is essential not to destroy this membrane, and therefore a Kocher maneuver should not be performed in this operation and the peritoneum on the lateral surface of the duodenum should not be divided. The dissection of the vascular tree should be undertaken with great care and diathermy of the monopolar type avoided. Bipolar diathermy can be used safely provided the dissection is accurate.

Indications

To justify duodenum preservation during a resection of the head of the pancreas, whether or not it is part of a total removal of the pancreas, requires most careful selection. It is necessary to determine first, that the patient requires pancreatic surgery to relieve the symptoms and second, that resection of the head is the correct procedure. To justify the operation of total pancreatectomy it is necessary to ensure that every other alternative management option has been exhausted. First, medical therapy must have failed after an adequate trial of conservative therapy including a period of inpatient management to ensure that the patient can be weaned off analgesics and is capable of the self-discipline to control the inevitable diabetes. Second, the patient's pain, which is the major indication for this type of conservative procedure, must be intractable and unrelieved by other therapy. Third, operations of a lesser severity such as drainage procedures or a partial resection must have been previously undertaken and deemed to have failed as a result of the persistence or recurrence of the symptoms. It is doubtful if a total pancreatectomy should be performed in the absence of either endocrine or exocrine insufficiency.

At operation it is essential to assess the disease carefully. If the duodenum is involved by the disease process, duodenum preservation is inappropriate. The ideal candidate for duodenum preservation is the patient who has severe fibrosis such that the pancreas has contracted away from the duodenum. It is preferable that the vessels of the arcade are clearly seen so that some if not all the arcade can be preserved.

Preoperative Preparation

Once the decision has been made to undertake a duodenum-preserving pancreatectomy, it is necessary to counsel the patient regarding the sequelae of the operation. If the patient is not a diabetic, then this aspect requires careful preoperative preparation. If the patient has steatorrhea, it is important to ascertain that he can control this adequately using enzyme replacement preparations. Because many of the patients are malnourished, it is preferable to improve their nutritional status preoperatively. It is also important to reassess the disease preoperatively by computed tomography (CT) scanning and an endoscopic retrograde cholangiopancreatography (ERCP) to ensure that no unexpected findings are encountered during the operation.

Results

Recent data on total pancreatectomy for chronic pancreatitis are sparse, and there are few large series from which to glean information. In a review by Frey and colleagues, the information on total pancreatectomy was limited as the original papers lacked information [10]. The largest recent study is a retrospective report describing collective data on 83 patients from six centers in the United Kingdom [11]; unfortunately the follow-up data in this article are deficient. The largest series is from Mannheim describing 52 patients who had a total pancreatectomy, but only 17 of these were for chronic pancreatitis [12]. Smaller series of 10 patients [13], 7 patients [14], and 4 patients [15] support the general conclusions from the larger studies that total pancreatectomy for benign disease is a safe operation with comparatively low morbidity, yet with major long-term problems. These long-term problems are emphasized by the recent paper from Flemming and Williamson, who reported that of 40 patients who underwent total pancreatectomy there were 15 late deaths (at 2.5–120 months after surgery), 11 of which were disease related [16].

Personal Results

Since 1976, 356 patients have undergone resection for chronic pancreatitis. Of these 167 had a proximal pancreatectomy, 174 had a distal pancreatectomy, and 15 had a total pancreatectomy primarily. Of the 167 patients who have had a proximal pancreatectomy, 17 have proceeded to a distal pancreatectomy, thus ablating the pancreas; of the 174 distal pancreatectomies (12 performed elsewhere), 33 patients have proceeded to a proximal completion pancreatectomy. Thus, 65 patients have had a total pancreatectomy and of these 33 have had a duodenum-preserving procedure; 32 have undergone a total pancreatectomy with excision of the duodenum.

In this presentation of the results, the outcome of the standard resections is given with those of the duodenum-preserving procedures so as to compare the merits of the two operations. Table 1 shows that the median age of the duodenum-preserving patients was similar to those who had a standard procedure. Alcohol-related pancreatitis was more common in the standard group (56%) than in the duodenum-preserving group (30%). In the duodenum-preserving group, there were 9 patients (27%) with minimal change pancreatitis [17] compared with only 1 (3%) in the standard group. All the patients whose pancreatitis was caused by drinking alcohol had been weaned off alcohol by the time they had their total pancreatectomy performed; indeed, this was a prerequisite for the patient. The indication for surgery for all patients in the duodenum-preserving group was unremitting pain. Five patients (16%) in the standard group underwent urgent surgery for complications of the

TABLE 1. Author's experience

Patient characteristics	Duodenum-preserving TP	Standard TP
Number		
All	33	32
Single stage	7	8
Two stage	26	24
Male:female ratio	13:20	20:22
Age (years)		
Median	33	39
Range	19–52	22–55
Etiology		
Acute: gallstone		1
Chronic:		
Alcohol	10	18
Divisum	5	3
Juvenile onset	3	1
Minimal change	9	1
Gallstone	1	2
Pregnancy onset		2
Idiopathic	2	4
Choledochal cyst	1	
Trauma	2	

TP, total pancreatectomy.

TABLE 2. Author's experience: indications for surgery

	Duodenum-preserving TP ($n = 33$)	Standard TP ($n = 32$)
Indication for operation		
Pain	33	27
Sepsis		1
Hemorrhage		2
Sepsis and hemorrhage		1
Fulminant pancreatitis		1
Preoperative status		
Weight loss	11	10
Diabetes present	12	17
Steatorrhoea present	21	19
Length of history (years)		
Median	6	6
Range	1–26	.1–16
Prior resection (number of patients)	26	24
Time interval (months)		
Median	16	17
Range	3–150	.1–141

disease; pain was the indication for surgery in the remaining 27 (Table 2). Fifteen patients who had a duodenum-preserving total pancreatectomy were diabetic preoperatively, and 19 of the standard group were already diabetic. Steatorrhea was present in 13 of the duodenum-preserving patients and 16 of the standard group. The median length of history at the time of total pancreatectomy was 6 years in both groups.

Perioperative Complications

The mortality for the 33 patients who underwent a duodenum-preserving total pancreatectomy was nil, while 3 patients who underwent standard total pancreatectomy died; in these 3 patients, surgery had been undertaken urgently for complications of chronic pancreatitis (hemorrhage, 1; sepsis, 1; fulminant pancreatitis, 1). One died of adult respiratory distress syndrome while the other 2 died as a consequence of sepsis. The complications of both procedures are outlined in Table 3, with sepsis being the most common complication. A duodenal leak occurred in 3 patients who had had the duodenum-preserving procedure, but in none was this serious and in each it settled with simple conservative management; no reoperation was necessary.

The single biliary fistula was transitory and resolved within a few days without intervention. Delayed gastric emptying was a problem and accounts for the prolonged inpatient stay in some patients. In time it invariably settles. The length of stay was similar in the two groups, with a mean of 21 days in the duodenum-preserving and 19 in the standard group. Frequently the reason for the prolonged postoperative stay was the policy not to discharge patients until their diabetes was under control, their steatorrhea treated with enzyme supplements, and their analgesic consumption reduced to nil or a minimal dose of a minor analgesic. It has been found that if patients are discharged on pethidine or similar analgesics they remain on those narcotics for life.

TABLE 3. Author's experience: morbidity

Complications	Duodenum-preserving TP ($n = 33$)	Standard TP ($n = 32$)
Uncomplicated recovery	14 (42%)	16 (50%)
Sepsis		
Chest	3	4
Cardiovascular	2	3
Urinary tract infection	1	1
Wound	1	2
Pyrexia (of unknown origin)	1	1
Bacteremia	1	
Biliary		2
Leak		
Biliary	1	
Enteric	3	
Delayed gastric emptying	7	2
Bleeding, minor	1	
Pneumothorax	2	
Air embolus	1	
60-day mortality	0	3
Length of hospital stay (days)		
Median	21	19
Range	10–49	8–98

TABLE 4. Author's experience: late deaths

	Duodenum-preserving TP ($n = 33$)	Standard TP ($n = 32$)
Total number of deaths	5	8
Months postoperative		
Median	80	45
Range	3–105	10–112
Etiology of pancreatitis		
Alcohol	3	6
Acute gallstone		1
Divisum	1	
Chronic post trauma		1
Idiopathic	1	
Cause of death		
Diabetic related	2	3
Ethanol intoxication		1
Gastrointestinal bleeding		1
Myocardial infarction		2
Carcinoma (breast)	1	
Sepsis	1	1
After unrelated surgery	1	

Outcome

Readmission is a simple way of assessing patients who have an unsatisfactory result from any operation. Unfortunately, only a few patients avoided readmission, and some required many hospital admissions because of their underlying disease.

Narcotic abuse, nutritional difficulties, and poor diabetic control have been the reason for these returns. Nevertheless, with better outpatient care through the appointment of a liaison sister (visiting nurse), such readmissions are now less frequent. Numbers of readmissions were similar in both groups of patients. There have been 13 late deaths, 8 in the standard group and 5 in the duodenum-preserving group (Table 4).

Bile Duct Stricture

The major late surgical complication associated with duodenum-preserving procedures has been the development of a bile duct stricture, which has occurred in seven patients. In two patients, an endoscopic sphincterotomy at 14 months and 29 months has been sufficient to control the problem. In another patient insertion of a stent was found to be suitable, and this remained patent until elective removal when the structure resolved. Four patients have required a choledochojejunostomy at 5, 12, 15, and 30 months after the original procedure. Predisposing factors to the formation of a bile duct structure included damage at the time of the original operation and ischemia. Subsequent follow-up of these patients has been good, with normal liver function tests.

Quality of Recovery

It is our standard practice to see all patients following pancreatic surgery in a special pancreatic clinic. At this clinic standard questions are asked about pain, analgesic consumption, bowel function, pancreatic enzyme requirement, diabetic control, and the level of activity. At the 6-month, 12-month, and 3-, 5-, 7-, and 10-year follow-ups (Table 5), it is noted that results are variable with approximately one-fourth to one-third of patients having poor results as long as 10 years after the operation. The anticipated improvement from duodenum preservation in terms of simple quality of recovery is not apparent.

Diabetic Status

Most patients are managed by twice-daily injection of a combination of rapidly absorbed and intermediate insulins. Patients routinely monitor their blood glucose level and report regularly to a consultant diabetologist attached to the clinic. Only two patients have had any of the sequelae of diabetes: one has a peripheral neuropathy, having been a diabetic since 1977, while the other, who has been a diabetic since 1984, has a peripheral neuropathy complicated by carpal tunnel syndrome. Hypoglycemic episodes tend to occur more frequently in patients following standard total pancreatectomy. Many of the mild episodes of hypoglycemia experienced are associated with steatorrhea-related malabsorption. It is of interest that the overall requirement of insulin is greater following duodenum-preserving total pancreatectomy than following standard total pancreatectomy. This is interpreted as being related to the improved nutrition associated with that group and is borne out by their better weight status.

Pancreatic Enzyme Replacement Therapy

In the management of patients following total pancreatectomy, control of steatorrhea is important, and many patients have a less than optimal outcome because they do not

TABLE 5. Author's experience: quality of recovery

Time after surgery	Number at follow-up	Visick I/II (%)	Visick III (%)	Visick IV (%)
6 months				
DPTP	32	50	16	34
STP	27	44	23	33
12 months				
DPTP	31	45	13	42
STP	26	42	16	42
3 years				
DPTP	31	35	22	42
STP	23	52	13	35
5 years				
DPTP	31	52	19	29
STP	16	62	25	13
7 years				
DPTP	25	48	24	28
STP	12	42	16	42
10 years				
DPTP	12	67	18	25
STP	6	50	17	33

DPTP, duodenum-preserving total pancreatectomy; STP, standard total pancreatectomy.
Visick I–IV indicate.

TABLE 6. Personal experience: comparison of ideal body weight at time of operation and at 1, 3, and 5 years postoperatively

	Percent of ideal body weight	
Time	Duodenum-preserving	Standard
At operation		
n	21	14
Median	99.5	83
Range	75–138	64–129
At 1 year		
n	21	14
Median	105	89
Range	72–143	70–112
At 3 years		
n	17	8
Median	108	88
Range	74–142	63–117
At 5 yeas		
n	3	6
Median	116	82
Range	106–121	67–103

master sensible control of their pancreatic enzyme requirements. The amount of enzyme replacement required varies markedly between individuals and is illustrated by the range of capsules taken daily by the duodenum-preserving group: 4–100 standard strength capsules, with a median of 60 per day. For those patients who have had a standard total pancreatectomy, the median requirement was only 30 capsules per day. The increased requirement of enzyme capsules in the duodenum-preserving group mirrors the increased requirement for insulin already noted, and is almost certainly associated with an improved absorption of food and an associated weight gain (Table 6). It is apparent that patients who had had a standard total pancreatectomy had a lower body mass index than those selected for duodenum-preserving pancreatectomy. These data support the concept that duodenum preservation improves nutritional status.

Conclusions

Duodenal preservation can be safely performed in appropriate patients. Selection is important, and the procedure should only be undertaken in those patients in whom the technical risks of performing the operation are reasonable. Whether this rather tedious dissection is appropriate and preferable to a standard total pancreatectomy is difficult to determine. Certainly, there are no more immediate complications, and the only specific complication related to duodenum preservation is an incidence of biliary stricture. This complication should be lessened with more awareness of the blood supply of the bile duct and an appreciation of the care required to dissect out the biliary tree from the dense fibrosis often associated with chronic pancreatitis. A reasonable guideline is to suggest that if there is any disruption of the bile duct during the dissection, then a choledochoduodenostomy should be undertaken rather than a repair of the bile duct.

The advantages of duodenum preservation appear to be fewer long-term complications with improved gastrointestinal function and diabetic control. The work of Linehan et al. has shown that pancreatectomized patients with duodenum preservation have a more normal weight than those who have had a standard procedure and a better control of their diabetes [18]. Further, these patients have no dumping or liability to this complication [19]. These factors suggest that gastrointestinal function is more normal in patients with duodenum preservation than those without preservation and strongly suggest that the patient may well have a better result in the long term. Perhaps a surprising finding of this experience is that well-selected patients can manage with a standard total pancreatectomy and that, for the right patient, this procedure should not be neglected as one of the alternatives in the management of the patient with chronic pancreatitis.

References

1. Whipple AO (1946) Radical surgery for certain cases of pancreatic fibrosis associated with calcareous deposits. Ann Surg 124:991–1006
2. Traverso LW, Longmire WP (1979) Preservation of the pylorus in pancreatico-duodenectomy. A follow-up evaluation. Ann Surg 190:312–316
3. Beger HG, Krautzberger W, Bittner R, Buchler M, Limmer J (1985) Duodenum-preserving resection of the head of the pancreas in patients with severe pancreatitis. Surgery (St Louis) 97:467–473
4. Harken AH, Filler RM, Auruskin TW, Crigler JF (1971) The role of total pancreatectomy in the treatment of unremitting hypoglycaemia of infancy. J Pediatr Surg 6:284–289
5. Gough MH (1984) The surgical treatment of hyperinsulinism in infancy and childhood. Br J Surg 71:75–78

6. Murphy JP, Russell RCG (1988) Operative treatment of nesidioblastosis. Br J Surg 75:930

7. Thomas LM, Langford RM, Russell RCG, Le Quesne LP (1978) The anatomical basis for gastric mobilisation in total oesophagectomy. Br J Surg 65:356–360

8. Lambert MA, Linehan IP, Russell RCG (1987) Duodenum preserving total pancreatectomy for end stage chronic pancreatitis. Br J Surg 74:35–39

9. Kimura W, Nagai H (1995) Study of surgical anatomy for duodenum-preserving resection of the head of the pancreas. Ann Surg 221:359–363

10. Frey CF, Suzuki M, Isaji S, Zhu Y (1989) Pancreatic resection for chronic pancreatitis. Surg Clin North Am 69:499–528

11. Cooper MJ, Williamson RCN, Benjamin IS, et al (1988) Total pancreatectomy for chronic pancreatitis. Br J Surg 74:912–915

12. Trede M, Schwall G (1988) The complications of pancreatectomy. Ann Surg 207:39–47

13. Kiviluotu T, Schröder T, Lempinen M (1985) Total pancreatectomy for chronic pancreatitis. Surg Gynecol Obstet 160:223–227

14. Keith RG, Saibil FG, Sheppard RH (1989) Treatment of chronic pancreatitis by pancreatic resection. Am J Surg 157:156–162

15. McAfee MK, van Heerden JA, Adson MA (1989) Is proximal pancreatoduodenectomy with pyloric preservation superior to total pancreatectomy? Surgery (St Louis) 105: 347–351

16. Flemming WR, Williamson RCN (1995) The role of total pancreatectomy in the treatment of patients with end stage chronic pancreatitis. Br J Surg 82:1409–1412

17. Walsh TN, Theis BA, Rode J, Russell RCG (1992) Minimal change chronic pancreatitis. Gut 33:1566–1571

18. Linehan IP, Lambert MA, Brown DC, Kurtz AB, Cotton PB, Russell RCG (1988) Total pancreatectomy for chronic pancreatitis. Gut 29:358–365

19. Linehan IP, Russell RCG, Hobsley M (1988) The dumping syndrome after pancreatoduodenectomy. Surg Gynecol Obstet 167:114–118

Reconstruction after Pancreatoduodenectomy

Pancreatojejunostomy by Duct-Insertion Method: Clinical and Experimental Study

Hiroshi Shimada, Koichiro Misuta, Kunio Kameda, Itaru Endo, and Akira Nakano

Summary. We have applied the duct-insertion method with complete drainage of pancreatic juice to patients with normal pancreatic tissue and an undilated pancreatic duct, and the duct–mucosal suture method to patients with hard pancreatic tissue and a dilated pancreatic duct. The safety and certainty of this duct-insertion method was examined by experiments with animals. There was no significant difference in bursting pressure of the anastomosis and hydroxyproline content between the two methods. In the histopathological findings, adhesion of the subserosal layer was found at 14 postoperative days and regenerative mucosa at 28 days after operation. In a clinical study, there was no significant difference in frequency of leakage. The value of pancreatic functional diagnostant (PFD) was maintained at a high rate 12 months after operation. It was considered that anastomotic patency was preserved. It is concluded the duct-insertion method is a safe and useful procedure, especially for patients with normal pancreatic tissue and an undilated pancreatic duct.

Key words. Pancreatojejunostomy—Duct-insertion method—Leakage of anastomosis—Bursting pressure—Hydroxyproline

Introduction

Pancreatic fistula caused by a leak or a fistula from the pancreatic anastomosis, a common complication following pancreatoduodenectomy, can lead to intra-abdominal abscess, hemorrhage, or death. Technical factors, such as invagination pancreatojejunostomy or the duct-mucosal suture method and the use or nonuse of an anastomotic stent, continue to be a matter of debate [1,2]. Compared with normal pancreatic tissue, a fibrotic pancreas with a dilated pancreatic duct resulted in a low rate of pancreas fistula. This fact indicated that the texture of the pancreas, the grade of pancreatic fibrosis, is more important than other factors in determining whether a pancreatic fistula develops postoperatively. Thus, we apply the duct-insertion method, with complete drainage of pancreatic juice by a stent tube, to patients with

Yokohama City University School of Medicine, Second Department of Surgery, Kanazawa-ku, Yokohama, Kanagawa 236, Japan.

normal pancreatic tissue and an undilated pancreatic duct, and use the duct-mucosal suture method with partial drainage of pancreatic juice for patients with hard pancreatic tissue and dilated ducts (Table 1). The safety and reliability of the duct-insertion method in pancreatojejunostomy was examined by experiments with animals. Also, the duct-insertion method was compared clinically with the duct-mucosal suture method in terms of the frequency of leakage of the anastomosis.

Technique of Duct-Insertion Method

After the pancreas body is dissected from the retroperitoneum, the pancreas is transected by a knife. Hemostasis is secured by a 4-0 prolene Z-suture to the pancreatic stump. The fishmouth suture is not used to prevent necrosis of the cut end of the distal pancreas. The pancreatic duct is exposed with a little pancreatic tissue about 1 cm in length from the cut end. After the duct is isolated, the duct is opened to insert a pancreatic duct tube with many side holes and double notches. The inserted tube is fixed to the pancreatic duct by ligation with 4-0 vicryl (Fig. 1). After a small opening at the jejunum is made, the pancreatic duct tube is passed through this opening. The pancreatic duct is brought into close contact with the jejunal mucosa, with the pursestring suture placed around the opening. Interrupted sutures with 3-0 prolene are placed between the pancreas parenchyma and the seromuscular layer of the jejunum and tied.

TABLE 1. Application of methods

Pancreatojejunostomy	Pancreatic duct	Pancreas tissue
Duct-insertion method	Undilated ($\phi \leqq 3\,mm$)	Soft
Duct-mucosal suture method	Dilated ($\phi > 3\,mm$)	Hard

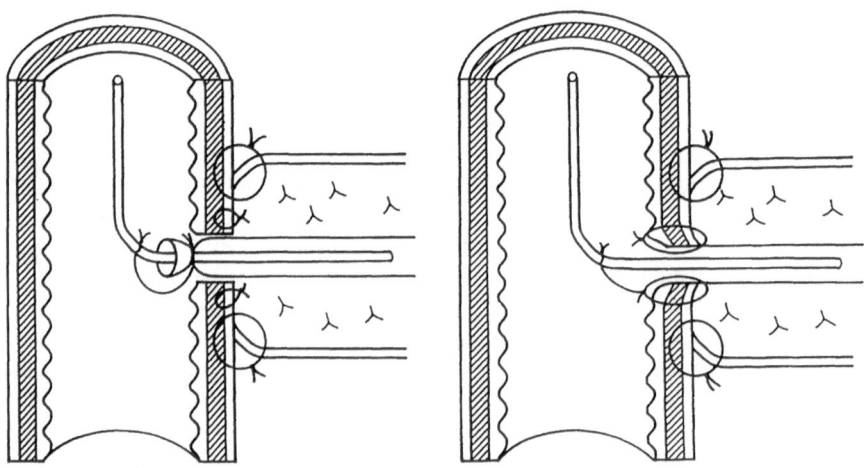

FIG. 1. Schematic illustration of two types of pancreatojejunostomy. *Left*: duct-insertion method; *right*, duct-mucosal suture method

Materials and Methods

Experimental Study

To compare wound healing of pancreatojejunostomy, we operated on mongrel dogs and studied the bursting strength of the anastomotic site [3], hydroxyproline content [4], and histopathological findings at the pancreatojejunostomy 2 and 4 weeks after operation. Bursting strength was studied by an air inflation leak test in which we pumped air into the removed specimen from the jejunal side underwater; the pressure is measured when air leaks from the anastomotic site.

Clinical Study

We studied 69 cases of pancreatojejunostomy between 1984 and 1995. We examined frequency of leakage of the anastomosis and the pancreatic functional diagnostant (PFD) test. Minor leakage is defined as seepage of pancreatic juice, and major leakage is defined as presence of intestinal contents in the excreta or demonstration of leakage from the anastomosis by radiological study.

Results

Experimental Study

In the duct-insertion method, bursting pressure was 288 mmHg at 2 weeks and 267 mmHg at 4 weeks after the anastomosis. In the duct-mucosal suture method, it was 290 mmHg at 2 weeks and 265 mmHg at 4 weeks after the anastomosis (Fig. 2). There was no significant difference in bursting strength of the anastomosis between the two methods.

Hydroxyproline content, which indicates the content of collagen fiber produced in the course of wound healing, was measured on the pancreas side of the anastomosis by high performance liquid chromatography. In the duct-insertion method, hydroxyproline content was 18.0 μmol/wg at 2 weeks and 21.0 μmol/wg at 4 weeks after operation. In the duct–mucosal suture method, it was 17.0 μmol/wg at 2 weeks and 16.0 μmol/wg at 4 weeks after operation (Fig. 3). There was no significant difference in hydroxyproline content.

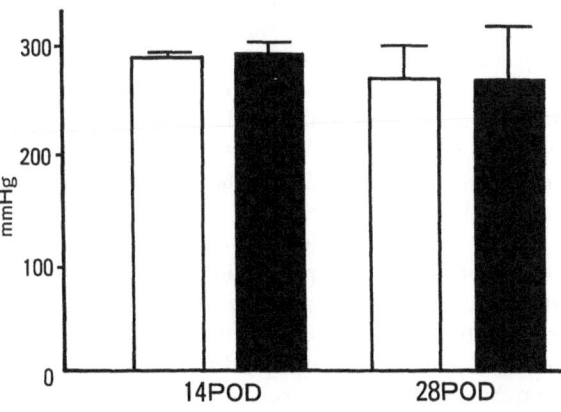

FIG. 2. Bursting strength of the anastomotic site (mmHg). Duct-insertion method (*n* = 4), *open bars*; duct-mucosal suture method (*n* = 4), *solid bars* (mean ± SD). *POD*, days after surgery

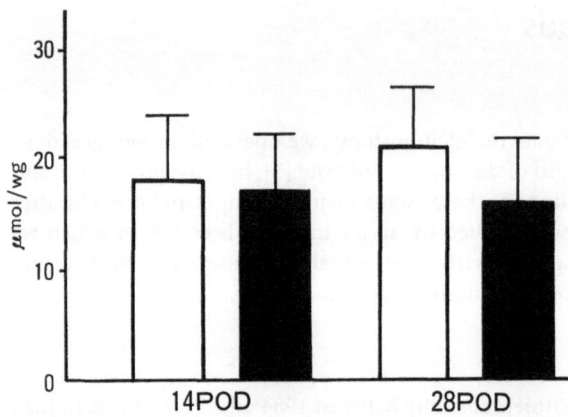

FIG. 3. Hydroxyproline content of the pancreas side of the anastomosis (μmol/wg). *Open bars*, duct-insertion; *solid bars*, duct-mucosal suture (mean ± SD)

TABLE 2. Anastomotic leakage (1984–1995)

Method	Minor	Major
Duct-insertion method ($n = 30$)	7 (23.3%)	3 (10.0%)
Duct-mucosal suture method ($n = 39$)	7 (17.9%)	2 (5.1%)

In the histopathological findings after the duct-mucosal suture method, adhesion of subserosal layer was complete 14 days after operation. Regenerative jejunal mucosa and joining of the epithelium was found after 14 days, and it was complete 28 days after operation (Fig. 4). In the duct-insertion method, acute inflammation had disappeared and adhesion of the subserosal layer was complete 14 days postoperatively (Fig. 5). Regenerative jejunal mucosa was found, although it was insufficient. Closure of the epithelium was complete 28 days postoperatively (Fig. 6).

Clinical Study

The duct-mucosal suture method was performed in 39 cases and the duct-insertion method in 30 cases. Minor leakage occurred in seven cases (23.3%) of the duct-insertion method and in seven cases (17.9%) of the duct-mucosal suture method. Major leakage occurred in three cases (10.0%) and two cases (5.1%), respectively, of each group (Table 2). There was no significant difference between the two groups in frequency of minor and major leakage.

When we compared the courses of drainage volume of pancreatic juice via stent tube of the duct-insertion method between patients with and without a major leakage, we found a sudden decrease of volume a few days before clinical presentation of a major leakage, which indicates that blockage or expulsion of the tube can induce a major leakage (Fig. 7).

We experienced five cases of major leakage; three cases were cured by conservative management including prohibition of oral intake, total parenteral nutrition, and irrigation by saline with protease inhibitor. Intraabdominal bleeding as a secondary complication following leakage of the pancreatojejunostomy occurred in two other cases. Reoperation was performed and hemostasis was obtained. In one case, bleeding from the stump of the pancreas was found and hemostasis by suture was obtained. In

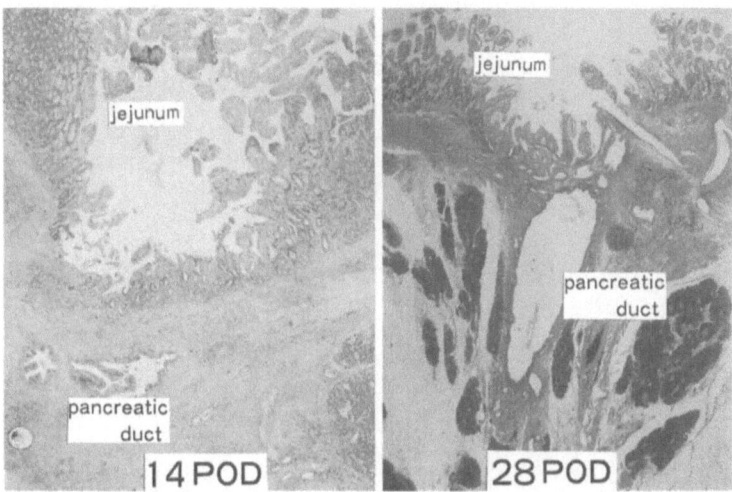

FIG. 4. Histological findings of anastomosis at 2 weeks (*left*) and 4 weeks (*right*) after duct-mucosal suture method. Adhesion of the subserosal layer is complete and regenerative jejunal mucosa is seen 2 weeks postoperatively. Closure of the epithelium is complete 4 weeks after operation

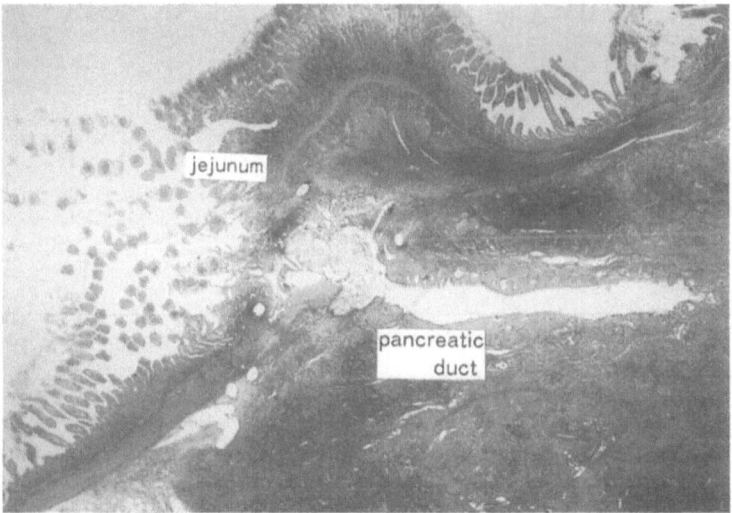

FIG. 5. Histological findings of anastomosis at 2 weeks after duct-insertion method. Adhesion of subserosal layer is complete but regenerative jejunal mucosa is insufficient

another case accompanied by bleeding caused by pseudoaneurysm of the superior mesenteric artery, (SMA), we made a bypass using the saphenous vein between the aorta and the peripheral SMA. Another secondary complication following leakage is intraabdominal abscess. Although we did not experience a case of abscess, if it does

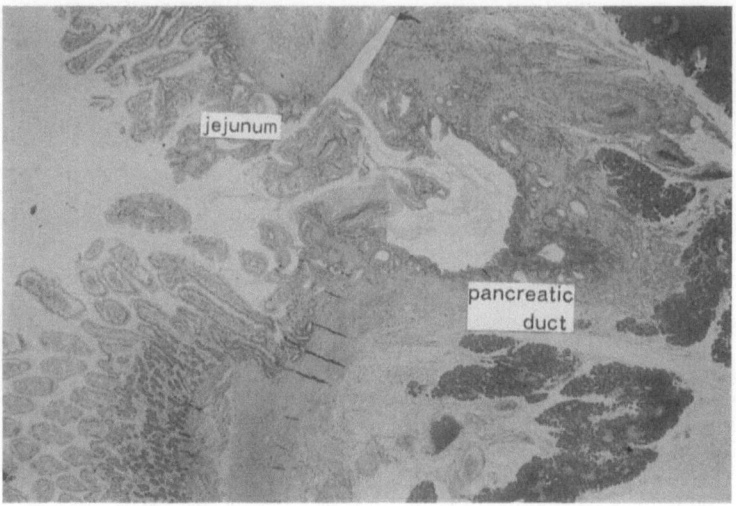

FIG. 6. Histological findings of anastomosis 4 weeks after duct-insertion method. Closure of
epithelium is complete

LEAKAGE(−)   LEAKAGE(+)

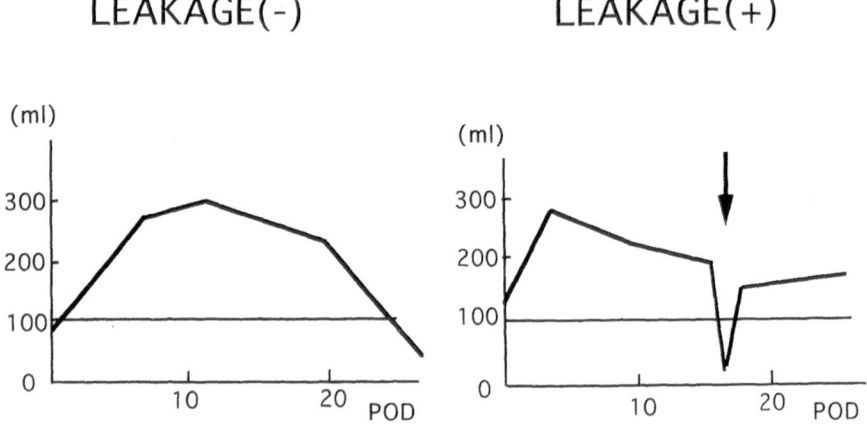

FIG. 7. Discharge of pancreatic juice compared with the course of drainage volume of pancreatic juice via complete drainage tube of the duct-insertion method patients, comparing patients
with (*right*) and without (*left*) major leakage. Sudden decrease of volume (*arrow*) was found a
few days before clinical presentation, which indicates that blockage or expulsion of the tube can
induce a major leakage

occur, drainage by puncture or reoperation is necessary. We did not have any operative deaths, so the mortality rate was 0%.

We studied the PFD test in 8 cases of duct-mucosal suture method and 12 cases of
duct-insertion method (Fig. 8). The value of the PFD test was slightly decreased until
6 months postoperatively in both methods, but no change was seen from 6 months to

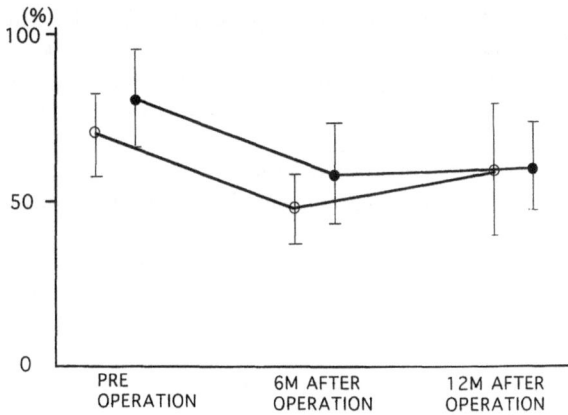

FIG. 8. Results of the pancreatic function diagnostant (PFD) test before surgery compared to values at 6 months and 12 months after operation. *Open circles*, duct-insertion method ($n = 12$); *solid circles*, duct-mucosal suture method

12 months. As the PFD test indicates exocrine function of pancreas, it was considered that patency of the anastomosis was preserved.

Discussion

Pancreatojejunostomy is the most important part of gastrointestinal reconstruction after pancreatoduodenectomy. In our department of surgery, in cases with hard pancreatic tissue or a dilated pancreatic duct ($\geqq 3$ mm), the mucosa of pancreatic duct and the jejunum are approximated with interrupted sutures. In cases having soft pancreatic tissue or an undilated pancreatic duct (<3 mm), however, this duct-mucosal suture method is difficult so we use the duct-insertion method. An advantage of the duct-insertion method is ease in performing even when the pancreatic duct is not dilated. Also, drainage of all secretion of pancreatic juice is an advantage, preventing abdominal abscess and hemorrhage [5,6].

Bursting strength indicates general evaluation of wound healing of anastomosis. It indicates completion of adhesion between the pancreas and jejunum. There was no significant difference in bursting pressure between the two methods 2 and 4 weeks after operation. Thus, it is considered that sufficient strength of anastomosis was obtained in the early phase after the duct-insertion method, equal to that with the duct-mucosal suture method.

Hydroxyproline is the amino acid of component of collagen fiber. Hydroxyproline content thus indicates restoration of tissue and the degree of fibrosis in the course of wound healing. Although there was no significant postoperative difference in hydroxyproline content between the two groups, its content in the duct-insertion method showed a tendency to be slightly high. The duct-mucosal suture method is expected to provide primary wound healing and the duct-insertion method is expected to cause secondary wound healing. Thus, the degree of granulation after the duct-insertion method has a tendency to increase.

In the histopathological findings, adhesion between pancreas parenchyma and the seromuscular layer of jejunum was almost complete 2 weeks after the operation in both methods. It took about 2 weeks for completion of mucosal continuity after the duct-mucosal suture method and, in contrast, about 3 or 4 weeks after the duct-insertion method (Fig. 9). In the duct-mucosal suture method, the pancreatic duct and jejunal mucosa are connected directly, but in the duct-insertion method, they are connected by secondary wound healing. Thus, more time is required for joining of the epithelium to be completed in the duct-insertion method. It is necessary therefore to perform drainage of all secretion of pancreatic juice during 4 weeks the after duct-insertion method.

In the clinical study, frequency of minor and major leakage after the duct-insertion method tended to be slightly greater than after the duct-mucosal suture method. The reason is that the duct-insertion method was applied in cases in which it was difficult to perform pancreatojejunostomy, such as those with soft pancreatic tissue and an undilated pancreatic duct. In comparison with the results of other institutions [7,8], it is considered that our result is equal or better in the case of normal pancreas tissue. The advantage of the duct-insertion method is complete drainage of pancreatic juice. The pancreatic duct tube is allowed to remain in the pancreatic duct for 3 or 4 weeks to avoid contact of pancreatic juice with the cut end of the pancreas.

If leakage of the pancreatojejunostomy occurs, it is necessary to prohibit oral intake, perform total parenteral nutrition, and maintain the drain position. Further, more continuous suction or lavage of a pancreatic fistula is performed. An abdominal computed tomography (CT) scan shoud be performed to exclude the presence of undrained fluid collections. Charles and Yeo reported that approximately 80% of patients with pancreatic fistulas following pancreatoduodenectomy heal with conservative measures [9].

Secondary complications following leakage of the pancreatojejunostomy are intraabdominal hemorrhage and abscess. If hemmorhage occurs, we must perform angiography to detect the bleeding point; hemostasis is obtained by transcatheter arterial embolization (TAE). When hemostasis by TAE fails, it is necessary to suture (ligature) the bleeding point or perform a complete pancreatectomy. Intraabdominal abscess is managed by percutaneous or operative drainage. Percutaneous catheter drainage using ultrasonographic and radiographic guidance is the preferred method of drainage.

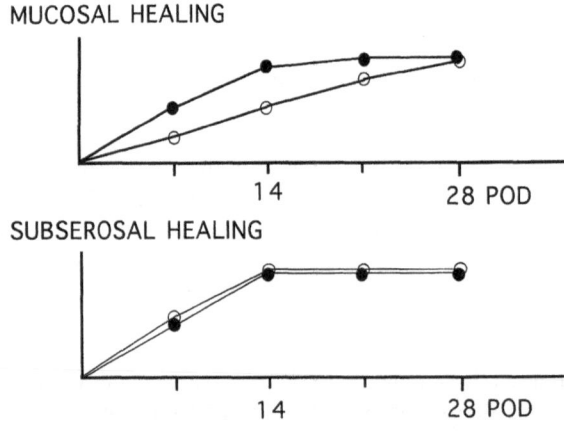

MUCOSAL HEALING

1 4   28 POD

SUBSEROSAL HEALING

1 4   28 POD

Fig. 9. About 2 weeks are required for completion of mucosal continuity after the duct-mucosal suture method is used (*solid circles*) about 3–4 weeks after using duct-insertion method (*open circles*)

The PFD test is useful for evaluation of pancreatic exocrine function and indirect evaluation of patency of the pancreatic duct and anastomosis [10]. Decrease of PFD rate 6 months after operation, in both methods, indicates the influence of the pancreatectomy or operation itself. The value of PFD was maintained at a high rate 12 months after surgery, which meant that the patency was maintained.

Conclusion

It is concluded that the duct-insertion method with a duration of 4 weeks of complete pancreatic juice drainage is a safe and useful procedure of pancreatojejunostomy, especially for patients with normal pancreas tissue.

References

1. Tashiro S, Murata E, Hiraoka T, et al (1987) New technique for pancreaticojejunostomy using a biological adhesive. Br J Surg 74:392–394
2. Spivack B, Wile AG (1984) Purse-string modification of the dunking pancreatojejunostomy. Br J Surg 81:431–432
3. Cronin K, Jackson DS, Dunphy JE (1968) Changing bursting strength and collagen content of the healing colon. Surg Gynecol Obstet 126:747–749
4. Palmerini CA, Fini C, Floridi A, et al (1985) High-performance liquid chromatographic analysis of free hydroxyproline and proline in blood plasma and peptidebound hydroxyproline in urine. J Chromatogr 339:285–292
5. Kojima Y, Shimada H, Katayama K, et al (1992) Pancreaticojejunostomy and pancreatic leakage after pancreaticojejunostomy. Int Surg 77:80–83
6. Hamanaka Y, Suzuki T (1994) Total pancreatic duct drainage for leakproof pancreatojejunostomy. Surgery (St Louis) 115:22–26
7. Grace PA, Pitt HA, et al (1986) Decreased morbidity and mortality after pancreaticoduodenectomy. Am J Surg 151:141–149
8. Trede M, Schwall G (1988) The complications of pancreatectomy. Ann Surg 207:39–47
9. Charles J. Yeo (1995) Management of complications following pancreaticoduodenectomy. Surg Clin North Am 75:913–924
10. Hall RI, Rhodes M, Isabel-Martinez L, et al (1990) Pancreatic exocrine function after a sutureless pancreaticojejunostomy following pancreaticoduodenectomy, Br J Surg 77:83–85

Isolated Pancreatoduodenectomy and Imanaga's Procedure for Carcinoma of the Pancreatic Head Region

AKIMASA NAKAO

Summary. We have been performing reconstruction of the alimentary tract using Imanaga's procedure after pancreatoduodenectomy. Between 1981 and 1995, 180 patients in Department of Surgery II, Nagoya University Hospital, underwent surgical resection for carcinoma of the pancreatic head region (119 ductal carcinoma of the pancreas, 28 distal bile duct carcinoma, and 23 duodenal papilla of Vater carcinoma). We performed 49 total pancreatectomies, 110 pancreatoduodenectomies, 3 pylorus-preserving total pancreatectomies, and 18 pylorus-preserving pancreato-duodenectomies. Portal vein resection was performed in 111 (62%) of the 180 resected cases using catheter bypass procedures of the portal vein. Reconstruction of the alimentary tract after pancreatectomy was performed using Imanaga's procedure in 168 of 180 resected cases. The perioperative death rate was 8% in 119 duct cell carcinomas of the pancreas, 0% in 28 distal bile duct carcinomas, and 0% in 33 duodenal papilla of Vater carcinomas. Perioperative death was observed only in extended resection. The postoperative quality of life after standard resection using Imanaga's procedure was quite good. Imanaga's procedure after pancrea-toduodenectomy is a physiological and safe surgical method.

Key words. Pancreatoduodenectomy—Imanaga procedure—Carcinoma of the pan creatic head region—Catheter bypass of the portal vein—Portal vein resection

Introduction

The basic radical surgery for carcinoma of the pancreatic head region is pancreatoduodenectomy, which has been a complex operation with a high postoperative mortality [1]. One of the serious complications after pancreatoduodenectomy is an anastomotic leak from the pancreatojejunostomy, which sometimes leads to fatal intraabdominal bleeding. Since the first report of pancreatoduodenectomy by Whipple et al. [2] in 1935, many different procedures for reconstruction of the alimentary tract after pancreatoduodenectomy have been reported [3–5]. In 1960, Imanaga [6] reported a new reconstruction method similar to a Billroth I type reconstruction

Department of Surgery II, Nagoya University School of Medicine, Showa-ku, Nagoya, Aichi 466, Japan.

after gastrectomy. His intention was to preserve liver and pancreatic function after pancreatoduodenectomy. The surgical technique of isolated pancreatoduodenectomy using catheter bypass of the portal vein [7–11] and Imanaga's procedure are described in this chapter.

Patients and Methods

Between 1981 and 1995, 178 patients with ductal carcinoma of the pancreatic head, 28 patients with distal bile duct carcinoma, and 36 patients with duodenal papilla of Vater carcinoma were operated on at our institution (Table 1). Of these, 180 (74%) underwent surgical resection. We performed 49 total pancreatectomies (TP), 110 pancreatoduodenectomies (PD), 3 pylorus-preserving total pancreatectomies (PpTP), and 18 pylorus-preserving pancreatoduodenectomies (PpPD). Portal vein resection was performed in 111 (62%) of the 180 resected cases using the catheter bypass procedure of the portal vein [7–10]. Reconstruction of the alimentary tract after TP, PD, PpTP, and PpPD was performed using Imanaga's procedure in 168 of the 180 resected cases. The perioperative death rate was 8% (9 patients) in the 119 resected cases of ductal carcinoma of the head of the pancreas, 0% in cases of distal bile duct carcinoma, and 0% in cases of duodenal papilla of Vater carcinoma.

Surgical Procedure

Isolated Pancreatoduodenectomy Using Catheter Bypass of the Portal Vein for Carcinoma of the Head of the Pancreas

Catheter Bypass of the Portal Vein

Using an antithrombogenic portal vein bypass catheter (Anthron, Toray, Tokyo, Japan) [7], mesenteric venous blood is bypassed to the systemic circulation to prevent portal congestion during portal obstruction [7–9] (Fig. 1). This catheter can also be used to bypass the mesenteric venous blood to the intrahepatic portal vein to avoid both portal congestion and hepatic ischemia during simultaneous obstruction of the portal vein and the hepatic artery [10,11] (Fig. 1).

TABLE 1. Resectability rate and operative procedures for carcinoma of the pancreatic head region

Carcinoma	Patients (n)	Operation	Resection	Operative deaths	TP	PD	PpTP	PpPD
Pancreatic head carcinoma	185	177	119 (67%)	9 (8%)	47 (47)	63 (51)	2 (2)	7 (4)
Distal bile duct carcinoma	29	28	28 (100%)	0 (0%)	1 (1)	21 (3)	1	5
Papilla of Vater carcinoma	36	36	33 (92%)	0 (0%)	1 (1)	26 (2)	0	6

TP, Total pancreatectomy; PD, pancreatoduodenectomy; PpTP, pylorus-preserving total pancreatectomy; PpPD, pylorus-preserving pancreatoduodenectomy. Numbers in parentheses indicate portal vein resection.

Fig. 1. Catheter bypass procedures of the portal vein. *A*, Bypass of mesenteric venous blood to systemic circulation; *B,C*, bypass to intra hepatic portal vein. *PV*, Portal vein; *SV*, splenic vein; *SMV*, superior mesenteric vein; *IVC*, inferior vena cava; *FV*, femoral vein; *GSV*, greater saphenous vein

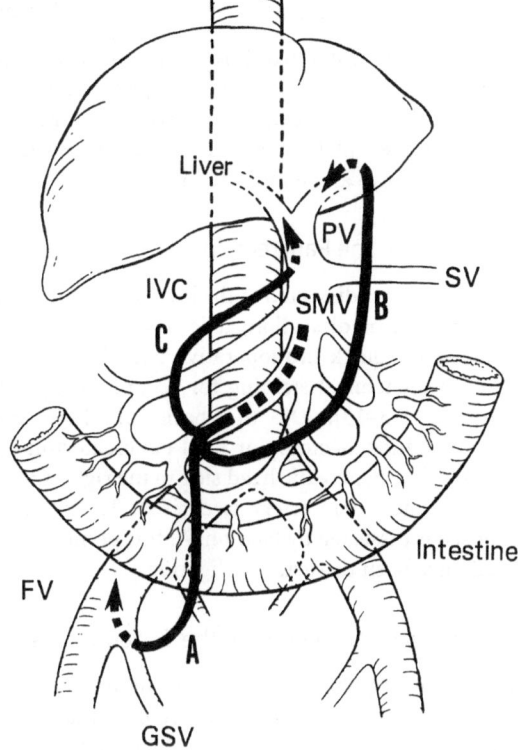

Mesenteric Excision

With this technique, the pancreatic head is not manipulated before ligating and dissecting the arteries supplying the pancreatic head and the veins leading from the pancreatic head. Therefore, Kocher's maneuver is not performed. First, the mesentery about 5 cm distal to the mesenteric root and the lower pancreatic margin is incised horizontally. The tissues other than the mesenteric veins and arteries are all excised toward the mesenteric root. During this manipulation, the mesenteric root lymph nodes and the nerve plexus around the superior mesenteric artery are excised; the lymph nodes of the mesocolon are also excised. The middle colic artery is usually dissected if cancer invasion is severe.

Excision of the Hepatoduodenal Ligament

The hepatic hilar region is next manipulated, and the gallbladder bed is freed. The common hepatic duct is dissected at its hepatic hilar side as far as possible. The stump is sampled for quick intraoperative pathological examination. Lymph node excision proceeds from the hepatic hilar region to the proper hepatic artery and to the area around the common hepatic artery. The right gastric artery and the gastroduodenal artery are dissected by ligation at their root. The lymph nodes around the left gastric artery and the splenic artery are also excised, followed by the lymph nodes around the portal vein. In this way, only the hepatic artery and the portal vein are left in the hepatoduodenal ligament.

Dissection of the Stomach and the Upper Jejunum

In general, the distal two-thirds of the stomach is resected, preserving the ascending branch of the left gastric artery. The jejunum is dissected at a point about 10 cm from ligament of Treitz. If carcinoma invasion of the serosa or duodenum and perigastric lymph node metastasis are not observed, pylorus-preserving pancreato-duodenectomy can be indicated [12].

Dissection of the Pancreas

The pancreas is dissected at the line between body and tail. The splenic vein is ligated at the point of dissection; it is not reconstructed. The stump of the pancreas is sampled for quick intraoperative pathological examination and instantaneous im-munohistochemical staining for accurate diagnosis of cancer invasion of the body and tail [13–15]. On the basis of these examinations, the indication for pancreatoduodenectomy or total pancreatectomy is determined. While turning the stump of the pancreatic head side to the right, the nerve plexus around the root of the superior mesentric artery is excised. The inferior pancreatoduodenal artery thus exposed is dissected by ligation. At this point, all the arteries supplying the pancreatic head have been dissected by ligation.

Simultaneous Dissection of the Superior Mesenteric Vein and the Portal Vein

While holding the intestinal side of the superior mesenteric vein with Satinsky clamps, the superior mesenteric vein is dissected by ligation at the lower border of the pancreas. While holding the hepatic side of the portal vein with the same clamps, the portal vein is also dissected by ligation at the upper border of the pancreas. In this way, all veins leading from the pancreatic head have now been dissected. Then the pancreatic head is resected together with mesenteric lymph nodes and the nerve plexus around the superior mesenteric artery.

Paraaortic Lymph Node Excision

The paraaortic lymph node excision extends to the right margin of the inferior vena cava, downward to the root of the inferior mesenteric artery, to the left margin of the aorta, and upward to the upper margin of the root of the celiac artery.

Reconstruction of the Portal Vein

As a rule, the portal vein is reconstructed by end-to-end anastomosis between portal and superior mesenteric veins, using 5-0 or 6-0 Prolene sutures (Fig. 2). On comple-tion of the anastomosis, the bypass catheter is withdrawn from the greater saphenous vein.

Standard Pancreatoduodenectomy for Distal Bile Duct Carcinoma and Duodenal Papilla of Vater Carcinoma

For distal bile duct carcinoma and duodenal papilla of Vater carcinoma, standard pancreateatoduodenectomy is performed. Pylorus-preserving pancrea-toduodenectomy is also indicated [12]. In standard resection, the portal vein is

FIG. 2. End-to-end anastomosis between portal and superior mesenteric veins in isolated pancreatoduodenectomy

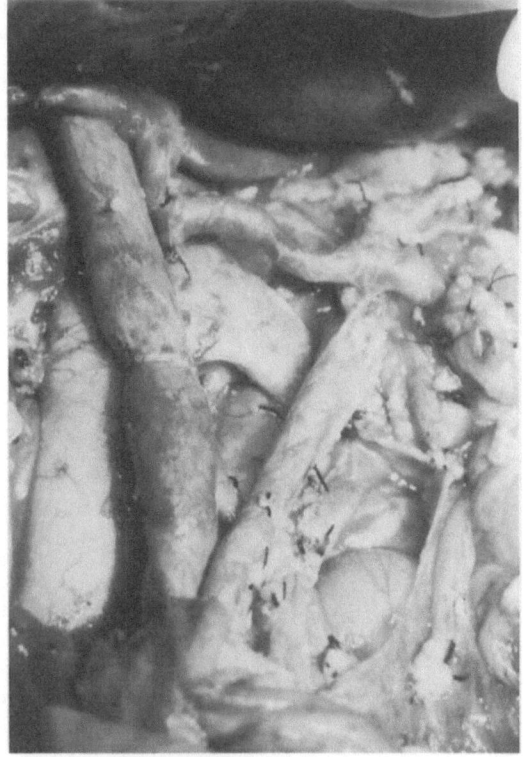

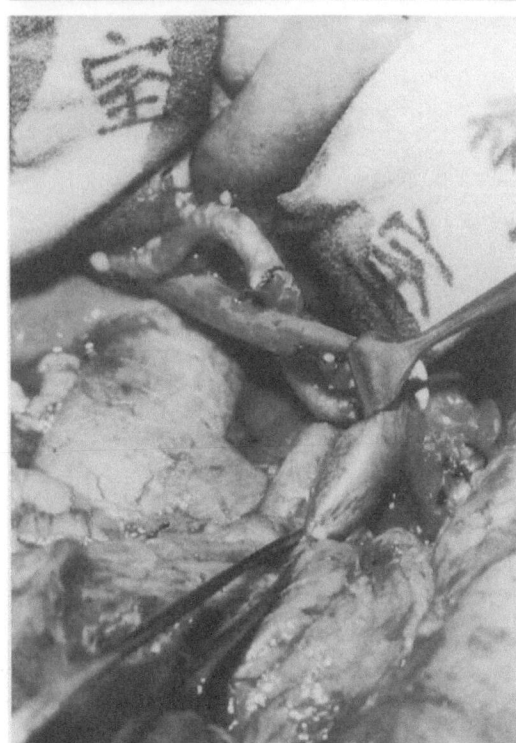

FIG. 3. Retroperitoneal cavity after standard pancreatoduodenectomy

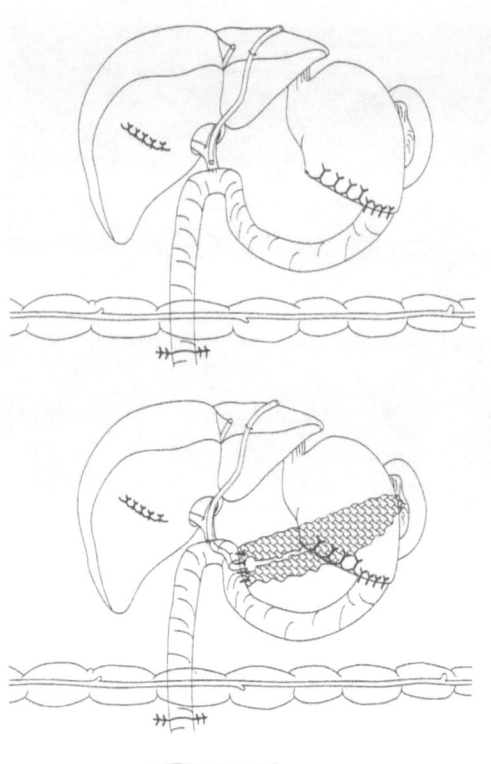

FIG. 4. Imanaga's procedure after total pancreatectomy (TP)

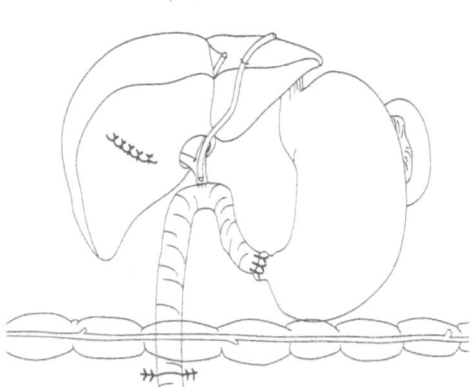

FIG. 5. Imanaga's procedure after pancreatoduodenectomy (PD)

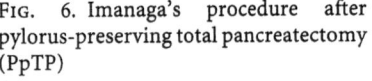

FIG. 6. Imanaga's procedure after pylorus-preserving total pancreatectomy (PpTP)

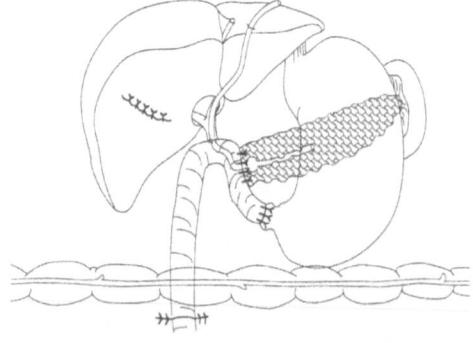

FIG. 7. Imanaga's procedure after pylorus-preserving pancreatoduodenectomy (PpPD)

preserved and the cut line of the pancreas is on a line with the portal vein. The mesenteric root lymph nodes are dissected, but the left side of the nerve plexus around the superior mesenteric artery is preserved (Fig. 3).

Reconstruction using Imanaga's Procedure

Reconstruction using Imanaga's procedure after TP, PD, PpTP, and PpPD is shown in Figs. 4, 5, 6, and 7, respectively. The jejunum is elevated from the right side of the mesocolon. At a point about 10–15 cm from the jejunal stump, an end-to-side pancreatojejunostomy is performed. A pancreatic tube is inserted into the main pancreatic duct. A mucosa-to-mucosa anastomosis between pancreatic duct and jejunum is then performed using 5-0 nylon. Subsequently, end-to-side choledochojejunostomy is performed with absorbable 4-0 sutures at a point 10 cm distal to the above-mentioned point. Finally, end-to-end gastrojejunostomy is performed (Fig. 5). A pancreatic duct tube is left inserted via the liver.

Discussion

The main factor contributing to perioperative death in patients with carcinoma of the head of the pancreas is not portal vein resection using the bypass procedure, but rather various postoperative complications, such as insufficiency of the pancreatojejunostomy and thrombosis of the hepatic artery or superior mesenteric artery, which develop after resection and reconstruction [16,17]. Although the diarrhea and malnutrition that follow resection of the nerve plexus around the superior mesenteric artery require strict management, patients who have undergone this extended pancreatoduodenectomy require no insulin therapy and can frequently resume their normal daily activities with time. Perioperative death was not observed in patients with distal bile duct carcinoma and duodenal papilla of Vater carcinoma. For these patients, the standard operation was indicated rather than an extended operation. No diarrhea or malnutrition was observed. The quality of life in standard pancreatoduodenectomy using Imanaga's procedure is quite good. Persistent reflux cholangitis has not yet been encountered in the use of Imanaga's procedure. Thus, Imanaga's procedure is a physiological and safe reconstruction method of the alimentary tract after pancreatoduodenecotmy.

References

1. Grace PA, Pitt HA, Tompkins RK, Den Besten L, Longmire WP (1986) Decreased morbidity and mortality after pancreatoduodenectomy. Am J Surg 151:141–148
2. Whipple AO, Parsons WB, Mullins CR (1935) Treatment of carcinoma of the ampulla of Vater. Ann Surg 102:763–779
3. Child CG III (1944) Pancreaticojejunostomy and other problems associated with the surgical management of carcinoma involving the head of the pancreas. Ann Surg 119:845–855
4. Cattell RB (1943) Resection of the pancreas; discussion of special problem. Surg Clin North Am 23:753–766
5. Whipple AO (1946) Observation on radical surgery for lesions of the pancreas. Surg Gynecol Obstet 82:623–631
6. Imanaga H (1960) A new method of pancreaticoduodenectomy designed to preserve liver and pancreatic function. Surgery (St Louis) 47:577–586

7. Nakao A, Horisawa M, Suenaga M, Yamamoto T, Kondo T, Kawase S, Nagaoka S, Mori Y (1982) Temporal portosystemic bypass with the use of the heparinized hydrophilic catheter. Jpn J Artif Organs 11:962–965
8. Nakao A, Kondo T (1983) New technique of radical pancreatectomy with the use of the heparinized hydrophilic bypass catheter of the portal vein. Jpn J Artif Organs 12:697–700
9. Nakao A, Horisawa M, Kondo T, Ando H, Kishimoto W, Ichihara T, Sako T, Takimoto H, Ito N (1983) Total pancreatectomy accompanied by portal vein resection using catheter-bypass between mesenteric and femoral veins (in Japanese). Shujutsu (Operation) 37:1–6
10. Nakao A, Nonami S, Harada A, Kasuga T, Takagi H (1990) Portal vein resection with a new antithrombogenic catheter. Surgery (St Louis) 108:913–918
11. Nakao A, Takagi H (1993) Isolated pancreatectomy for pancreatic head carcinoma using catheter bypass of the portal vein. Hepato-Gastroenterology 40:426–429
12. Nakao A, Harada A, Nonami T, Kaneko T, Murakami H, Inoue S, Takeuchi Y, Takagi H (1995) Lymph node metastases in carcinoma of the head the pancreas region. Br J Surg 82:399–402
13. Ichihara T, Nakao A, Sakamoto J, Nonami T, Harada A, Watanabe T, Nagura H, Takagi H (1989) Application of the immunoperoxidase method for rapid intraoperative pathological diagnosis of pancreatic cancer. J Surg Oncol 40:8–16
14. Nakao A, Ichihara T, Nonami T, Harada A, Koshikawa T, Nakashima N, Nagura H, Takagi H (1989) Clinicohistopathologic and immunohistochemical studies of intrapancreatic development of carcinoma of the head of the pancreas. Ann Surg 209:181–187
15. Ichihara T, Nakao A, Suzuki Y, Sakamoto J, Nonami T, Harada A, Nagura H, Takagi H (1989) Improvement of the rapid immunoperoxidase staining method for intraoperative pathological diagnosis of pancreatic cancer using microwave irradiation. J Surg Oncol 42:209–214
16. Nakao A, Harada A, Nonami T, Kaneko T, Inoue S, Takagi H (1995) Clinical significance of portal invasion of carcinoma of the head of the pancreas. Surgery (St Louis) 117:50–55
17. Nakao A, Harada A, Nonami T, Kaneko T, Takagi H (1995) Regional vascular resection using catheter bypass procedure for pancreatic cancer. Hepato-Gastroenterology 42:734–739

Pancreaticojejunostomy After Normal Soft Pancreaticoduodenectomy: A Study of the No-Stent Method

Toshihide Imaizumi, Toshiaki Nakasako, Nobuhiko Harada, Takashi Hatori, Akira Fukuda, and Fujio Hanyu

Summary. There is high risk for anastomotic leakage after pancreaticojejunostomy in pancreaticoduodenectomy (PD) of the normal pancreas because the pancreas is soft and its exocrine activity is high. In this type of PD, a procedure with stent tubing is generally performed (stent method). In recent years, we have performed pancreaticojejunostomy after PD using a procedure without stent tubing (no-stent method) and obtained good results. The intent of this anastomotic technique is to preserve adequate patency of the pancreatic duct by carefully picking up the pancreatic duct wall with a fine atraumatic needle and monofilament sutures. The results of pancreaticojejunostomy after normal soft PD were compared between the no-stent method (group A, 28 cases) and the stent method (group B, 20 cases). There were no differences between the groups in background characteristics of patients, including underlying diseases and age. The mean operative time was 258 min in group A and 283 min in group B; mean pancreaticojejunostomy time was 27.2 and 23.0 min, respectively. Mean perioperative blood loss was less in group A (1075 ml) than in group B (1280 ml). The morbidity rate of early postoperative complications was 32% and 30%, with a frequency of pancreatic–enteric anastomotic leakage of 14% and 15%, respectively, showing no substantial differences. Mean time to postoperative intake of solid food was 15.1 and 17.7 days, and mean postoperative hospital stay 27.3 and 31.3 days, respectively, showing a slight tendency toward fewer days in group A. As shown, we could perform pancreaticojejunostomy safely after normal soft PD without using a stent tube and with no major postoperative complications.

Key words. Whipple operation—Pancreaticoduodenectomy—Pancreaticojejunostomy—Pancreaticojejunostomy without stent tube—Leakage of pancreaticojejunostomy

Department of Gastroenterological Surgery, Tokyo Women's Medical College, Shinjuku-ku, Tokyo 162, Japan.

Introduction

In early complications after pancreaticoduodenectomy (PD), anastomotic leakage at pancreaticojejunostomy is most frequently involved. In addition, serious secondary complications such as intraabdominal abscess or bleeding are likely to occur. In particular, it is said that there is high risk for these complications in the soft pancreas without a dilated pancreatic duct. In general, pancreaticojejunostomy performed without stent tubing has been chosen for patients with a dilated pancreatic duct such as in cases of chronic pancreatitis. Since November 1992, we have performed mucosa-mucosa pancreaticojejunostomy after PD in patients involving a soft pancreas without a dilated pancreatic duct using a procedure without stent tubing (no-stent method) and obtained good results. In this chapter, we present our surgical technique and results.

Operative Procedure

The pancreas is sharply transected with a scalpel together with the pancreatic duct without leaving the longer parts of the duct wall. The pancreatic stump is sutured only at bleeding spots with electrocautery or 4-0 or 5-0 nonabsorbable sutures, but no other treatment of the stump such as mattress suturing or fishmouth-shaped suturing is performed. Usually the gastrointestinal tract is reconstructed according to Child's procedure with alignment of the pancreas, choledochus, and stomach (duodenum). A pancreaticojejunostomy is created by end-to-side anastomosis in almost all cases. Only a small opening is made in the jejunal wall, but excision of the jejunal seromuscularis or scarification is not performed.

The end-to-side anastomosis is created in two layers as follows: anastomosis of the capsular parenchyma of the pancreatic stump and jejunal seromuscularis, and anastomosis of the pancreatic duct and parenchyma and the entire jejunal muscularis. In the outer layer, an anterior row of interrupted sutures and a posterior row of continuous sutures are placed with 4-0 nonabsorbable sutures, and continuous sutures are placed in the inner layer with 6-0 absorbable sutures. These operations are performed with a fine atraumatic needle and monofilament sutures. The point of this anastomotic technique is to preserve adequate patency of the pancreatic duct by carefully picking up the pancreatic duct wall to avoid injury or constriction of the pancreatic duct. It is advantageous to place a fine stay suture in the middle anterior stump of the pancreatic duct and to pull it slightly to the left, so that, in the soft undilated pancreatic duct, the inside of the duct lumen is adequately expanded to set a needle suture on the pancreatic wall. The suture is performed with a posterior row of five stitches and an anterior row of three stitches. If patency of the duct is preserved adequately, stent tubing is unnecessary (Figs. 1, 2).

Patients

We classified 48 patients undergoing normal soft PD during the 3 years since November 1992 into two groups: 28 patients in the no-stent group (group A) and 20 patients in the stent group (group B), in which a stent tube was retained irrespective of mucosa-to-mucosa pancreaticojejunostomy. The results of the operation were compared between the two groups. A pancreas with no decreased pancreatic function

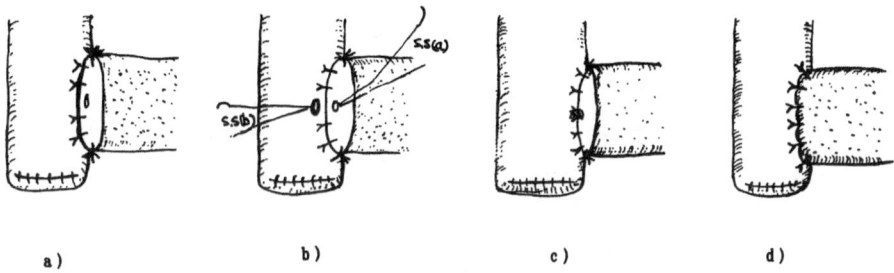

a)   b)   c)   d)

FIG. 1a–d. Pancreaticojejunostomy after normal soft pancreaticoduodenectomy with no stent. Dorsal surface of pancreas is sutured to proximal jejunum in end-to-side anastomosis. Interrupted sutures (nylon 4-0) attach the seromuscular layer of the jejunum to the capsule and parenchyma of the pancreas posteriorly 1 cm from resection borders of both organs (a). A stay suture (s.s.(a)) is put in the middle anterior wall of the pancreatic duct using absorbable fine 6-0 Polydioxanone (PDS); small opening of same size as the pancreatic duct is made in the jejunal wall (b). This stay suture helps to see inside the pancreatic duct and the jejunum (s.s.(b)) and to anastomose the pancreaticojejunostomy. The second row of posterior sutures, placed between the full thickness of the jejunum and the duct including the pancreatic parenchyma, without a microscope, uses interrupted fine absorbable suture (6-0) from posterior to anterior wall (c). Anteriorly placed continuous or interrupted sutures between capsule and resection surface of the pancreas and jejunal seromuscular layer complete the pancreaticojejunostomy (d). s.s.(a), Stay suture in middle anterior pancreatic duct wall; s.s.(b), Stay suture in middle anterior jejunal wall

before the operation, with no intraoperative induration, and with a main pancreas duct diameter of 3 mm or less was defined as a normal pancreas.

Patient diagnoses included cancer of the pancreatic head in 11 patients in group A and in 4 in group B, papilla cancer in 5 and 4, bile duct cancer in 1 and 4, gastric cancer in 2 and 1, and other (islet cell tumor, pancreaticobiliary maljunction, mucin-producing pancreatic tumor, etc.) in 9 and 7 patients, respectively. Mean age was 58.5 years in group A and 59.5 years in group B. The male-to-female ratio was 16:12 in group A and 10:10 in group B. There was no significant difference in these background factors between the two group.

The PD-II method, with alignment of the pancreas, choledochus, and stomach (duodenum) for reconstruction of the gastrointestinal tract, was used in 23 patients in group A and 16 patients in group B. The PD-III method, with alignment of the stomach (duodenum), pancreas, and choledochus, was used in 1 patient in group A and none in group B. Other methods of alignment were used in 4 patients each in the two groups. Items to be evaluated included mean operative time, mean pancreaticojejunostomy time, mean perioperative blood loss, morbidity rate of early complications, frequency of anastomotic leakage at pancreaticojejunostomy, mortality rate, mean time to postoperative intake of solid food, and mean postoperative hospital stay.

Results

The mean operative time was 258 min in group A and 283 min in group B; mean pancreaticojejunostomy time was 27.2 min and 23.0 min; and mean perioperative blood loss was 1075 ml and 1280 ml, respectively. There was no significant difference

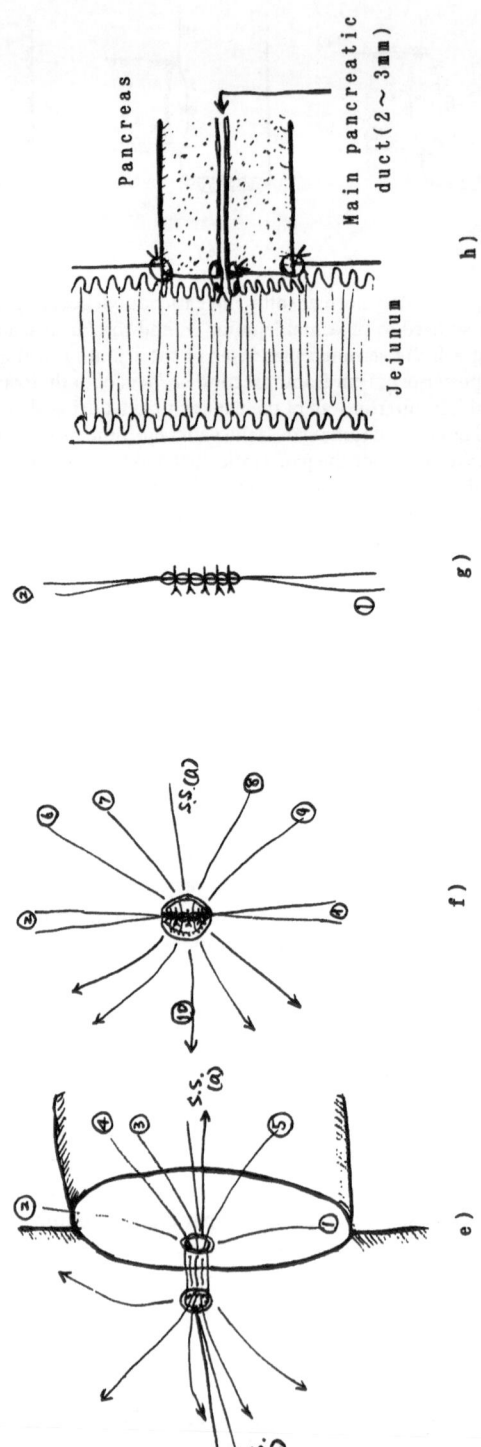

FIG. 2e–h. Mucosa-to-mucosa pancreaticojejunostomy without stent tube. Posterior sutures of the pancreaticojejunostomy, placed between the full thickness of the jejunum and the duct including the pancreatic parenchyma, without a microscope, use interrupted fine absorbable suture (6-0) (e; 1–5). Sutures must be tied with extreme care to avoid cuts in normal glandular tissue and thin non-dilated pancreatic duct. Anteriorly placed interrupted sutures are placed as in the posterior wall; anastomosis is then complete by means of the first stay suture (a) (f; 6–10). All sutures are placed first and then tied (g). Stent tube to bridge the anastomosis is not placed (sectional view, h) because anastomosis is complete and patency of the pancreatic duct is preserved

in these parameters, but the mean perioperative blood loss tended to be less in Group A.

The morbidity rate of early postoperative complications was 32% and 30%, with a frequency of pancreatic anastomotic leakage of 14% and 15%, respectively, showing no substantial differences. There was no operative or hospital death after surgery. The mean time to postoperative intake of solid food was 15.1 days and 17.7 days, and the mean postoperative hospital stay was 27.3 days and 31.3 days, respectively, showing a slight tendency toward fewer days in group A (Table 1). In patients followed-up for 1 year, the pancreatic endocrine and exocrine functions were satisfactorily preserved in both groups, and no significant difference was found.

Discussion

Since PD was established by Whipple et al. [1], various innovations or improvements of this procedure have been made through many modifications [2–4]. Along with the development of various diagnostic procedures, the application of this procedure has increased and the procedure has become widely used with little risk. In cases of malignant diseases, in which a radical operation is required, various PD techniques range from an extended operation to the functional preservation operation including the PD preserving the whole stomach and pylorus ring [5] to retain ingestion ability.

In general, a high morbidity rate of complications in PD is found at 18%–52%, and in particular pancreatic fistula is reported in 5%–19% [6–11]. Serious complications such as intraabdominal abscess and bleeding are associated with anastomotic leakage at the pancreaticojejunostomy, and these complications will directly influence the results of the operation. Because the pancreas is very vulnerable to ischemia and has an active exocrine function, pancreatic fistula, bleeding, autolysis, or necrosis can easily occur after surgical treatment. Therefore, the various serious complications associated with pancreaticojejunostomy are different from anastomotic leakage in gastrointestinal tract anastomosis, and pancreaticojejunostomy is the most difficult technique in reconstruction after PD.

The frequency of complications associated with pancreaticojejunostomy and the difficulty of the surgical technique are influenced greatly by the pathology of the pancreas where anastomosis is required, or by consistency of the remaining pancreas and dilatation of the pancreatic duct. In many cases of cancer of the pancreatic head with pronounced chronic pancreatitis or concomitant pancreatitis, the pancreas is

TABLE 1. Pancreaticojejunostomy after normal soft pancreaticoduodenectomy: September 1992–September 1995

Operative results	No stenting ($n = 28$)	Stenting ($n = 20$)
Mean operative time (min)	258	283
Mean time of pancreaticojejunostomy (min)	27.2	23.0
Mean blood loss (ml)	1075	1280
Morbidity rate (%)	32	30
Leakage of pancreaticojejunostomy (%)	14	15
Mortality rate (%)	0	0
Mean duration before intake of solid food (days)	15.1	17.7
Mean hospital stay (days)	27.3	31.7

hardening and the pancreatic duct is dilated. Because the exocrine activity is decreased, the anastomosis is not difficult to perform, and the frequency of complications is low. In contrast, in bile duct cancer or gastric cancer, the pancreas is normal and soft, the pancreatic duct is narrow at 2–3 mm, the anastomosis is difficult to perform, and the frequency of complications is very high.

It has been thought that pancreaticojejunostomy should be applied only to cases of a dilated pancreatic duct but not to cases of undilated pancreatic duct, instead allowing spontaneously formation of an internal fistula of pancreatic fluid with stent tubing. In contrast, there is another suggestion that pancreaticojejunostomy should be performed irrespective of stent tubing or no stent tubing. When a stent tube is inserted, lost tubing is used to maintain patency of the pancreatic duct, or external pancreatic drainage established through the intestine or through the liver is carried out to form a complete internal drainage for pancreatic juice; however, external drainage through the intestine is commonly used.

Our experience in 1000 cases of PD shows an frequency of early complications of 24% and an in-patient mortality rate of 8%; 34% of these events were associated with anastomotic leakage at the pancreaticojejunostomy. In particular, the frequency of anastomotic leakage at the pancreaticojejunostomy was 11% in cases of a soft and undilated pancreas and only 4% in cases of a hard and dilated pancreas ($P < .001$). To prevent anastomotic leakage, a procedure in which an external drainage tube through the pancreatic duct or a stent tube such as a lost tube has been used in conventional procedures. It has been frequently reported that frequency of anastomotic leakage at the pancreaticojejunostomy was decreased by these procedures.

In pancreaticojejunostomies involving a normal pancreas previously carried out in our department, interrupted sutures were placed in the pancreatic stump and an opening was made in the jejunal wall contralateral to the pancreatic duct corresponding to the diameter of the duct in early cases. Neither mucosa-to-mucosa anastomosis nor a stent tube was used, expecting spontaneous formation of an inner fistula. The frequency of anastomotic leakage at the pancreaticojejunostomy was more than 50%, and mortality was also high. We have used a pancreatic external drainage tube since about 1976, and adopted pancreaticojejunostomy in 1979 because, to prevent anastomotic leakage, it was considered essential to decrease the pressure in the anastomotic site and preserve patency in the opening of the anastomosis or to carry out drainage of pancreatic fluid and stent tubing. After introduction of the pancreatic external drainage tube and pancreaticojejunostomy, the frequency of anastomotic leakage decreased markedly but was still approximately 15%. Because anastomotic leakage at the pancreaticojejunostomy is not avoidable in patients with a normal pancreas, we began to perform thorough abdominal drainage surrounding the pancreaticojejunostomy. Thus, the number of deaths from anastomotic leakage at the pancreaticojejunostomy was drastically decreased.

We however experienced some complications associated with stent tubing. Using a pancreatic external drainage tube, we experienced two cases in which stenosis of the pancreatic duct occurred by injury to the pancreatic duct wall because a suture used to support the tube and the duct wall did not come off when the tube was drawn out. There were some cases with damage caused by pancreatic leakage by bending and stenosis at the area where the tube was fixed to the skin. Pancreatitis occurred in two cases after high-pressure imaging through the tube for examination of patency in the pancreaticojejunostomy. Similar complications have been reported from other medical institutions. In patients with a lost stent tube, we experienced cases with damage caused by a pancreatic leak from an obstructed tube or from long-term retention of the tube. Because we experienced these complications associated with retention of the stent tube, we finally concluded that stent tubing would be unnecessary if patency of the pancreatic duct were satisfactorily preserved by adequate anastomosis of the pancreatic duct wall and jejunal wall. The point of the procedure of this operation is to satisfactorily preserve patency of the pancreatic duct by carefully picking up the pancreatic duct wall to prevent injury and stenosis of the pancreatic duct.

This study is based on the results from a controlled randomized study in which a particular surgeon performed all operations by a standardized procedure. According to the results obtained for the past 3 years, there was no significant difference in mean operative time or in mean pancreaticojejunostomy time. While it seems that the anastomosis of the fine pancreatic duct and jejunum is more troublesome and a longer operative time is necessary, there is actually no significant difference. If surgeons master this surgical technique, the operative time may be shortened further. There is no significant difference in the mean perioperative blood loss, but there a tendency for the loss to be about 200 ml less in the no-stent method than that in the stent method. The reason may be that not only the anastomosis but also the whole course of this operation was performed carefully. The morbidity rates of early complications and anastomotic leakage at the pancreaticojejunostomy are about 30% and about 15%, respectively, showing no significant difference. No patient died as a result of the operation. There is no significant difference in the mean time to postoperative food intake and the mean postoperative hospital stay, but the number of days was slightly less in the no-stent method. In patients followed-up for 1 year, the pancreatic endocrine and exocrine functions were preserved.

In conclusion, this operative procedure is considered a basic procedure of pancreaticojejunostomy because it can be performed with little risk and the pancreatic functions are preserved. This procedure is applicable to operations after pancreatectomy and to reconstruction such as pancreaticojejunostomy involving the Roux-en-Y-elevated jejunal crus after pancreatic segmental resection.

References

1. Whipple AO, Parsons WB, Mullins CR (1935) Treatment of carcinoma of the ampulla of Vater. Ann Surg 102:763–779
2. Cattell RB (1943) Resection of the pancreas; discussion of special problem. Surg Clin N Am 23:753–766
3. Child CG III (1944) Pancreaticojejunostomy and other problems associated with the surgical management of carcinoma involving the head of the pancreas. Ann Surg 119:845–855
4. Imanaga H (1960) A new method of pancreaticoduodenectomy designed to preserve liver and pancreatic function. Surgery (St Louis) 47:577–586
5. Traverso LW, Longmire WP Jr (1978) Preservation of the pylorus in pancreaticoduodenectomy. Surg Gynecol Obstet 146:959–962
6. Crist DW, Sitzmann JV, Cameron JL (1987) Improved hospital morbidity, mortality, and survival after the Whipple procedure. Ann Surg 206:358–365
7. Grace PA, Pitt HA, Tompkins RK, DenBesten L, Longmire WP Jr (1986) Decreased morbidity and mortality after pancreatoduodenectomy. Am J Surg 151:141–149
8. Cameron JL, Pitt HA, Yeo CJ, Lillemoe KD, Kaufman HS, Coleman J (1993) One hundred and forty-five consecutive pancreaticoduodenectomies without mortality. Ann Surg 217:430–438

9. Castillo CF, Rattner DW, Warshaw AL (1995) Standards for pancreatic resection in the 1990s. Arch Surg 130:295–300
10. Trede M, Schwall G, Saeger H (1990) Survival after pancreatoduodenectomy—118 consecutive resections without an operative mortality. Ann Surg 211:447–458
11. Andersen HB, Baden H, Brahe NEB, Burcharth F (1994) Pancreaticoduodenectomy for periampullary adenocarcinoma. J Am Coll Surg 179:545–552

Reconstruction after Pancreatoduodenectomy

Hans-Bernd Reith[1], Waldemar Kozuschek[2], and Wilhelm Haarmann[2]

Summary. The Whipple procedure is improved by preservation of a functioning pylorus. Indications for this procedure are malignancies of the head of pancreas and chronic pancreatitis. The reconstruction after this substantial operation depends on tissue formation and the personal experience of the surgeon. Gastroduodenostomy is performed in the right-upper abdomen or in an antecolic way. Hepaticojejunostomy is carried out in the triangle technique described by A. Gütgemann and J.P.W. Longmire. The pancreatojejunostomy we perform is an end-to-end technique in cases of fibrotic or hard pancreatic tissue and an end-to-side technique with ventral plication of the anastomosis for the soft pancreas remnant. The response of cytokines after duodenopancreatectomy is demonstrated for the pylorus-preserving procedure (PPPD) and compared to standard Whipple and PPPD in jaundiced patients. The results showed no significant differences in these three groups.

Key words. Pylorus preservation—Reconstruction techniques—End-to-side pancreatojejunostomy with plication—Cytokine response

Background of Pancreatoduodenectomy

It appears that Friedrich Trendelenburg (1844–1924) was the first, in 1882, to successfully excise a solid tumor of the pancreas that turned out to be a spindle cell carcinoma involving the body and tail of the pancreas. In 1889, Guiseppe Ruggi (1844–1906) removed a solid tumor of the pancreas [1]. In 1894 D. Biondi removed a tumor of papilla vateri with a two-thirds resection of the head of the pancreas [2].

An important point in this history is the year 1898. Two surgeons, Allessandro Codivilla (1861–1912) in Bologna and also William Stewart Halsted (1852–1922) in New York, excised successfully a malignant tumor of the ampullary region. Codivilla [3] performed a block excision of a major part of the duodenum and head of the

---

[1] Department of Surgery, University Würzburg, D-97080 Würzburg, Germany.
[2] Department of Surgery, Ruhr-University Bochum, Knappschaftskrankenhaus, D-44892 Bochum, Germany.

pancreas. The pylorus was closed and the termination of the duodenum invaginated. Reconstruction with gastroenterostomy and cholecystojejunostomy was carried out. Halsted [4] performed the duodenopancreatectomy in a very similar way. In 1909 Walter Kausch (1867–1928) in Berlin performed a radical duodenopancreatectomy with preservation of the gastric antrum and the pylorus region [5]. Kausch performed the operation in two stages. For years he was the only one to be successful with this procedure and only a few cared to copy the method. O. Tenani in 1922 resected two-thirds of the pancreas head and performed a duodenoduodenal anastomosis with choledochoduodenostomy.

The surgical procedure developed for lesions of the duodenum and pancreas by Allen Oldfather Whipple (1881–1963) and colleagues in 1935 [6] did not intend partial gastric resection. In the procedure the duodenum was transected, the stump blindly closed, and the antropyloric passage bridged by a gastroenterostomy; it was indeed the same method as Kausch performed 24 years earlier. K. Watson reported in 1942 a case in which he preserved the antrum, the pylorus, and 2.5 cm of the duodenum. Watson believed that preservation of an intact stomach would be beneficial for digestion and thus improve the nutritional status [7].

Chronic Pancreatitis

Excision of the head of the pancreas was required in patients with chronic pancreatitis for abdominal pain resulting from one of two situations: progressive disease in the pancreatic head (pseudocyst, duct blowout, or arteriovenous fistula) or significant fibrosis in the pancreatic head resulting in an enlarged, usually extensively calcified, head with duct obstruction with or without bile or duodenal obstruction [8].

According to the different intraoperative situations, we performed, between 1975 and 1994, 144 operations in patients with chronic pancreatitis (Fig. 1); 85 patients underwent a resection in this period (Fig. 2). The standard Whipple procedure and pylorus-preserving pancreatoduodenectomy (PPPD) were carried out in 27 and 28

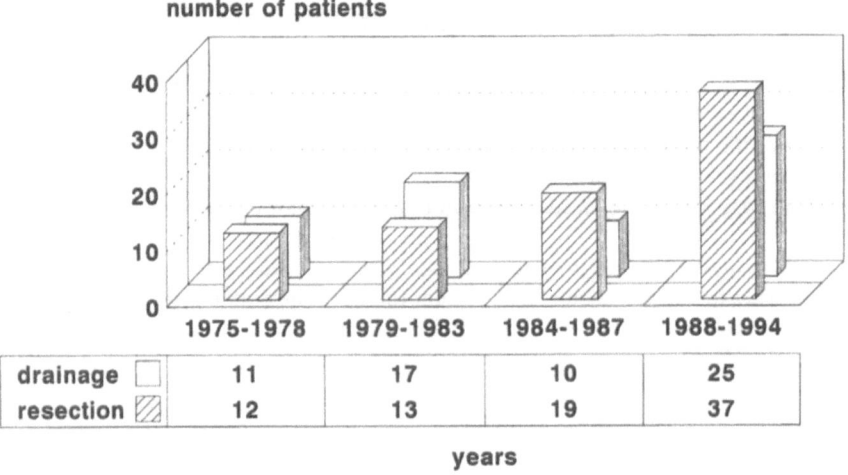

number of patients	1975-1978	1979-1983	1984-1987	1988-1994
drainage ☐	11	17	10	25
resection ▨	12	13	19	37

years

FIG. 1. Number of operations for chronic pancreatitis between 1975 and 1994 with resection (*shaded bars*) and drainage (*unshaded bars*) operations

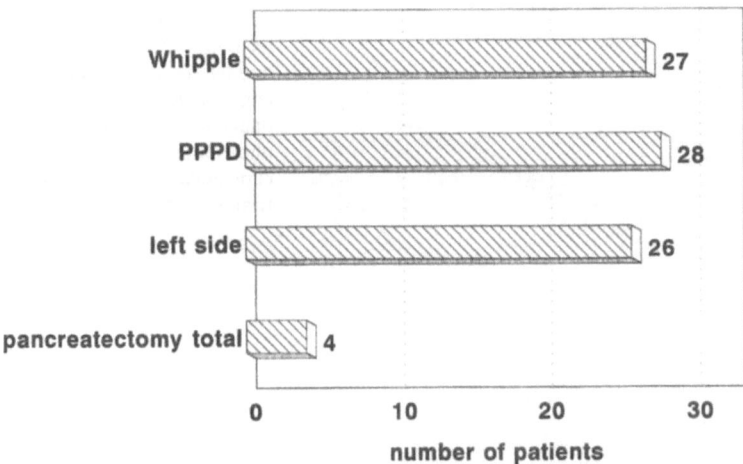

FIG. 2. Number of patients undergoing various resections resulting from chronic pancreatitis. PPPD, Pylorus-preserving pancreatoduodenectomy

patients. The ability to gain weight was much better in the PPPD; however, all the patients have had a more or less aggressive chronic pancreatitis of the remnant pancreas, so the results are at least not comparable.

Reconstruction Techniques

The different techniques of reconstruction are described elsewhere. We would like to point out our modifications from the bile duct–jejunostomy and the pancreaticojejunostomy.

Choledochojejunostomy or Hepaticojejunostomy

The biliary anastomosis in the Whipple procedure may be either a choledocho- or a hepaticojejunostomy. This is governed to a certain extent by the level of division of the bile duct at resection. The common hepatic duct has a better blood supply and is, on a theoretical basis, the anastomotic site of choice.

For the biliary anastomosis, we prefer the end-to-side triangle anastomosis from the technique of Gütgemann et al. [9]. We never use stents or T-tubes; however, the triangle technique leads also, for normal-caliber bile ducts, to a wide-open anastomosis. Every bile duct anastomosis has some tendency of shrinking, so this technique is a safe method. In the situation with dilatated bile ducts, this technique is also important.

Pancreaticojejunal Anastomosis

The two most frequently employed types of pancreaticojejunal anastomosis are end-to-end invagination and the end-to-side technique. The invaginated end-to-end anastomosis is made in such a way that the pancreatic remnant is telescoped into the lumen of the jejunum. This is achieved by using two long-stay sutures; the anastomo-

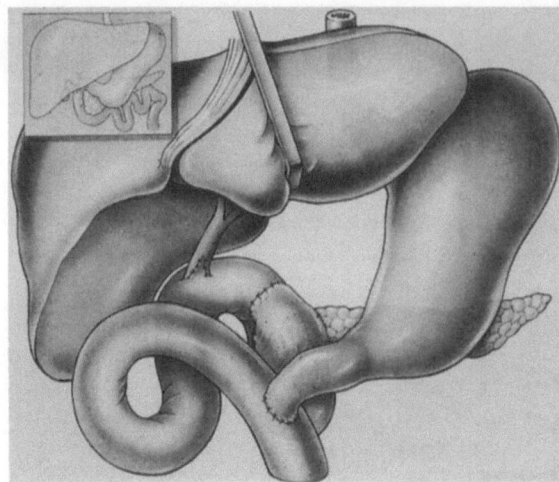

FIG. 3. Reconstruction technique after duodenopancreatectomy; end-to-side pancreatojejunostomy with plication, end-to-side choledochojejunostomy with triangle procedure

sis is completed with sutures between the pancreas and the full thickness of the jejunal wall.

The end-to-side technique with the principle of duct-to-mucosa anastomosis is the other often-used way. In our own experience we prefer the end-to-end technique only if a fibrotic pancreas exists; however, with a soft-tissued pancreas we perform a end-to-side technique with a plication of the blind ending loop to the ventral surface. This is a protection for the abdominal cavity and also prevents postoperative fistulas (Fig. 3).

Cytokine Response After Duodenopancreatectomy

Trauma, shock, and infection initiate a complex inflammatory response in which proinflammatory cytokines, tumor necrosis factor-α (TNF-α), and interleukin-6 (Il-6) are thought to play a pivotal role [10,11]. The role of these cytokines has been studied almost exclusively in relation to pathogenesis of infection and septic shock; only a few studies consider cytokinemia after trauma or hemorrhagic shock. In some new references there have been reported investigations of cytokine patterns in patients after major vascular surgery and major operations. The role of cytokines in patients having operations still is not completely understood. Serum concentrations of routinely used indicators of inflammatory response, i.e., C-reactive protein, often are difficult to interpret when measured postoperatively and give little guidance about differentiation between infective inflammation and inflammation caused by the operation [12,13].

We studied 19 patients undergoing a duodenopancreas head resection, 10 patients with preservation of the pylorus (PPPD), 4 patients with standard Whipple procedure (SW), and 5 patients with PPPD who were jaundiced at the time of operation (JP), but only with slow depression of liver function (Quick, >50%; albumin, >4.5 g%; bilirubin, <10 mg%). We investigated the kinetics of serum concentrations of TNF-α, Il-6, and C-reactive protein (CRP), and also leukocytes and urea nitrogen.

Methods

Serum samples were drawn preoperatively, 2 h after the end of the operation, and postoperatively on days 1, 2, 3, 5, 7, and 10. The samples were immediately centrifuged and then stored at −20°C until the assays were done. Immunoassay measurements were made using an EASIA (enzyme-amplified sensitivity immunoassay) for Il-6 and TNF (Medgenix Diagnostics, Ratingen, Germany). CRP was assayed by an immunoturbidimetry method in routine use (Boehringer Mannheim GmbH, Mannheim, Germany). The routinely used laboratory data were also measured and correlated. All data are mean ± SEM. For statistic analysis we used the Mann–Whitney U-test to evaluate differences with $P < .05$ (P = n.s. means without statistical significance).

Results

In all 19 patients who underwent duodenopancreatectomy there was an increase in serum Il-6 concentration after the operation. Il-6 reached a mean serum concentration of 332 ng/ml (±113) for PPPD, 364 ng/ml (±109) for SW, and 388 ng/ml (±124) for JP (P = n.s.). A decrease followed in the next days in all groups. None of the patients had infective complications, and none of the patients required support with vasoactive amines, adrenalin or noradrenalin infusion, or prolonged treatment in the intensive care unit (Fig. 4).

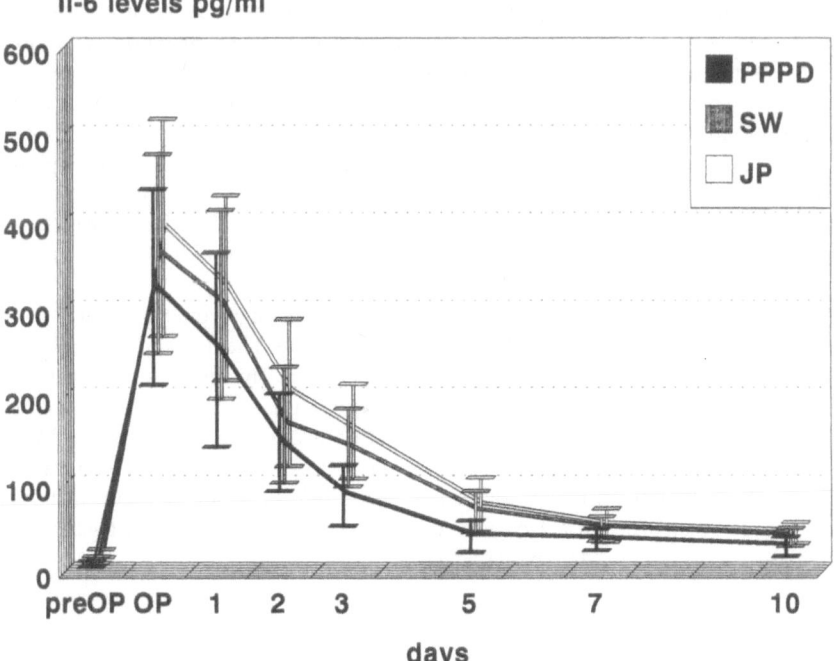

FIG. 4. Interleukin-6 levels of different groups with duodenopancreatectomy. *PPPD*, Pyloruspreserving group (*black symbols*); *SW*, standard Whipple group (*shaded symbols*); JP, jaundiced patients with PPPD (*unshaded symbols*). All levels are mean ± SEM; no statistical differences

TNF-α levels in all groups remained low. The mean levels were in the normal range preoperatively in the PPPD and SW groups; however, in the JP group there was a slight increase. Levels were 15.4 ng/ml (±3.7) for PPPD, 16.2 ng/ml (±3.2) for SW, and 34.2 ng/ml (±4.7) for the JP group (P = n.s. for all groups). All levels without differences after day 2. CRP concentrations rose 48–96 h after the operation without differences among the three groups. After peaking the levels decreased slowly and did not reach a normal range until day 10. There were no statistically significant differences.

All other measured data of blood samples such as leukocytes, thrombocytes, and urea nitrogen showed no significant differences from the pre- to postoperative course. For example, the mean values of leukocytes ranged from 8700 mm^3 (±1400) pre-operatively to 13 100 mm^3 (±1300) maximum value after the operation.

Discussion

After an operation, macrophages are thought to have a pivotal role in the process of tissue remodeling and repair, and they may be responsible for the initial secretion of cytokines, such as Il-6. C-Reactive protein production is induced mainly by Il-6, while other cytokines such as TNF-α have only an accessory function in this respect. As all patients with duodenopancreatectomy have had no periods of hemorrhagic shock or ischemia, it seems to be clear that no increase of TNF blood serum concentrations were found [14–16].

In the present study, concentrations of Il-6 increased immediately after the operation in all patients undergoing this substantial procedure. Without any infective episode or complication in the postoperative period, Il-6 levels decreased within the next 48 h. The extent of the operation is correlated with Il-6 concentrations, as shown by the fact that the patients who have the longest operation times have the highest Il-6 response. These findings are in agreement with other reports [17]. There was no correlation to the Il-6 response for jaundiced patients.

The C-reactive concentrations reached a maximum at 48–96 h after surgery and then slowly declined over a few days. In view of the slow reaction of C-reactive protein this acute-phase reaction may be of limited help when predicting the occurrence of early postoperative infective complications. These results are similar to the findings of other groups [13,17].

To summarize, even during uncomplicated operations high concentrations of Il-6 are produced, which results in high concentrations of CRP. The Il-6 values returned to low concentrations within a mean of 48 h after operation. This indicates that patients who were jaundiced could also undergo a duodenopancreatectomy, without a complete recovery of their liver function if the function is only slightly depressed. Every preoperative manipulation in the bile duct system, e.g., stenting or a nasobiliary tube, increases the risk of inflammatory tissue reaction and this excluded patients from the pylorus-preserving procedure. However, it is necessary to have a cytokine baseline for major operations like duodenopancreatectomy.

References

1. Ruggi G (1890) Intorno ad uno caso di carcinoma primitivo del pancreas. G Int Scienz Med 12:81

2. Biondi D (1896) Contributio clinico esperimentals alla chirurgia del pancreas. Clin Chir 4:131
3. Codivilla A (1898) Chirurgia del pancreas. Bull Soc Med Bologna 9:651
4. Halsted WS (1899) Contributions to the surgery of the bile passages. Boston Med Surg J 141:645
5. Kausch W (1912) Das Karzinom der Papilla duodeni und seine radikale Behandlung. Bruns' Beitr Klin Chir 78:439
6. Whipple AO, Parson WB, Mullins CR (1935) Treatment of carcinoma of the ampulla of Vater. Ann Surg 102:763
7. Watson K (1944) Carcinoma of the ampulla of Vater. Successful radical resection. Br J Surg 31:515–526
8. Traverso LW (1993) The pylorus-preserving Whipple procedure for severe complications of chronic pancreatitis. In: Beger HG, Büchler M, Malfertheiner P (eds) Standards in pancreatic surgery. Springer, Berlin Heidelberg New York, pp 369–413
9. Gütgemann A, Schriefers KH, Philip R, Wülfing D (1965) Zur rekonstruktiven Chirurgie des verletzten und strikturierten Gallenganges. Bruns' Beitr Klin Chir 210:129–138
10. Cerami A (1992) Inflammatory cytokines. Clin Immunol Immunpathol 62:3–10
11. Dianrello CA, Mier JW (1987) Current concepts—lymphokines. N Engl J Med 317:940–945
12. Roumen RMH, Hendriks T, van der Ven-Jongekrijg, Nieuwenhuijzen GAP, Sauerwein RW, van der Meer JWM, Goris RJA (1993) Cytokine patterns in patients after major vascular surgery, hemorrhagic shock and severe blunt trauma. Ann Surg 218:769–776
13. Kragsbjerg P, Holmberg H, Vikerfors T (1995) Serum concentrations of interleukin-6, tumor necrosis factor alpha and C-reactive protein in patients undergoing major operations. Eur J Surg 161:17–22
14. Ayala A, Wang P, Ba ZF, Perin MM (1991) Different alterations in plasma Il-6 and TNF levels after trauma and hemorrhage. Am J Physiol 260:167–171
15. Caty MG, Guice KS, Oldmann KT (1990) Evidence for tumor necrosis factor-induced pulmonary microvascular injury after intestinal ischemia-reperfusion injury. Ann Surg 21:694–700
16. Ghezzi P, Dinarello CA, Bianchi M (1991) Hypoxia increases production of interleukin-1 and tumor necrosis factor by human mononuclear cells. Cytokine 3:189–194
17. Baigrie RJ, Lamont PM, Kwiatkowski D, Dallman MJ, Morris PJ (1992) Systemic cytokine response after major surgery. Br J Surg 79:757–760

Quality of Life After Pancreatoduodenectomy

A Comparison of Quality of Life: Standard Versus Pylorus-Preserving Pancreatoduodenectomy

Makoto Sunamura, Masao Kobari,
Kazunori Takeda, and Seiki Matsuno

Summary. Pylorus-preserving pancreatoduodenectomy (PPPD) has been adopted for patients with disease of the periampullary region as an alternative to the standard pancreatoduodenectomy. To qualify the exact effect of PPPD, we evaluated early postoperative condition and nutritional status 12 months after surgery in patients suffering from periampullary disease without pancreatic ductal carcinoma and chronic pancreatitis. Fifteen patients underwent PPPD and 16 patients, PD. The type of resection had no influence on postoperative condition and nutritional status. There was no significant difference in length of hospital stay and in medical expenses. Although it is suggested that PPPD is a useful procedure for patients with pancreatic ductal carcinoma, further studies are required to estimate the advantage of PPPD for pancreatic ductal carcinoma.

Key words. Pylorus-preserving pancreatoduodenectomy—Standard pancreatoduodenectomy—Periampullary carcinoma—Cystic disease of the pancreatic head

Introduction

Since Whipple et al. [1] in 1953 described the first resection of the head of the pancreas, intestinal disturbances such as dumping, diarrhea, dyspeptic complaints, and ulcer at the gastroenterostomy site have been involved in this procedure. In 1978, pancreatoduodenectomy entered the current era of pylorus preservation. Traverso and Longmire [2] reasoned that preservation of an intact stomach would eliminate the complications of a reduced gastric reservoir and improve the nutritional status of patients. It is now apparent that the morbidity and mortality rates of pylorus-preserving pancreatoduodenectomy (PPPD) do not exceed those of the conventional Whipple resection [3–5]. It is reasonable to assume, however, that preservation of an intact stomach will improve postoperative nutrition and weight gain.

Department of Surgery 1, Tohoku University School of Medicine, Aoba-ku, Sendai, Miyagi 980-77, Japan.

It is important to evaluate this alternative of pancreatoduodenectomy to determine if its promise of better gastrointestinal function has been accomplished. To qualify the advantage of PPPD, studies were conducted to estimate the postoperative condition of patients after pancreatoduodenectomy (PD) for not only benign disease but also maliganant disease. The aim of this study was to establish whether PPPD brings about a better quality of life compared with the standard Whipple's procedure. We excluded patients with pancreatic cancer and chronic pancreatitis from this study.

Patients and Methods

Between 1987 and 1995, 15 and 16 patients underwent PPPD or PD, respectively, for cancer of the papilla of Vater, cystic tumor of the pancreas, pancreatic endocrine tumor, and noninvasive bile duct cancer. The two modalities of treatment were compared with respect to operative complications, early postoperative recovery, and nutritional status. Medical costs were also compared between PPPD and PD.

The results reported represent the mean ± SEM for multiple determinations. Differences between groups were evaluated using the unpaired t-test with significant differences defined as those associated with a probability value of <.05.

Results

Patients and Operative Complications

PPPD and PD groups had one and two major leakages of the pancreatojejunostomy, respectively, and both cases resorted consequently to operations for drainage. The PPPD group had a case complicated with bleeding from the duodenojejunostomy, followed by distal gastrectomy. One patient in the PD group underwent reoperation because of an adhesional ileus. These five patients were excluded from the following studies related to postoperative conditions. There were five and seven patients, re-

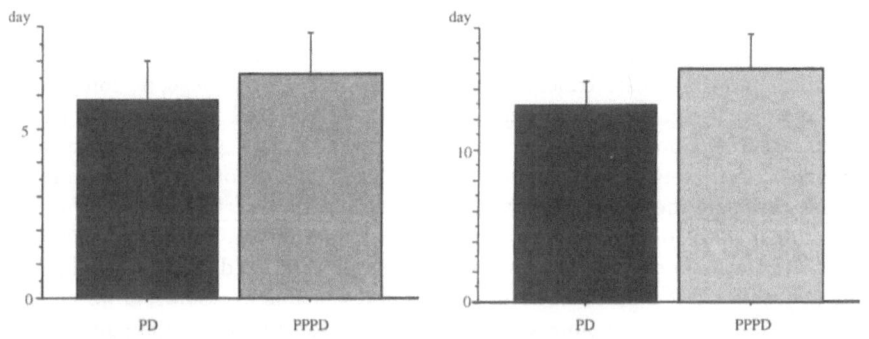

FIG. 1. Duration of nasogastric intubation. The period in the pylorus-preserving pancreatoduodenectomy (PPPD) group was about 6.6 days (*shaded bar*), showing no significant difference as compared with 5.8 days in the PD (*black bar*) group

FIG. 2. Date of oral intake after operation. The patients in the PD (*black bar*) group started their fluid meals on average 13 days after operation with earlier recovery than those in PPPD group (*shaded bar*), who began fluid meals on the fifteenth day; however, there was no significant difference

spectively, who suffered from cancer of the papilla of Vater in the PPPD group and the PD group. Five cases in the PPPD group and one case in the PD group underwent operations for cystic tumor of the pancreas.

Early Postoperative Recovery

To evaluate early postoperative recovery, duration of gastric suction and postoperative date of oral intake of the first fluid meal were analyzed. Duration of nasogastric suction in the PPPD group was about 6.6 days, showing no significant difference as compared with 5.8 days in the PD group (Fig. 1). The patients in the PD group started their fluid meals on average 13 days after operation, with earlier recovery than those in PPPD group, who started on or after the fifteenth day; however, there was no significant difference between the two groups (Fig. 2).

Nutritional Status After Surgery

Patients were not rendered anemic after surgery, with a tendency toward a gradual increase in red blood cell numbers (Fig. 3). The levels of serum proteins in both groups elevated gradually after operation without a significant difference between the two groups (Fig. 4). The values in the PPPD and PD groups increased from 6.8 and 6.7 mg/dl to 7.3 and 7.1 mg/dl, respectively, 12 months later. Increases in serum albumin values were also detected in both groups, with no significant difference (Fig. 5). Loss of body weight was noted 6 months after the surgery (Fig. 6); however, body weight gradually recovered and reached preoperative values 12 months after the surgery.

Hospital Stay and Medical Costs

Neither intensive chemotherapy nor irradiation was adopted for patients in this study. Mean duration of the hospital stay after operations was about 46 days in the PPPD group, a shorter period as compared with that of the PD group, 50 days (Fig. 7).

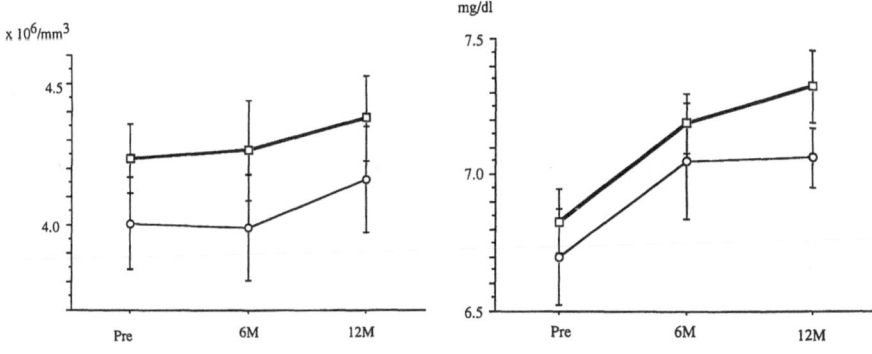

FIG. 3. Changes of red blood cell numbers. Patients (*squares*, PPPD; *circles*, PD) were not rendered anemic after surgery, with a tendency toward gradual increase in numbers of red blood cells

FIG. 4. Changes of serum protein levels. The levels in both groups (*squares*, PPPD; *circles*, PD) elevated gradually after operation without significant difference. The values in the PPPD and PD groups increased from 6.8 and 6.7 mg/dl to 7.3 and 7.1 mg/dl, respectively, 12 months later

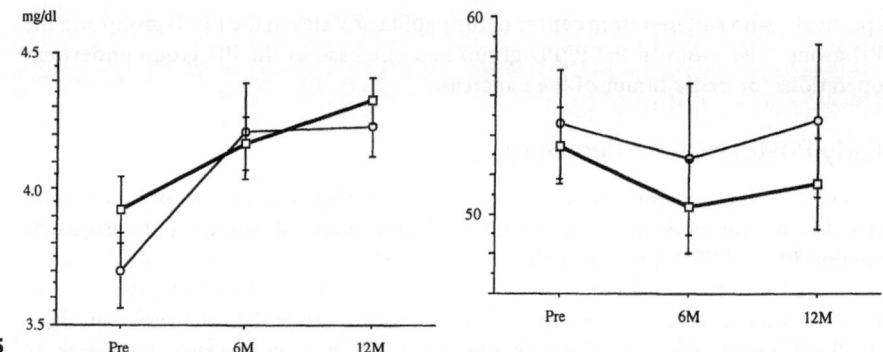

Fig. 5. Changes of serum albumin levels. The increases in serum albumin values were also detected in both groups (*squares*, PPPD; *circles*, PD), showing no significant difference

Fig. 6. Postoperative ability to gain weight. Loss of body weight was noted 6 months after surgery. Body weight gradually recovered and reached preoperative period values 12 months after surgery. *Circles*, PD; *squares*, PPPD

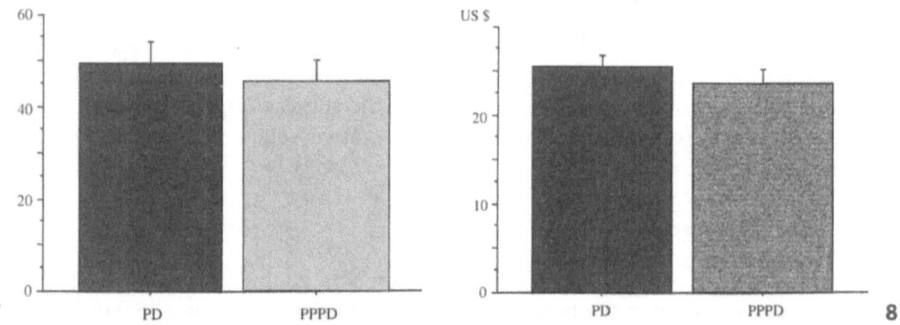

Fig. 7. Length of hospital stay. Mean duration of the hospital stay after operations was about 46 days in the PPPD group (*shaded bar*), a shorter period as compared with that of PD group (*black bar*), 50 days

Fig. 8. Medical costs for PD and PPPD. Mean expenses in the PPPD (*shaded bar*) and PD (*black bar*) groups were about $23 665 and $25 474, respectively, during their hospital stay

Medical costs during hospital stay were calculated; the mean expenses in the PPPD and PD groups were about $23 665 and $25 474, respectively (Fig. 8).

Discussion

It is presumed that the nutritional status of patients with pancreatic ductal carcinoma is poorer than that of those with carcinoma of ampulla and cystic neoplasms of the pancreas because patients with pancreatic cancer are vulnerable to recurrence and subject to malnutrition after extended radical operations accompanied by retroperitoneal dissection and resection of the neural plexus. Furthermore, we adopted combined interventions such as irradiation therapy and chemotherapy after pancreatoduodenectomy. These factors affect the quality of life (QOL) of the patients in addition to the effect of the operation. In this study, we excluded the factors that are not brought about by the resection of organs. Fibrotic changes of pancreatic parenchyma in chronic pancreatitis are responsible for diabetes mellitus, resulting in worsening of the nutritional status after resection of the pancreas. We excluded the patients with pancreatic ductal carcinoma and chronic pancreatitis to estimate the nutritional conditions following the operations of PPPD and standard PD.

PPPD did not show delayed gastric emptying or delayed oral intake. It is observed that leakage of the pancreatojejunostomy disturbed intestinal motility, resulting in delayed recovery of the alimentary tract. It was considered that PPPD was a suitable operation for carcinoma of the papilla of Vater and cystic disease of the pancreatic head in which the pancreatic parenchyma is normal. The softer parenchyma had a higher frequency of leakage from pancreatojejunostomy, followed by delayed gastric emptying. This is speculated to result from the lengthy time of nasogastric suction employed in PPPD. In this study, the data did not show any disadvantages of PPPD in the aspect of early recovery of oral intake.

Regarding nutritional condition, PPPD showed no advantage over conventional PD 1 year after surgery for patients who suffered from low-grade malignant disease or benign disease. The patients in the PD group could recover postoperatively to a stable nutritional condition as quickly as those in the PPPD group. One patient underwent PD for carcinoma of the papilla of Vater 12 years ago. His body weight was stable, between 70 and 72 kg, and his serum protein levels were maintained at more than 6.8 mg/dl during this period. He did not experience any inconvenience in his daily work.

It is suggested that PPPD is a useful alternative for patients with pancreatic ductal carcinoma. We routinely treat these patients not only by surgery but also by chemotherapy, irradiation therapy, and immunotherapy, exposing the patients to conditions of malnutrition. PPPD plays a role for these patients by maintaining the volume of oral intake and by providing a better QOL during intensive therapies.

There is still controversy about the indication of PPPD for pancreatic cancer. The histological analysis in our department demonstrated that the positive ratio of metastatic lymph nodes was 11.1% and 10.5% in the upper portion and lower portion of the pyloric ring, respectively. Roder et al. [6] reported that patients with pancreatic carcinoma who underwent PD had a significantly better survival rate than those who underwent PPPD. Further controlled studies are necessary to quantify the usefulness of PPPD for pancreatic carcinoma.

References

1. Whipple AO, Parsons W, Mullins CR (1935) Treatment of carcinoma of the ampulla of Vater. Ann Surg 102:763–779
2. Traverso LW, Longmire WP Jr (1978) Preservation of the pylorus in pancreaticoduodenectomy. Surg Gynecol Obstet 146:959–962
3. Klinkenbijil JHG, van der Schelling GP, Hop WCJ, et al (1992) The advantage of pylorus-preserving pancreatoduodenectomy in malignant disease of the pancreas and periampullary region. Ann Surg 216:142–145
4. Itani KMF, Coleman RE, Akwari OE, Meyers WC (1986) Pylorus-preserving pancreatoduodenectomy. A clinical and physiologic appraisal. Ann Surg 204:655–664

5. Kozuschek W, Reith HB, Waleczek H, et al (1994) A comparison of long term results of the standard Whipple procedure and the pylorus preserving pancreatoduodenectomy. Am Coll Surg 178:443–453
6. Roder JD, Stein HJ, Huttle W, Siewert JR (1992) Pylorus-preserving versus standard pancreaticoduodenectomy: an analysis of 110 pancreatic and periampullary carcinomas. Br J Surg 79:152–155

Assessment of Quality of Life After Pancreatoduodenectomy

Masahiro Yamamoto, Hidehumi Ishida, Osamu Ohashi,
Takashi Kamigaki, Taichi Kanamaru,
Hirohiko Onoyama, and Yoichi Saitoh

Summary. The quality of life (QOL) after pancreatoduodenectomy (PD) was assessed by symptom scale scores related to physical and emotional aspects, performance status (PS) as social activity, and the Cornell Medical Index (CMI), related to psycho-physiological aspects. Complete sets of data were obtained from 33 patients. A follow-up period after PD varied from 1 to 16 years. The incidence of the emotional symptoms was relatively higher than the physical symptoms. The symptom scale scores showed highest correlations with PS and CMI. Problems in the psychological condition might be related to significant differences in QOL. It is necessary to make a long-term evaluation for postoperative cholangitis, for which alkaline phosphatase levels in the blood and biliary scintigraphy are useful for diagnosis even in a symptom-free period.

Key words. Pancreatoduodenectomy—Quality of life—Cholangitis

Introduction

Pancreatoduodenectomy (PD), also termed the Whipple procedure, has been a standard surgery for patients with periampullary and pancreatic head carcinoma and with pancreatic head complications in chronic pancreatitis. Recently, the pylorus-preserving PD (PPPD) as an organ-preserving procedure has been also applied with the intention of better long-term outcome. As the procedure has come to be very successful with low morbidity and mortality, the number of patients who do survive for a long-term period are increasing, with the consequence that more attention is paid to the quality of this longer life. Quality of life (QOL) is, however, hard to assess and seldom measured, especially in patients having had undergone PD. The present study investigated QOL up to 16 years after PD with regard to physical and emotional symptoms, social activity, psychological distress, and postoperative cholangitis.

First Department of Surgery, Kobe University School of Medicine, Chuo-ku, Kobe, Hyogo 650, Japan.

Patients and Methods

Postoperative results were evaluated from patients who had been followed for more than 1 year. Patients who had residual or recurrent disease were excluded.

The quality of postoperative life was assessed by hospital visit, phone call, or questionnaire. The 12 items related to physical and emotional symptoms were chosen, and each item was scored on a four-point rating scale, with alternatives from "no complaint at all" (score = 0) to "severe complaint" (score = 3). The symptom scale scores could range from 0 (not impaired at all) to 36 (strongly impaired). The level of social activity was assessed by using the Eastern Cooperative Oncology Group (ECOG) performance status (PS) scale. Additionally, the Cornell Medical Index (CMI) was used to measure psychophysiological alterations.

A clinical assessment of nutritional status was performed by assessing body weight change. Body weight was expressed as a percentage of the preillness weight. Analysis of body composition was performed using dual-energy X-ray absorptiometry (DXA), and changes in bone mineral content, lean body mass, and fat mass were measured. Glucose tolerance was examined by 75-g oral glucose tolerance test (OGTT) or judged from insulin dependency. Fatty liver was diagnosed as a reference of the findings obtained by laboratory test and ultrasonography (US).

Evaluation of cholangitis used the following items: (1) clinical symptom (a episode of fever or chills), (2) laboratory test (elevation of the biliary enzymes in the blood), and (3) US or cholangiography (dilation of the hepatic bile duct or stenosis of the bilioenteric anastomotic region). When at least two of these factors were present, the diagnosis of cholangitis was made. If only one item was present, the case was considered to be a suspected condition. Dynamic findings of the bile flow were obtained by means of biliary scintigraphy; the scintigram was taken up to 120 min after ^{99m}Tc-PMT (-pyridoxyl-5-methyl triptophan) intravenous injection.

Complete sets of data were obtained from 33 patients. Survival after operation ranged from 1 to 16 years (mean, 5.6 years). Of those, 27 patients had undergone a standard PD and 6 had a PPPD; 22 patients had neoplastic diseases for which pancreatic resection had been required, and 11 had chronic pancreatitis.

Results were expressed as mean and standard deviation, and differences were evaluated by Student's t-test for unpaired values. $P < .05$ was taken as the criterion of statistical significance. In addition, the chi-square test with Yates' correction and Spearman rank correlations were used to compare groups.

Results

Assessment of QOL and Relations Between QOL Indicators

With regard to social activity level, the PS scale proposed by ECOG was examined. About half the patients were fully active and had returned to their previous work or were capable of working without any restrictions after surgery (PS 0). About one-third of the patients were unable to carry out any work activities or were incapable of any self-care (PS 3 or 4) (Fig. 1).

Table 1 lists the 12 items related to physical and emotional symptoms. The percentages of patients who complained of the emotional symptoms such as feelings of illness and anxiety were relatively higher than the physical symptoms such as fatigue, thirstiness, sleep disturbance, and loss of appetite. As a result of scoring each item according

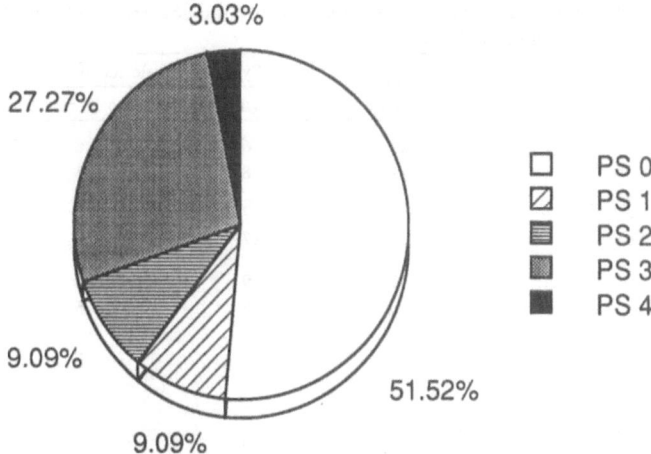

FIG. 1. The level of social activity assessed by Eastern Cooperative Oncology Group (ECOG) performance status (PS) scale in 33 patients who had undergone a standard pancreatoduodenectomy (PD) or pylorus-preserving PD (PPPD). PS 0, Fully active, able to carry on all predisease performance without restrictions; PS 1, restricted in physically strenuous activity but ambulatory and able to carry out work of a light or sedentary nature; such as light housework, office work; PS 2, ambulatory and capable of total self-care but unable to carry out any work activities, up and about more than 50% of waking hours; PS 3, capable of only limited self-care, confined to bed or chair more than 50% of waking hours; PS 4, completely disabled, incapable of any self-care; totally confined to bed or chair

TABLE 1. Assessment of quality of life (QOL): distribution of 33 patients under study on 12 survey items related to physical and emotional symptoms

Symptom	None (score = 0)	Mild (score = 1)	Moderate (score = 2)	Severe (score = 3)
Ill feeling	8	22	3	0
Loss of appetite	21	10	2	0
Sleep disturbance	14	12	7	0
Abdominal pain	25	6	2	0
Fever/chills	27	3	3	0
Nausea/vomiting	29	2	2	0
Fullness	24	7	2	0
Diarrhea	29	3	1	0
Constipation	26	7	0	0
Fatigue	12	17	3	1
Thirst	18	14	1	0
Anxiety	9	21	1	2

Each number indicates number of patients.
These symptoms were rated as none/mild/moderate/severe complaint and scored with alternatives as none (scace = 0) to severe (score = 3).

to the methods described in *Materials and Methods*, the symptom scale scores of each patient did not correlate with gender, age at time of assessment, duration of postoperative period, or type of operative procedure, but did correlate significantly with the disease for which pancreatic resection had been required such as neoplastic diseases

TABLE 2. Correlation between patient characteristics and the degree of symptom scale scores related to physical and emotional aspects

| Characteristic | No. of patients | Symptom scale scores | | P value |
		0 to 7 ($n = 24$)	8 to 18 ($n = 9$)	
Male	22	16	6	.65
Female	11	8	3	
Less than 60 years old	12	7	5	.16
More than 60 years old	21	17	4	
Within 5 years postoperative	13	9	4	.71
More than 5 years postoperative	20	15	5	
Neoplastic disease	22	20	2	<.001
Chronic pancreatitis	11	4	7	
Standard PD	27	20	7	.71
PPPD	6	4	2	

PD, Pancreatoduodenectomy; PPPD, pylorus-preserving PD. P value indicates the significance for chi-square test.

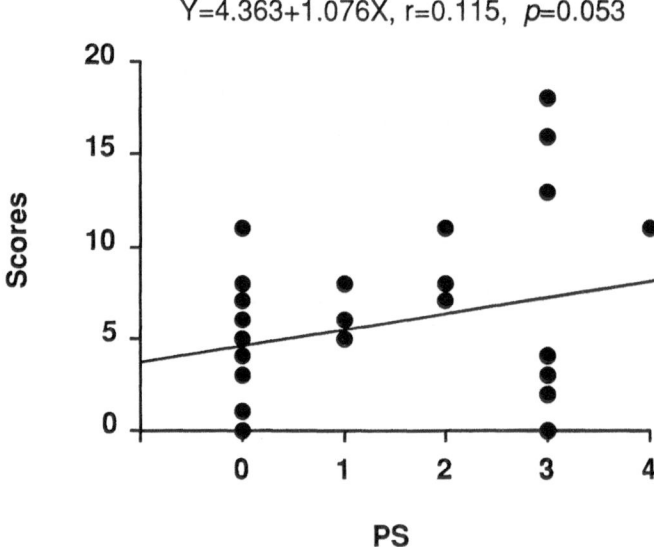

$Y=4.363+1.076X$, $r=0.115$, $p=0.053$

FIG. 2. Intercorrelation (Spearman rank correlations) between symptom scale scores and PS. Average scores were 4.17 ± 2.47 in PS 0 ($n = 17$) vs. 7.25 ± 5.37 in PS 1 to 4 ($n = 16$) ($P < .05$)

and chronic pancreatitis (neoplastic disease, 4.27 ± 3.46 vs. chronic pancreatitis, 8.45 ± 5.10; $P < .01$). There was a significant correlation between the degree (high or low) of the scores and the diseases (chi-square test for independence; $P < .001$) (Table 2).

The patients who scored high or low on physical and emotional symptoms tended to have a PS similarly high or low (Spearman rank correlations; $P = .053$) (Fig. 2). In the patients classed as PS 0, the mean symptom scores were 4.17 ± 2.87 ($n = 17$), while those with PS 1 to 4 were 7.25 ± 5.37 ($n = 16$) ($P < .05$).

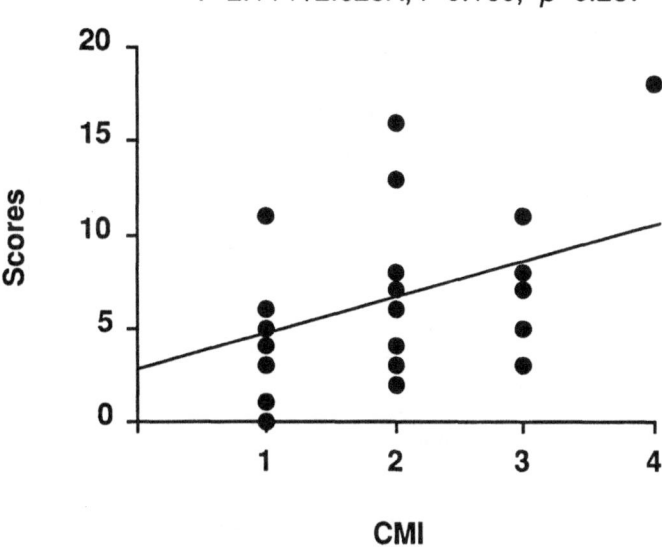

$Y=2.114+2.028X$, r=0.160, p=0.287

FIG. 3. Intercorrelation (Spearman rank-correlations) between symptom scale scores and Cornell Medical Index (CMI). Average scores were 4.00 ± 3.69 in CMI 1 ($n = 13$) vs. 7.35 ± 4.72 in CMI 2 to 4 ($n = 17$) ($P < .05$)

Results with regard to CMI showed 56.7% of the patients had some psychophysiological alterations such as being easily offended or melancholic, or having a dispairing nature and compulsive ideas. The patients who had some psychological distress tended to have symptom scale scores similarly high (Spearman rank correlations; $P = .028$) (Fig. 3). However, the CMI did not reflect disease-specific characteristics; that is, the psychological problems in most patients with chronic pancreatitis were negative ($P = .889$). Moreover, no significant correlations were found between CMI and PS ($P = .415$).

Clinical Symptoms and Factors Influencing QOL

Clinical symptoms such as body weight changes, impaired glucose tolerance, and postoperative cholangitis had been observed in a high frequency of patients during a long-term follow-up period (Table 3).

From the standpoint of postoperative nutritional status, differences of body weight changes were found between PD and PPPD. Patients who had undergone a PPPD experienced an increase in body weight, although patients who had undergone a standard PD had decreased body weight postoperatively, and no improvement was even observed during a follow-up period as long as 10 years. The average weight gain was 104% in the PPPD group but 90% in the PD group at 1 year after surgery ($P < .05$).

Impaired glucose tolerance and episode of postoperative cholangitis were not significantly related to patient characteristics such as disease and operative procedure. However, impaired glucose tolerance, including borderline-type diabetes evaluated by OGTT, resulted in significant correlation with a lower level of activity on PS scores (chi-square test for independence; $P < .05$) (Table 4).

TABLE 3. Clinical symptoms observed for a long-term follow-up period in relation to patient characteristics

	Disease		Type of surgery	
Characteristic	Neoplastic diseases	Chronic pancreatitis	PD	PPPD
Decreased body weight				
Less than 10% ($n = 19$)	14	5	14	5
More than 10% ($n = 14$)	8	6	13	1
Glucose tolerance				
Normal ($n = 20$)	15 5	5	17	3
Border or diabetes ($n = 13$)	7	6	10	3
Cholangitis				
None ($n = 19$)	13	6	15	4
Suspected or definite ($n = 14$)	9	5	12	2

Each number indicates number of patients.

TABLE 4. Intercorrelations (chi-square test for independence) between clinical symptoms observed for a follow-up period and QOL indicators

Symptom	Symptom scale scores	PS	CMI
Body weight change	.08	.11	.88
Glucose tolerance	.71	<.05	.34
Cholangitis	.35	.57	.43

PS, performance status (social activity); CMI, Cornell Medical Index.

TABLE 5. Expectation of cholangitis based on laboratory data in a symptom-free period during long-term follow-up

Factor	Cholangitis group ($n = 14$)	Noncholangitis group ($n = 19$)	P value
ALP(IU/l)	575.5 ± 368.1	257.4 ± 93.3	<.05
Total bilirubin (mg/ml)	.67 ± .29	.85 ± .3	.19
LAP (IU/l)	140.2 ± 85.3	95.5 ± 85.2	.31
γ-GTP (IU/l)	125.4 ± 106.8	69.3 ± 12.7	.29
GOT (IU/l)	35.3 ± 13.7	29.6 ± 7.6	.27

ALP, alkaline phosphatase; LAP, leusin aminopeptidase; γ-GTP, γ-glutamyl transferase; GOT, glutamic oxaloacetic transaminase.
Cholangitis group, patients who had experienced cholangitis; noncholangitis group, no episode of cholangitis during follow-up period.
Each value indicates mean and standard deviation of the data in a symptom-free period. P value evaluated by Student's t-test.

Postoperative Cholangitis

Of the patients enrolled in this study, 42.4% had been suspected or determined to have experienced cholangitis during long-term follow-up. In patients who had experienced cholangitis, alkaline phosphatase (ALP) levels in the blood tended to maintain high values even in a symptom-free period. There was a significant difference in ALP level

TABLE 6. Findings of biliary scintigraphy in a symptom-free period in patients with and without cholangitis

	Cholangitis	Noncholangitis	P value
Bilioenteric anastomotic region/whole liver	.273 ± .029	.130 ± .094	<.05
Enteric loop region/whole liver	.957 ± .729	.729 ± .246	.24

Each value indicates mean and standard deviation of the ratio, which was calculated by the scintillation count obtained at 60 min after ^{99}mTc-PMT (-pyridoxyl-5-methyl triptophan) injection. Results are data of patients in a symptom-free period. P value evaluated by Student's t-test.

in the blood between patients who had an episode of cholangitis and those who had not had cholangitis ($P < .05$), while no significant differences were observed in the other biliary enzymes such as bilirubin, leusin aminopeptidase (LAP), and γ-glutamyl transferase (γ-GTP) (Table 5).

In addition, characteristic findings by means of biliary scintigraphy were observed in the patients who had an episode of cholangitis; the bile duct was dilatated and excretion of the bile from the liver was remarkably retarded as long as 60 min after isotope injection even in a symptom-free period (data not shown). The ratio of the scintillation count in the bilioenteric anastomotic region to that in the whole liver was significantly higher in patients with cholangitis than in those without cholangitis ($P < .05$) (Table 6).

Discussion

Although more attention has recently been directed to quality of postoperative life as one criterion of therapeutic success, little is known of the results following PD [1–4]. A study of the patient's QOL, even though still controversially discussed in terms of the relevance, feasibility, and reliability of such investigations, has been performed using a QOL measurement system that consisted of a functional scale, a working ability scale, a general symptom scale, scales on cognitive, emotional, and social functioning, a financial strain scale, a global QOL scale, and so on [5,6]. This QOL measurement system was generally supplemented by a diagnosis-specific questionnaire module, e.g., concerning a pain score for chronic pancreatitis [7]. Moreover, it was recently reported that the psychosocial aspects have gained importance in patients who have undergone surgery [8].

The present study on the QOL of patients who had undergone PD was performed depending on the following indicators: symptom scale scores related to physical and emotional aspects, PS as social activity level, and CMI related to psychological aspects.

The symptom scale scores used in this study covered physical and emotional aspects of QOL and showed the highest correlation with PS. The activity level of many patients probably decreased as a consequence of the physical and emotional symptoms. It is surprising that a moderate correlation was observed between the symptom scores and CMI as these were investigated in a different manner. Problems in psychological alterations might lead to significant differences or changes in QOL. It is suggested that more attention be paid to psychological support, resulting in a better postoperative QOL.

With regard to the disease for which surgery had been required, patients with chronic pancreatitis experienced more distress after surgery. Both the symptom scale scores and PS scales were higher in patients with chronic pancreatitis than in those with other diseases. In patients with clinically suggested chronic pancreatitis, wrong ideas about the disease, anxiety, and a depressed nature often influence the body and exacerbate the symptoms, forming a vicious cycle [9]. On the contrary, no significant correlations have been reported between the disease-specific functional and physical problems and psychoneurotic complaints in the quality of postoperative life [10]. The results of this study did not suggest frequent symptoms after surgery of chronic pancreatitis with consequences for psychosomatic disease.

When comparing standard PD and PPPD, the results demonstrated malnutrition and postgastrectomy syndrome in some patients after a standard PD but not in those with PPPD. The QOL was better in the latter group [11]. In this study, however, there were no significant differences in the QOL indicators between PD and PPPD, except in nutritional status. The patients who had undergone a PPPD in most cases definitely experienced an increase in body weight, which did not lead to better QOL. However, some of the patients who had undergone a standard PD ate less and weighed less, but most appeared to be well adjusted. There were also no significant differences in the incidence of fatty liver and postoperative diabetes between the two groups. Recently, a newer organ-preserving procedure, duodenum-preserving partial pancreatic head resection, has been developed in chronic pancreatitis and has demonstrated superiority with regard to postoperative QOL and glucose metabolism [12].

Analysis of body composition is valuable in the assessment of nutritional status. The recent development of dual-energy X-ray absorptiometry (DXA) made it possible to measure bone mineral content, lean body mass, and fat mass more precisely and easily [13]. According to the measurements of body composition by DXA, the loss of body weight after PD tended to be mainly dependent on the decrease of lean tissue (data not shown). DXA seems to be accurate and useful for nutritional assessment, and a worthwhile method for investigating the quality of life of the patients receiving surgery.

As a problem we should not ignore, patients who had experienced cholangitis were often found during long-term follow-up, although it is necessary to define a certain diagnostic criterion for postoperative cholangitis. Whether the episodes of cholangitis were sequelae related to the operation was retrospectively examined. The experience of postoperative cholangitis was not correlated with the preoperative choledochal status (dilated or not dilated) or choledochojejunostomy leakage (present or absent) (data not shown). A precise cause could not be determined, but it is necessary to make a long-term evaluation and projection and take a positive preventative approach.

In patients who had experienced cholangitis. ALP levels in the blood tended to maintain high values even in a symptom-free period and showed even higher values during an episode of cholangitis. On the other hand, the values usually changed within normal ranges in patients without cholangitis. Other biliary enzymes, such as bilirubin and leusin aminopeptidase (LAP), were not observed to be useful in predicting such episodes. In addition, in the patients who had episodes of cholangitis, the characteristic findings as observed by means of biliary scintigraphy in a symptom-free period were a remarkably dilated bile duct and marked retardation of excretion of bile from the liver for as long as 60 min after isotope injection. Patency of the bilioenteric anastomosis was documented by biliary scintigraphy [14]. Should such laboratory data be observed, the existence of cholangitis should be seriously suspected, suggesting careful consideration during a long follow-up.

In conclusion, QOL data obtained by self-estimation of the patient did not necessarily lead to precise evaluation of treatment. More research on psychological factors as determinants of QOL is needed to provide an objective view of the assessment. It is necessary to make a long-term projection with regard to nutritional status, glucose tolerance, and postoperative cholangitis and to take a positive preventive approach.

References

1. Lygidakis NJ, Brummelkamp WH, Tytgat GH, Huibtegtse KH, Lubbers MJ, van der Meer AD, Schenk KE, van Gulik TM, Roesing H (1986) Periampullary and pancreatic head carcinoma: facts and factors influencing mortality, survival, and quality of postoperative life. Am J Gastroenterol 81:968–974
2. Patti MG, Pellegrini CA, Way LW (1987) Gastric emptying and small bowel transit of solid food after pylorus-preserving pancreaticoduodenectomy. Arch Surg 122:528–532
3. Matsno S, Takeda K, Miyashita E, Miyagawa K, Imamura M, Sato T (1988) Pancreatic function and rehabilitation after pancreaticoduodenectomy. Jon J Surg 18:23–30
4. McLeod RS, Taylor BR, O'Connor BI, Greenberg GR, Jeejeebhoy KN, Royall D, Langer B (1995) Quality of life, nutritional status, and gastrointestinal hormone profile following the Whipple procedure. Am J Surg 169:179–178
5. Aaronson NK, Bullinger M, Ahmedzai S (1988) A modular approach to quality of life assessment in cancer clinical trials. Recent Results Cancer Res 111:231–249
6. Donovan K, Sanson-Fisher RW, Redman S (1989) Measuring quality of life in cancer patients. J Clin Oncol 7:959–968
7. Bloechle C, Izbicki JR, Knoefel WT, Kuechler T, Broelsch CE (1995) Quality of life in chronic pancreatitis—results after duodenum-preserving resection of tthe head of the pancreas. Pancreas 11:77–85
8. Knippenberg FCE, Out JJ, Tilanus HW, Mud HJ, Hop WCJ, Verhage F (1992) Quality of life in patients with resected oesophageal cancer. Soc Sci Med 35:139–145
9. Nakai Y, Mine K, Nakagawa T (1989) Psychosomatic medicinal view of mild chronic pancreatitis. Biomed Res 10:71–76
10. Petrin P, Andreoli A, Antoniutti M, Zaramella D, Da Lio C, Bonadimani B, Garbin L, Pedrazzoli S (1995) Surgery for chronic pancreatitis: what quality of life ahead? World J Surg 19:398–402
11. Zebri A, Balzano G, Patuzzo R, Calori G, Braga M, DiCarlo V (1995) Comparison between pylorus-preserving and Whipple pancreatoduodenectomy. Br J Surg 82:975–979
12. Büchler MW, Friess H, Muller MW, Wheatley AM, Beger HG (1995) Randomized trial of duodenum-preserving pancreatic head resection versus pylorus-preserving Whipple in chronic pancreatitis. Am J Surg 169:65–69
13. Inoue K, Shiomi K, Higashide H, Kan N, Nio Y, Tobe T, Shigeno C, Konishi J, Okumura H, Yamamuro T, Fukunaga M (1992) Metabolic bone disease following gastrectomy: assessment by dual energy X-ray absorptiometry. Br J Surg 79:321–324
14. Zimmermann H, Reichen J, Zimmermann A (1992) Reversibility of secondary biliary fibrosis by biliodigestive anastomosis in the rat. Gastroenterology 103:579–589

Quality of Life of Recurrence-Free Patients After Pancreatoduodenectomy for Periampullary Cancer: A Statistical Comparison with Healthy People Without Surgery and Patients After Subtotal and Total Gastrectomy for Early Gastric Cancer

HIDEO NAGAI, KATSUMI KURIHARA, JUN OHKI, YASUO KONDO,
TOSHIHIKO YASUDA, KOGORO KASAHARA, and KYOTARO KANAZAWA

Summary. Quality of life (QOL) of recurrence-free patients after pan-creatoduodenectomy (PD) for periampullary cancer was investigated employing nutritional parameters and QOL instruments to evaluate health- and non-health-related aspects of patients' lives. The study focused on comparison of post-PD patients with a control group without surgery and with patients after subtotal and total gastrectomy performed for early gastric cancer, matching pairs according to age, gender, and date of surgery. The results suggested that the long-term, health-related QOL of patients after PD for advanced periampullary cancer would be the same as that of healthy people without surgery, somewhat better than that after subtotal gastrectomy for early gastric cancer, and much superior to that after total gastrectomy for early gastric cancer. Assessment of total life did not reveal any difference among the individual groups. The present study failed to advocate the advantage of the pylorus-preserving PD over the conventional PD (Whipple) in postoperative QOL of five closely matched pairs. A prospective randomized study with a larger sample is needed to clarify the rationale of pylorus preservation.

Key words. Quality of life—Pancreatoduodenectomy—Periampullary cancer—Gastrectomy

Introduction

Pancreatoduodenectomy (PD) has been considered to be one of the most invasive operations in gastrointestinal surgery. When performed for periampullary malignacy, the procedure can be more extensive than in cases of benign disease of the region.

Although the prognosis of periampullary cancer still remains poor, we have come to encounter an increasing number of long-term survivors without recurrence after PD for periampullary malignancy owing to recent development of advanced techniques for diagnosis and treatment. These disease-free patients seem to live a surprisingly satisfactory life with no or very few gastrointestinal symptoms, despite the fact

Department of Surgery, Jichi Medical School, Minami-Kawachi, Tochigi 329-04, Japan.

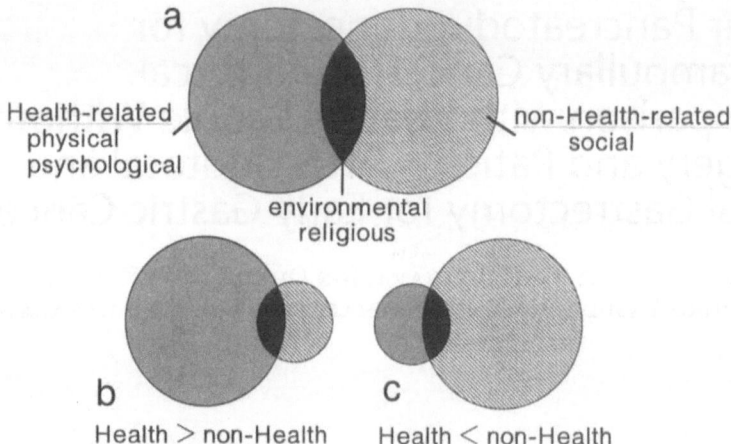

FIG. 1a–c. The authors' basic concept of quality of life (QOL). **a** QOL consists of health-related and non-health-related domains. The area overlapped by the two domains involves environmental and religious aspects. **b** The health-related domain predominates the QOL of patients after major surgery. **c** The non-health-related domain occupies most of the QOL of people who are too healthy to worry about health

that they spent the convalescent period with a certain amount of difficulty. Not a few even look like healthy persons who have not had surgery. We have had the impression that this situation appears to be the same as or even better than that after other major upper abdominal operations, such as radical resection of the stomach performed for gastric cancer.

We therefore analyzed the quality of life (QOL) of recurrence-free patients after PD with special reference to a statistical comparison with healthy people without surgery as well as with other patients after curative gastrectomy for early gastric cancer. Because lifestyle and philosophy may differ with gender and age, we attempted to make a sex- and age-matched comparison. Postoperative time was adjusted as similarly as possible for surgical cases of PD and gastrectomy.

QOL is a complex concept and has been variously defined. The authors concur with Gill and colleagues that QOL is a reflection of the way that individuals perceive and react to their health status as well as to nonmedical aspects of their lives [1]. Thus, QOL can be divided into two domains, health-related and non-health-related. The former includes physical and psychological aspects, and the latter usually refers to social life including family, occupation, income, position, etc. (Fig. 1); the area overlapped by the two domains includes environmental and religious aspects, for example. Generally speaking, those who underwent major surgery are more concerned with the health-related domain rather than the non-health-related aspects. This investigation, therefore, focused mainly on assessment of health-related QOL.

Materials and Methods

PD was performed at our institution for 61 patients with periampullary cancer between October 1990 and April 1995. At the time of investigation of the current study, in November 1995, 5 of the patients had died of other causes than recurrence and 39 were dead of or alive with recurrence. The remaining 17 were alive and had been recurrence-free for more than 6 months. We subjected these 17 patients (8 men and 9 women, ages 51–81 years, with a mean of 65) to the comparative study of QOL after PD. The postoperative time ranged from 6 to 61 months, with an average of 28 months. The resected primary tumors included 7 ampullary cancers, 5 common bile duct cancers, and 5 pancreatic cancers (adenocarcinoma 4, islet cell cancer 1). All the tumors except 1 mucosal cancer of the common bile duct had been shown to have invaded the surrounding tissues on postoperative histological sections. Five of the 17 patients had undergone a conventional Whipple procedure with resection of the distal one-third to two-thirds of the stomach, preserving half of the greater and lesser omenti. The procedure of the other 12 had been a pylorus-preserving PD (PPPD). Both procedures had involved dissection of peripancreatic tissues and lymph nodes and gastrointestinal reconstruction with Roux-en-Y. The residual pancreas had been anastomosed to the stomach in cases in which the pancreas was soft and fragile, and to the jejunum if the pancreas had been fibrotic. Five patients had had duct-to-mucosa anastomosis for pancreatic reconstruction, while the other 12 had undergone an invagination method. Two patients had received post-operative irradiation to the upper abdomen and the other 2 had been put on chemotherapy after surgery.

As surgical procedures compared to PD, we selected subtotal and total gastrectomy curatively performed for early gastric cancer, with patients matched as closely as possible to the PD cases according to sex, age (within 1–5 years), and date of surgery (within 1–6 months). No patient had received chemotherapy or irradiation postoperatively. Although we have a large number of gastrectomy cases every year (approximately 120 for early and advanced gastric cancer), we were not able to find matched pairs for all 17 cases of PD. However, 12 pairs of subtotal gastrectomy and PD, and 11 pairs of total gastrectomy and PD, were finally matched according to sex, age, and date of surgery. The standard procedure of subtotal gastrectomy for early gastric cancer had involved resection of the distal three-fourths to four-fifths of the stomach and wide dissection of the perigastric tissues and lymph nodes as well as all of the greater and lesser omenti plus vagal trunks. Total gastrectomy had involved splenectomy in 4 cases for an en bloc dissection of the splenic hilus in addition to the above-mentioned wide dissection.

As a control group compared to the surgical groups, we chose 17 citizens who visited our health checkup facility (the Center of Jichi Medical School for Multiphasic Health Testing and Services) between July and September 1995. The 17 persons were completely matched to the PD group according to age and sex. The examination of these health-conscious "healthy" people revealed several minor illnesses including hypertension (4 persons), diabetes mellitus (1), asymptomatic gallstone (1), and gout (1).

We evaluated the QOL of these four groups, i.e., control (healthy people), PD, subtotal gastrectomy, and total gastrectomy, mainly focusing on the health-related aspects, including objective assessment of nutritional parameters such as total protein and albumin in the serum, hemoglobin and HbA1c in the peripheral blood, body weight, and body mass index (BMI) (Table 1).

As instruments for measurement of both subjective and objective aspects of health-related QOL, we employed the Japanese version (translated by the authors) of the Gastrointestinal Quality-of-Life Index (GIQLI) proposed by Eypasch and colleagues [2] and the Quality of Well-Being (QWB) originally designed by Bush and later modified by Kaplan and associates [3]. For comprehensive assessment of QOL cover-

TABLE 1. Evaluation of quality of life (QOL)

1. Nutritional parameters
   Total protein (serum)
   Albumin (serum)
   Hemoglobin (peripheral blood)
   Hb A1c (peripheral blood)
   Body weight
   Body mass index (BMI)
2. Questionnaire investigation
   Gastrointestinal (GI) tract:
      Gastrointestinal Quality-of-Life Index (GIQLI) [2]
   General health:
      Quality of Well-Being (QWB) [3]
      Satisfaction Scale for Total Life (authors)

ing both health-related and non-health-related domains, we conceived the Satisfaction Scale for Total Life (SSTL), which consisted of questions asking patients how much they were satisfied with their own health (satisfaction scale ranging from 0 [not at all] to 10 [completely satisfied]), how much they were satisfied with non-health-related aspects of life, and how much health occupied their everyday life (health ratio ranging from 0 [no interest in health] to 1 [completely occupied by concerns of health]). The score of SSTL was calculated from the equation:

$$SSTL = (\text{satisfaction scale for health}) \cdot (\text{health ratio}) +$$
$$(\text{satisfaction scale for life not related to health}) \cdot (1 - \text{health ratio})$$

All those in the four groups were interviewed by the same person (H.N.).

Results

Nutritional Parameters

Serum total protein and albumin did not show any difference among the four groups (Tables 2, 3). Hemoglobin in the peripheral blood decreased in the order of control, PD, subtotal gastrectomy, and total gastrectomy (Table 4). The PD group had significantly more hemoglobin than the subtotal gastrectomy group according to the pair-matched comparison. Data of HbA1c were available in the control and PD groups; there was no statistically significant difference (Table 5).

Alterations in body weight after surgery showed loss of weight to be significantly less in the PD (2.41%) than in the subtotal and total gastrectomy groups (13.18%, 19.41%) (Table 6). BMI was also higher in the PD group than the subtotal and total groups, although the control had a higher index than the PD group (24.67 vs. 21.65) (Table 7). The high value of BMI in the control, however, reflected a tendency to obesity, because the ideal BMI is supposed to be about 22. Thus, the post-PD status could be said to induce a near-ideal BMI.

When changes of BMI were separated according to the preoperative values of more than 23.00 (fat patients) and less than 22.99 (lean patients), the former tended to lose more weight than the latter after surgery. Of special note is that the lean patients in the PD group did not lose weight after surgery and even slightly increased their preoperative index, while the fat patients lost weight considerably, approaching the

TABLE 2. Total protein in serum

Group	Overall		Pair-matched	
Control	7.37 ± .37 ⎤			
PD	7.28 ± .61 ⎥ NS	7.49 ± .56 ⎤ NS	7.33 ± .60 ⎤	
Sub Gx	7.25 ± .41 ⎥	7.25 ± .41 ⎦		NS
Tot Gx	7.37 ± .61 ⎦		7.37 ± .61 ⎦	

PD, pancreatoduodenectomy; Sub Gx, subtotal gastrectomy; Tot Gx, total gastrectomy.
Data are in g/dl, mean ± SD.

TABLE 3. Albumin in serum

Group	Overall		Pair-matched	
Control	4.22 ± .29 ⎤			
PD	4.23 ± .43 ⎥ NS	4.35 ± .36 ⎤ NS	4.28 ± .27 ⎤	
Sub Gx	4.17 ± .41 ⎥	4.20 ± .43 ⎦		NS
Tot Gx	4.23 ± .34 ⎦		4.26 ± .35 ⎦	

Data are in g/dl, mean ± SD.

TABLE 4. Hemoglobin in peripheral blood

Group	Overall		Pair-matched	
Control	14.64 ± 1.53 ⎤ * ⎤ ⎤			
PD	13.09 ± 1.15 ⎦ * ⎥ * ⎥ *	13.37 ± .99 ⎤ *	13.38 ± .45	
Sub Gx	12.39 ± .92 ⎦ * ⎥ *	12.39 ± .92 ⎦		
Tot Gx	12.72 ± 1.51 ⎦		12.72 ± 1.52	

Data are in g/dl, mean ± SD.
*, $P < .05$; **, $P < .01$; ***, $P < .001$.

TABLE 5. Hb A1c in peripheral blood

Group	Overall
Control	5.05 ± .41 ⎤ NS
PD	5.26 ± .53 ⎦

Data are %, mean ± SD.

TABLE 6. Body weight changes after surgery

Group	Overall		Pair-matched	
PD	−2.41 ± 6.63 ⎤		−3.13 ± 6.57	−3.7 ± 8.2
	**	*	*	
Sub Gx	−13.18 ± 11.45	*	−13.18 ± 11.45	***
		*		
Tot Gx	−19.41 ± 6.21 ⎦			−19.41 ± 6.21

Data are %, mean ± SD.
*, $P < .05$; **, $P < .01$; ***, $P < .001$.

TABLE 7. Body mass index (BMI)

Group	Overall		Pair-matched	
Control	24.67 ± 3.55			
PD	21.65 ± 1.83		21.76 ± 1.64	21.41 ± 2.06
Sub Gx	19.93 ± 2.34		19.93 ± 2.34	
Tot Gx	19.08 ± 2.21			19.08 ± 2.21

BMI, body weight (kg)/height (m)^2.
*, $P < .05$; **, $P < .01$; ***, $P < .001$ (mean ± SD).

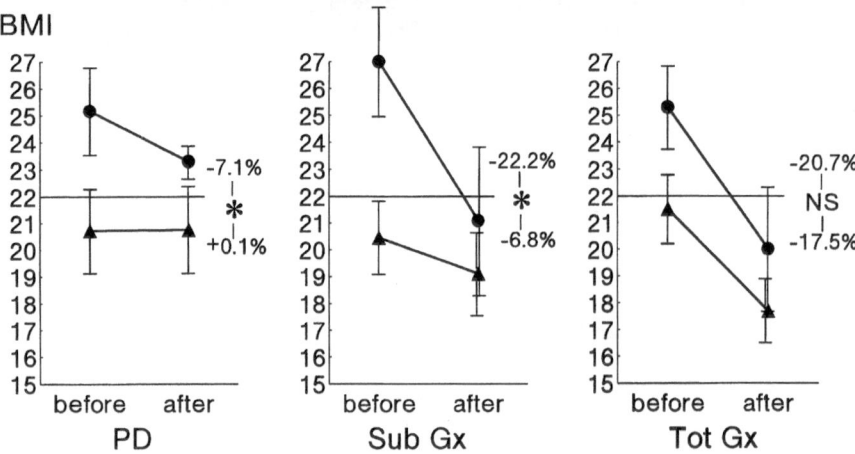

FIG. 2. Changes of body mass index (BMI) after pancreatoduodenectomy (PD), subtotal gastrectomy (Sub Gx), and total gastrectomy (Tot Gx) according to preoperative levels of BMI greater than 23 (*circles*) and less than (*triangles*) 23. PD patients with preoperative BMI below 23 did not lose weight after surgery, while those above 23 lost weight considerably, approaching the ideal BMI level of 22. *, $P < .05$

ideal index of 22 (Fig. 2). This tendency could not be observed in the subtotal and total gastrectomy groups.

Assessments with QOL Instruments

GIQLI scores decreased in the order of control, PD, subtotal gastrectomy, and total gastrectomy, although a significant difference was observed only between PD and total gastrectomy and between subtotal and total gastrectomy (Table 8). QWB showed a similar tendency with higher values in the order of control, PD, subtotal, and total gastrectomy; nonetheless, the differences were not statistically significant (Table 9).

The SSTL revealed that the satisfaction scale was more in the PD than in the subtotal and total gastrectomy groups (Table 10). The ratio of concerns about health in total life was extremely high in the total gastrectomy group, .73 (Table 11). Other

TABLE 8. Gastrointestinal quality-of-life index (GIQLI)

Group	Overall	Pair-matched	
Control	−6.43 ± 3.69		
PD	−8.29 ± 5.02	−6.41 ± 2.19	−7.70 ± 4.27
Sub Gx	−11.08 ± 7.70	−11.08 ± 7.70	***
Tot Gx	−21.90 ± 8.20		−21.90 ± 8.20

**, P < .01; ***, P < .001 (GIQLI-140, mean ± SD).

TABLE 9. Quality of well-being (QWB)

Group	Overall	Pair-matched	
Control	.67 ± .15		
PD	.65 ± .19	.66 ± .19	.69 ± .20
Sub Gx	.58 ± .28 NS	.58 ± .28 NS	NS
Tot Gx	.35 ± .74		.35 ± .74

Mean ± SD.

TABLE 10. Satisfaction scale for health:

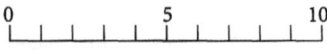

(How much are you satisfied with your health?)

Group	Overall	Pair-matched	
Control	7.71 ± 1.12		
PD	8.03 ± 1.12	8.38 ± .88	7.95 ± 1.30
Sub Gx	7.33 ± 1.13 *	7.33 ± 1.13 *	*
Tot Gx	6.80 ± 1.14		6.80 ± 1.14

*, P < .05 (mean ± SD).

TABLE 11. Health ratio:

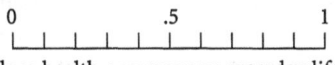

(How much does health occupy your everyday life?)

Group	Overall	Pair-matched	
Control	.51 ± .17		
PD	.54 ± .19	.54 ± .19	.45 ± .18
Sub Gx	.54 ± .16	.54 ± .16	**
Tot Gx	.73 ± .14		.73 ± .14

*, P < .05; **, P < .01 (mean ± SD).

TABLE 12. Satisfaction scale for total life (SSTL)[a]

Group	Overall		Pair-matched	
Control	8.06 ± .90			
PD	8.15 ± .84	NS	8.45 ± .69 ⌐ NS	8.02 ± .88 ⌐
Sub Gx	7.74 ± 1.00		7.74 ± 1.00 ⌐	
Tot Gx	7.23 ± 1.04			7.23 ± 1.04 ⌐ NS

[a] SSTL, satisfaction scale for health × health ratio + satisfaction scale for life not related to health × (1 − health ratio).
Data are mean ± SD.

TABLE 13. Conventional PD versus pylorus-preserving PD

Factor	PD[a]	PPPD[b]
Total protein	7.0	7.3
Albumin	3.9	4.2
Hemoglobin	12.6	12.7
HbA1c	5.4	5.3
Weight change	−5.6	1.2
BMI	21.8	20.7
GIQLI	−8.4	−10.2
Satisfaction with health	8.0	7.8
QWB	.71	.64
Satisfaction with total life	7.8	8.0

NS (mean).
[a] Conventional PD; 5 patients, 24–61 months (mean, 45 months) after surgery; age range, 68 ± 9 years; M:F, 2:3.
[b] PPPD; 5 patients, 22–46 months (mean, 32 months) after surgery; age range, 67 ± 13 years; M:F, 1:4.

groups remained the same, slightly above .5. The PD group had the highest mean score of SSTL followed by control, subtotal, and total gastrectomy (Table 12). However, no statistical difference was observed among the four groups.

QOL of Whipple procedure and PPPD

We could not obtain adequately matched pairs to compare QOL after Whipple and PPPD because of the preferential selection of PPPD during the recent 3 years. However, based on similar backgrounds, five pairs were compared that had undergone resection in the period of transition from Whipple to PPPD. There was no statistically significant difference between the two procedures in nutritional parameters or in questionnaire-based assessment of QOL (Table 13).

Discussion

On taking into account the complexity and vagueness of its concept, QOL seems to be inadequate for quantitative measurement with a single score or a configuration pattern [4]. Nevertheless, QOL measurement has been reported to be helpful in assessing the impact of treatments on patients' personal perception of life [5,6].

The current study investigated nutritional conditions with medical methodology outputting definitive figures related to objective evaluation of general physical status. Then, we proceeded with the task of learning individuals' reaction to their own health as well as to the nonmedical aspects of their life. Three instruments were chosen for this purpose: GIQLI, as an assessment of gastrointestinal (GI) tract-associated conditions; QWB, as comprehension of general physical status; and SSTL, as an overall estimation of medical and social features.

Among the nutritional parameters measured in this study were body weight and BMI shown to be the best methods to detect distinctive features between the surgical groups. The weight loss rate after PD was a remarkably low 2.41%, while patients undergoing subtotal and total gastrectomy lost weight by 13.18% and 19.41%, respectively. These data overwhelm us in that the PD group included a large number of advanced cancer cases and several patients on postoperative irradiation and chemotherapy, while none of the gastrectomy patients had advanced cancer or received stressful adjuvant therapies. Thus, the superiority of PD to subtotal and total gastrectomy may be indicated in terms of less weight loss after surgery.

The BMI calculation revealed a similar inclination among surgical groups with significantly higher values in the PD. The BMI of the PD, although lower than that of the nonsurgical people, was nearly equivalent to the standard or ideal value of 22. It could be said that the control group may have a tendency to obesity, while the PD group downsized to the ideal body weight.

The breakdown of the PD group according to preoperative BMI above and below 23 disclosed that fat patients lost more weight, approaching the standard BMI of 22. Lean patients, on the other hand, maintained their weight just below the ideal value. This adjusting characteristic is unique, because subtotal or total gastrectomy does not seem to have the same effects on BMI.

Other parameters such as serum albumin and total protein appear nonspecific in distinguishing the nutritional status among individual groups, except for hemoglobin in the peripheral blood, which showed a significant decrease after surgery, in either PD, subtotal, or total gastrectomy groups. The lack of significant difference of HbA1c between "healthy" people and the PD group might suggest slight derangement of glucose tolerance following pancreatectomy or a slight diabetic disposition in the control.

QOL indices derived from the GI-tract-specific questionnaire (GIQLI) revealed the superiority of PD to subtotal and total gastrectomy. QWB, aiming at comprehension of general health, did not, however, produce any significant distinction among the surgical groups and even between the controls without surgery and the patients after major operations. This may imply inadequacy of this instrument for QOL assessment of upper abdominal surgery.

The "satisfaction scale for health," a part of our SSTL instrument, showed a significantly higher score in the PD than in the subtotal and total gastrectomy groups. Although not statistically significant, the health satisfaction rate after PD was even higher than that of the "healthy" people without surgery. The total score of SSTL, including not only health status but nonmedical aspects, failed to reveal any statistically significant difference among the groups. This could be attributed in part to inadequacy of the instrument for comprehensive evaluation of total life, or more probably to the immeasurable complexity of individual perception of social life and philosophy.

McLeod and co-workers reported the excellency of QOL in patients following PD, equaling that in age- and sex-matched postcholecystectomy patients [7]. They commented that the assessments of subjects in the PD group are biased compared with those of the postcholecystectomy group by the fact that most PD patients are grateful and relieved to have survived a major operation and, in most cases, a potentially lethal disease. Still inevitable also in the current study, this bias could be lessened by choosing a more invasive and extensive operation such as subtotal and total gastrectomy as compared groups instead of cholecystectomy.

The pylorus-preserving procedure has gained wide recognition since the report of Traverso and Longmire in 1978, surpassing the conventional PD (Whipple procedure) in terms of alleged greater physiological function and better postoperative nutrition [8]. The apparent failure to prove this allegation in the present QOL measurement study may or may not be a reflection of sample size. A prospective randomized study of a much larger sample should clarify the clinical and psychosocial significance of pylorus preservation.

Besides the issue of pylorus preservation, the post-PD QOL may depend on other methodological factors including how and where the remnant pancreas is anastomosed, as well as the fashion of reconstructing the gastrointestinal continuity. Although use of various methods of pancreatic anastomosis in the current study made an investigation of individual procedures almost impossible, a new QOL measurement of post-PD patients from these viewpoints will be mandatory.

Conclusion

Based on the age-, sex- and date-of-surgery-matched investigation of QOL utilizing nutritional parameters and health-related questionnaires as well as total life self-assessment, we could conclude that, so long as there is no evidence of recurrence of the tumor, the long-term, health-related QOL of PD for advanced periampullary cancer would be the same as that of "healthy" people without surgery, somewhat better than that of subtotal gastrectomy for early gastric cancer, and much superior to that of total gastrectomy for early gastric cancer. The superiority of PD to subtotal and total gastrectomy should be applauded by pancreatologists, but on the other hand it seems to raise questions concerning the suitability of the presently standardized surgery in Japan for early gastric cancer involving resection of the omentum, vagal trunks, and spleen (in total gastrectomy). As for the rationale of pylorus preservation, further study is needed to prove or deny the advantage of PPPD over the conventional PD in postoperative QOL.

Acknowledgments. The authors are grateful to Dr. Masato Sasaki, Director of the Center of Jichi Medical School for Multiphasic Health Testing and Services, for his cooperation in investigating the data of the healthy control.

References

1. Gill TM, Feinstein AR (1994) A critical appraisal of the quality of quality-of-life measurements. JAMA 272:619–626
2. Eypasch E, Williams JI, Wood-Dauphinese S, Ure BM, Schmulling C, Neugebauer E, Troidl H (1995) Gastrointestinal quality of life index: development, validation and application of a new instrument. Br J Surg 82:216–222
3. Kaplan RM, Bush JW, Berry CC (1976) Health status: types of validity for an index of well-being. Health Serv Res 11:478–507

4. Perneger TV, Hudelson PM (1995) The quality of quality-of-life measurements. Letter. JAMA 273:843–844
5. WHOQOL Group (1993) Study protocol for the World Health Organization project to develop a quality of life assessment instrument (WHOQOL). Qual Life Res 2:153–159
6. Sprangers MAG, Taal BG, Aaronson NK, te Velde A (1995) Quality of life in colorectal cancer: stoma vs. nonstoma patients. Dis Colon Rectum 38:361–369
7. McLeod RS, Taylor BR, O'Connor BI, Greenberg GR, Jeejeebhoy KN, Royall D, Langer B (1995) Quality of life, nutritional status, and gastrointestinal hormone profile following the Whipple procedure. Am J Surg 169:179–185
8. Traverso LW, Longmire WP (1994) Preservation of the pylorus during pancreaticoduodenectomy: evolution and current indications. J Jpn Biliary Pancr Surg 4:329–334

Pylorus-Preserving Pancreatoduodenectomy for Severe Complications of Chronic Pancreatitis*

L. William Traverso[1] and Richard A. Kozarek[2]

Summary. Anatomical changes around or within the head of the pancreas, resulting from chronic pancreatitis that is frequently alcohol induced, can be associated with abdominal pain. In symptomatic patients we follow the Longmire principle, i.e., that the head of the pancreas acts as a pacemaker for the pathological inflammatory process and thus must be removed. Using the pylorus-preserving pancreatoduodenectomy (PPPD) technique we have alleviated clinical symptoms of benign disease with few sequelae, permitting long-term follow-up. Careful selection of patients according to pathological criteria, and the requirement for a *functioning* pylorus, are emphasized. Selection criteria, anatomical anomalies, surgical techniques, and hospital data for 42 patients undergoing surgery between 1986 and 1995 are reviewed in this chapter. Commonly encountered were pancreatic pseudocysts, obstructions of pancreatic or biliary ducts or the duodenum, arteriovenous fistula, and abnormalities of the upper abdominal blood supply. Development of a seromuscular envelope with contained end-to-end mucosa-to-mucosa pancreaticojejunostomy has recently eliminated the problem of anastomosis leakage. Abdominal pain is completely relieved for most patients. Nearly all the patients in this series returned to their normal lifestyle. The 5-year survival rate in patients over five years after surgery was 88%.

Key words. Pancreatitis—Pylorus-preserving pancreatoduodenectomy—Selection criteria—Anastomoses—Pancreaticojejunostomy

Introduction

Severe or potentially fatal complications of chronic pancreatitis commonly occur inside or around the head of the pancreas. These anatomical changes are always associated with abdominal pain. The vexing and sometimes critical clinical problems

[1] Department of General Surgery and [2] Department of Gastroenterology, Virginia Mason Medical Center, Seattle, WA 98111, U.S.A.
* This chapter is a slightly adapted version of a chapter by the same title originally published in *Advances in Pancreatic Diseases*, Stuttgart, George Thieme Verlag, 1996. Used by permission of the publisher.

can seem insurmountable; however, our approach has been successful after utilizing an integrated multimodality approach. We use specific diagnostic maneuvers to pattern the pathological anatomy of the disease, and therapeutic endeavors are then targeted toward those pathological patterns through the expertise of the interventional radiologist, therapeutic endoscopist, and pancreatic surgeon.

In many of these complicated cases we follow the Longmire principle that the head of the pancreas acts as the "pacemaker" for the pathological inflammatory process and thus must be removed. We have used pylorus-preserving pancreatoduodenectomy (PPPD) for removal of the head and have observed amelioration of the clinical problem with few gastrointestinal sequelae [1]. The patients resumes a normal lifestyle and remains in this improved condition if the etiology for the disease (usually alcohol) remains eliminated. Long-term follow-up after pancreatoduodenectomy (PD) is unknown because reports of this surgical technique involve periampullary cancer; these patients succumb to their disease and long-term follow-up is thus not possible. Our patients, with benign disease, have provided the first opportunity for an in-depth long-term follow-up after any type of PD. These patients are routinely contacted on a yearly schedule to observe how they are living after PPPD for benign disease.

Our results with PPPD have been pain relief in all patients, but these superlative results cannot be achieved unless two criteria have been met: the patients have been *properly selected* and the *preserved pylorus is functioning*. After these criteria have been met, the postoperative long-term problems focus away from the abdominal pain and are mainly related to the patient taking responsibility for their health, i.e., abstinence from alcohol and coping with the progressive and insidious sequelae of chronic pancreatitis that may smolder in the pancreatic remnant. Slow and progressive loss of exocrine and endocrine function results. Although uncommon, the pancreatic remnant may become symptomatic, causing episodic left-sided abdominal pain. The alternative would have been total PD and diabetes; the latter is already common in these patients before surgery. After surgery relief of abdominal pain is obtained in all these patients, and the majority have refocused themselves on diabetes control; unfortunately, some do return to alcohol use. Preservation of endocrine tissue during surgery is an important judgment decision, and we have learned to avoid total PPPD. Medical assistance for these patients with complications of chronic pancreatitis is not only by means of a surgical procedure but entails a long-term commitment by physicians from many specialties.

The purpose of this chapter is to outline the selection criteria for PPPD and to describe the technique for preserving a functioning pylorus while removing the head of the pancreas. Because the technique of PD with hemigastrectomy is familiar to abdominal surgeons, only a few modifications are required to preserve a functional pylorus. This chapter then continues with a description of in-hospital and long-term follow-up after the integrated approach that has culminated with PPPD.

Selection Criteria

Not all patients with chronic pancreatitis have symptoms. When symptoms develop, the most common type is abdominal pain. Some of the patients who develop symptoms have specific pathological alterations in pancreatic anatomy. Patients with both abdominal pain and pathological changes can be helped with a variety of therapeutic

TABLE 1. Selection criteria for resection in 42 cases of pancreaticoduodenectomy

Criteria/Symptoms	No. of cases
Expanding pseudocyst(s) in pancreatic head; pain	9
Pancreatic duct blowout (6)	
Common bile duct to pancreatic duct fistula (3)	
Pleural fistula (1)	
Biliary obstruction (4)	
Arteriovenous fistula bleeding into cyst (3)	
Duodenal obstruction (1)	
Multiple pseudocysts in pancreatic head; pain	9
Pancreatic and bile duct obstruction (6)	
Pancreatic duct blowout (5)	
"Pseudotumors," 6–12 cm (3)	
Biliary and pancreatic duct obstruction; pain	15
Diffuse calcified and enlarged pancreatic head (6)	
Pancreatic duct blowout with cutaneous fistula (5)	
Duodenal obstruction (2)	
Pancreatic duct obstruction; pain	9
Diffuse calcified and enlarged pancreatic head (7)	
Uncinate obliterated with stones/sand (6)	
Pancreatic duct blowout (2)	
"Pseudo tumors," 5–6 cm (2)	

approaches. In the absence of pathological changes, any attempt to treat the abdominal pain of a chronic pancreatitis patient with surgery will *not* result in pain relief. Therefore, strict criteria must be met before a patient is a candidate for resective or drainage procedures.

When severe pathological changes are observed in a chronic pancreatitis patient, these are frequently detected in the head of the pancreas, and surgical removal of the head is required to eliminate the pain. Specific examples of these pathological changes are best described with the information obtained from dynamic bolus CT scanning (computerized axial tomography or, more recently, helical tomography) and endoscopic retrograde cholangiopancreatography (ERCP). Examples are a expanding pseudocyst in the pancreatic head, with or without a contained or leaking arteriovenous fistula; pancreatic duct blowout at the genu with pancreatic juice leaking ventrally into the lesser sac or leaves of omentum, or dorsally over the portal vein into the retroperitoneum or pleural cavity; a giant pseudotumor of coalescing macro- or micro-pseudocysts; or calcified fibrosis with bile duct, pancreatic duct, or duodenal obstruction. These anatomical criteria for PPPD for our last 42 patients, divided into four groups, are listed in Table 1.

Case Profiles

All operations were performed by a single surgeon between 1986 and 1995. Ten of these 42 patients (24%) required *total* PD during their PPPD for extensive fistulous disease or an obliterated ductal system throughout the pancreas. Fortunately almost all these 10 patients were diabetic preoperatively (90%). Of the 42 patients, 4 had a prior partial gastrectomy with Billroth II anastomosis for pain presumed to have been caused by peptic ulcer disease. In retrospect, several of these cases may have had pain from chronic pancreatitis rather than ulcer disease. These patients were converted to a Roux-en-Y gastrojejunostomy during their PD. Therefore, 38 of the 42 patients had PPPD in this series: total PPPD ($n = 10$), PPPD ($n = 28$), and PD after prior antrectomy ($n = 4$).

The patients were predominatly male (64%) or abusers of alcohol (78%); their average age was 45 years (range, 19–81). Chronic pancreatitis was well established in these patients, as 40% were already diabetic. A previous pancreatic operation (Puestow or pseudocyst drainage, internal or external) had been performed in 31%. Preoperatively all patients were studied with ERCP and CT scans, and some received preoperative endoscopic placement of bile duct (43%) or pancreatic duct stents (29%) to decrease inflammation and facilitate surgical dissection. Percutaneous drainage of pancreatic fluid collections was also utilized in 19%. The average anatomy profile included calcified pancreas (50%), biliary obstruction (69%), pancreatic duct obstruction (93%), gastric outlet (duodenal) obstruction (7%), single or multiple pseudocysts in the head (48%), and pancreatic duct blowout with or without pancreatic fistula to the skin or other organs (40%).

Upper abdominal arterial and venous anatomy was assessed in 41 patients by visceral arteriography with portal venous phase ($n = 40$) or helical CT with hepatic artery reconstruction ($n = 1$). The importance of understanding the frequent presence of hepatic artery anomalies under the pancreatic head and their significance to prevent biliary fistula cannot be overemphasized when PD is performed [2]. When chronic pancreatitis is present, knowledge of the blood supply to the structures of the upper abdomen provides information for preoperative planning and avoidance of major complications inherent to PD [3].

Fifty percent of our cases were associated with at least one abnormality: pseudoaneurysm or arteriovenous fistula in the mesenteric vessels around the pancreas (7%), occluded splenic vein (14%), or thrombosed or compressed portal vein with venous collaterals (12%). These vascular findings led us to preoperatively occlude the pseudoaneurysm or arteriovenous connection with arteriographically placed coils or to remove the spleen at the beginning of the procedure to decrease blood loss [3]. Hepatic artery anomalies, such as a replaced common hepatic artery or an accessory or replaced right hepatic artery coursing under the pancreatic head, were observed in 26% of the patients. These aberrant vessels originate from the superior mesenteric artery and travel dorsal to the pancreas to enter the hepatoduodenal ligament just dorsal to the common bile duct as it emerges from the superior border of the pancreas. During PD these aberrant vessels can be erroneously divided as the common bile duct is divided. This accident devascularizes the common bile duct as the blood supply is derived through a watershed of anastomosing channels between the gastroduodenal artery (divided during PD) and the right hepatic artery. Biliary fistula results because the biliary portion of the bilioenteric anastomosis is ischemic. We have observed another vessel that courses under the common bile duct. An early bifurcation of a common hepatic artery near the celiac axis will send the right hepatic artery component under the common bile duct to enter the hepatoduodenal ligament in the same area as the replaced right hepatic artery.

Another anomaly should be mentioned. We have observed a replaced common hepatic artery from the superior mesenteric artery that coursed ventral (not dorsal) to the pancreas in the area where the pancreas is traditionally divided over the portal vein during PD [4]. Only with the preoperative knowledge of the presence of this aberrant artery were we able to determine that this large artery on the head of the pancreas mimicked a large anterosuperior pancreaticoduodenal artery but actually represented the entire blood supply to the liver.

Surgical Technique of PPPD

The goal of PPPD is to preserve a *functioning* pylorus, the entire stomach, and the first part of the duodenum (approximately 5 cm). Therefore, during the procedure the neurovascular supply to the pylorus is protected and preserved by wide dissection. An intact vagal innervation to the distal stomach is mandatory to preserve a functioning pylorus. Therefore, PPPD is not possible if a truncal vagotomy has been performed.

Instead of antrectomy or hemigastrectomy during PD, the pylorus and antrum are preserved by widely dissecting them free of the hepatoduodenal ligament (Fig. 1). The following blood vessels to the pylorus are divided at their origins away from the pylorus: the right gastric artery (if present) in the hepatoduodenal ligament at the superior pancreatic border, and the right gastroepiploic artery and vein at the inferior border of the pancreas. With this wide dissection technique the neurovascular supply to the pylorus is protected and preserved. Dissection of the duodenal bulb is continued until the area where the first and second parts of duodenum join has been

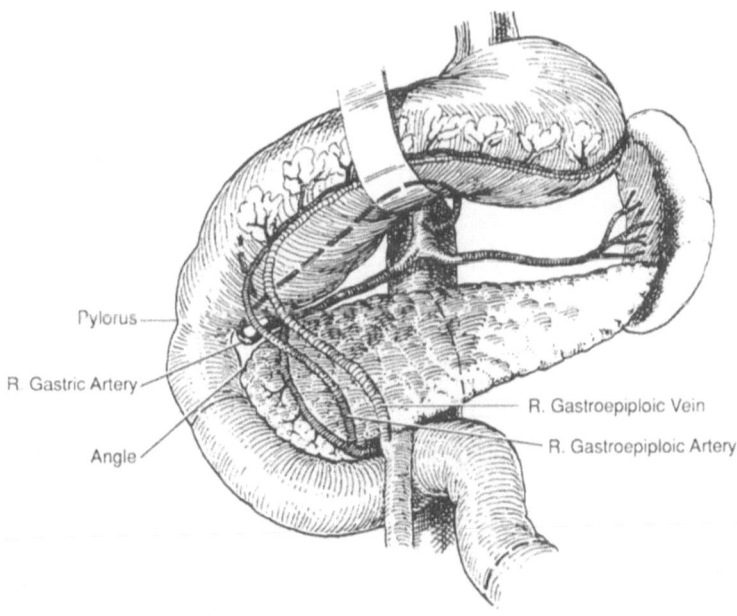

FIG. 1. *Dashed lines* indicate the area of the pancreas, duodenum (parts 2, 3, 4), and jejunum resected during the pylorus-preserving Whipple procedure. The stomach has been elevated off the pancreas. Ligation of the right (R.) gastric (superior pancreatic border) and right gastroepiploic vessels (inferior pancreatic border) at their origin preserve the vascular arcade on the lesser and greater curvatures of the stomach. An intact neurovascular supply to the antrum, pylorus, and first portion of the duodenum is mandatory for a functioning pylorus. A vagotomy or history of vagotomy precludes pylorus preservation. (From [5], with permission)

reached. This area is also where the duodenum and pancreas merge, forming an "angle" (see Fig. 1). Many tiny shared blood vessels between pancreas and duodenum are observed at this point and about 5 cm of duodenum will have been freed. The GIA stapling device (U.S. Surgical, Norwalk, CT, USA) is used to divide the duodenum at the junction of the first and second parts. Wide dissection of the pylorus and duodenum adjacent to the head of the pancreas makes PPPD of speculative value for en bloc resection of duodenal or pancreatic cancer but uniquely suited for chronic pancreatitis. The stomach and stapled-over first part of the duodenum are now mobile and together are placed in the left-upper quadrant until reconstruction.

After excision of the pancreatic head, remaining duodenum, and distal common bile duct, the anastomoses are positioned to isolate potential leakage of the bile ad pancreatic duct connections from the duodenojejunostomy. This maneuver may help to prevent delayed gastric outlet function. In our experience, delayed gastrointestinal function is almost always caused by a retrogastric amylase-rich collection of fluid [1]. Therefore, the proximal jejunum is directed toward the pancreatic ad bile duct remnants by a retrocolic route, and the stomach with preserved pylorus and duodenum is brought antecolic to the left transverse colon, allowing for a remote duodenojejunostomy (Fig. 2).

The chain-of-lakes type of ductal dilatation may be present in the pancreatic remnant. These areas may contain sigificat strictures. If so, the pancreatic anastomosis should be constructed with a longitudinal side-to-side technique. Intraoperative fluo-

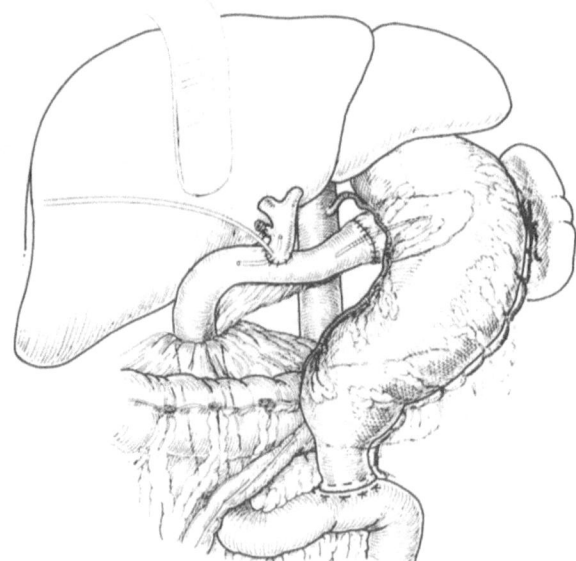

Fig. 2. Reconstruction with retrocolic anastomosis of the pancreatic duct and the bile duct. The pancreatic duct connection should be made with a side-to-side technique if a "chain-of-lakes" type of ductal dilatation is present. Otherwise, a seromuscular envelope containing an end-to-end mucosa-to-mucosa stented pancreaticojejunostomy is utilized, as shown. The end-duodenal-to-side-jejunal anastomosis is made antecolic over the left transverse colon to isolate the duodenal anastomosis from the other anastomoses that have leakage potential and could cause temporary gastric outlet dysfunction. (From [5], with permission)

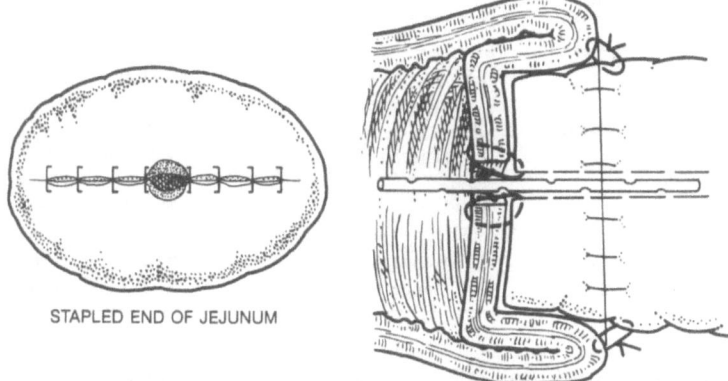

STAPLED END OF JEJUNUM

FIG. 3. The proximal jejunum has previously been divided from the surgical specimen with the GIA stapling device (U.S. Surgical). A staple is removed from the middle of the staple line (*left side of figure*), and an end-to-end mucosa-to-mucosa pancreaticojejunostomy is performed with 5-0 Maxon (Davis and Geck). A polytetrafluoroethylene 3-Fr. radiodense stent (Wilson-Cook Medical) is attached to the anastomosis with absorbable suture. The outer layer is completed with 3-0 silk providing a seromuscular envelope to prevent pancreatic fluid leakage. (From [6], with permission)

roscopic pancreatography will help in deciding which type of anastomosis to use if the preoperative ERCP is not sufficient. Many patients will have a normal duct in the pancreatic remnant with a diameter of 1–2 mm because the patient's abdominal pain is caused by a focal problem in the pancreatic head, i.e., an expanding or leaking pseudocyst or arteriovenous fistula in the head. These small pancreatic ducts are more prone to leak after pancreaticojejunostomy. We reconstruct them with a seromuscular envelope containing a stented end-to-end mucosa-to-mucosa pancreaticojejunostomy (Figs. 2 and 3). This anastomosis, developed in experimental animals [4], has been shown to be effective in preventing pancreaticojejunostomy leakage without the assistance of somatostatin. We use a 3-Fr. polytetrafluoroethylene radiodense stent that has multiple holes throughout (Wilson-Cook Medical, Winston-Salem, NC, USA). Our study indicated that the technique for a successful nonleaking anastomosis was *exact* placement of mucosa-to-mucosa sutures. This suture placement could be accomplished by using a surgical microscope or loops, while the stent allowed the tiny duct to remain expanded and its wall visualized. In our animal study the stent was removed in one group after the anastomosis was completed with the same results as in the group with the stent left in place, i.e., none leaked.

Hospital Results

Hospital data are divided as presented in Table 2. Except for a slight decrease in blood loss and transfusion requirements, the data for the 42 patients had not changed since our previous report when 28 patients were analyzed [1]. During that earlier analysis, we compared the values for hospital data between PPPD versus total PPPD patients and found no significant differences.

Morbidity, defined as any complication that occurred during a 45-day postoperative period, was seen in 14 of 42 (33%) patients. The most common complication,

TABLE 2. Hospital data

Variable	$n = 28$	$n = 42$
Time of operation	9.8 h (range, 7–19)	9.7 h (range, 6–19)
Estimated blood loss	1474 ml (range, 300–10 000)	1347 ml (range, 300–10 000)
Percent of blood transfused	68%	57%
Units	2.5 (range, 0–20)	2.0 (range, 0–20)
Epidural catheter	85%	83%
Mortality	None	None
Morbidity	36%	33%
Gastrointestinal function	12 d (range, 8–36)	11 d (range, 5–36)
Days in hospital	17 d (range, 8–68)	17 d (range, 7–68)

which resulted in delay of hospital discharge, was gastric outlet dysfunction (oral intake not resumed by 14 days postoperatively). This observation was seen in 7 of 42 (17%) of patients (4 with PPPD, 2 with total PPPD, and 1 with PD after prior antrectomy). Four of these 7 cases were associated with a retrogastric amylase-rich fluid collection that required percutaneous drainage. Within several days after drainage, the gastric outlet dysfunction resolved. Percutaneous drainage was temporary and eliminated the fluid collection; pancreatic fistula did not result. Three patients developed adult respiratory distress syndrome and ventilator dependence for 10, 12, and 30 days, respectively. There were 2 cases of wound infection. One patient was readmitted on the 13th postoperative day for control of pre-existing diabetes; he had been discharged prematurely after surgery. Finally, 1 patient developed primary bile duct sludge 6 weeks postoperatively as a result of use of monofilament absorbable sutures with delayed absorption time at the bilioenteric anastomosis. The stones and sutures were removed endoscopically.

Long-Term Follow-Up

Four of the 42 patients died during follow-up: a 40-year-old man at 3 months postoperative (suicide), a 30-year-old woman at 4 months postoperative (mixed connective tissue disorder, steroids, renal failure, sepsis), a 55-year-old woman at 9 months postoperative (lung cancer), and a 54-year-old man at 6 years and 4 months postoperative (AIDS). Eight patients were beyond 5 years postoperative with an actual 5-year survival rate of 88%.

Long-term results are meaningful after the patient has resumed regular physical activity and diet. This stage usually begins at approximately 3 months postoperatively. Certainly by 1 year after surgery a new steady state has been reached. Of the 42 patients, 36 were more than 1 year past surgery, and 35 (97%) were contacted. Therefore, subsequent data for "long-term follow-up" represent 35 patients interviewed by telephone or at an office visit after an interval of at least 1 year following their operation. These patients represented a 97% follow-up rate with an average follow-up of 46 (14–112) months.

All except two patients (94%) had returned to full physical activity, work, or school. The first of the two exceptions is a 37-year-old man with severe morning diarrhea not related to eating and with variable improvement after oral enzyme replacement. Workup suggested a colonic etiology for his diarrhea. He had two large cysts replacing the pancreatic head and multiple small cysts throughout the remaining pancreas secondary to alcohol-induced chronic calcific pancreatitis. He had been an insulin-dependent diabetic for a year before his total PPPD. At 52 months follow-up, his severe preoperative continuous pain is gone but he remains tired and unable to work, and is taking oral codeine-based analgesics for mild continuous abdominal pain that worsens with eating and could be related to diabetic gastroparesis. The second exception is a 41-year-old man with alcohol-induced chronic calcific pancreatitis 14 months following a PPPD for a chronic pain secondary to inspissated stones and sand throughout the pancreas and especially in the pancreatic head and uncinate process. The right-sided pain was absent after surgery, but left-sided pain is so disabling that he has not been able to return to normal activity because of presumed remnant chronic pancreatitis. He is not diabetic.

All patients have markedly decreased abdominal pain and 86% are pain free (85% of PD cases and 90% of total PD cases). Five patients with residual pain include the 2 patients just described plus 3 others with presumed remnant pancreatitis, all of whom describe their preoperative pain as improved but not absent. For example, a 19-year-old woman 34 months after PPPD and after three prior Puestow operations still complained of epigastric pain; however, she has been able to return to college although before her PPPD she had been totally disabled. She is not diabetic. Preoperatively all 35 patients were taking pain medication while during follow-up only 3 (9%) reported continuing to do so. A return to alcohol use was found in 25% of the patients with an alcohol etiology.

No patient had symptoms of dumping while most indicated they were eating from "everything" to "eating like a horse." Twenty-seven patients (77%) had gained weight, and many were worried about being overweight. Among the 8 patients without weight gain, 6 have resumed alcohol intake and 5 of these are diabetic. The average operative weight of the 35 patients was 69 (46–166) kg. Mean percent of their operative weight for 1, 2, 3, 4, and 5 years after surgery was 104%, 106%, 102%, 107%, and 103%, respectively. Diarrhea was noted to be prominent among 14% of these patients and, except in the case of colonic diarrhea mentioned earlier, was ameliorated by restarting pancreatic enzymes or increasing the dosage taken. Oral exocrine enzymes were being taken by 80% of the 35 patients in a successful attempt to prevent diarrhea.

Diabetes was present preoperatively in 43% of the patients, but during postoperative follow-up diabetes was present in 54%. There were 9 patients in the follow-up group that required total PPPD, and all these patients were diabetic preoperatively. The remaining 26 patients had a Whipple procedure (PPPD = 22, PD with previous hemigastectomy = 4) and 6 were diabetic preoperatively. Therefore, 20 patients were at risk for diabetes in the postoperative period from either the resection or the progressive fibrosis of chronic pancreatitis. None became diabetic during the first year, and 4 of the 20 (20%) converted to hyperglycemia at 12, 24, 36, and 40 months, respectively, after surgery. In these 4 patients, the diabetes was most likely caused by the progressive fibrosis and not the resection for the following three reasons: onset was delayed in those who did develop diabetes; only a minority of patients developed diabetes on an average of 46 months after resection; and there was a significant correlation ($P < .05$, Fisher's exact test) of pancreatic calcifications in those who developed diabetes (100%) versus those who did not (31%).

During follow-up, gastrointestinal bleeding was presumed to be present because of anemia, melena, or guaiac-positive stools in five (14%) of these patients. Ulcerations were observed in three (9%) of these patients, all of whom had undergone total PPPD, while the other endoscopic workups were inconclusive. One patient developed a marginal ulcer 9 months after PPPD associated with chronic small bowel obstructions that ultimately had to be treated by lysis of adhesions. This patient had a history of peptic ulcer disease and was successfully treated with omeprazole. Another patient developed an ulcer in the duodenal bulb 3 years after total PPPD, requiring blood transfusions. He had a prior history of peptic ulcer and was successfully treated with ranitidine. The third patient, who required multiple transfusions at 34 months after total PPPD for a marginal ulcer, is being treated with omeprazole. No patient has required antrectomy or any other peptic ulcer operation.

Six patients have required seven operations for PD-related problems: small bowel obstruction secondary to adhesions (2 patients), ventral hernia repair (2 patients), exploratory laparotomy for gastrointestinal bleeding with the source not found, and a stitch abscess in the abdominal wall that formed heterotopic bone. Finally, an end-to-end pancreaticojejunostomy was revised to a lateral variety after the anastomosis could not be demonstrated during ERCP. However, this revision was an unsuccessful attempt to reverse left-sided abdominal pain thought to be secondary to remnant pancreatitis in a man who continued to abuse alcohol after PPPD. Twelve patients (34%) have required rehospitalization 4 for diabetes control, 2 for small bowel obstruction, 2 for elective operation (stitch abscess and revision of pancreatic anastomosis), 2 for gastrointestinal bleeding, and 1 each for recurrent remnant pancreatitis and cholangitis.

Discussion

Pain Relief After Excision of the Pacemaker

Even the best surgical approach in patients with chronic pancreatitis will not be successful if patients are not properly selected or the cause of the disease is not removed.

Excision of the head and uncinate process of the pancreas was successful in all our patients because they had abdominal pain resulting from strict anatomical causes. At least one of two pathological situations was present in the pancreatic head and uncinate process: *progressive disease* (expanding pseudocyst, duct blowout, arteriovenous fistula) or *significant fibrosis* causing an enlarged, usually extensively calcified head and uncinate process that resulted in pancreatic duct obstruction with or without biliary or duodenal obstruction.

This review indicates that excision of the head and uncinate process of the gland relieved disabling symptoms in all patients and provided complete pain relief in 86%. This superlative result was achieved with zero mortality and resulted in little gastrointestinal dysfunction. In patients with a follow-up of more than 5 years, the actual 5-year survival rate was 88%. Pain relief was immediate. A return to physical activity, work, or school was observed in 94%. There were no complaints of dumping. Diarrhea (14%) was related to inadequate exocrine enzyme replacement. Between the first and fifth postoperative years, the average weight of all patients always exceeded their operative weight (from 102% to 106%). In the few patients who could not gain weight, the cause was alcohol abuse or diabetes.

In addition, PPPD solved distressing clinical problems of sepsis, jaundice, or dependence on parenteral nutrition. These cases emphasize that the head of the pancreas is the pacemaker of chronic pancreatitis. A continuous smoldering inflammatory process within the head of the gland will result in persistent symptoms even after major ductal decompression procedures. The latter procedure is incapable of draining the multiple ductal connections within the pancreatic head or uncinate process and therefore cannot interrupt the process. If the selection criteria shown in Table 1 are present, the patient will benefit from head resection rather than a drainage procedure.

Even if patients with chronic pancreatitis have been properly selected for operation the results can be compromised if the cause of the disease is not removed. Eighty percent ($n = 28$) of our patients in the follow-up group were believed to have an alcohol etiology, and at interview 25% of them were currently consuming alcohol while 50% had drunk alcohol at some time after their operation. Of the 28 patients, 21 had a remnant of pancreas remaining, i.e., they had not undergone a total PD, and were at risk for remnant pancreatitis. The incidence of remnant pancreatitis in this group of 21 patients was 50% if they were currently drinking alcohol and 20% if they had not drunk alcohol after their operation. Previous experience with pain relief following PD has been superior if patients abstained from alcohol abuse [7]. In the earlier study, the patients also had statistically superior results (as compared to pseudocyst drainage) with fewer readmissions for recurrent pancreatitis. Follow-up in the previous study was 3.2 years and in this series is 3.8 years.

In our experience, total PPPD may eliminate the possibility of remnant pancreatitis but this operation is not a good trade for insulin-dependent diabetes. A better option is the 85% chance of complete pain relief with PD rather than diabetes in a patient who may return to alcohol use.

In-Hospital Results

This series showed a significant morbidity, as with any series of PD. Generally the major complications can be divided into two categories: (1) the pulmonary complication of adult respiratory distress syndrome (ARDS) secondary to prolonged dissection through inflamed and infected tissue and (2) the leaking pancreatic anastomosis. In contrast to excision of the pancreatic head for periampullary tumors, the patient with chronic pancreatitis has a marked inflammatory or fibrotic process. Portal venous compression or thrombosis and splenic vein occlusion are not uncommon. An obligate intraoperative blood loss results. Blood transfusions were, therefore, the rule in treating with excisional procedures when significant peripancreatic inflammation was present. The operative difficulty with this inflammatory process is demonstrated by the prolonged operating time. Advances in anesthesia, radiology, and endoscopy kept the sequelae at a minimum for pulmonary complications or dissecting through inflammation. Therefore these advances also helped keep the mortality rate at zero.

Specifically, advances in anesthesia through the use of epidural catheters have significantly decreased the amount of inhalation anesthetics needed to obtain adequate anesthesia. The epidural catheter is utilized for excellent pain control in the postoperative period, although it may prolong postoperative ileus. Improved postoperative pain control with regional administration of narcotics improves the patients' respiratory function in these chronically debilitated individuals, who usually are smokers of tobacco. No episodes of persistent atelectasis or pneumonia were seen in these patients. The three pulmonary complications of ARDS were related to large intravascular volume changes associated with the operative blood loss. We believe this complication would have been more frequent without the use of prolonged preoperative drainage or embolic procedures from interventional radiology and therapeutic endoscopy.

Preoperatively, 8 patients underwent percutaneous drainage of pseudocysts while 2 underwent embolization of an arteriovenous fistula contained within a pseudocyst. Biliary obstruction was seen in 69%, and 18 of these individuals underwent preoperative biliary stent placements, either endoscopically or transhepatically. Biliary decompression was allowed to occur for at least 2 weeks before surgery. Pancreatic duct obstruction was common (84%), with 8 patients having endoscopically placed pancreatic stents. The PD stent allows time for nutritional support while inflammation subsides [8]. For example, 1 patient underwent endoscopic transduodenal decompression of a large pseudocyst in the leaves of the transverse mesocolon. A pancreatic stent was placed from the duodenum through the pancreatic duct in the body of the gland and then through a duct blowout into the cyst. The stent allowed resolution of the pseudocyst and ultimate operative management with much less inflammation. Finally, as is discussed later, 4 patients required postoperative percutaneous drainage of fluid collections around the pancreatic anastomosis.

Patients with standard PD or PPPD resume gastromtestinal (GI) function later than those undergoing other biliary or gastric procedures. A pancreatic anastomotic leak is probably present when return of GI function is delayed after any type of PD. If a delay did no occur, then our patients resumed a diet on the 11th postoperative day on average. Gastric outlet dysfunction developed in 7 of our 42 patients: in 6 after PPPD in 1 patient who had a previous antrectomy. In 3 of the 6 PPPD patients with gastric outlet dysfunction, a CT scan showed a retrogastric or peri-pancreaticojejunostomy fluid collection, which was percutaneously drained. All collections were associated with an elevated amylase level, and the patients began eating within several days of percutaneous drainage. None developed a pancreatic fistula. The patient with prior antrectomy had a similar CT finding of peripancreatic fluid collection. Effective drainage resulted after repositioning a nearby drain on the 22nd postoperative day; however, he did not resume a diet until the 36th postoperative day. Therefore, gastric outlet dysfunction after PPPD in our patients was attributable not to preserving the pylorus but rather to a subclinical inflammation from pancreatic juice.

The pancreatic anastomosis techniques associated with gastric outlet dysfunction were reviewed. One side-to-side 8-cm pancreaticojejunostomy and two end-to-side pancreaticojejunostomy procedures leaked. The latter two were performed with silicone rubber stents, a technique I have found in the dog pancreas to be associated with a 40% leak rate as compared to no leaks using the Wilson-Cook stent. After development in the laboratory of the seromuscular envelope with contained end-to-end mucosa-to-mucosa pancreaticojejunostomy (described in Fig. 3), we have not observed a leak or abscess in the last 20 anastomoses. The stent facilitates exact placement of mucosa-to-mucosa sutures and probably does not have to remain in place. The use of somatostatin analogue in patients with PD should be considered to decrease the incidence of pancreatic fistula from a leaking anastomosis, although many of the patients in a multicenter study addressing this pharmacological maneuver did not have a pancreatic anastomosis [9].

Long-Term Outcome

The main goal of PD is to relieve abdominal pain while preserving gastrointestinal performance, and also to salvage what might remain of endocrine and exocrine function. Pain relief after PD is superlative and with few gastrointestinal sequelae, as discussed earlier. Our long-term follow-up allowed us to also look at two specific items that are important for evaluating PPPD: marginal ulceration and the development of diabetes.

Marginal ulceration was observed in two PPPD patients (6%). A duodenal ulcer was found in another. Two of these three patients had a preoperative history of peptic ulcer disease. Another predisposition may have been that all three had undergone total PPPD with its associated lack of bicarbonate and therefore acid neutralization. These rates of ulceration are similar to a 5-year follow-up study after PD by Grant and Van Heerden [10]. They also found total PD to be more ulcerogenic and thought 60 months was necessary to assess the incidence of GI ulceration after PD. It seems fair to state that no higher incidence has been observed after PPPD when compared to the standard PD [11,12]. During PD for benign disease, antrectomy seems unnecessary as its only role is prevention of marginal ulceration. Also, antrectomy is accompanied by other gastrointestinal-emptying sequelae.

Marginal ulceration has been observed after standard PD in as many as 20% of cases when hemigastrectomy had not been performed to decrease acid production. Preservation of the metering function of the pylorus seems to prevent this incidence of marginal ulceration. PPPD allows for both preservation of the antral pyloric pump and the reservoir capacity of the stomach. Patients with a prior history of peptic ulcer disease should be just as susceptible to acid-associated ulceration after PPPD as before this surgery. If this history is present preoperatively, then the advantages and disadvantages of postoperative H_2-blockers versus antrectomy should be considered. When ulceration has developed in our PPPD cases, oral medications to prevent acid production has sufficed and no patient has required surgical therapy.

Diabetes was frequent in our patients because they were selected with severe complications of long-standing chronic pancreatitis. The presence of calcifications was also a sign of long-standing fibrosis caused by this inflammatory disease. Not surprising in this series was the incidence of preoperative diabetes (43%) and calcifications (50%). After the 46-month (on average) postoperative follow-up, 54% of these patients were diabetic. Was this 9% increase in diabetes caused by the PD or by progressive fibrosis in the pancreatic remnant? Others have suggested that PD promotes diabetes because approximately 40% of the pancreas is removed or that lack of a duodenum (as part of the enteroinsular axis) interferes with postprandial insulin release [13]. Actually, the first part of the duodenum, which is rich in enteric hormones, is preserved during PPPD.

In our series 20 patients were not diabetic before PD and were at risk for developing postoperative diabetes. None became diabetic during the first year, suggesting that excision of the pancreatic head removed nonfunctional endocrine tissue replaced by scar. In a patient with a normal pancreas, PD would also not be expected to result in diabetes. After the first year, 4 patients (20%) became diabetic at 12, 24, 36, and 40 months, respectively, after PD. All these patients had pancreatic calcifications while only 31% of the remaining 16 nondiabetic patients' pancreata were with calcification. This statistically significant finding confirms that diabetes after PD is caused by progressive fibrosis replacing endocrine tissue in the pancreatic remnant because it occurs years after PD, appears in a minority of cases, and is associated with the calcification of chronic inflammation.

Various Techniques to Remove the Pacemaker

Several methods can be utilized to remove the pancreatic head. These procedures include the standard Whipple operation with hemigastrectomy [14], the pylorus-preserving Whipple (PPPD) procedure [15], the Beger procedure, excision of most of the pancreatic head with duodenal and common bile duct preservation [16], or the Frey procedure, resection of the ventral pancreatic head [17].

Beger and colleagues [16] reported the same rate of remnant pancreatitis as ours (14%). They did so after a median follow-up of 24 months in 56 patients following duodenal and common bile duct preservation plus excision of almost all the pancreatic head. Partial or complete relief of chronic pain was observed in 34% and 59%, respectively. As the results of this operation approach those of PPPD, a randomized comparison study to PPPD was begun; however, only a 6-month follow-up is available and, even though PPPD removes all the pancreatic head, this latter group had more residual pain [13]. The criteria for removal of the head therefore need to be clarified as their preliminary results with PPPD do not agree with our experience. The Beger procedure preserves the pylorus, entire duodenum, and common bile duct while removing most of the pancreatic head.

The potential sequelae of PPPD, which removes all the pancreatic head, the common bile duct, and most of the duodenum (except duodenal bulb) were assessed in our series by histories of our PPPD patients with 46-month follow-up. All described pain relief without episodes of biliary stenosis, biliary fistula, dumping, or postprandial diarrhea. In our patients, we did not believe the Beger procedure to be indicate because of significant inflammation, fibrosis, and pancreatic ductal blowout in the head of the gland. An intrapancreatic cyst spontaneously disrupted into the bile duct in two cases [18]. This condition caused stenosis of the duodenum or common bile duct, and we believed these structures should be removed. Therefore, a procedure that preserved the duodenum and distal common bile duct did not seem to be indicated. Further, PPPD was performed without mortality. In this series, no significant or permanent sequelae from removal of the second through fourth parts of the duodenum or preserving the pylorus were seen, while all patients experienced relief of symptoms.

Pancreatic surgeons should assess the concept of preserving portions of the gastrointestinal tract traditionally removed during PD. Future studies with long-term follow-up are required to compare the results of PPPD to other resective operations such as the duodenal-preserving resection of the pancreatic head, a procedure that also removes the "pacemaker of pancreatitis."

References

1. Traverso LW, Kozarek RA (1993) The Whipple procedure for severe complications of chronic pancreatitis. Arch Surg 128:1047–1053
2. Traverso LW, Freeny PC (1989) Pancreaticoduodenectomy: the importance of preserving hepatic blood flow to prevent biliary fistula. Am Surg 55:421–426

3. Biehl TR, Traverso LW, Hauptmann E, Ryan JA (1993) Preoperative visceral arteriography alters intraoperative strategy during the Whipple procedure. Am J Surg 165:581–586
4. Woods MS, Traverso LW (1993) Sparing an anterior replaced common hepatic artery during a pylorus-preserving pancreatic duodenectomy. Am Surg 59:719–721
5. Traverso LW (1993) The pylorus-preserving Whipple procedure for severe complications of chronic pancreatitis. In: Beger HG, Buchler MW, Malfertheiner P (eds) Standards of pancreatic surgery. Springer-Verlag, Berlin, pp 397–398
6. Biehl TA, Traverso LW (1992) Is stenting necessary for a successful pancreatic anastomosis? Am J Surg 163:530–532
7. Traverso LW, Tompkins RK, Urrea PT, Longmire WP (1979) Surgical treatment of chronic pancreatitis. Twenty-two years experience. Ann Surg 190:312–319
8. Kozarek RA, Patterson DJ, Ball TJ, Traverso LW (1989) Endoscopic placement of pancreatic stents and drains in the management of pancreatitis. Ann Surg 209:261–266
9. Buchler M, Friej H, Hermanek P, Sulkowsky U, Becker H, Klemps I, Schafmayer A, Dennler HJ, Beger HG, et al (1992) Role of octreotide in the prevention of postoperative complications following pancreatic resection. Am J Surg 163:125–131
10. Grant CS, Van Heerden JA (1979) Anastomotic ulceration following subtotal and total pancreatectomy. Ann Surg 190:1–5
11. Itani KM, Coleman RE, Akwari OE, Meyers WC (1986) Pylorus-preserving pancreaticoduodenectomy. Ann Surg 204:655–665
12. Traverso LW, Longmire WP (1980) Preservation of the pylorus in pancreaticoduodenectomy. A follow-up evaluation. Ann Surg 192:306–310
13. Buchler MW, Freiss H, Muller MW, Wheatley AM, Beger HG (1995) Randomized trial of duodenum-preserving pancreatic head resection versus pylorus-preserving Whipple in chronic pancreatitis. Am J Surg 169:65–70
14. Child CG, Frey CF (1996) Pancreaticoduodenectomy. Surg Clin North Am 46:1201–1213
15. Traverso LW, Longmire WP (1978) Preservation of the pylorus during pancreaticoduodenectomy. Surg Gynecol Obstet 146:959–962
16. Beger HG, Krautzberger W, Bittner R, Buchler M, Limmer J (1985) Duodenum-preserving resection of the head of the pancreas in patients with severe chronic pancreatitis. Surgery (St Louis) 97:467–473
17. Frey CF, Smith GJ (1987) Description and rationale of a new operation for chronic pancreatitis. Pancreas 2:701–702
18. Miller BM, Traverso LW (1988) Intrapancreatic communication of bile and pancreatic ducts secondary to pancreatic necrosis. Arch Surg 123:1000–1003

The Comparison of Long-Term Results of Pylorus-Preserving Pancreatoduodenectomy Versus Standard Whipple

Waldemar Kozuschek[1], Hans-Bernd Reith[2], and Wilhelm Haarmann[1]

Summary. The standard Whipple procedure involves intestinal disturbances such as dumping, diarrhea, dyspeptic complaints, and the occurrence of ulcera of the anastomoses. A postoperative weight loss was observed, ranging between 10 and 40 kg. Only a few patients were able to compensate and only after several months. In keeping with several other authors we suggest that preservation of the stomach, the pylorus, and small portions of the duodenum improve postoperative digestive parameters. It was thought that preservation of the intact stomach would prevent the complications arising from a loss of gastric reservoir function and thus the malnutrition could be improved postoperatively. Between 1985 and April 1995 we performed the pylorus-preserving Whipple procedure and treated a total of 98 patients, 81 patients with basic malignancies, with this method. In the same period a total of 34 patients were operated on with the standard Whipple procedure. The present evaluation of the according patient collectives, including extensive functional studies, led to the following results: better capacity for food uptake, no occurrence of gastric or jejunal ulcera was observed, no clinical signs of digestive disorders were apparent, the postoperative exocrine function was only slightly decreased, and the glucose metabolism after surgery was influenced only slightly by preservation of the pylorus. Taking all examination results into consideration, it can be said that the restricted organ loss in the Whipple procedure with pylorus preservation left the incretoric capacity of the upper gastrointestinal tract almost unchanged.

Key words. Pylorus-preserving pancreatoduodenectomy—Standard Whipple—Long-term results—Comparison

Introduction

The standard Whipple procedure involves intestinal disturbances such as dumping, diarrhea, dyspeptic complaints, and the occurrence of ulcera of the anastomoses. Fish

---

[1] Department of Surgery, Ruhr-University Bochum, Knappschaftskrankenhaus, D-44892 Bochum, Germany.
[2] Department of Surgery, University Würzburg, D-97080 Würzburg, Germany.

TABLE 1. Distribution of malignant diseases in both operative groups

Disease	Pylorus-preserving pancreatoduodenectomy (PPPD)	Standard Whipple
Adenocarcinoma	56	34
Carcinoma of papilla vateri	19	0
Duodenal carcinoma	4	0
Islet-cell carcinoma	1	0
Carcinoid	1	0

et al. [1] observed postoperative weight losses ranging between 10 and 40 kg, which only 3 of 49 patients were able to compensate only after several months. In keeping with Watson [2], Traverso and Longmire [3] suggested preservation of the stomach, the pylorus, and small portions of the duodenum to improve postoperative digestive parameters. It was thought that preservation of the intact stomach would prevent the complications arising from a loss of gastric reservoir function and thus malnutrition could be improved postoperatively. The long-term results, in regards to digestive and endocrine function, for the standard versus pylorus-preserving Whipple procedure were first compared in 1994 [4].

Material and Methods

The basis for the present study were 98 patients treated with the pylorus-preserving modified Whipple procedure (pancreaticoduodenectomy) (PPPD), 81 patients for a malignant disease, at the University Surgical Clinic, Bochum-Langendreer, between 1985 and April 1995. The constitution and postoperative results of this patients were compared with a group of 34 patients treated with the standard Whipple procedure during the same time period (Table 1). No ductal occlusion techniques were used in either group. The operative procedure was similar to the standard operation, with the exception that the duodenum was dissected 2-4 cm from the pylorus. On average, it was possible to preserve 3 cm of the duodenal part.

Similar to the documentation of Braasch et al. [5], eating habits, i.e., the frequency and the number of meals were recorded, 3-4 meals per day being considered normal. The postoperative body weight was documented. The pre- and postoperative blood glucose levels were also documented. Determination of a fasting blood glucose under defined dietary measures (light diet, full diet, 150- or 180-g CHO-diabetes diet) permits subclinical or manifest postoperative onset of diabetes mellitus to be ruled out. Late results were obtained by out- or in-patient follow-up examinations. One test was performed to determine the maximal possible endocrine B-cell activity in the remainder of the pancreas causing maximal insulin and C-peptide liberation.

Results

The average age of the 45 men and 36 women treated with PPPD was 62.7 years (range, 42-84 years). The average age of the 21 men and 13 women treated with the standard Whipple procedure in the same time period was 61.2 years (37-78 years). The long-term results of all patients with an adenocarcinoma in the PPPD group showed a

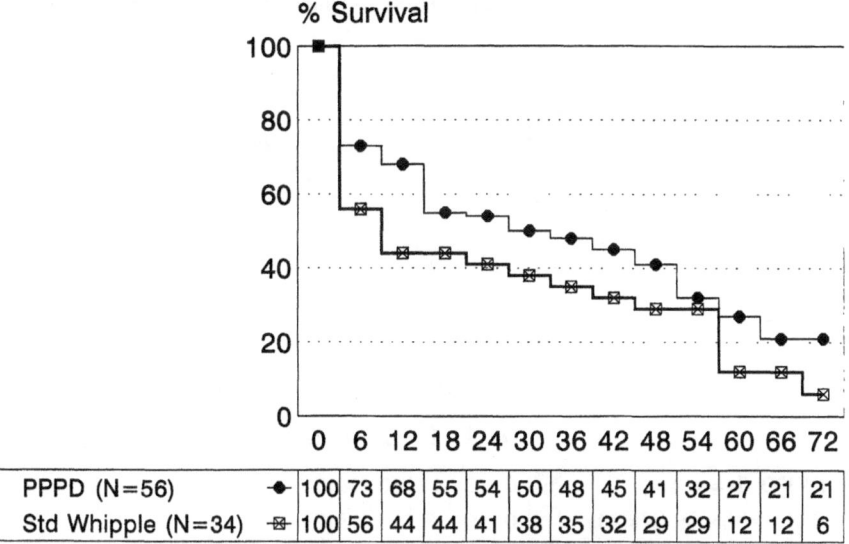

FIG. 1. Survival rates of patients with adenocarcinoma of the head of the pancreas: 56 patients after pylorus-preserving pancreatoduodenectomy (PPPD) and 34 after standard Whipple procedure

1-year survival rate of 68% versus 44% and a 5-year survival rate of 27% versus 12% (Fig. 1).

In the PPPD group, which included only patients with adenocarcinoma, during the first 6 postoperative months body weight before operation was regained by 33 of the 46 examined patients (72%) and by 40 (87%) after 12 months. The postoperative body weight of 21 patients of the Whipple group was recorded. The preoperative body weight was reached by 34% after 6 months and by 47% after 1 year. The statistical analysis showed a significant difference after 6 and 12 months ($P < .05$) (Fig. 2).

In the fasting blood glucose values of the 81 patients of the PPPD group, there were 23 cases (28.3%) of preoperative insulin-dependent diabetes mellitus; 9 patients were treated with dietary methods and drugs either before or after surgery. Seven patients who required oral hypoglycemic agents before PPPD required insulin after surgery. Thus, 31 patients (32%) were manifest diabetics before surgery, of which only 1 suffered an increase in severity after surgery. Average follow-up time of the PPPD group was 44.5 months.

In the standard Whipple group, there were 10 patients (29%) with diabetes mellitus preoperatively, 6 treated with insulin. In 2 patients with diabetes not requiring insulin and in 1 nondiabetic patient, insulin treatment became mandatory. Average follow-up time for these standard Whipple patients was 46.1 months. All alterations of the blood glucose metabolism became manifest in the early postoperative phase and showed no further long-term changes.

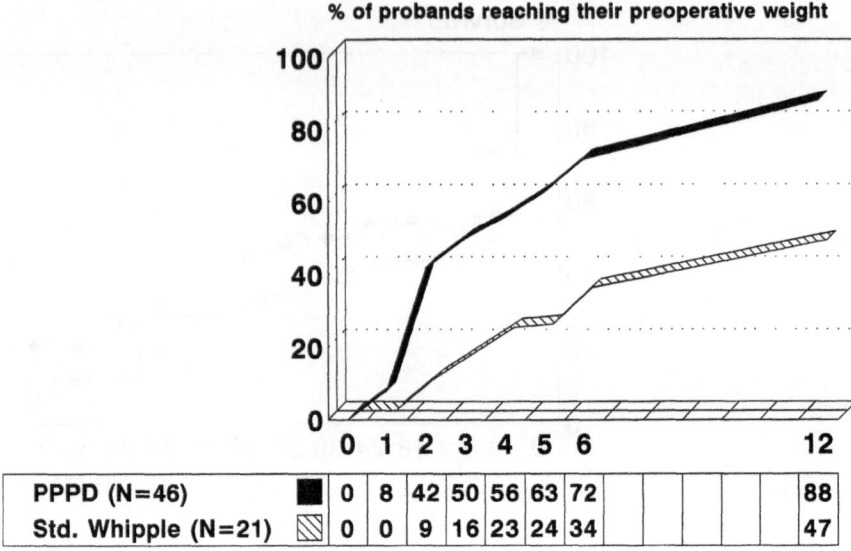

% of probands reaching their preoperative weight

		0	1	2	3	4	5	6				12
PPPD (N=46)	■	0	8	42	50	56	63	72				88
Std. Whipple (N=21)	▨	0	0	9	16	23	24	34				47

Time in months

FIG. 2. Postoperative weight gain of patients with adenocarcinoma of the head of the pancreas: 46 patients after PPPD and 21 after standard Whipple procedure. Differences after 6 and 12 months are significant

Eight patients underwent maximum beta cell stimulation investigations after PPPD, 12 after standard Whipple (6–42 months postoperative). There was a 9-patient control group. Before maximal stimulation but after oral glucose, the control group showed a gradual increase in blood glucose concentrations. Immediately following bolus administration of glucagon and sulfonylurea, an immediate drop in blood glucose occurred, causing the initial blood glucose levels to be regained within 150 min in all groups. The course of curves were identical for PPPD and the control group and slightly decreased for the standard Whipple, but without statistical signifi-cance. The commencing drop in blood glucose was simultaneous to the maximal insulin concentration and can thus be considered an indisputable effect of insulin, values peaking at 35 min in each group. In the Whipple group a continous decrease thereafter was observed in each patient, whereas after PPPD and in the control group several following peaks up to 90 min after maximal beta cell stimulation were ob-served. The space integral under the insulin curve was significantly different ($P = .05$) for PPPD and control versus Whipple group, indicating a better secretory function of the pancreas after PPPD.

Discussion

Forty-six patients (57%) in the PPPD and 21 (62%) in the standard collective, only adenocarcinoma, were older than 60 years. Our application of this modification in malignancy cases was above the average of other authors; Itani et al. [6] applied it in 21%, Braasch et al. [7] in 17%, McAfee et al. [8] in 18%, and Grace et al. [9] in 30% of the cases. In view of the high average age and the high portion of malignancies in our collective group, the mortality of 5 of 81 patients (6.1%) for PPPD and 4 of 34 patients (11.7%) for the standard Whipple was entirely acceptable and agrees with the experience of other authors [7–10].

In our experience, the standard Whipple group showed in correlation to Cubillas' results less lymph node involvement to the lesser and greater curve of the stomach. The 5-year survival rate of 27% for PPPD and 12% for the standard Whipple in cancer patients of all tumor stages shows comparable statistical results.

A comparison of our groups showed that the quality of life was much better in the patients treated with PPPD, although other investigators have speculated that PPPD allowed better weight gain compared to the standard Whipple procedure [4,5]. Digestion was described as normal in 86% of the PPPD group but 50% in the standard Whipple group after 1 year. At the end of 1 year almost all the PPPD group had regained their weight while in the standard Whipple group only 43% had regained their preoperative weight. One reason for this better regain is in our opinion the orocecal transit time of food, so a better nutrition time for PPPD patients is one of the favorable results.

Studies examining the long-term course of the remaining endocrine pancreatic function subsequent to the standard Whipple procedure are infrequently reported in the literature [11,12]. The registration in the intravenous glucose tolerance test of insulin levels showed an initial increase in insulin liberation in all the patients. The degree of increase was variable, but it was present in all groups. The insulin and C-peptide levels also showed an increase on stimulation; the insulin levels peaked after 20 min and then gradually decreased slightly, while C-peptide levels continued to increase after a 20-min peak. Although without statistical significance because of the small number of patients, the absolute values of insulin and C-peptide secretion obtained in the group with pylorus preservation were only slightly lower than those obtained from the controls. Both are superior to the standard Whipple group.

It is also important to remark that pylorus preservation does not inhibit secretion of insulin and C-peptide. Furthermore, comparing the pre- and postoperative results of the glucose tolerance tests, it is obvious that no difference in postoperative function exists. We assume that blood glucose metabolism in the PPPD group is maintained by the preserved part I of the duodenum; however, we cannot compare preoperative to postoperative results in the standard Whipple group. To diagnose endocrine insufficiency, differentiated investigations extending beyond the intravenous glucose tolerance test are necessary.

Conclusions

1. Survival differences were not observed.
2. After documenting a functioning pylorus in the PPPD group, we observed improved eating habits, less dependence on an enzyme supplement, and ability to gain weight as compared to the standard Whipple group.
3. There are no clinical signs of digestive disorders such as different forms of dumping in the PPPD group. Transit time was preserved because of the preserved pylorus, which showed unaltered function but was increased significantly after standard Whipple.
4. Glucose metabolism after surgery was not altered after PPPD but was depressed in the standard Whipple group.

References

1. Fish JC, Smith LB, Williams RD (1969) Digestive function after radical pancreaticoduodenectomy. Am J Surg 117:40–45
2. Watson K (1942) Carcinoma of ampulla of Vateri: successful radical resection. Br J Surg 31:515–526
3. Traverso LW, Longmire WPJ (1978) Preservation of the pylorus in pancreaticoduodenectomy. Surg Gynecol Obstet 146:959–962
4. Kozuschek W, Reith HB, Waleczek H, Haarmann W, Edelmann M, Sonntag D (1994) A comparison of long-term results of the standard Whipple procedure and the pylorus-preserving pancreatoduodenectomy. J Am Coll Surg 178:443–453
5. Braasch JW, Gongliang J, Rossi RL (1984) Pancreatoduodenectomy with preservation of the pylorus. World J Surg 8:900–905
6. Itani KMF, Coleman RE, Akwari OE, Meyers WC (1986) Pylorus-preserving pancreatoduodenectomy. A clinical and physiological appraisal. Ann Surg 204:655–664
7. Braasch JW, Rossi RL, Watkins E, Deziel D, Winter P (1986) Pyloric and gastric preserving pancreatic resection. Experience with 87 patients. Ann Surg 204:411–417
8. McAfee MK, van Heerden JA, Adson MA (1987) Is proximal pancreatoduodenectomy with pyloric preservation superior to total pancreatectomy. Surgery (St Louis) 105:347–351
9. Grace PA, Pitt HA, Longmire WPJ (1986) Pancreatoduodenectomy with pylorus preservation for adenocarcinoma of the head of the pancreas. Br J Surg 73:647–650
10. Kozuschek W (1989) Duodeno-Kephalopankreatektomie mit Pyloruserhaltung. Zentralbl Chir 114:745–754
11. van Heerden JA (1984) Pancreatic resection of carcinoma of the pancreas: Whipple versus total pancreatectomy—an institutional perspective. World J Surg 8:880–888
12. Mielke F, Beger HG, Schirop T (1975) Digestive undinkretorische Funktion nach partieller Duodeno-Pankreatektomie. Dtsch Med Wochenschr 100:171–176

Experience of Pancreatoduodenectomy in Various Countries

Pancreaticoduodenectomy in the United States

Karen E. Todd[1,2] and Howard A. Reber[1,2]

Summary. Pancreatic cancer afflicts 27000 patients each year and is the second most common cause of death from gastrointestinal malignancy in the United States. The historical experience of pancreaticoduodenectomy is reviewed, as well as the criteria for resection and the technical aspects of the procedure. The morbidity of pancreaticoduodenectomy including pancreatic fistula and delayed gastric emptying is addressed, and management is discussed. Mortality statistics for pancreaticoduodenectomy in the United States and factors influencing survival are reviewed.

Key words. Pancreas—Surgery—Pancreaticoduodenectomy—Whipple—Pancreatic cancer

Introduction

In the United States, 27000 new cases of pancreatic cancer will be diagnosed in 1997, and almost as many patients will die of the disease. Pancreatic cancer is now second only to colon and rectal cancer as the cause of death from gastrointestinal malignancies in this country.

The management of pancreatic cancer has had an interesting and controversial history. Halstead performed the first successful local resection of a periampullary carcinoma in the United States in 1898, with reimplantation of the biliary and pancreatic ducts directly into the duodenum. The patient survived the procedure, but died 7 months later of tumor recurrence [1]. A more extensive resection for periampullary cancer was performed first by the German surgeon W. Kausch in 1909 and reported in 1912 [2]. Nevertheless, until 1935 most patients with periampullary malignancies were managed by transduodenal local excision of the tumor as described by Halstead [3,4]. In 1935, 76 patients were reported who had undergone transduodenal resection, with

---

[1] Department of Surgery, Sepulveda Veterans Administration Medical Center, Sepulveda, CA, U.S.A.
[2] Department of Surgery, University of California School of Medicine, Los Angeles, CA 90024-6904, U.S.A.

381

an operative mortality rate of 40%. Hemorrhage was the most serious postoperative complication [3–5].

The pancreaticoduodenal resection used today was described by Dr. Alan O. Whipple in 1935 for carcinoma of the ampulla of Vater [6]. It was performed originally as a two-stage operation. The first stage decompressed the duodenal and biliary obstruction with a gastrojejunostomy and cholecystogastrostomy. The second operation consisted of a limited resection of the duodenum and pancreas; the pancreatic remnant was oversewn. In 1937, Brunschwig performed a pancreaticoduodenectomy for cancer of the head of the pancreas [7]. By 1941, the procedure was perfected to a one-stage resection much like the operation associated with Whipple's name today. In 1945, Whipple further modified the procedure to include a pancreaticojejunostomy, which was described as a two-layered end-to-side anastomosis by Cattell in 1948 [8,9].

In 1953, Cattell and Warren published their experience with 102 Whipple resections, 88 performed for periampullary cancers and the rest for benign diseases. Of the 88 patients, 46 had pancreatic cancer, and 19 of the 46 underwent one-stage resections for their disease. The mortality rate in these 46 patients was 17%, a significant accomplishment at the time [10]. Mortality rates for the operation remained at 15%–20% until the last decade [11].

The wisdom of performing the Whipple resection for pancreatic cancer has been debated in the United States. Indeed, in the early 1970s, some suggested that the operation be abandoned because the high operative morbidity and mortality rates and the small chance of curing the disease [12,13]. These issues are no longer relevant. Today, the operative mortality rate is less than 5% in the hands of surgeons experienced with the operation, and short- and long-term morbidity is quite low [1,2,14–17]. There is evidence that patients are living longer after resection, even if cure of the cancer has not been achieved. The operation still represents the only chance to cure the disease.

Criteria for Resection

In the United States, the Whipple procedure is performed if there appears to be a chance of curing the disease. Thus, distant metastases (e.g., liver, peritoneum) or direct extension of the tumor to adjacent organs such as the colon, stomach, or spleen preclude resection. Involvement of the superior mesenteric vessels, the portal vein, the hepatic artery, and the vena cava also are generally viewed as contraindications to resection. Regional lymph node involvement or extension of the tumor to the duodenum or common bile duct are not contraindications.

In 1991, Livingston and associates reviewed the U.S. experience with the resection of pancreatic cancer [18]. When 36 pancreatic surgeons, members of the Pancreas Club, were questioned about their experience with biopsy-proven adenocarcinoma of the pancreas, excluding other periampullary tumors, 72% of the surgeons did not believe that the size of the tumor was an important determinant of resectability. Only 40% of surgeons performed a formal lymph node dissection as part of the resection. Of those who did do a node dissection, only 29% indicated that their pathologists made a detailed assessment of the site and distribution of the lymph nodes in the operative specimen.

Technical Aspects of Pancreaticoduodenectomy

Pancreaticoduodenectomy is the standard procedure for carcinoma of the pancreatic head. This operation involves resection of the distal stomach, gallbladder, distal common bile duct, head of the pancreas, duodenum, proximal jejunum, and regional lymphatics. Details of the conduct of the resection have been outlined in many texts and are not given here. Certain more controversial aspects of the techniques of reconstruction are reviewed, and the authors' approach is outlined. To restore continuity of the gastrointestinal tract, a pancreaticojejunostomy, choledochojejunostomy, and gastrojejunostomy are performed.

Pancreaticojejunostomy

A variety of technical modifications of the pancreaticojejunostomy have been described. We prefer a two-layer telescoping anastomosis in which the end of the pancreatic remnant is "dunked" inside the jejunal lumen. The inner layer of the anastomosis is performed with a continuous 3-0 absorbable suture (e.g., Maxon). This layer incorporates the full thickness of both the jejunum and the pancreas, including the lumen of the pancreatic duct. The outer layer consists of interrupted 3-0 silk sutures, which are seromuscular on the jejunal side and placed deeply enough into the pancreas so that the tissue does not tear when the suture is tied. The anastomosis can be fashioned either to the end of the jejunum, if the size of the pancreatic remnant is appropriate, or to the side of the jejunum if it is not. Recently, we have begun to use the side of the jejunum in all cases because the opening in the jejunum always can be made to fit the pancreas exactly.

Although a pancreatic duct stent to protect this anastomosis is advocated by many surgeons [1,19], we never use a stent regardless of the size of the duct. It is simpler to not use one, and the incidence of pancreatic fistula (6%) has not been increased over that reported from other centers with experience. A closed silastic suction drain is placed next to the pancreaticojejunal anastomosis, so that if a fistula occurs the juices will be rapidly evacuated. In the absence of a fistula, the drain is generally removed on about the ninth or tenth postoperative day, after the patient has begun eating and just before discharge from the hospital.

Pancreaticogastrostomy has also been used to restore continuity between the pancreas and the gastrointestinal tract. The pancreatic remnant is mobilized sufficiently from the retroperitoneum and anastomosed to the posterior wall of the stomach, using a two-layer technique. It has been said that this is a safer anastomosis than pancreaticojejunostomy, and less likely to leak. The results of a prospective randomized trial comparing the two operations has recently been published [20]. There was no difference in fistula rate or any other complication between the two groups. Thus, the operations appear to be equivalent.

Hepaticojejunostomy

Biliary continuity is restored with a single-layer end-to-side hepaticojejunostomy about 10–15 cm distal to the pancreatic anastomosis. We use interrupted 4-0 absorbable suture (e.g., Maxon). The sutures are placed through the anterior wall of the duct first, which is elevated to expose the posterior wall. The posterior row of sutures are then placed through both the duct and the full thickness of the opened jejunum and then tied after all the sutures are in place; these knots are on the inside of the ductal lumen. Finally, the anterior row of sutures are placed through the anterior wall of the jejunum, and these sutures are tied with the knots on the outside. The sutures are placed 2–3 mm apart and 2–3 mm back from the duct edge.

Some surgeons advocate stenting the biliary anastomosis with either the preoperatively placed transhepatic biliary catheter, if one has been used, or with an operatively placed T-tube [1,19]. We use a stent (T-tube) only when the bile duct is 1 cm or less in diameter. The T-tube is clamped in 1 week and removed 3 weeks after that, at an office visit. We generally do not obtain a cholangiogram before either clamping the tube or removing it. Whether or not a T-tube is used, we place a closed-suction drain near the biliary anastomosis. This is usually removed after 5 or 6 days, once the patient begins to take food by mouth and there is no evidence of a leak at this site.

Gastrojejunostomy

The gastrojejunostomy (or duodenojejunostomy, if a pylorus-preserving operation has been done) is performed last. This ensures that bile and pancreatic juices neutralize the gastric acid and minimizes the risk of marginal ulceration [21]. We prefer a retrocolic isoperistaltic anastomosis, using 4–5 cm of the cut edge of the stomach on the greater curvature side (i.e., a Hoffmeister reconstruction, rather than a Polya). We do not routinely use a feeding gastrostomy or jejunostomy. The nasogastric tube is removed on the first postoperative morning; the patient is given nothing by mouth until peristaltic activity returns, usually on the fifth or sixth day.

Most American surgeons no longer perform a truncal vagotomy as part of the Whipple pancreaticoduodenectomy. The patient is maintained on acid antisecretory medication during the perioperative period, but unless there are symptoms of acid peptic disease later, we do not continue this treatment once a normal diet is resumed.

Morbidity

Significant postoperative morbidity follows pancreaticoduodenectomy in 20%–30% of patients. The most common problems directly related to the operation are pancreatic fistula and delayed gastric emptying.

Pancreatic Fistula

There is evidence that the incidence of pancreatic fistula is decreasing. A recent meta-analysis showed that the incidence of pancreatic fistula was 15% before 1975 but dropped to 11% after 1975 [22]. The mortality rate also decreased from 26% before 1975 to 16% after that time. A decrease in the incidence of pancreatic fistula has also been seen at the University of California, Los Angeles (UCLA). Between 1975 and 1984, fistula complicated 14% of pancreatic resections for cancer; from 1989 to 1993, the incidence fell to 6% [11]. There have been no fistula-related deaths since 1985.

The lower frequency and mortality of this complication may be explained by the fact that the Whipple procedure is being performed by more experienced pancreatic surgeons at major medical institutions. Adequate drainage of a fistula and avoidance of infection are both important to minimize the mortality associated with this complication. The newer closed-suction drains also probably evacuate the fluid more effectively and are less likely to introduce bacteria than the older drains that were used earlier. Parenteral nutrition also represents a significant improvement in the overall management of this group.

Delayed Gastric Emptying

The complication of delayed gastric emptying (DGE) has been reported in as many as one-third of patients after pancreaticoduodenectomy [23]. The definition of DGE is arbitrary, but commonly it is described as the inability to tolerate at least liquids orally beyond 7-10 days after operation [23]. The problem has been most commonly seen after the pylorus-preserving modification of the standard Whipple resection. In a recent retrospective review at UCLA, delayed gastric emptying (unable to tolerate oral intake by the seventh postoperative day) was seen in 41% of patients after the standard Whipple and in 61% after the pylorus-preserving operation [24]. In a subsequent prospective study investigating various aspects of the two types of operations, both performed by the same surgeon, the incidence of DGE was 10% (1/11 patients) after the standard Whipple and did not occur in any of 12 patients who had the pylorus-preserving operation. Thus, the problem needs to be investigated further in prospective studies with larger numbers of patients.

The causes of delayed emptying are often unclear. Obviously, the operation must be performed well technically, with good vascular supply to the duodenal segment. Sometimes, delayed emptying may be a sign of another problem (abscess, fistula) that has been overlooked and must be treated. When delayed emptying occurs in the absence of another treatable condition, it is managed by nasogastric decompression and nutritional support. Once obstruction has been ruled out as a cause, various prokinetic agents (e.g., metoclopropamide) may be useful.

Mortality

Livingston et al. reported survival data on 1681 resections for biopsy-proven adenocarcinoma of the pancreas in the United States [18]. Of the cases, 73% (1234) were Whipple procedures, 16% (275) were pylorus-preserving Whipple operations, and 10% (175) were total pancreatectomy; there was 1 extended Whipple procedure. There were 158 five-year survivors, corresponding to a 9% 5-year survival rate. However, 40% of the 5-year survivors still died later of recurrent cancer. In node-negative patients, 5-year actuarial survival was 20%-30%. A study by Cameron et al. reported 82 patients undergoing pancreaticoduodenectomy. The 5-year actuarial survival rate for 22 patients with no lymph node involvement was 57%; it was 5% for the 59 patients with tumor in the lymph nodes [17].

In a recent retrospective analysis from Memorial Cancer Center, the survival of patients following resection for pancreatic cancer was assessed according to the degree of histologic differentiation of the tumor. Regardless of lymph node involvement, there was a strong correlation. Patients with poorly differentiated tumors had a 10% 5-year survival; those with moderately differentiated tumors had a 25% 5-year survival. Patients with well-differentiated tumors had about a 50% chance to survive 5 years [25].

The overall resectability rate of pancreatic cancer in the United States has increased from about 15% in the early 1980s to 25% in the early 1990s [26]. This is not attributable to any single factor. Diagnosis is made about 2 months earlier now than in the past, so patients may come to operation with less advanced disease. With the low operative mortality rates now being achieved, a more aggressive approach may be used in some centers. Thus some patients may be resected today who would not have been in the past. Finally, many patients who are judged preoperatively to have unresectable disease can be palliated nonoperatively today; they never reach the operating room.

Conclusions

The standard Whipple pancreaticoduodenectomy remains the gold standard for the treatment of potentially curable pancreatic cancer, although the pylorus-preserving pancreaticoduodenectomy is being performed often. The operative mortality rate is 2%–3% at major U.S. institutions where at least 15–20 resections per year are performed. While the resectability rate has increased in the past decade and survival has increased by greater than 6 months after resection, the *actual* 5-year survival rate remains dismal at 5%–10%. At least 40% of 5-year survivors will die of recurrence of the tumor. In lymph node-negative patients, the 5-year survival rate is 20%–30%, but most patients have lymph node metastases by the time they are treated. Although the Whipple procedure provides the only hope for cure, it probably palliates many patients effectively while curing almost no one.

References

1. Crist DW, Sitzman JV, Cameron JL (1987) Improved hospital morbidity, mortality, and survival after the Whipple procedure. Ann Surg 206:358–365
2. Trede M, Schwall G, Saeger HD (1990) Survival after pancreaticoduodenectomy: 118 consecutive resections without an operative mortality. Ann Surg 211:447–458
3. Cohen I, Colp R (1927) Cancer of periampullary region of the duodenum. Surg Gynecol Obstet 45:332–346
4. Hunt VC (1941) Surgical management of carcinoma of the ampulla of Vater and of the periampullary portion of the duodenum. Ann Surg 114:570–602
5. Hunt VC, Budd JW (1935) Transduodenal resection of the ampulla of Vater for carcinoma of the distal end of the common duct with restoration of continuity of the common and pancreatic ducts with the duodenum. Surg Gynecol Obstet 61:651–661
6. Whipple AO, Parsons WB, Mullins CR (1935) Treatment of carcinoma of the ampulla of Vater. Ann Surg 102:763–779
7. Brunschwig A (1937) One-stage pancreaticoduodenectomy. Surg Gynecol Obstet 65:681–684
8. Whipple AO (1945) Pancreaticoduodenectomy for islet carcinoma. Five-year follow-up. Ann Surg 121:847–852
9. Cattell RB (1948) A technique for pancreaticoduodenal resection. Surg Clin North Am 28:761–775
10. Cattell RB, Warren KW (1953) Surgery of the pancreas. Saunders, Philadelphia, p 374
11. Reber HA (1994) The classic Whipple operation for pancreatic cancer. Dig Surg 11:387–389
12. Crile G Jr (1970) The advantages of bypass operations over radical pancreaticoduodenectomy in the treatment of pancreatic carcinoma. Surg Gynecol Obstet 130:1049–1053
13. Shapiro TM (1975) Adenocarcinoma of the pancreas: a statistical analysis of bypass vs. Whipple resection in good risk patients. Ann Surg 182:715–721
14. Grace PA, Pitt HA, Tompkins RK, DenBensten L, Longmire WP Jr (1986) Decreased morbidity and mortality after pancreaticoduodenectomy. Am J Surg 151:141–149

15. Braasch JW, Deziel DJ, Rossi RL, Deziel DJ, Rossi RL, Watkins E Jr, Winter PF (1986) Pyloric and gastric preserving resection: experience with 87 patients. Ann Surg 204:411–418
16. Cameron JL, Pitt HA, Yeo CJ, Lillemoe KD, Kaufman HS, Coleman J (1993) One hundred and forty-five consecutive pancreaticoduodenectomies without mortality. Ann Surg 217:430–438
17. Cameron JL, Crist DW, Sitzmann JV, Hruban RH, Boitnott JK, Seidler AJ, Coleman J (1991) Factors influencing survival after pancreaticoduodenectomy for pancreatic cancer. Am J Surg 161:120–125
18. Livingston EH, Welton ML, Reber HA (1991) Surgical treatment of pancreatic cancer: the United States experience. Int J Pancreatol 9:153–157
19. Lillemoe KD (1995) Current management of pancreatic carcinoma. Ann Surg 221:133–148
20. Yeo CJ, Cameron JL, Maher MM, Sauter PK, Zahurak ML, Talamini MA, Lillemoe KD, Pitt HA (1995) A prospective, randomized trial of pancreaticogastrostomy versus pancreaticojejunostomy after pancreaticoduodenectomy. Ann Surg 222:580–592
21. Ashley SW, Reber HA (1993) Surgical management of exocrine pancreatic cancer. In: Go VLW, et al (eds) The pancreas: biology, pathobiology, and disease, 2nd edn. Raven Press, New York, pp 913–929
22. Bartoli FG, Arnone GB, Ravera G, Bachi V (1991) Pancreatic fistula and relative mortality in malignant disease after pancreaticoduodenectomy. Review and statistical meta-analysis regarding 15 years of literature. Anticancer Res 11:1831–1848
23. Yeo CJ (1995) Management of complications following pancreaticoduodenectomy. Surg Clin North Am 75:913–924
24. Patel AG, Toyama MT, Kusske AM, Alexander P, Ashley SW, Reber HA (1995) Pylorus-preserving Whipple resection for pancreatic cancer—is it any better? Arch Surg 130:838–843
25. Geer RJ, Brennan MF (1993) Prognostic indicators for survival after resection of pancreatic adenocarcinoma. Am J Surg 165:68–73
26. Nitecki SS, Sarr MG, Colby TV, van Heerden JA (1995) Long-term survival after resection for ductal adenocarcinoma of the pancreas. Is it really improving? Ann Surg 221:59–66

Pancreatic Cancer: A London Perspective: The British Experience of Pancreatic Surgery for Cancer

R.C.G. Russell

Summary. Pancreatic cancer in the U.K. is a disease of aging, and one that is decreasing slightly in incidence. Consequently, few patients are suitable for radical surgery. In a survey of the West Midlands Region, a 2.5% resection rate was found with an operative mortality rate of 27.6% in 145 patients undergoing resection. However, in a postal survey of specialist centers in the U.K. documenting 663 resected patients, the operative mortality rate was 5.3%, similar to personal experience. The long-term outlook (5-year survival rate) for patients who were resected for a ductal carcinoma was only 9% compared to 28% for those who underwent resection for a malignant neuroendocrine tumor. These low resection rates and poor results following resection has convinced the U.K. oncologist to adopt a nihilistic approach to the surgical treatment of this disease.

Key words. Pancreatic cancer—Pancreatectomy

Introduction

Carcinoma of the pancreas remains a common disease within the United Kingdom and is the seventh most common cause of cancer death. The incidence of pancreatic cancer is approximately the same as its death rate. Throughout the 1970s there was a steady increase in its incidence, but since 1985 there has been a decrease in incidence. In 1985 there were 6390 deaths; in 1990 there were 6145 deaths, in 1991, 6009 deaths, and in 1993, 5874 deaths. It is interesting to speculate whether this decrease is related to any external factor or if the previous rise merely reflected the aging of the population and the fact that there were more people in the right age group exposed to the disease process.

Certainly, pancreatic cancer in the U.K. is a disease of ageing (Fig. 1). Fewer than 5% of patients are less than 50 years of age, and 45% of such patients are more than 75 years of age. This incidence of elderly patients means that many patients will have coexistent disease at the time of presentation that will render them unsuitable for a radical surgical approach. The implications of the incidence and age in the commu-

The Middlesex Hospital, London, W1N 8AA, U.K.

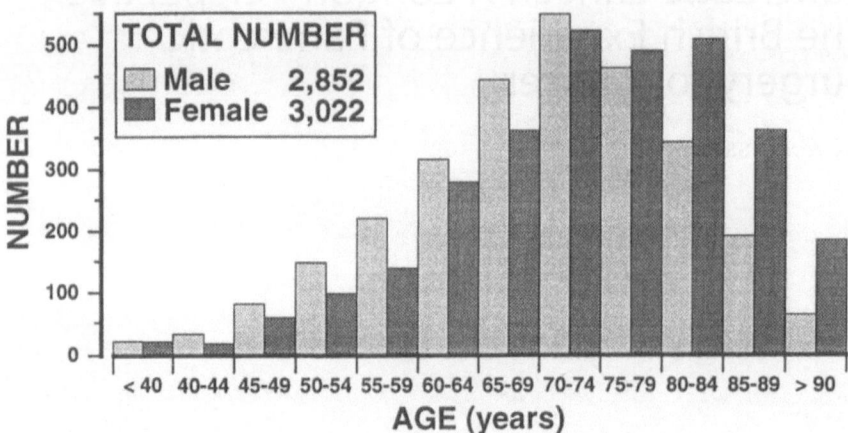

FIG. 1. Deaths from pancreatic cancer in England and Wales in 1993: A histogram of age at death of men and women [1]

nity at large is that the average hospital serving a quarter of a million people will see no more than 14 such patients per year, of whom only 3 will be less than 70 years of age and only 1 per year, at most, is likely to be suitable for a radical surgical approach.

Regional Review

Professor Neoptolemos undertook a review of the incidence and trends in the management of pancreatic cancer in the West Midlands, an industrial zone of the U.K. in which the health region cares for approximately 3.5 million people [2]. A careful Cancer Registry has been kept in this area since the early 1950s. In this survey, the trends in treatment and outcome of 13 560 patients with pancreatic cancer were determined between 1957 and 1986, using data from the West Midlands Cancer Registry. Patients were divided into those diagnosed in the first 20 years (1957–1976; $n = 7888$) and the most recent 10 years (1977–1986; $n = 5672$). The disease was more common in men, and the incidence increased until 1970 after which time it leveled off. In 1977–1986, a smaller proportion of patients had a laparotomy alone, 825 (14.5%) versus 1552 (19.7%) between 1957 and 1976.

A similar proportion had bypass surgery, 2010 (35.4%) versus 2760 (35%), while a greater proportion had supportive care, 2710 (47.8%) versus 3368 (42.7%), but the resection rates were the same, 145 (2.6%) versus 208 (2.6%). The 30-day mortality rates between the periods improved for resection, 40 (27.6%) versus 94 (45.2%), bypass surgery, 436 (21.7%) versus 691 (25%), and laparotomy, 37 (45.1%) versus 873 (56.3%). The 12-month survival rate for bypass did not significantly differ during the study periods (14.9% versus 12.4%), but there was significant improvement in the 5-year survival rate following resection (9.7% versus 2.6%) (Table 1). The resection rates were low and the 30-day mortality rates were high compared with those of other published series. Nevertheless, these data include every operation performed within a region, and the only similar data come from a study from New York in which a similar mortality rate was found for New York State compared with those who had undergone specialized surgery within the city institutions of New York [3].

Current Mortality

During the past 20 years, there has been a trend toward managing surgical disease of the pancreas in fewer, more centralized units, usually those associated with the advantages of better radiology and endoscopy within the university centers in the United Kingdom. To determine whether the mortality rate for the U.K. as a whole is the same as that occurring in specialized centers, a postal survey was undertaken of 13 centers well known for their pancreatic surgical work. The total number of resected patients documented was 663, with a Whipple procedure being performed in 539 (81%), a total pancreatectomy in 44 (7%), and a distal pancreatectomy in 50 (7.5%). The operative mortality rate in this group was 5.3%, which agrees with the major centers worldwide, as was the median length of stay of 17 days (range, 7–180). Unfortunately, in this survey we were unable to gather data concerning long-term outlook.

TABLE 1. Regional review: West Midlands Survey of 5672 cases, 1977–1986

Operation	Patients (%)	Mortality (%)
Laparotomy alone	14.5	45
Bypass surgery	35.4	21.7
Supportive care	47.8	
Resection	2.6	27.6
30-day mortality	27.6	
5-year survival	9.7	
1-year survival	30.6	
Median survival (months)	6.1	

Data from [2].

TABLE 2. Author's experience with resection

Tumor location	Resection				
	All	Proximal	Total	Distal	Local
Total	268	197	3	45	23
Ampullary	78	71			7
Pancreatic duct	70	60	3	7	
Bile duct	19	19			
Neuroendocrine					
Malignant	26	17		6	3
Benign	27	2		15	10
Miscellaneous					
Malignant	18	10		8	
Benign	30	18		9	3
Mortality					
n	12	11	1	0	0
Percent	4.5	5.6	33.3		
Pancreatitis	395	167	65	162	1	(Pancreatitis figures quoted for comparison)
Mortality					
n	11	3	3	5	0
Percent	2.8	1.8	4.6	3.0	

TABLE 3. Author's experience: major morbidity and mortality

Tumor location	n	Leakage			Delayed gastric emptying	Bleeding		Patients with major morbidity (%)	Reoperated		Mortality 60-day	
		P	B	G		≥4g	<4g		n	%	n	%
Ampullary	78	7	1	2	11	3		25	3	4	3	3.8
Pancreatic duct	70	1	5	1	13	5	2	32	3	4.5	5	7.1
Bile duct	19	0	0	0	2	3	0	33	1	5.6	3	15.8
Neuroendocrine												
Malignant	26	1	0	0	5	1	0	20	1	4	1	3.8
Benign	27	1	0	0	1	1	1	13	1	6.7	0	
Miscellaneous												
Malignant	18	0	1	0	1	1	0	12.5	1		0	
Benign	30	0	0	2	2	1	2	20	0		0	
Total												
n	268	10	7	5	35	15	5		10		12	
Percent		3.7	2.6	1.9	13.0	5.6	1.9	22.2	3.7		4.5	

P, pancreatic; B, biliary; G, gastric.

TABLE 4. Author's experience: survival rates

Tumor	Survival (%)	
	3 years	5 years
Ampullary	36	21
Ductal carcinoma	17	9
Bile duct	17	17
Neuroendocrine malignant	44	28
Miscellaneous malignant	56	24

Personal Experience

Since 1976, I have worked at the Middlesex Hospital where I have undertaken the surgical management of patients with pancreatic cancer. The Middlesex Hospital had one of the first units interested in interventional endoscopy, which was set up by Dr. P.B. Cotton and attracted a large number of patients with pancreatic cancer. During this period I have resected 268 patients, 197 of whom have had a proximal pancreatectomy (Table 2).

My own experience has been tempered with a number of complications, as shown in Table 3. There has been little evidence that the complication rate has decreased with time. Emphasis has been laid on the importance of pathology, and great care has been taken to differentiate the types of pancreatic cancer. Thus, the miscellaneous tumors in the group have been carefully separated from other cancers, and the outcome shows improved prognosis with both the neuroendocrine and malignant miscellaneous group compared to primary ductal cell carcinoma (Table 4). The disappointing 5-year survival rate, 9% for ductal carcinoma is in keeping with experience from other groups who have carefully differentiated the rarer tumors from the duct cell carcinoma [4].

Conclusion

The poor results shown in this review illustrate much of the experience within the U.K. Few centers undertake chemotherapy combined with surgical resection, although there is a national trial examining surgery alone versus surgery and radiotherapy with or without chemotherapy. On the basis of current experience, it is unlikely that this will improve the outcome by more than 5% improvement in the 5-year survival rate and an improved median survival of approximately 6 months. Such results are a reminder that until a new and different approach is adopted, no great improvement in survival in pancreatic cancer will occur. It should be remembered that the resection rate in the U.K. remains low, probably no more than 5%, because the attitude to this disease is that of nihilism, possibly justified by the poor long-term outlook associated even with resection for cure.

References

1. Office of Population Consenses and Surveys (1994) Mortality statistics: cause. Deaths: underlying cause, sex, age. England and Wales 1993. Series DH2, no 20. HMSO, London

2. Bramhill SR, Allum WH, Jones AG, Allwood A, Cummins C, Neoptolemos JPN (1995) Treatment and survival in 13560 patients with pancreatic cancer, and incidence of the disease, in the West Midlands: an epidemiological study. Br J Surg 82:111–115
3. Lieberman MD, Kilburn H, Lindley MF (1995) Relation of perioperative deaths to hospital volume among patients undergoing resection for malignancy. Ann Surg 222:638–645
4. Nitecki SS, Sarr MG, Colby TV, van Heerden JA (1995) Long-term survival after resection for ductal adenocarcinoma of the pancreas; is it really improving? Ann Surg 221:59–66

Total Pancreatectomy and Subtotal Duodenopancreatectomy for the Management of Carcinoma of the Head of the Pancreas: An Institutional Experience and Evolving Trends

B. Launois[1], E. Bardaxoglou[1], S. Landen[1], G.J. Maddern[2], J.L. Buard[1], B. Meunier[1], J.P. Campion[1], and J. Terblanche[3]

Summary. This retrospective study includes 88 consecutive patients treated by surgical resection for adenocarcinoma of the head of the pancreas between January 1973 and December 1992. Since 1973, total pancreatectomy has been the treatment of choice. Our policy changed after a review of 47 consecutive total pancreatectomies in 1986, which showed no benefit. We reintroduced the Whipple procedure as our standard operation, and for the following 41 patients, the Whipple procedure was performed 19 times; a total pancreatectomy was performed 22 times, however, because of positive resection margins or a friable pancreatic remnant. After total pancreatectomy, the 5-year survival rate was 7.8%. For lymph node-negative patients, the 1-, 3-, and 5-year survival rates were 54%, 24%, and 15%, respectively. For lymph node-positive patients, the 1- and 3-year survival rates were 46% and 4%, respectively, and there were no survivors at 54 months. This difference was not statistically significant. After the Whipple procedure, the 5-year survival rate was 12.5%. For lymph node-negative patients, the 1-, 3-, and 5-year survival rates were 50%, 59%, and 25%. For lymph node-positive patients, the 1-year survival rate was 21%; this difference was significant ($P = .007$). This study highlights the fact that extended radical surgery does not improve overall survival, but stages 2 and 3 disease (Hermreck classification) was associated with prolonged survival.

Key words. Adenocarcinoma—Pancreas—Whipple—Total pancreatectomy—Surgery

[1] Surgical Department and Transplantation Unit, Bloc Hôpital Pontchaillou, University of Rennes, 35033 Rennes Cedex, France.
[2] Department of Surgery, Queen Elizabeth Hospital, University of Adelaide, Woodville, South Australia 5011, Australia.
[3] Department of Surgery, University of Cape Town, Medical School Observatory, Cape Town 7925, South Africa.

Introduction

Cancer of the pancreas is generally considered to have a dismal prognosis, the principal reasons being inability to diagnose the disease at an early stage and the lack of effective adjuvant treatment [1]. Currently the only chance of cure lies in surgical resection of the tumor. However, the choice between a Whipple procedure and total pancreatectomy remains a subject of controversy. Although total pancreatectomy is conceptually a better procedure for the eradication of possible multifocal disease and allows wider lymph node clearance, this advantage has not been demonstrated to lead to improved survival. This study reports a surgical referral unit's experience with cancer of pancreas during the last two decades, with particular attention to evolving trends concerning surgical treatment.

Materials and Methods

Between January 1973 and December 1992, 445 patients were treated in our department for cancer of the pancreas. Cancer was localized in the head ($n = 310$), body ($n = 78$), or tail ($n = 26$) of the pancreas, and in 31 patients the lesions were diffuse, involving two or more segments of the pancreas. The overall resectability rate was 30.6% (136 cases). Among the group of patients with pancreatic head carcinoma, 100 underwent resection (69 total pancreatectomies, 25 Whipple procedures, and 6 tumorectomies).

A subgroup of 88 patients with adenocarcinoma of the head of the pancreas treated by total pancreatectomy ($n = 69$) or the Whipple procedure ($n = 19$) was analyzed to compare the two procedures. This subgroup contained 61 men and 27 women with a mean age of 60 years.

Operative Procedure

Total pancreatectomy was carried out with en bloc removal of the pancreas and skeletonization of the celiac axis, hepatic artery, superior mesenteric artery, and portal vein with complete retroperitoneal node dissection. Cholecystectomy was performed with high transection of the common bile duct. Portal vein resection was necessary in 14 patients. Direct suture by an end-to-end anastomosis was possible in 8 patients; in 4, a saphenous vein graft (2 cases) or a vascular prosthesis (2 cases) was used for venous repair. In 2 patients, only a lateral portal vein resection was done, followed by a lateral suture without narrowing of the vein. Postoperative diabetes was managed by administration of regular insulin for the first 2 weeks, then by neutral protamine Hagedorn (NPH) insulin. Exocrine insufficiency was compensated by 20–35 g of pancreatic extract per day and begun as soon as oral feedings became possible. Antacids were given to prevent stomal ulceration. Truncal vagotomy was not performed.

Subtotal pancreaticoduodenal resection was performed using the Child technique with transection of the pancreas to the left of the superior mesenteric artery. The end-to-side pancreaticojejunostomy utilized nonabsorbable sutures and included intubation of the pancreatic duct with a drain in ten cases. A pylorus-preserving procedure was performed in two patients.

TABLE 1. Classifications used for pancreatic carcinoma

Hermreck classification

I.	Local disease only
II.	Invasion into surrounding tissue (duodenum, portal vein and mesenteric vessels)
III.	Lymph node metastases
IV.	Generalized carcinoma (liver metastases and peritoneal implants)

Tumor node metastasis (TNM) classification

T1.	No direct extension of the primary tumor beyond the pancreas
T2.	Limited direct extension to the duodenum, bile ducts, or stomach, still possibly permitting tumor resection
T3.	Further direct extension, incompatible with surgical resection
N0.	Regional nodes not involved
N1.	Regional nodes involved
M0.	No (known) distant metastasis
M1.	Distant metastasis present
Stage I.	T1, T2, N0, M0
Stage II.	T1–T3, N0 (direct extension of tumor that precludes surgical resection)
Stage III.	T1–T3, N1, M0
Stage IV.	T1–T3, N0–N1, M1

Lymph node extension

N0.	None
N1.	Preduodenopancreatic group
	Retroduodenopancreatic group
	Splenic group
	Inferior body group
N2.	Mesenteric root group
	Transverse mesocolon group
	Hepatic group
N3.	Celiac group
	Interaorticocaval group
	Left subrenal group

Postoperative mortality was defined as death occurring during the hospital stay. Standard statistical methods (the Kaplan–Meier method, chi-square analysis) were used to evaluate differences in patient survival. Wherever it is stated that groups are not significantly different, the P value always exceeds .05. Patients were staged according to the Hermreck and tumor node metastasis (TNM) classifications and lymph node extension outlined in Table 1.

Results

Pathology

Intraoperative transduodenal needle aspiration cytology was performed 34 times. Cytology was positive 25 times, negative 7 times, and uninterpretable in 2 cases. The sensitivity of aspiration cytology was 78%. Median tumor diameter was 3 cm (range, 1–9 cm) after total pancreatectomy and 2.6 cm (range, 1–9 cm) after the Whipple procedure. Duodenal involvement was found in 30 specimens following total pancreatectomy (43.5%) and in 11 specimens following Whipple procedures (57.9%). The nerve sheaths were seen to be involved in 33 cases following total pancreatectomy (47.8%) and in 8 cases following Whipple procedures (42.1%). Following total pancreatectomy, lymph node extension was present in 31 patients; it involved juxtatumoral nodes in 17 specimens (55%), peripancreatic nodes in 8 specimens (26%), and distal nodes in 6 specimens (19%). Following Whipple procedures, lymph node extension was found to be juxtatumoral in 4 cases (57.1%) and peripancreatic in 3 cases (42.9%). Tumors were multifocal in 15 of 69 total pancreatectomy specimens (21.7%).

Total Pancreatectomy

Survival According to Hermreck Staging

Among the 69 patients, tumors were staged as follows: 21 were stage I, 17 stage II, 29 stage III, and 2 stage IV (Fig. 1). The 5-year survival rate for patients with stage I tumors was 25%. There were no survivors at 54 months for patients with stage II tumors, at 48 months for stage III tumors, or at 24 months for patients with stage IV tumors. There was no significant difference in actuarial survival for stage I tumors as compared with stage II, III, and IV tumors ($P = .016$; $\chi^2 = 7.37$). The median survival time for patients with stage I tumors was 22 months, versus 11 months for patients with stage II and III tumors and 6 months for patients with stage IV tumors.

Survival According to Portal Vein Resection
(Fortner's type I extended procedure)

En bloc resection of the portal vein and pancreas was performed 14 times (Fig. 2). The 5-year survival rate was 8.2% without vein resection versus 15% at 34 months when portal vein resection was necessary ($P = .032$; $\chi^2 = 4.5974$). The median survival time was 15 months versus 5 months when portal vein resection was done.

Survival According to Lymph Node Status

For patients without node involvement (N0), the 1-, 3-, and 5-year survival rates were 54%, 24%, and 15%, respectively (Fig. 3). In the presence of node involvement, the 1-

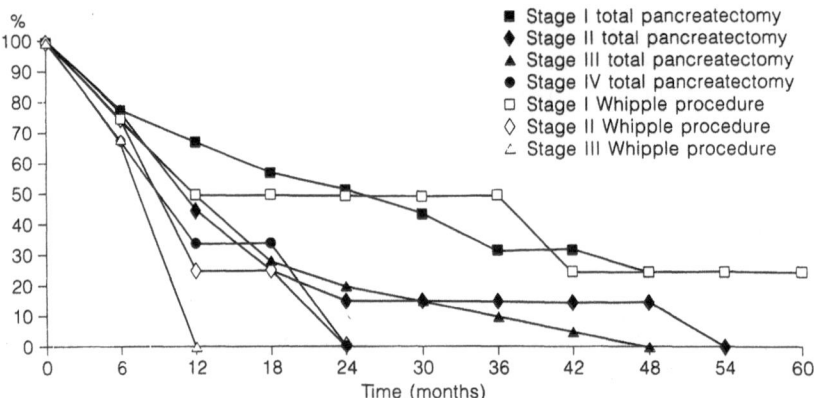

FIG. 1. Survival (%) according to Hermreck classification after total pancreatectomy or Whipple procedure

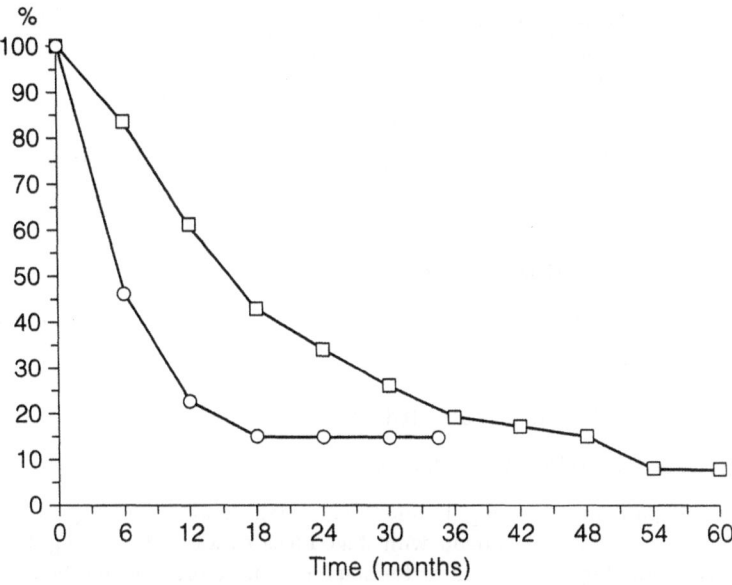

FIG. 2. Long-term survival (%) with (*circles*) or without (*squares*) portal vein resection

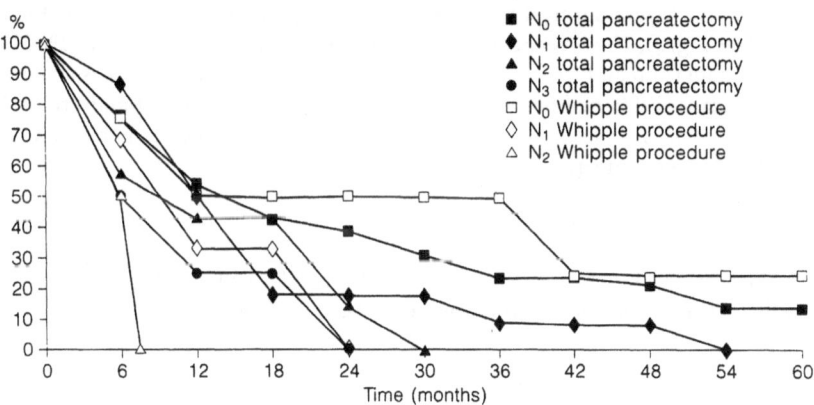

FIG. 3. Long-term survival (%) related to lymph node status after total pancreatectomy or Whipple procedure

and 3-year survival rates were 46% and 4%, respectively, and there were no survivors at 54 months. The median survival times for node-negative and node-positive patients were not statistically significant. When various stages of nodal involvement were considered (Table 2), the 1- and 3-year survival rates were 50% and 9%, respectively, for the N1 subgroup, 43% and 0%, respectively, for the N2 subgroup, and 25% and 0%, respectively, for the N3 subgroup.

TABLE 2. Lymph node extension

Stage	Total pancreatectomy	Whipple
N0	38	12
N1	17	4
N2	8	3
N3	5	—

Survival According to TNM Staging

The 5-year survival rate for patients with stage I was 15%; there were no survivors at 5 years for patients with stages II, III, and IV (Fig. 4).

Subtotal Duodenopancreatectomy

Survival According to Hermreck Staging

Among the 19 patients, 6 had stage I tumors, 7 had stage II, and 6 had stage III tumors. The 5-year survival rate for patients with stage I lesions was 25% (see Fig. 1). There were no survivors beyond 24 months for stage II tumors or, as would be expected, beyond 12 months for stage III tumors. The median survival time for patients with stages I, II, and III tumors was 11, 7, and 7 months, respectively.

Survival According to Lymph Node Status

The 1-, 3-, and 5-year survival rates were 50%, 50%, and 25%, respectively, for N0 patients (see Fig. 3). The 1-year survival rate for node-positive patients was 21% (33% for the N1 subgroup and 0% for the N2 subgroup; see Table 2). There was a statistically significant difference between the survival times of group N0 and group N+ patients ($P = .007$; $\chi^2 = 9.9$). The median survival time for N0 and N+ patients was 11 and 5 months, respectively.

Survival According to TNM Staging

The 5-year survival rate for patients with stage I was 22%, with no survivors at 5 years for patients with stages II and III disease ($P = .02$; $\chi^2 = 7.7892$) (see Fig. 4).

Global Survival

The 5-year survival rate following total pancreatectomy was 7.8% and was 12.5% following subtotal duodenopancreatectomy (Fig. 5). The difference is not statistically significant.

Hospital Mortality

Eighteen patients (26%) died in hospital after total pancreatectomy: 9 died within 30 days of operation. These deaths were caused by septicemia (8 patients), gastrointestinal hemorrhage (2), uncontrollable hemorrhage (2), hypoglycemic coma (2), hyperosmolar coma (2), and cardiopulmonary failure (2 patients). The mean hospital stay was 26.5 days (up to 3 months) after total pancreatectomy. Hospital mortality was highest in the period between 1978 and 1982, reaching 43% (Fig. 6). During the last

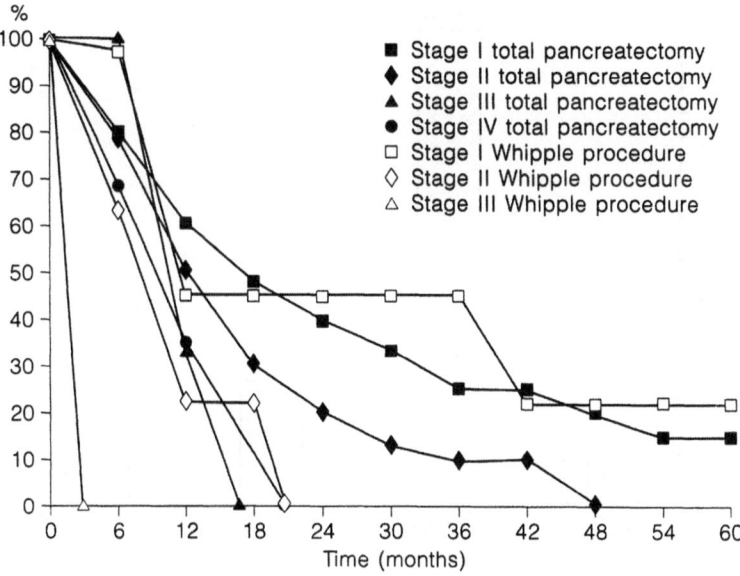

FIG. 4. Long-term survival (%) related to tumor node metastasis (TNM) classification after total pancreatectomy or Whipple procedure

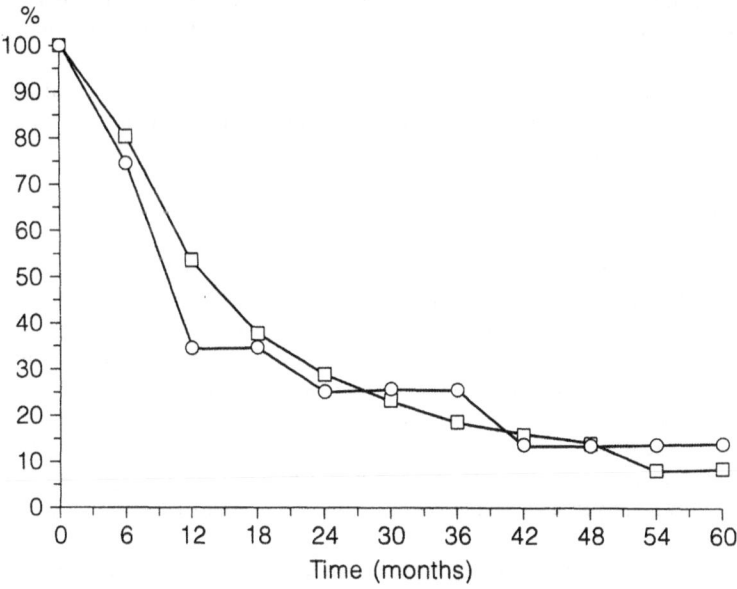

FIG. 5. Actuarial survival related to total pancreatectomy (*squares*) versus Whipple procedure (*circles*)

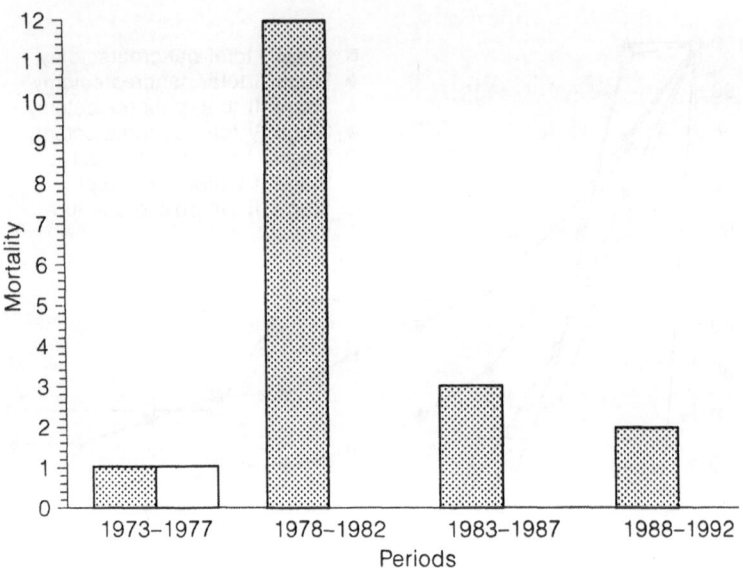

FIG. 6. Hospital mortality: *shaded bars*, total pancreatectomy; *white bars*, Whipple procedure

decade mortality decreased to 13%, largely because of progress in postoperative management. Following a Whipple procedure, 1 patient died 34 days postoperatively. The mean hospital stay was 19.4 days.

Patient's age, preoperative serum bilirubin level, and the duration of jaundice were not correlated to hospital mortality. Hypoalbuminemia was associated with a higher operative mortality rate ($P < .01$; Table 3).

Morbidity

Morbidity was higher following total pancreatectomy (Table 4), with 25 patients (36%) presenting with surgical complications: 3 biliary fistulas, 5 digestive fistulas, 6 gastrointestinal hemorrhages (anastomotic ulceration in 3 cases, erosive gastritis in 1, and anastomotic bleeding from the ileal loop in 2 cases), 13 septicemias, 8 intraperitoneal abcesses, and 3 cases of postoperative hemoperitoneum. Three patients had pulmonary complications and cardiac failure. Reoperation was necessary 19 times in 14 patients, including fistulas (3 cases), hemoperitoneum (3 cases), gastrointestinal hemorrhage (3 cases), septicemia of unknown origin (4 cases), subphrenic abcess (3 cases), pleural empyema (1 case), intestinal obstruction (1 case), and evisceration (1 case).

Following total pancreatectomy, brittle diabetes was noted during the postoperative period with enhanced insulin sensitivity resulting in oscillating blood glucose levels. Seven patients developed severe hypoglycemia, five patients presented with hyperosmolar coma, and one patient had ketoacidosis. These metabolic disorders were observed during our early experience. After Whipple procedures, surgical complications were noted in six patients (one biliary fistula, one digestive fistula, three pancreatic fistulas, and one gastrointestinal hemorrhage), which required two

TABLE 3. Nonparametric tests for continuous data analysis of bilirubin, length of jaundice, age, and hypoalbuminemia

Factor	Amount	Fisher's test
Serum bilirubin	<6 mg/dl	NS
	>6 mg/dl	NS
Length of jaundice	<3 days	NS
	>3 days	NS
Age	<65 years	NS
	>65 years	NS
Hypoalbuminemia	<35 mg/dl	$P < .01$
	>35 mg/dl	$P < .01$

TABLE 4. Morbidity

Complication	Total pancreatectomy (n)	Whipple procedure (n)
Biliary fistula	3	1
Digestive fistula:		
Gastroenteroanastomosis	1	1
Colonic fistula	1	0
Enteric fistula	3	0
Pancreatic leak	0	3
Gastrointestinal bleeding	6	1
Intraabdominal hemorrhage	3	0
Intraabdominal abscess	8	0
Generalized sepsis	3	1
Severe hypoglycemia	7	0
Hyperosmolar coma	5	0
Reoperation	14	2

reoperations (Table 4). Two pancreatic leaks healed spontaneously, and one necessitated a reoperation. No deaths resulted from pancreatic fistulas.

Discussion

The therapy of choice for cancer of the head of the pancreas is resection because it represents the only chance of cure [2]. One of the major controversies regarding radical resection is the role of total pancreatectomy for ductal adenocarcinoma. As the results of the Whipple procedure were disappointing, some surgeons converted to total pancreatectomy [3–5].

When the study commenced in 1973, we advocated total pancreatectomy as the treatment of choice for cancer of the pancreas. This seemed justified because of the possible spread to the left of the mesenteric vessels by cancer situated in the head of the pancreas; the procedure achieved a wider lymphadenectomy as well as ensuring removal of multicentric malignant foci. Furthermore, it avoided performance of a pancreaticojejunostomy, the Achilles heel of the Whipple procedure. The major criticisms leveled against total pancreatectomy have been the high postoperative morbidity and mortality rates observed in most series. Thus in 1986 we reviewed the results of 47 consecutive total pancreatectomies for carcinoma of the head of the pancreas of which 9 were associated with portal vein resection [4]. Resectability rates increased from 15% to 32%, because patients with tumor spread beyond the usual margin of division for the Whipple procedure were excluded. However, we found this extended procedure to be of no benefit when portal vein resection was necessary or when multicentric cancer or neoplastic emboli were present in the operative specimen.

As a result of our study, and in accordance with attitudes adopted by other authors, we reverted to the Whipple procedure as the operation of choice for the treatment of pancreatic carcinoma. Since 1986, Whipple procedures have been performed in 19 patients, and total pancreatectomy was done of necessity in 22 patients with adenocarcinoma of the pancreas because the pancreatic resection margin contained residual tumor or because the pancreatic remnant was considered too friable for anastomosis. The 5-year survival rate after total pancreatectomy was 7.8% versus 12.5% after the Whipple procedure. In the group having undergone total pancreatectomy, patients with nodal involvement had a median survival time of 12 months versus 11 months for patients without nodal involvement. There was no significant difference in 3-year cumulative survival rates between the group with peripancreatic node involvement and the group with distant node involvement.

It is noteworthy that pancreatic cancer is often found to have extension of cancer cells via lymph node metastases and infiltration within lymphatic vessels, nerves, or connective tissue [6]. Lymphatic metastases of pancreatic cancer were studied by Cubilla et al. [7], who reported that cancer situated in the head of the pancreas often metastasized to the superior head (45%), posterior pancreaticoduodenal (45%), superior body (27%), and inferior (23%) lymph node groups. These authors noted extension to the inferior body, midcolic, pyloric anterior pancreaticoduodenal, and mesenteric node groups in only 5%–9% of specimens. Nagai et al. [8] found lymph involvement of the inferior head group in all their patients presenting with T2 pancreatic cancer. A few lymph nodes of the paraaortic group were found to have micrometastases in 50% of patients, and distribution of the metastatic nodes ranged between the origin of the renal artery and that of the inferior mesenteric artery.

The high incidence of cancer spread via lymphatics and nerves suggests that wide resection of the peritumoral and nervous tissue is required for complete eradication of cancer cells. Although most node-positive patients treated by total pancreatectomy died of local recurrence and distant metastases, the median survival rate was comparable with the survival of patients with node-negative status. This is likely to result from the extended dissection of regional lymph nodes and en bloc tissue excision associated with total pancreatectomy. These findings were not observed after the Whipple procedure.

When comparing actuarial survival rates of node-positive patients after total and subtotal pancreatectomy, we found no significant difference. In accordance with the findings of van Heerden et al. [9], nodal involvement did not seem to bear any prognostic significance. However, other studies have shown an improved 5-year survival rate when lymph nodes were not invaded by tumor [10–14]. In our experience, subtotal pancreatectomy was superior to total pancreatectomy when operative mortality, morbidity, and duration of hospital stay were considered, confirming the findings of others [15,16]. Total pancreatectomy was associated with higher operative mortality and morbidity rates, but these have improved significantly during the past 10 years in most series, mainly as a result of advances in intensive care monitoring and nutrition and increased experience in pancreatic surgery [17].

In conclusion, extended radical surgery, aimed at eradicating possible mutifocal disease and achieving wider lymph node clearance, did not lead to improved survival. However, patients with Hermreck stages 2 and 3 tumors undergoing this extended operation had prolonged survival and acceptable palliation. Surgery alone will probably not solve the problem of pancreatic cancer. Whether a Whipple procedure or a total pancreatectomy is the ideal procedure is debatable. Multimodal treatment combining surgery, adjuvant radiation therapy, and chemotherapy may break the current deadlock in the management of pancreatic carcinoma [11,18-20].

References

1. Warshaw AL, Castillo CFD (1992) Pancreatic carcinoma. N Engl J Med 326:455–465
2. Moossa AR (1982) Pancreatic cancer. Approach to diagnosis, selection and choice of operation. Cancer (Phila) 50:2689–2698
3. Fortner JG, Kim DK, Cubilla A, Turnbull A, Pahnke LD, Shils ME (1977) Regional pancreatectomy: en bloc pancreatic portal vein and lymph node resection. Ann Surg 186:42–50
4. Launois B, Franci J, Bardaxoglou E, Ramée MP, Paul JL, Malledant Y, Campion JP (1993) Total pancreatectomy for ductal adenocarcinoma of the pancreas with special reference to resection of portal vein and multicentric cancer. World J Surg 17:122–127
5. Ihse I, Arnesjö B, Bengmark S (1977) Total pancreatectomy for cancer. An appraisal of 75 cases. Ann Surg 186:675–680
6. Ishikawa O, Ohhigashi H, Sasaki Y, Kabuto T, Fukuda I, Furukawa H, Imaoka S, Iwanaga T (1988) Practical usefulness of lymphatic and connective tissue clearance for the carcinoma of the pancreas head. Ann Surg 208:215–220
7. Cubilla AC, Fortner J, Fitzgerald PJ (1978) Lymph node involvement in carcinoma of the pancreas area. Cancer (Phila) 41:880–887
8. Nagai H, Kuroda A, Marioka Y (1986) Lymphatic and local spread of T1 and T2 pancreas cancer: a study of autopsy material. Ann Surg 204:65–71
9. van Heerden JA, McIlrath DC, Ilstup DM, Weiland LH (1988) Total pancreatectomy for ductal adenocarcinoma of the pancreas: an update. World J Surg 12:658–662
10. Crist DW, Sitzmann JV, Cameron JL (1987) Improved hospital morbidity, mortality and survival after the Whipple procedure. Ann Surg 206:358–365
11. Kalser MH, Ellenberg SS (1985) Pancreatic cancer. Adjuvant combined radiation and chemotherapy following curative resection. Arch Surg 120:899–903
12. Cameron JL, Crist DW, Sitzmann JV, Hruban RH, Boitnott JK, Seidler AJ, Coleman J (1991) Factors influencing survival after pancreaticoduodenectomy for pancreatic cancer. Am J Surg 161:121–125
13. Andrén-Sandberg A, Ihse I (1983) Factors influencing survival after total pancreatectomy in patients with pancreatic cancer. Ann Surg 198:605–610
14. Mannell A, Weiland LH, van Heerden JA, Ilstrup DM (1986) Factors influencing survival after resection for ductal adenocarcinoma of the pancreas. Ann Surg 203:403–407
15. Trede M, Schwall G, Saeger HD (1990) Survival after pancreatoduodenectomy. 118 consecutive resections without an operative mortality. Ann Surg 211:447–459
16. Cooperman AM, Herter FP, Marboe CA, Helmreich ZV, Perzin KH (1981) Pancreatoduodenal resection and total pancreatectomy. An institutional review. Surgery (St Louis) 90:707–712
17. Brooks JR, Brooks DC, Levine JD (1989) Total pancreatectomy for ductal cell carcinoma of the pancreas. An update. Ann Surg 209:405–410

18. Dobelbower RR Jr, Konski AA, Merrick HW III, Bronn DG, Schfeling D, Kamen C
   (1991) Intraoperative electron beam radiation therapy (IOEBRT) for carcinoma of the
   exocrine pancreas. Int J Radiat Oncol Biol Phys 20:113–119
19. Heijmans HJ, Hoekstra HJ, Mehta DM (1989) Is adjuvant intraoperative radiotherapy
   (IORT) for resectable and unresectable pancreatic carcinoma worthwhile? Hepato-
   Gastroenterology 36:474–477
20. Arbuck SG (1990) Overview of chemotherapy for pancreatic carcinoma. Int J
   Pancreatol 7:209–222

Complications After Pancreaticoduodenectomy: Analysis of Risk Factors, Their Incidence, and Possible Prevention in Italy

M. Falconi[1], C. Bassi[1], R. Salvia[1], A. Bonora[1], N. Sartori[1], E. Caldiron[1], G. Talamini[2], P. Pederzoli[1], and the Italian Study Group

Summary. Pancreaticoduodenectomy is unquestionably the most difficult operation in major pancreatic surgery as the result of both problems posed by perioperative management of the patients and the particular anatomical relationships of the pancreas. Over the years, many studies have analyzed the factors influencing the success or failure of this procedure, but all of these are retrospective and inevitably reflect the particular experience of single centers. It may be noted that pancreatic enzymes are separated biologically and physically from their activators. The surgical operations performed in this sector, and particularly pancreaticoduodenectomy, thus disrupt the normal anatomical situation and increase the risk of postoperative complications. One distinct possibility, irrespective of the surgeon's experience and expertise, the degree of fibrosis of the pancreas, and the metabolic status of the patient, hinges upon the feasibility of intervening by specifically reducing pancreatic exocrine secretion. To assess this aspect, a prospective Italian multicenter study has evaluated the occurrence of complications in the course of treatment with Octreotide at subcutaneous doses of $100\,\mu g$ three times daily versus a placebo. This study reveals that the use of Octreotide induces a significant mean reduction, roughly 50%, in the risk of pancreatic fistula formation as compared to placebo. All in all, however, the results are still disappointing, as the post-pancreaticoduodenectomy morbidity rate ranges from 16% to 32% of the various case series analyzed.

Key words. Pancreatic neoplasms—Pancreaticoduodenectomy—Complications— Octreotide

Introduction

Ever since 1934, when Whipple performed his first resection of the head of the pancreas and the patient died 48 h later of the ensuing complications [1], surgeons throughout the world have been only too familiar with the high morbidity and mortality rates associated with subtotal pancreatectomy.

---

[1] Surgical Department and [2] Gastroenterological Department, University of Verona, 37134 Verona, Italy.

Although the mortality rates reported over the years by some authors are less than 5% [2–5], the associated morbidity, even in specialized centers, is still high, with incidences ranging from 30% to 40% [3,6–10]. These complications are mainly related to the risk of dehiscence of an anastomosed intestinal loop, the formation of a pancreatic fistula, or sterile fluid collections and abscesses, with the risk of triggering acute pancreatitis. When this later eventuality occurs, the presence of active enzymes in the blood-stream may also cause not only the development of local complications but also the onset of systemic complications such as kidney and respiratory insufficiency and even shock. The risk of hemorrhage, which is common to all surgical interventions, is higher in pancreatic resections because of the rich and very particular vascularization of the pancreas resulting from its close relationships with the main vessels of the abdominal region. What makes pancreatic surgery so difficult and singular, apart from the anatomical relationships, is the presence of pancreatic juice with its very high content of proteolytic enzymes; these enzymes, once activated, are capable of digesting almost all biological substrates.

In the normal anatomy of the pancreas, these enzymes are "compartmentalized" both biologically and physically from their activators, mainly bile and enterokinases of intestinal origin. Surgical operations on the pancreas, which give rise to a new anatomical situation with the artificial breaching of some of these barriers, brings the pancreatic juice in direct contact with these enzymes. This is all the more true in the case of pancreaticoduodenectomy in which resection of the head of the pancreas and duodenum eliminates perhaps the most important barrier between the intestinal contents and pancreatic juice, consisting of the periampullary region and its elements. Further decisive factors in the development of complications appear to be related to the surgeon's experience, to the degree of fibrosis of the pancreas [11], and to the patient's nutritional and metabolic status, as well as to the use of substances capable of reducing pancreatic secretion [12a].

Unfortunately, there are very few studies in the literature that analyze these factors in pancreaticoduodenectomy alone; such studies as there are mostly retrospective and very often report data from a single, inevitably "expert" center. In Italy, however, although there are no published reports on this specific subject, a recent study [12] that is not dissimilar to the one conducted in Germany [11] was aimed at assessing the efficacy of the pancreatic secretion inhibitor Octreotide in preventing the onset of postoperative complications after pancreatic surgery. Patients suffering from pancreatic and periampullary tumours or from chronic pancreatitis were prospectively recruited into this study. The patients were allocated, according to a randomized double-blind design, to one of two groups, the first treated with active drug and the other with placebo.

The reelaboration of the study, although not specifically aimed at analyzing the complications of pancreaticoduodenectomy, provides us with some important data on their effective incidence in this type of operation and the factors conditioning their occurrence. In addition, comparison of the various pancreatic operations allows us to assess the effective risk of complications related to pancreaticoduodenectomy and the impact that therapy with the pancreatic secretion inhibitor Octreotide has on their incidence. Moreover, the fact that this is a multicenter study overcomes the drawback inherent in single expert center studies, thus conferring a broader significance upon the data obtained.

The aim of the present study is therefore to assess, through a re-analysis of this study, the effective incidence of postpancreaticoduodenectomy complications in Italy, quantifying the impact of the various risk factors.

Patients and Methods

The study, the characteristics of which are described elsewhere [12], was conducted from March 1990 to January 1992. On the day surgery was performed and for 7 days postoperatively, the patients received either Octreotide, at subcutaneous doses of .1 mg three times daily, or an identical amount of placebo. The patients were stratified into two subgroups: a high-risk group (those with tumors of the pancreas or periampullary region) and a low-risk group (those suffering from chronic pancreatitis).

All patients were monitored clinically on the day before the operation, on the day of the operation itself, on days 1, 3, 4, 5, and 7 postoperatively, and thereafter at weekly intervals. This monitoring consisted of blood tests (including serum albumin, glucose, and bilirubin) and of monitoring of drainage fluid, when present in significant amounts, with quantification of the volume and amylase and lipase contents. In addition, patients underwent routine echotomography and abdominal computed tomography (CT) scans.

The complications monitored, which are better defined elsewhere [12], were death, dehiscence of the pancreatic anastomosis, formation of pancreatic fistulas, sterile abdominal fluid collections and abscesses, acute pancreatitis, shock, sepsis, kidney or respiratory insufficiency, and hemorrhage. In the reelaboration of the data for the present study, however, these complications were divided into pancreatic fistulas and all other nonfistular complications in general. The surgical operations were grouped as pancreaticoduodenectomies. pancreaticojejunostomies, left pancreatectomies, and atypical resections including enucleations, duodenum-preserving head resections, and intermediate resections.

Statistical Analysis

The differences between complication rates were analyzed using the chi-square test or Fisher test, when required by sample size. The other variables were compared by means of appropriate parametric and nonparametric tests. In the univariate analysis, we considered the following variables as potential predictors of occurrence of postoperative complications (fistulas or other complications in general): sex, age, risk status, type of operation performed, and preoperative blood test values (serum albumin, bilirubin, and glucose).

For the odds ratio estimates, multivariate logistic analysis was carried out with backward stepping of variables and evaluations of the model using three goodness-of-fit chi-squared statistics. Preassigned P values equal to .05 controlled the stepping removal. The BMDP (BMDP Inc., Los Angeles, CA, USA) and SPSS (SPSS Inc., Chicago, IL, USA) statistical programs were used.

No patients dropped out.

Results

Of the 303 patients recruited, 51 were not evaluable, in most cases because the lesions proved unresectable at surgery. Of the 252 evaluable patients, 130 were treated with placebo and the other 122 with Octreotide. The two treatment groups were comparable for all significant variables.

Of the patients, 162 were considered at high risk (tumors) and 90 at low risk (chronic pancreatitis) (Table 1). Subsequently, 186 patients (73.8%) underwent pancreatic resections (100 pancreaticoduodenectomies, 60 left pancreatectomies, and 26 atypical resections); 66 of 84 patients with chronic pancreatitis (78.6%) were submitted to a pancreaticojejunosotomy (Table 2).

Overall, 57 patients presented one or more complications, 38 (29.7%) in the placebo group and 19 (15.6%) in the group treated with Octreotide ($P = .01$). In particular, 33% of the patients undergoing pancreaticoduodenectomy presented complications, 24.2% of patients undergoing atypical resections, 19% of those treated by left pancreatectomy, and only 8.2% of patients undergoing pancreaticojejunostomy (chi-squared test; $P = .003$).

The univariate analysis revealed bilirubinemia as a possible risk factor for the onset of complications in general (mean value, 3.02 ± 5.9 mg/dl in the group without complications vs. 5.5 ± 6.7 mg/dl in the group with complications; $P = .01$), as well as risk status (high-risk stratum, 29% of patients with complications; low-risk stratum, 11%; $P = .001$).

Age, sex, and serum albumin and glucose levels did not prove significantly different in patients with complications as compared to those without. A different and significantly longer period of postoperative hospitalization was observed in patients with

TABLE 1. Distribution of 252 evaluable patients in terms of treatment and risk status

Status	Placebo (n)	Octreotide (n)	Total (n)
High-risk	86	76	162
Low-risk	44	46	90
Total	130	122	252

TABLE 2. Types of operation performed in 252 evaluable patients subdivided according to treatment

Operation	Placebo		Octreotide		Total	
	n	%[a]	n	%[a]	n	%[b]
Pancreaticoduodenectomy	50	(50)	50	(50)	100	(39.7)
Left pancreatectomy	34	(56.7)	26	(43.3)	60	(23.8)
Atypical resection	16	(61.5)	10	(38.5)	26[c]	(10.3)
Pancreaticojejunostomy	30	(45.4)	36	(54.6)	66	(26.2)
Total	130		122		252	

[a] Row percentage.
[b] Column percentage.
[c] Fourteen enucleations, 7 intermediate resections, 5 duodenum-preserving head resections.

TABLE 3. Univariate analysis of factors associated with development of complications in general and of pancreatic fistulas

Group	Complications in general: 57/252 patients (22.6%)	Pancreatic fistulas: 35/252 patients (13.9%)
Placebo	$P = .01$	$P = .02$
High-risk stratum	$P = .001$	$P = .01$
Serum bilirubin elevation	$P = .01$	NS

TABLE 4. Multivariate analysis of risk of nonfistula complications in general

Variable	Relative risk (odds ratio)	95% confidence limits LL	UL	P
Octreotide	.43	.22	.82	.011
High-risk stratum	3.11	1.47	6.59	.003

LL, lower limit; UL, upper limit.
N.B.: The baseline risk considered with regard to the risk stratum corresponds to that of nonfistula complications in general following pancreaticojejunosotomy, i.e., 8.2% in the study, while the baseline risk with regard to treatment is that of the patients treated with placebo.

complications compared to those with no complications (35.4 ± 20.9 days vs. 18.1 ± 8.8 days; $P = .0001$) (Table 3).

As regards the formation of pancreatic fistulas, 35 patients presented this complication, 24/130 (18.5%) in the placebo group and 11/122 (9%) in the group treated with Octreotide ($P = .02$). Development of a pancreatic fistula was observed in 20 (20%) of the 100 patients undergoing pancreaticoduodenectomy, in 8 (30.8%) of the 26 patients undergoing atypical resections, in 4 (6.7%) of the 60 left pancreatectomy cases, and in 3 (4.5%) of the 66 pancreaticojejunostomies (chi-squared test; $P = .005$). Fistula formation correlated in univariate analysis not only with treatment, but also with the risk stratum, being higher in the high-risk group, i.e., in those in whom the pancreas was softer (high-risk stratum, 17.9% of patients with fistulas vs. 6.7% in the low-risk stratum; $P = .01$). Formation of pancreatic fistulas also entailed a significantly longer period of hospitalization (37.6 ± 23 days vs. 19.2 ± 10.2 days for patients not developing pancreatic fistulas; $P = .0001$). Age, sex, serum bilirubin, albumin, and glucose did not prove significantly different in patients developing pancreatic fistulas compared to those not presenting this complication (Table 3).

Of all the variables considered, our multivariate analysis indicated that, as regards the risk of onset of general complications other than fistula, the only point worthy of note was that belonging to the high-risk stratum was associated with a risk of developing such complications roughly three times greater than that associated with pancreaticojejunostomy, which is regarded as an operation usually indicating the low-risk category. The use of Octreotide induces a significant (roughly 50%) mean reduction in the risk of developing complications other than fistula compared to placebo (Table 4).

For development of pancreatic fistulas, the multivariate analysis indicates that, of all the variables considered, only treatment with Octreotide and the type of operation performed are associated with pancreatic fistula formation. In the odds ratio analysis,

TABLE 5. Multivariate analysis of risk of pancreatic fistula formation

Variable	Relative risk (odds ratio)	95% confidence limits		P
		LL	UL	
Octreotide	.38	.17	.84	.01
Type of operation				.01
Left pancreatectomy	1.26	.27	5.95	.77
Pancreaticoduodenectomy	4.95	1.39	17.6	.01
Atypical resection	5.14	1.21	21.8	.02

LL, lower limit; UL, upper limit.
N.B.: The baseline risk considered with regard to the type of operation is that of pancreatic fistula formation after pancreaticojejunostomy, i.e., 4.5% in the study, while the baseline risk with regard to treatment is that of the patients treated with placebo.

as far as treatment is concerned, once again the baseline risk we considered was that of placebo-treated subjects; the baseline risk was that of subjects undergoing pancreaticojejunosotomy, this being the operation associated with the least risk of pancreatic fistula formation (4.5%). The data reported in Table 5 indicate that Octreotide produces a significant mean reduction (roughly 50%) in the risk of fistula formation. As regards the type of operation, the relative risk figures show that left pancreatectomy carries a risk of fistula formation comparable to that of pancreaticojejunostomy. By the same token, both pancreaticoduodenectomy and atypical resections carry much higher risks (roughly fivefold) than pancreaticojejunostomy.

In the case of analysis of the risk both of fistula formation and of developing complications other than fistula, interactions between variables were not all significant. Analysis of residues revealed that the model used was adequate.

Discussion

Pancreatic surgery, despite the major advances made during the past few years in perioperative patient management, still remains distinctly difficult. Several factors contribute to the surgeon's difficulties. Some of these, such as the rich vascularization of the pancreas, its very particular anatomical relationships, and the management of complications once they have occurred, may be counteracted by the skill and experience of the surgeon performing the operation and monitoring of the patient's progress postoperatively [2,13,14]. There are, however, other factors whose effects are only partly amenable to the surgeon's expertise and which are to some extent interrelated: (1) the presence of pancreatic juice and the enzymes it contains; (2) the type of operation; and (3) the degree of fibrosis of the pancreas. It is well known that when surgery is performed on a fibrotic pancreas, which therefore possesses a reduced degree of exocrine secretion, dehiscence of the anastomosis is less frequent [11,15,16]. This finding is also confirmed in our series where the multivariate analysis showed that the risk of complications was three-fold higher when the surgeon had to perform an operation for a malignancy and thus when the pancreas, outside the area affected, was of soft consistency with intact exocrine capacity. The degree of fibrosis of the pancreas, however, is not something that the surgeon can choose, just as, within certain limits, he has no choice as to the type of intervention.

It is well known, in fact, that pancreatic fistulas are less frequent after left pancreatectomy, this being an operation which preserves the natural outflow of pancreatic juice to the duodenum, as opposed to pancreaticoduodenectomy where the pancreatic juice will come into contact with any anastomosis constructed [17–21]. Once again the results of the multivariate analysis conducted in our center confirm the truth of this observation, and indeed the risk of developing a pancreatic fistula after left pancreatectomy is comparable to that after a pancreaticojejunostomy. This risk, however, is 4 times greater when the operation performed is a pancreaticoduodenectomy.

To reduce the risk, a number of surgeons have suggested the possibility of performing a total pancreatectomy, in the presence of a "soft" pancreas, rather than a procedure involving an anastomosis with a high risk of dehiscence [19]. This solution, if not strictly related to the nature of the disease, appears highly incapacitating and disproportionate, particularly in terms of the development of diabetes, for which it is very hard to compensate.

Perhaps the decisive factor, however, in the genesis of most complications after pancreatic surgery is the presence of pancreatic juice with its proteolytic enzymes [21]. Surgical trauma may, in fact, activate proteolytic enzymes within the pancreas that, via a cascade mechanism, bring about the digestion of cellular membranes, edema, and necrosis. The proportions of these events correspond to the different types and degrees of complications, which may go right across the board in clinical terms from partial anastomotic dehiscence, with corresponding conditions ranging from pancreatic fistula development to the formation of peripancreatic collections, to the more dramatic situations of pancreatitis of the pancreatic remnant [Al Sharaf, Ihse, Dawskiba et al. (to be published); 21–23].

The surgeon's experience undoubtedly plays an important role in the prevention of these events, but only within certain limits, because in all the case series, these complications are reported with incidences ranging from 20% to 40% [3,6–10]. In an attempt to counteract the risks associated with the presence and activation of pancreatic juice, two types of approach have been implemented, one related to surgical technique and the other pharmacological.

A variety of technical modifications of the original Whipple resection have been adopted for managing the pancreatic duct. In addition to total pancreatectomy [19], other techniques proposed have been pancreaticogastrostomy, dunk anastomosis, muco-mucosal anastomosis with the temporary insertion of a transanastomotic stent, and procedures involving the occlusion of Wirsung's duct by means of ligation, neoprene, and fibrin sealant [17–20,24–26]. None of these, however, has shown indisputable superiority over the others, as their efficacy depends largely on the experience of the surgeons performing them.

The pharmacological approach, based on temporary inhibition of pancreatic exocrine secretion, would appear to offer more objective and widely applicable advantages. Klempa et al. [27,28] were the first to report that the intravenous use of naturally occurring somatostatin at a dose of 250 µg/h for 6 days in the postoperative period reduces the complication rate after pancreaticoduodenectomy.

Two multicenter trials [11,12], one of which has been reelaborated in the present study, have demonstrated that Octreotide administered at subcutaneous doses of 100 µg three times daily from 1 h before surgery until postoperative day 7 is capable of significantly reducing the number of complications after pancreatic surgery. The multivariate analysis reported here shows that the use of the drug is the only independent factor capable of inducing a 50% reduction in the risk of non-fistula complications in general and in the risk of pancreatic fistula formation.

Even with this type of approach, the number of complications remains high, ranging from 16% [11] to 32% [12]. From this standpoint, it may seem advisable to administer a combination of an exocrine secretion inhibitor such as naturally occurring somatostatin or Octreotide and a protease inhibitor such as gabexate mesilate, which has already yielded promising results in the prophylaxis of complications after endoscopic retrograde cholangiopanereatography (ERCP) [29]. The reduction of secretion in conjunction with proteolytic enzyme inhibition might, in fact, substantially decrease the incidence of complications, particularly for operations such as pancreaticoduodenectomy, which still constitutes the finest and most difficult operation in the field of pancreatic surgery.

Further studies, however, are needed to test the soundness of this hypothesis.

Acknowledgments. The Italian multicenter prospective study reported here was supported by a grant from Sandoz Prodotti Farmaceutici S.p.A., Milan, Italy. The physicians and centers participating in the study are M. Battistoni (Borgo Trento Hospital, Verona); S. Pedrazzoli, C. Pasquali (University of Padua); R. Dionigi, G. Carcano (Varese Hospital); V. Di Carlo, A. Zerbi (University of Milan); G.P. Marzoli, F. Martin (Bolzano Hospital); U. Valente, V. Casolino (University of Genoa); G. Uomo, D. Molino (Cardarelli Hospital, Naples); P. Mascagni (S. Filippo Neri Hospital, Rome); C. Prior (University of Genoa); G. Flati (La Sapienza University, Rome); F. Mazzeo, L. Gaeta (Policlinico II, Naples); M. Rubino (University of Bari); P. Bazzan, I. Demma (University of Palermo); G. Rodolico, S. Puleo (University of Catania); S. Becelli, M. Coletti (La Sapienza University, Rome); F. Orcalli (Villafranca Hospital, Verona); A. Bano, M. Ferrari (Hospital of Thiene, Vicenza); G. Ludovisi (Le Scotte Hospital, Siena); G. Di Matteo (La Sapienza University, Rome); and M. Di Gregorio (Sandoz Prodotti Farmaceutici SpA, Milan).

References

1. Mizuma K, Lee PC, Howard JM (1977) The disintegration of surgical suture to pancreatic juice. Ann Surg 186:718
2. Crist DW, Sitzman JV, Cameron JL (1987) Improved hospital morbidity, mortality and survival after the Whipple procedure. Ann Surg 206:358–365
3. Grace PA, Pitt HA, Tompkins RK (1987) Decreased morbidity and mortality after pancreaticoduodenectomy. Am J Surg 151:141–149
4. Pelligrini C, Heck CH, Raper S, Way LW (1989) An analysis of the reduced morbidity and mortality rates after pancreaticoduodenectomy. Arch Surg 124:778–781
5. Trede M, Schwall G, Saeger H (1990) Survival after pancreaticoduodenectomy. Ann Surg 211:447–458
6. Peters JH, Carey LC (1991) Historical review of pancreaticoduodenectomy. Am J Surg 161:219–225
7. Neoptolemos JP, Talbot IC, Carr-Locke DL, et al (1987) Treatment and outcome in 52 consecutive cases of ampullary carcinoma. Br J Surg 74:957–961
8. Robertson JFR, Imrie CW, Hole DJ, Carter DC, Blumgart LH (1987) Management of periampullary carcinoma. Br J Surg 74:816–819
9. Moossa AR (1987) Surgical treatment of chronic pancreatitis: an overview. Br J Surg 74:661–667
10. Rossi RL, Rothschild J, Braasch JW, et al. (1987) Pancreatoduodenectomy in the management of chronic pancreatitis. Arch Surg 122:416–420

11. Buechler M, Firees H, Klempa I, et al. (1992) Role of Octreotide in the prevention of postoperative complications following pancreatic resection. Am J Surg 163:125–131
12. Pederzoli P, Bassi C, Falconi M, et al. (1993) Efficacy of Octreotide in preventing complications related to elective pancreatic surgery. Br J Surg 81:265–269
12a. Alsmaraf K, Ihse I, Dawiskiba S, Andrew-Sandberg A (1997) Characteristics of the gland remnant predict complications after subtotal pancreatectomy. Dig Surg 14:101–106
13. Andrén-Sandberg A, Ihse I (1983) Factors influencing survival after total pancreatectomy in patients with pancreatic cancer. Ann Surg 198:605–610
14. Bramhall SR, Allura WH, Jones AG, et al. (1995) Treatment and survival in 13 540 patients with pancreatic cancer, and incidence of disease in the West Midlands: an epidemiological study. Br J Surg 82:101–105
15. Aston JS, Longmire WP (1973) Pancreaticoduodenal resection. Arch Surg 106:813–817
16. Lerut JP, Giannello PR, Otte JB, et al. (1984) Pancreaticoduodenal resection. Ann Surg 199(suppl 4):432–437
17. Papachristou DN, D'Agostino H, Fortner JC (1980) Ligation of the pancreatic duct in pancreatectomy. Br J Surg 67:260–262
18. Edis AJ, Kiernan PD, Taylor WF (1980) Attempted curative resection of ductal carcinoma of the pancreas: review of Mayo Clinic experience, 1951–1975. Mayo Clin Proc 55:531–536
19. Longmire WP (1984) Cancer of the pancreas: palliative operation. Whipple procedure or total pancreatectomy. World J Surg 8:872–879
20. Warshaw AL, Swanson RS (1988) What's new in general surgery. Pancreatic cancer in 1988. Possibilities and probabilities. Ann Surg 208:541–553
21. Pederzoli P, Falconi M, Bassi C, Briani G, Camboni MG (1996) Octreotide in preventing complications from pancreatic surgery. Octreotide: from basic science to clinical medicine. Prog Basic Clin Pharmacol 10:192–200
22. Miedema BW, Sarr MG, Van Heerden JA, et al. (1992) Complications following pancreaticoduodenectomy. Current management. Arch Surg 127:945–950
23. Trede M, Schwall G (1988) The complications of pancreatectomy. Ann Surg 207:39–47
24. Morris DM, Ford RS (1993) Pancreaticogastrostomy: preferred reconstruction for Whipple resection. J Surg Res 54:122–125
25. Mason GR, Freerak RJ (1995) Current experience with pancreaticogastrostomy. Am J Surg 169:217–219
26. Marczell AP, Stiere M (1992) Partial pancreaticoduodenectomy (Whipple procedure) for pancreatic malignancy: occlusion of nonanastomosed pancreatic stump with fibrin sealant. Hepato Pancr Biliary Surg 5:254–260
27. Klempa J, Schwedes U, Usadel KH (1979) Verhütung von postoperativen pankreatitischen Komplikationen nach Duodenopankreatektomie durch Somatostatin. Chirurg 50:427–432
28. Klempa J, Schwedes U, Encke A, Usadel KH (1989) Somatostatin therapy in pancreatic surgery. In: Raptis S, Rosenthal J, Gerich JE (eds) Proceedings of the 2nd International Symposium on somatostatin, Tübingen, 1989
29. Cavallini G, Tittobello A, Frulloni L, et al. (1996) Gabexate mesilate for prevention of pancreatic damage related to endoscopic retrograde cholangiopancreatography. New Engl J Med 335;13:919–923

10. Beckham CB, Flora J, Kienzle J, et al. (1997) Role of Octreotide in the prevention of postoperative complications following pancreatic resection. Am J Surg 16:125–131.

11. Pederzoli P, Bassi C, Falconi M, et al. (1994) Efficacy of Octreotide in prevention of complications related to elective pancreatic surgery. Br J Surg 81:265–269.

12. Lowy AM, Lee J, Pisters PW, Andrews S, Rodriguez S, et al. (1997) Intraoperative and early treatment pyloric complications after pancreaticoduodenectomy. Dig Surg 14:310–.

13. Andren-Sandberg A, Ihse I (1983) Factors influencing survival after total pancreatectomy in patients with pancreatic cancer. Ann Surg 198:605–610.

14. Trimble IR, Adham N, Jones CA, et al. (1941) Early treatment and survival in 151–30 patients with pancreatic carcinoma: the dose of cancers in the ... Oklahoma study. Br J Surg 42:161–166.

15. Bottger TC, Junginger T (1999) Factors influencing morbidity and mortality after...

16. Martin TR, Callery PG, Lillemoe KD (1995) Pancreatoduodenectomy. Preoperative ... Surg 222:638–.

17. Crist DW, Sitzmann JV, Cameron JL (1987) Improved hospital morbidity, mortality, and survival after the Whipple procedure. Ann Surg 206:358–365.

18. Kairaluoma MI, Kiviniemi H, Stahlberg M (1989) Pancreatic resection for carcinoma of the pancreas and the periampullary region in patients over 70 years of age. Br J Surg 74:116–.

Pattern of Recurrence After Pancreaticoduodenectomy for Exocrine Pancreatic Cancer: Correlation with Survival

Åke Andrén-Sandberg and Ingemar Ihse

Summary. The results of radical surgery for pancreatic cancer depend, like all other cancer surgery, on the technique used and the biology of the disease. We have analyzed the site and time of recurrence after pancreaticoduodenectomy for exocrine pancreatic cancer in 99 patients who died more than 6 months postoperatively. All patients had recurrent disease; 87 had local recurrence in the pancreatic bed and 93 had liver metasases. Local recurrence without liver metastases was found in 6 patients, and 12 had liver metastases but no local recurrence. Both the time from operation to clinically evident recurrence and the postoperative survival time were significantly longer for patients with local recurrence only. None of those with small tumors (≤2 cm) had liver metastases only and none of them was in stage I. Although not statistically significant, there was a tendency (4 in 5) for smaller, well-differentiated tumors without spread outside the pancreas to be associated with local recurrence without liver metastases. We conclude that, in retrospect, the surgical procedures used were inappropriate and inadequate. To cure these patients, a more radical operation or effective adjuvant treatment is needed.

Key words. Pancreaticoduodenectomy—Pancreatic cancer—Radical—Recurrence—Surgery

Introduction

Removal of the tumor is the only chance for cure in exocrine pancreatic cancer. The type of resection to be used in an attempted radical surgery has been discussed ever since the reports of pancreaticoduodenectomy by Whipple et al. [1] and total pancreatectomy by Rockey [2]. For more than 20 years, total pancreatectomy was the routine method in our hospital for resective surgery in patients with exocrine pancreatic cancer. However, since 1985 we have been using a modified technique for resection, subtotal pancreatectomy, leaving about 5 cm of the pancreatic tail and the spleen. Whatever type of operation used, cure continues to be rare. These unfavorable results may be the result of inappropriate patient selection criteria or preoperative

Department of Surgery, Lund University Hospital, S-221 85 Lund, Sweden.

workup, or may reflect the fact that too many surgeons—each one with too little experience in pancreatic surgery—carried out the operations. On the other hand, it may also be that the surgical technique so far does not meet the demands for local and distant control of the cancer. We earlier reported on an analysis of the site and time of recurrence after pancreatic resection for exocrine pancreatic cancer [3] and have now exended this study.

Patients and Methods

The study comprises 97 patients with adenocarcinoma of the pancreatic head undergoing total pancreatectomy between 1959 and 1985 and 53 patients operated on with subtotal pancreatectomy between 1985 and 1995 at Lund University Hospital. During the 37-year period, a total of 1164 patients with carcinoma of the exocrine pancreas were treated at the hospital, and the resectability rate was 13% (150/1164). Except for 3 patients who had a Whipple operation (i.e., resection of the pancreatic head and duodenum followed by a pancreaticojejunostomy), no other type of surgical procedure was done as an attemped cure of pancreatic cancer during the study period. In addition, 31 patients had a total pancreatectomy and 48 patients a subtotal pancreatectomy for cancer of the papilla of Vater, intrapancreatic bile duct, the juxtapapillary part of the duodenum, or endocrine pancreas during the same period. These patients are not included in the present study.

Between 1959 and 1985 the resective procedure was done as previously described [4] with en bloc removal of the pancreas, the greater omentum, duodenum, common

TABLE 1. Clinical data in patients with either local recurrence or liver metastases following pancreatectomy for exocrine pancreatic cancer

Factor	Evaluable patients	Liver metastases ($n = 12$)	Local recurrence ($n = 6$)
Age, >65 years	48	5	2
Women	40	3	3
Jaundice as first symptom	76	6	6
Preoperative diabetes, >3 months	19	2	1
Preoperative weight loss, >8 kg	68	5	3
Preoperative bile drainage procedure	61	5	4
Year of operation:			
1959–1985	49	7	1
1986–1995	50	5	5
Stage of tumor:			
I	21	0	2
II	20	3	2
III	55	9	2
Tumor size according to the pathologist:			
≤2 cm	25	0	2
<2 cm	74	12	4
Grade of differentiation:			
High	18	0	2
Moderate	42	4	4
Low	39	8	0
Radical resection according to the surgeon	45	6	2

TABLE 2. Pattern of recurrence in 99 patients operated on for exocrine pancreatic cancer by total or subtotal pancreatecomy

Factor	Total pancreatectomy	Subtotal pancreatectomy	All patients
Number of evaluable patients	54	45	99
Number of patients with liver metastases and local recurrence	42	39	81
Number of patients with liver metastases only	8	4	12
Number of patients with local recurrence only	4	2	6

bile duct, gallbladder, spleen, and at least 50% of the stomach. Because a total of 29 surgeons were involved in the 97 operations there was considerable variation in surgical technique. During the period 1985–1995 the operative technique was more standardized, all but one of the operations being done by 3 surgeons. During this later period a technique similar to the one described was used, except that the spleen and distal 5 cm of the pancreas were preserved [5,6], and since 1992 pancreaticogastrostomy has been chosen in most cases. The cancer disease was staged in accordance with a slightly modified Hermreck classification [7]: stage I means that the tumor is localized within the pancreatic "capsule"; stage II, that the tumor has invaded the duodenum; stage III, that there is invasion of any of the superior mesenteric vessels, the portal vein, or regional lymph nodes; and stage IV, that there is distant spread (e.g., liver metastases). The first 88 patients, operated on during the period 1959–1985, have already been decribed in detail elsewhere [4]. Seventeen different variables (11 of which are listed in Table 1) were evaluated for each patient in the current study.

The records of 4 of the earliest patients were incomplete, but adequate data were available for 146 patients. Of these patients, 31 died after the operation without leaving the hospital ("in-hospital mortality"). Of the remaining patients, 4 were cured (i.e., long-term survival with no signs of recurrence at least 7 years postoperatively), and 3 are still alive and are not discussed further here (Table 2). Thus, 108 patients remained to be analyzed. The presence or absence of local recurrence or liver metastases was verified by laparotomy or autopsy in 81 of these patients and demonstrated by computerized tomography (CT), ultrasonography, or arteriography in another 18. In the records of the remaining 9 patients, it was not clear whether there was a local recurrence. Thus, the data given here are based on the findings in 99 patients. The statistical analyses utilized the generalized Wilcoxon's test when comparing factors affecting long-term survival.

Results

Of the 99 patients, 87 patients developed local recurrence of the cancer in the pancreatic bed. Ninety-three patients had liver metastases, 6 patients had local recurrence without liver metastases, and 12 patients had liver metastases with no signs of local recurrence; 81 patients thus had both local recurrence and liver metastases. There was no statistically significant difference between the number of patients with or without local recurrence after total, as compared with subtotal, pancreatectomy (Table 2). The

TABLE 3. Time from operation to clinical recurrence and from operation to death in 99 patients who underwent pancreatectomy (total or subtotal) for pancreatic cancer

Recurrence	Number of patients	Time to clinical recurrence (months)		Postoperative survival (months)	
		Mean	Median	Mean	Median
Liver metastases only	12	8	4	13	7
Local recurrence and liver metastases	81	10	6	20	9
Local recurrence only	6	30*	15*	44*	23*

* $P < .001$ compared with patients in each of the other two groups.

median time from operation to clinical recurrence and postoperative survival time, respectively, were significantly longer in patients with local recurrence only ($P < .001$) as compared both to patients with liver metastases only and to those with recurrence at both sites (Table 3). There were no statistically significant differences in potentially prognostic factors in the 6 patients with local recurrences only as compared to the 12 with liver metastases only. None of the patients with small tumors (≤ 2 cm) died of liver metastases only and none of them was in stage I. Although not statistically significant, there was a tendency (4 of 5) for smaller, well-differentiated tumors without spread outside the pancreas to be associated with local recurrence without liver metastases (Table 1).

Discussion

A review of the world literature involving a total of approximately 37000 patients revealed 4100 pancreatic resections for pancreatic cancer but only 156 survivors [8]. The authors seldom gave information on the site of recurrence of the disease. However, in a series of regional pancreatectomy published in 1977, Fortner et al. [9] concluded that "most patients developing recurrence did so due to an inadequate margin of resection." According to Herter and co-workers [10] the inherent biological nature of ductal carcinoma of the pancreas is (negatively) distinct from that of other epithelial tumors arising in the same region (periampullary and islet cell tumors). They stated that this dictates the ultimate fate of most of the patients, regardless of the type of surgical resection done, and that the operative procedure is of importance in a few patients only. Thus, it may be considered whether survival after resection for ductal pancreatic cancer—being so rare—may be a biological aberration rather than a result of radical surgery. Surgery with a curative intent for exocrine pancreatic cancer can be done by either regional, total, or subtotal pancreatectomy. The operative mortality rate for these procedures was in the past substantial [4,8,11], but today it ranges between 0% and 4% [5,6,12-17]. Despite earlier hopes that total pancreatectomy by avoidance of the pancreaticojejunal anastomosis, wider lymphadenectomy, and eradication of multicentric disease would be a superior operation to the Whipple procedure, it has thus far failed to satisfy the expectations. There is no evidence from the experience with total pancreatectomy today that complete resection of the pancreas leads to longer survival than subtotal resection [8,18,19].

Our current results are in accordance with those of Griffin et al. [20] concerning resection of primary pancreatic carcinoma. They found that almost one-fifth of their patients had recurrent disease in the local tumor bed only and that 73% had a component of local failure present at death. Tepper et al. [21] also pointed out that local recurrence is a significant problem after curative resection. However, their lower rate of local and intraabdominal failures as compared to our findings may reflect the meticulous documentation of recurrence we have practiced. If anything, our results favor a subtotal procedure over a total pancreatectomy, because the long-term results are about the same [19] and the metabolic sequelae following subtotal resection are less problematic. Our findings are comparable to the cumulative experience after pancreaticoduodenectomy in the English literature as reported by Connolly et al. [22]. They found 27 5-year survivors among 455 patients altogether (69). However, improved 5-year survival has lately been reported following partial pancreatectomy with or without extended lymph node dissection [23–27]. In institutions in which both total and subtotal pancreatectomies have been practiced no difference in survival between the two operations has been found (12,28,29]. However, taken together it appears that both subtotal and total pancreatectomy are inadequate operations for cure in most cases, even when combined with an extensive lymphadenectomy.

Logically, a still more radical operation ought to be preferable. Regional resection [30] refers to the en bloc removal of the pancreas (and the cancer), together with the pancreatic segment of the portal vein and sometimes the superior mesenteric artery [31,32]. However, published results [33] do not appear to favor these major operations. Of 51 patients with exocrine pancreatic cancer operated on by means of regional pancreatectomy over a period of 14 years, the results of 40 have been presented: only 9 (23%) survived to the end of follow-up; 23 (58%) died of recurrent cancer and 8 (20%) of other causes [33]. The median survival time for those who lived was 13 months (range, 1–52 months), which is in accord with most other series of attempted radical operations [8]. Thus, at present it would seem that extending the operation does not improve the results, unless it is combined with additional treatment such as intraoperative chemotherapy [34] or radiation [35].

The significance of multicentricity in the case of pancreatic cancer is difficult to assess, but according to Klöppel et al. [36] it seems to occur less frequently than previously reported. Moreover, Motojima et al. [37], using a polymerase chain reaction (PCR) technique, found different mutations in the K-ras gene in only 3 of 53 patients with pancreatic cancer, giving strong evidence for the existence of multicentric disease but at a much lower rate than previously reported. It seems as if the term "multicentric" has been used too uncritically in earlier studies by also including tumor extension and free-floating cells in the pancreatic duct. However, of some interest also are the findings by Forrest and Longmire [38], who biopsied the transected, preserved remnant after Whipple resections. The 31 patients who were histologically "clear" had an average survival time of 20 months, while the 8 patients in whom cancer cells were found in the remnant survived on average only 13 months.

Despite these current results, we believe that resective pancreatic surgery must be done also in the future, provided the patients can be properly selected. This opinion is based on the low hospital mortality associated with resection in recent years, the possible prolongation of life among surgical survivors, and a small, but growing, number of long-term survivors. Further support for this strategy comes from the fact that many of the small carcinomas in the pancreatic head cannot be distinguished grossly from periampullary cancers, which have a more favorable prognosis. Finally, one cannot in all conscience deny a patient the only currently existing chance of a cure, provided that the risks and possibilities are fully understood by the patient.

In summary, the present study shows a very high rate of local recurrence after total and subtotal pancreatectomy for pancreatic cancer. Therefore, better surgical techniques, improved selection of patients, and effective adjuvant treatment options are mandatory. However, it is obvious that any treatment aiming at a cure must include surgical removal of the tumor as its primary modality.

References

1. Whipple AO, Parson WP, Mullins CR (1935) Treatment of carcinoma of the ampulla of Vater. Ann Surg 102:763–779
2. Rockey EW (1943) Total pancreatectomy for carcinoma. Ann Surg 118:603–608
3. Westerdahl J, Andrén-Sandberg Å, Ihse I (1993) Recurrence of exocrine pancreatic cancer—local or hepatic? Hepato-Gastroenterology 40:384–387
4. Andrén-Sandberg Å, Ihse I (1983) Factors influencing survival after total pancreatectomy in patients with pancreatic cancer. Ann Surg 198:605–610
5. Gall FP, Hermanek P, Gebhardt C, Meier H (1981) Erweitere Resektion der Pankreas- und periampullären Karzinome: Regionale, totale und partiell Duodenopankreatektomie. Leber Magen Darm 11:179–184
6. Ihse I, Andrén-Sandberg Å, Permerth J, Larsson L (1993) Early results of subtotal pancreatectomy for cancer—an interim report. In: Beger H, Büchler M, Malfertheiner P (eds) Standards in pancreatic surgery. Springer, Berlin Heidelberg New York, pp 641–645
7. Hermreck AS, Thomas CY, Friesen SR (1974) Importance of pathological staging in the surgical management of adenocarcinoma of the exocrine pancreas. Am J Surg 127:653–657
8. Gudjonsson B (1995) Carcinoma of the pancreas: critical analysis of costs, results of resections, and the need for standardized reporting. J Am Coll Surg 181:483–503
9. Fortner JG, Kim DK, Cubilla A, Turnbull A, Pahnke LD, Shils ME (1977) Regional pancreatectomy: en bloc pancreatic, portal vein and lymph node resection. Ann Surg 186:42–50
10. Herter FP, Cooperman AM, Ahlborn TN, Antinori C (1982) Surgical experience with pancreatic and periampullary cancer. Ann Surg 195:274–281
11. Van Heerden JA (1984) Pancreatic resection for carcinoma of the pancreas: Whipple versus total pancreatectomy—an institutional perspective. World J Surg 8:880–888
12. Crist DW, Sitzmann JV, Cameron JL (1987) Improved hospital morbidity, mortality, and survival after the Whipple procedure. Ann Surg 206:358–365
13. Cooper MJ, Wiliamson RCN, Benjamin IS, Carter DC, Cuschieri A, Linehan IP, Russel RC, Torrace MB (1987) Total pancreatectomy for chronic pancreatitis. Br J Surg 74:912–915
14. Lygidakis NJ, Van der Hyde MN, Houthoff HJ, Schipper ME, Huibregtse K, Tytgat GN, Lubber MJ, Reeders JW, Bosey MM, Oosting J (1989) Resectional surgical procedures for carcinoma of the head of the pancreas. Surg Gynecol Obstet 168:157–165
15. Pellingrini CA, Heck CF, Raper S, Raw LW (1989) An analysis of the reduced morbidity and mortality rates after pancreaticoduodenetomy. Arch Surg 124:778–781
16. Brooks JR, Brooks DC, Levine JD (1989) Total pancreatectomy for ductal cell carcinoma of the pancreas—an update. Ann Surg 209:405–410
17. Trede M, Schwall G, Saeger HD (1980) Survival after pancreatoduodenectomy. 188 consecutive resections without operative mortality. Ann Surg 211:447–458
18. Trede M (1993) The surgical options. In: Trede M, Carter DC (eds) Surgery of the pancreas. Churchill Livingstone, Edinburgh, pp 433–442
19. Ihse I, Andrén-Sandberg Å, Andersson R, Axelson J, Kobari M (1994) The role of total pancreatectomy in pancreatic cancer. J Hepato Biliant Pancr Surg 1:546–551

20. Griffin JF, Smalley SR, Jewell W, Paradelo JG, Reymond RD, Hassanein RE, Evans RG (1990) Patterns of failure after curative resection of pancreatectomy carcinoma. Cancer (Phila) 66:56–61
21. Tepper J, Nardi G, Sutt H (1976) Carcinoma of the pancreas: review of MGH experience from 1963 to 1973. Analysis of surgical failure and implications for radiation therapy. Cancer (Phila) 37:1519–1524
22. Conolly MM, Dawson PJ, Michelassi F, Moossa AR, Lowenstein F (1987) Survival in 1001 patients with carcinoma of the pancreas. Ann Surg 206:366–373
23. Tsuchiya R, Noda T, Harada N, Miyamoto R, Tomioka T, Yamamoto K, Yamaguchi T, Izawa K, Tsunoda T, Yoshino R, Eto T (1986) Collective review of small carcinomas of the pancreas. Ann Surg 203:77–81
24. Ishikawa O, Ohigoshi H, Sasaki Y, Kabuto T, Fukuda J, Furukawa H, Imaoka S, Iwanaga T (1988) Practical usefulness of lymphatic and connective tissue clearance. Ann Surg 208:215–220
25. Cameron JL, Crist DW, Sitzman JV, Hruban RH, Boitnott JK, Seidler AJ, Coleman JA (1991) Factors influencing survival after pancreaticoduodenectomy for pancreatic cancer. Am J Surg 161:120–125
26. Gall FP, Kessler H, Hermanek P (1991) Surgical treatment of ductal pancreatic carcinoma. Eur J Surg Oncol 17:178–181
27. Geer RJ, Brennan MF (1993) Prognostic indicators of survival after resection of pancreatic adenocarcinoma. Am J Surg 165:68–73
28. Grace A, Pitt HA, Tompkins RK, Den Besten L, Longmire WP (1986) Decreased morbidity and mortality after pancreatoduodenectomy. Am J Surg 151:141–149
29. Edis AJ, Kiernan PD, Taylor WF (1980) Attempted curative resection of ductal carcinoma of the pancreas. Review of Mayo Clinic experience, 1951–1975. Mayo Cinic Proc 55:531–536
30. Fortner JG (1973) Regional resection of cancer of the pancreas: a new surgical approach. Surgery (St Louis) 73:307–320.
31. Dardik H, Dardik II, Spreyregen S, Becker N, Gliedman ML (1975) Total pancreatectomy with primary mesenteric vascular reconstruction. Am J Surg 129:691–693
32. Norton L, Eiseman B (1975) Replacement of portal vein during pancreatectomy for carcinoma. Surgery (St Louis) 77:180–184
33. Fortner JG (1986) Results of treating cancer of the pancreas and peripancreatic sites by regional pancreatectomy. Front Gastrointest Res 12:273–277
34. Wils JA (1991) Chemotherapy in pancreatic cancer: a rational pursuit? Anticancer Drugs 2:273–277
35. Dobelbower RR, Konski AA, Merrich HW, Bronn DG, Schifeling D, Kmer C (1991) Intraoperative electron beam radiation therapy (IOEBRT) for carcinoma of the exocrine pancreas. Int J Radiat Oncol Biol Phys 20:113–119
36. Klöppel G, Lohse T, Bosslet K, Rückert K (1987) Ductal adenocarcinoma of the head of the pancreas: incidence of tumor involvement beyond the Whipple resection line. Histology and immunocytochemical analyses of 37 total pancreatectomy specimens. Pancreas 2:170–175
37. Motojima K, Urano R, Nagata Y, Hiroshi S, Tsurifune T, Kanematsu T (1993) Detection of point mutations in the Kirsten-ras oncogene provides evidence for the multicentricity of pancreatic carcinoma. Ann Surg 217:138–143
38. Forrest JF, Longmire WP (1979) Carcinoma of the pancreas and periampullary region: a study of 279 patients. Ann Surg 189:129–138

Results of Pancreaticoduodenectomy for Periampullary Carcinoma and Analysis of Prognostic Factors for Survival

MIIN-FU CHEN, CHIA-SIU WANG, YI-YIN JAN, LONG-BIN JENG, TSANN-LONG HWANG, SHIN-CHEH CHEN, TZU-CHIEH CHAO, HAN-MING CHEN, CHIH-CHI WANG, WEI-CHEN LEE, TA-SEN YEH, and YUNG-FENG LO

Summary. A retrospective review of 131 pancreaticoduodenectomies was performed and the prognostic factors were analyzed. In the 11-year period between 1981 and 1991, 297 patients with periampullary tumor were referred to our surgical department; 131 pancreaticoduodenectomies were performed, including 79 for ampullary carcinoma, 22 for pancreatic head tumor, 18 for distal common bile duct carcinoma, and 12 for duodenal tumor. Patients who underwent pancreaticoduodenectomy included 78 women and 53 men with a mean age of 55.8 years (range, 21–82 years). The overall mortality of the 131 pancreaticoduodenectomy patients was 7.63%; it was 4.76% in the past 5 years. The complication rate was as high as 38.9%. Anastomotic leakage (15.3%) was the leading cause of hospital mortality. Analysis of several factors indicated that advanced age, abdominal pain, duration of symptoms, levels of serum bilirubin, albumin, and serum alkaline phosphatase, and operative blood loss did not influence the survival rate. However, female patients and patients with no lymph node metastasis and well-differentiated tumor had a better survival rate. Excluding papillary cystoadenocarcinoma of the pancreatic head, leiomyosarcoma of the duodenum, and benign disease, the actual 5-year survival rates of patients with ampullary, pancreatic head, distal common bile duct, and duodenal carcinoma were 47.4%, 20%, 30.8%, and 33%, respectively. Pancreaticoduodenectomy is a major operation in hepatogastrointestinal surgery. Although the complication rate is still high, hospital mortality could be controlled to less than 5% in our hospital. Female patients, patients without lymph node metastasis, and patients with well-differentiated carcinoma had a better prognosis.

Key words. Pancreaticoduodenectomy—Ampullary carcinoma—Pancreatic carcinoma—Distal bile duct carcinoma—Duodenal carcinoma

Department of Surgery, Chang Gung Medical College, Chang Gung Memorial Hospital, Taipei, Taiwan.

Introduction

Of all malignancies of the periampullary region, pancreatic carcinoma, distal bile duct carcinoma, ampullary carcinoma, and duodenal carcinoma are the most frequent tumors [1–3]. Pancreaticoduodenectomy (PD) with or without pylorus preservation is the first treatment choice for these malignant tumors, and although the resectability rate is high for patients with ampullary carcinoma (80%), it is still disappointingly low for those with pancreatic carcinoma (20%) [1–7]. The mortality rates of this procedure have decreased drastically from more than 20% to about 5% in specialized centers during the last decade [5–10]. Five-year survival after PD has been low for pancreatic carcinoma (0%–10% in most series) but between 30% and 50% for ampullary carcinoma [1,3–6,11–16].

The aim of this study was to determine the results of PD for patients with periampullary carcinoma by evaluating mortality, hospital morbidity, and survival. Prognostic factors with impact on survival were analyzed in an attempt to identify patients who are good candidates for curative resection.

Patients and Methods

From 1981 until 1991, 131 consecutive patients underwent pancreaticoduodenectomy (PD) for ampullary carcinoma ($n = 79$), pancreatic carcinoma ($n = 22$), distal bile duct carcinoma ($n = 18$), or duodenal carcinoma ($n = 12$). These 131 patients had a mean age of 55.8 years (range, 21–82 years), and the female:male ratio was 1.5:1 (78 women and 53 men). In the same period of time, 297 patients with periampullary tumors underwent surgical treatment. The overall resection rate was 48.2% (Table 1).

Jaundice was the most frequent symptom, occurring in 80% of the patients, and 46% had abdominal or back pain. The median duration of symptoms before surgery was 6 weeks (range, 1–48 weeks), with a median weight loss of 5 kg (range, 0–20 kg).

All patients underwent a standard diagnostic imaging workup that included conventional ultrasonography, computed tomographic scanning, endoscopic retrograde cholangiopancreaticography, percutaneous transhepatic cholangiography, and selective angiography. Endoscopic ultrasonography has been used since 1989. In jaundiced patients, preoperative biliary drainage with insertion of a nasobiliary tube or percutaneous transhepatic tube was attempted in all patients with serum total bilirubin greater than 10 mg%.

Patients with a tumor size of greater than 5 cm on diagnostic imaging, with complete obstruction of the portal vein, or with distant metastases were excluded from

TABLE 1. Resection rate of ampullary carcinoma, pancreatic carcinoma, distal bile duct carcinoma, and duodenal carcinoma, 1981–1991

Tumor type	Total	Resected	Not resected	Resection rate (%)
Ampullary carcinoma	121	87 (79)[a]	34	71.9
Pancreatic head carcinoma	133	23 (22)	110	17.3
Distal common bile duct carcinoma	23	18 (18)	5	78.3
Duodenal carcinoma	20	13 (12)	7	65.0
All types	297	143 (131)	156	48.2

[a] Numbers in parentheses are pancreaticoduodenectomies.

laparotomy with intention to resect and underwent palliative treatment. Standard subtotal PD, including hemigastrectomy, was the first-choice treatment if the tumor was macroscopically resectable. If intraoperative biopsy of the pancreatic resection margin showed tumor or if the pancreatic remnant was too friable for a safe pancreaticojejunostomy, total PD was performed. If limited macroscopic invasion of the portal vein or superior mesenteric vein was encountered, partial resection of the vein was performed, followed by reconstruction.

Histology examination was performed emphasizing the following parameters: determination of the epithelium of origin of the carcinoma, tumor size, lymph node involvement, capsular invasion, differentiation, and involvement of resection margins.

At follow-up, special attention was given to specific late morbidity such as diabetes mellitus and steatorrhea. The median time of follow-up until death was 8 months (range, 0–60 months), and the median survival was 32 months (range, 2–72 months).

For comparison of observed proportions the chi-square test was applied, and for comparison of means the analysis of variance or Mann–Whitney test was used. For univariate analysis of the Kaplan–Meier survival curves, the log rank test and the chi-squared test were used. The multivariate survival analysis utilized Cox's regression model. For all tests, a P value less than .05 was considered to be significant.

Results

The 30-day hospital mortality was 7.63% (10/131); it became 4.76% (3/63) in the past 5 years. Causes of death were intraabdominal sepsis from anastomotic leakage (7 patients), and heart failure, seizure, and postoperative cholangitis in 1 patient each.

Overall surgical morbidity was 38.9% (Table 2). Anastomotic leakage, a major complication, was seen in 21 patients (15.3%). Wound infection was found in 16 patients (12.2%), intraabdominal abscess and pancreatic fistula in 5 patients each (3.82%), hemorrhage in 3 patients (2.29%), and diabetes mellitus in two patients (1.73%).

The 1-, 3-, and 5-year survival rates for the total series were 80%, 52%, and 40%, respectively. The 5-year survival for patients with ampullary carcinoma was 47.4%,

TABLE 2. Morbidity in 131 patients who underwent pancreatico-duodenectomy for periampullar carcinoma

Complication	Number of patients	Percent
Anastomotic leakage	21	15.30
Intraabdominal abscess	5	3.82
Upper gastrointestinal bleeding	2	1.53
Cerebral hemorrhage	1	0.77
Pancreatitis	1	0.77
Wound infection	16	12.20
Pancreatic fistula	5	3.82
Superior mesenteric artery injury	1	0.77
Hemorrhage	3	2.29
Colonic injury	1	0.77
Diabetes mellitus	2	1.73
Total:	51/31	38.9

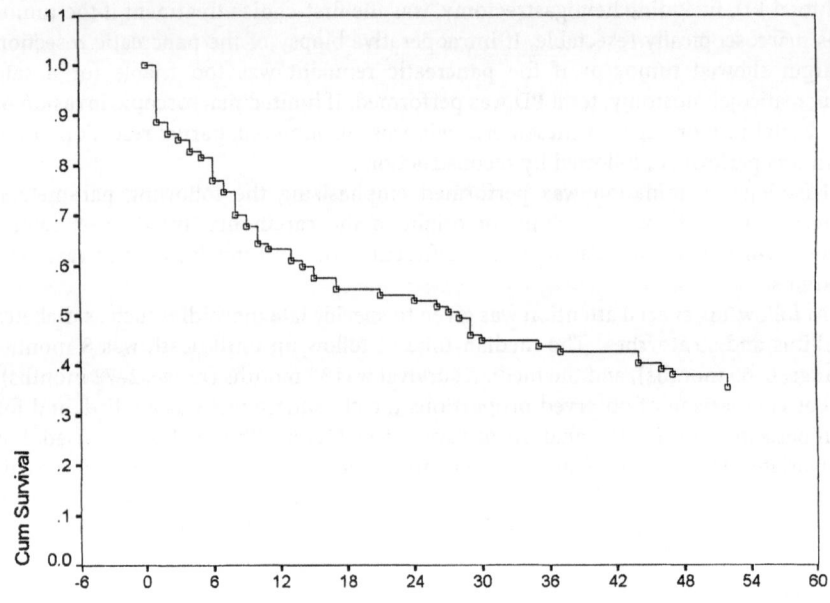

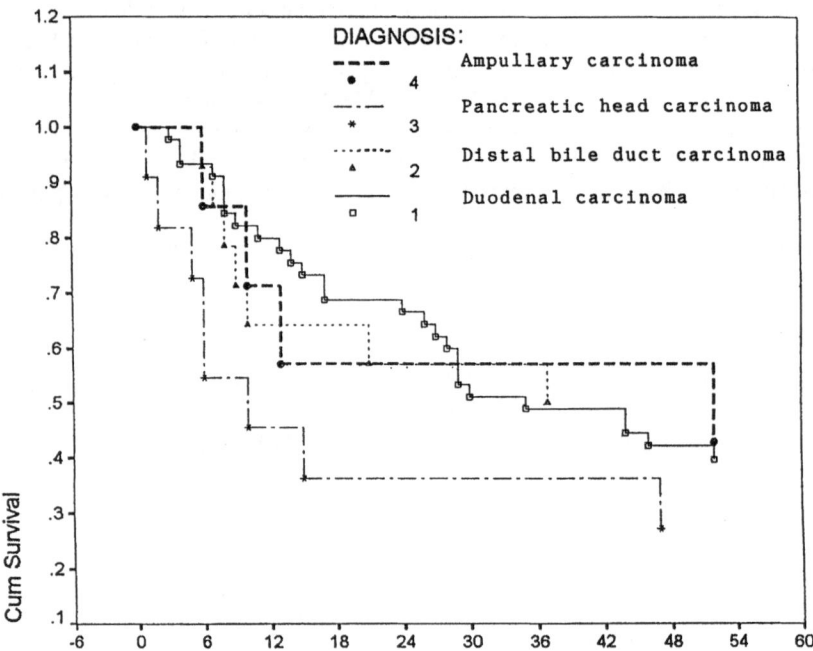

FIG. 1. Cumulative (*cum*) survival (Kaplan–Meier curve) after pancreaticoduodenectomy for all 131 patients with periampullary carcinoma (1981–1991)

FIG. 2. Cumulative survival (Kaplan–Meier curve) after pancreaticoduodenectomy for the subgroups of ampullary carcinoma, distal bile duct carcinoma, pancreatic carcinoma, and duodenal carcinoma

TABLE 3. Prognostic relationship of preoperative and perioperative data to survival rate after pancreaticoduodenectomy for periampulla carcinoma

Factor	Amount	Number	Five-year survival (%)	P Value
Age	≦70 Years	81	33	0.542
	>70 Years	6	38	
Sex	Female	48	48	0.003*
	Male	39	22	
Bilirubin	≦2 g/l	21	22	0.069
	>2 g/l	66	40	
	≦3 g/l	27	29	0.157
	>3 g/l	60	39	
Alkaline phosphatase	≦120 μ/l	13	38	0.170
	>120 μ/l	74	31	
Pain	No	39	25	0.072
	Yes	48	42	
Albumin	≦3.0 g/l	41	40	0.214
	>3.0 g/l	46	26	
Origin of carcinoma	Ampullary	52	47	0.808
	Pancreas	16	20	
	CBD	11	30	
	Duodenum	8	33	
Preoperative biliary drainage	Yes	37	40	0.05
	No	50	32	
Perioperative blood loss	≦1000 ml	34	28	0.663
	>1000 ml	53	38	
Lymph nodes	Involved	32	24	0.035*
	Free	53	49	
Differentiation grade	Moderate or good	63	34	0.027*
	Poor	24	12	
Complication	No	50	40	0.462
	Yes	27	34	
Macroscopic vascular invasion	Yes	7	0	0.000*
	No	80	44	
Resection margin	Involved	25	4	0.002*
	Free	52	44	

*, Statistically significant.

for pancreatic carcinoma, 20.0%, for distal bile duct carcinoma, 30.8%, and for duodenal carcinoma, 33.3%. The Kaplan–Meier curves for survival in the total group and in the four subgroups of patients with carcinoma are shown in Figs. 1 and 2, respectively.

Prognostic Factors for Survival: Univariate Analysis

The overall 5-year survival rate for women was significantly better than for men (48% vs. 22%). Age and preoperative symptoms were not significantly related to survival. Preoperative laboratory results had no statistical effect on survival rate (Table 3).

Preoperative biliary drainage was performed with percutaneous transhepatic biliary drainage (31 patients), with nasobiliary drainage (4 patients), or with T-tube drainage (2 patients); 50 patients did not undergo preoperative drainage. There was no significant difference in survival among these subgroups.

Macroscopic major vessel involvement was correlated with poor survival in the overall series. Total PD was associated with poor survival (compared with subtotal PD) in the total series. Pancreaticoduodenectomy with partial resection of the portal vein or superior mesenteric vein was correlated with poor survival also. Intraoperative blood loss (>1000 ml) was a negative prognostic factor in the total series, but was not significant (Table 3).

Survival after PD for ampullary carcinoma (5-year survival, 47.4%) was better than that for other types of carcinoma, but not significantly. Survival after PD for pancreatic carcinoma (5-year survival, 20%) was poorer than survival in the rest of the series. The strongest negative histological factor for survival was tumor involvement of the resection margins (5-year survival, 4% vs. 44%; P < .002). Involvement of one or more lymph nodes was a negative prognostic factor in the overall series. A poor tumor differentiation grade was associated with a lower survival rate in the overall group (Table 3).

Discussion

Mortality of patients after subtotal or total PD in this study was 7.63% (10/131), but has decreased to 4.76% (3/63) in the past 5 years, which agrees with reports in the literature. In collected series of the past decade, average mortality after PD was 12% for patients with ampullary carcinoma, 11% for those with distal bile duct carcinoma, and 10% for those with pancreatic carcinoma [1–16]. In most specialized treatment centers, mortality now is well below 10% [8,12,13]. Mortality after total PD was higher than after subtotal PD, as has been reported by others. The selection of more advanced tumors for total PD played a causative role in our study, with a larger tumor mass and more chance for involved resection margins. Although there was no problem with anastomotic leakage, intraabdominal sepsis developed more often after total PD than after subtotal PD [1,3–10,12–16].

Despite the decrease of mortality in recent years, PD remains a major surgical procedure with a high complication rate, between 25% and 70% [1–17]. In our series, 38.9% (51/131) of the patients had one or more complications, and some patients required relaparotomy. Intraabdominal sepsis, often caused by anastomotic leakage, was the most important problem. All 7 patients who died of complications had suffered intraabdominal sepsis, and 3 had experienced hemorrhage as well. Late morbidity can be very limited after subtotal PD. Diabetes mellitus is not a frequent problem; in our series, diabetes developed in only 2 of 131 patients after operation. Steatorrhea was often seen during follow-up but responded well to pancreatic enzyme supplementation.

The overall 5-year survival rate in this study was 37.5%. Although survival for patients with ampullary carcinoma was better than survival for the other types of carcinoma, and survival for patients with pancreatic carcinoma was poorer, the difference was not statistically significant. In a recent collected series of PD (1982–1993), we found an average 5-year survival of 11% (range, 0%–27%) for patients with pancreatic carcinoma, 24% (range, 0%–52%) for those with distal bile duct carcinoma, and 38% (range, 16%–61%) for those with ampullary carcinoma [1–16].

Age and preoperative symptoms were not significant negative factors with survival in this series, in concordance with most other reports [17,18]. The preoperative laboratory results did not show any influence on survival [17–20]. The correlation of female patients with better survival has not been reported previously, precluding any conclusion. Perioperative macroscopic involvement of the major vessels predicted poor outcome after resection in univariate and multivariate analyses. Still, most surgeons confronted with vascular involvement decide not to resect. In seven patients in this series, partial resection of a macroscopically involved portal vein or superior mesenteric vein was associated with high mortality and poor survival (no 5-year survivors). These results agree with recent reports in the literature [17,21–23].

As was expected, the strongest histological prognostic factor for survival was involvement of the resection margins. The key histological feature of a carcinoma, lymph node involvement, and differentiation grade all correlated significantly with survival in the univariate analysis [1–14,17–21,24–26]. This study showed no correlation between perioperative blood loss (>1000 ml) and survival. The negative effect of blood transfusions on survival has been reported previously for patients with pancreatic carcinoma and colorectal cancer; immunosuppression may play a causative role [24,27].

Evaluating the results of this study, we concluded that the overall 5-year survival was 37.5% for patients with periampullary carcinoma after subtotal or total PD, with a surgical mortality of 7.63% (4.76% in the past 5 years); survival was better after PD for patients with ampullary carcinoma but this was not statistically significant. Independent negative prognostic factors were gender, lymph node involvement, involvement of resection margins, histological differentiation grading, and macroscopic vascular involvement.

References

1. Peters JH, Carey LC (1991) Histological review of pancreaticoduodenectomy. Am J Surg 161:219–225
2. Warshaw AC, Fernandez-del Castillo C (1992) Pancreatic carcinoma. N Engl J Med 326:455–465
3. Forrest JF, Longmire WP Jr (1979) Carcinoma of the pancreas and periampullary region. Ann Surg 189:129–138
4. Lerut JP, Gianello PR, Otte JB, Kesteus PJ (1984) Pancreaticoduodenal resection: surgical experience and evaluation of risk factors in 103 patients. Ann Surg 199:432–437
5. Michelassi F, Erroi F, Pawson PJ, Pietrabissa A, Noda S, Handkock M (1989) Experience with 647 consecutive tumors of the duodenum, ampulla, head of the pancreas and distal common bile duct. Ann Surg 210:544–556
6. Gudjonsson B (1987) Cancer of the pancreas: 50 years of surgery. Cancer (Phila) 60:2284–2289
7. Hayes OH, Bolton JS, Willis GW, Bocoen JC (1987) Carcinoma of the ampulla of Vater. Ann Surg 206:572–577
8. Crist DW, Sitzmann JV, Cameran JC (1987) Improved hospital mortality, morbidity and survival after the Whipple procedure. Ann Surg 206:358–365
9. Miedema BW, Sarr MG, van Heerden JA, Nagorney DM, McIlrath DC, Ilstrup D (1992) Complications following pancreaticoduodenectomy: current management. Arch Surg 127:945–950
10. Grace PA, Pitt HA, Tompkins RK, DenBesten L, Lengmire WP Jr (1986) Decreased morbidity and mortality after pancreaticoduodenectomy. Am J Surg 151:141–149
11. Funovics JM, Karner J, Pratschner TH, Fristch A (1989) Current trends in the management of carcinoma of the pancreatic head. Hepato-Gastroenterology 36:450–455
12. Cohen JR, Kuchta N, Geller N, Shires T, Dinnen P (1982) Pancreaticoduodenectomy. A 40-year experience. Ann Surg 195:608–617

13. Herter FP, Cooperman AM, Ahlborn TN, Antinori C (1982) Surgical experience with pancreatic and periampullary cancer. Ann Surg 195:274–281
14. Knox RA, Kingston RD (1986) Carcinoma of the ampulla of Vater. Br J Surg 73:72–73
15. Robertston JFR, Imirie CW, Hole DJ, Carter DC, Blumgart LH (1987) Management of periampullary carcinoma. Br J Surg 74:816–819
16. Delcore R Jr, Connor CS, Thomas JH, Friesen SR, Hermreck AS (1989) Significance of tumor spread in adenocarcinoma of the ampulla of Vater. Am J Surg 158:593–597
17. Allema JH, Reinders ME, VanGulik TM, Koelemay MJ, Van Leeuwen DJ (1995) Prognostic factors for survival after pancreaticoduodenectomy for patients with carcinoma of the pancreatic head region. Cancer (Phila) 75:2069–2076
18. Kalser MH, Barkiu J, MacIntyre JM (1985) Pancreatic cancer—assessment of prognosis by clinical presentation. Cancer (Phila) 56:397–402
19. Kairaluoma MI, Kiviniemi H, Stahlberg M (1987) Pancreatic resection for carcinoma of the pancreas and the periampullary region in patients over 70 years of age. Br J Surg 74:116–118
20. Spencer MP, Sarr MG, Nagorvey DM (1990) Radical pancreatectomy for pancreatic cancer in the elderly—is it safe and justified. Ann Surg 212:140–143
21. Fortner JG (1984) Regional pancreatectomy for cancer of the pancreas, ampulla, and other related sites: tumor staging and results. Ann Surg 199:418–425
22. Ishikawa O, Ohigashi H, Imaoka S, Furukawa H, Sasaki Y, Fugita M (1992) Preoperative indication for extended pancreatectomy for locally advanced pancreas cancer involving the portal vein. Ann Surg 215:231–236
23. Tashiro S, Uchino R, Hiraoka T, Tsuji T, Kawamoto S, Saitoh N (1991) Surgical indication and significance of portal vein resection in biliary and pancreatic cancer. Surgery (St Louis) 109:481–487
24. Cameron JL, Crist DW, Sitzmann JV, Hruban RH, Boitnott JK, Seidler AJ (1991) Factors influencing survival after pancreaticoduodenectomy for pancreatic cancer. Am J Surg 161:120–125
25. Marcus SG, Cohen H, Ranson JH (1995) Optimal management of the pancreatic remnant after pancreaticoduodenectomy. Ann Surg 221:635–648
26. Reinders ME, Allema JH, VanGulik TM, Karsten TM (1995) Outcome of microscopically nonradical, subtotal pancreaticoduodenectomy (Whipple's resection) for treatment of pancreatic head tumor. World J Surg 19:410–415
27. Chung M, Steinmetz OK, Gordon PH (1993) Perioperative blood transfusion and outcome after resection for colorectal carcinoma. Br J Surg 80:427–432

Clinical Analysis of 100 Cases of Pancreaticoduodenectomy

JIA ZHENGENG, ZHOU ZHENG, CHEN PING, LI XIAOPING,
and ZHANG YUANCHUN

Summary. We have reviewed retrospectively a 10-year experience (1984–1994) with pancreaticoduodenectomy (PD) in which 100 patients underwent PD for ampullary carcinoma ($n = 39$), distal bile duct carcinoma ($n = 21$), pancreatic carcinoma ($n = 28$), or duodenal carcinoma ($n = 12$). The pylorus-preserving modification of the Whipple procedure (PPPD) was used for 15 patients and the conventional Whipple operation for 85 patients. In this group, 30-day mortality was 5% and hospital mortality was 9%. Negative prognostic factors were involvement of resection margins, lymph node metastasis, poorly differentiated tumor, and tumor size. In this group, 5-year survival for patients with ampullary carcinoma was significantly better (55%) than survival for duodenal carcinoma (40%) or for distal bile duct carcinoma (30%). The survival for patients with pancreatic carcinoma was significantly poorer. The 5-year survival following PPPD is similar to that following PD.

Key words. Pancreaticoduodenectomy—Ampullary carcinoma—Distal bile duct carcinoma—Pancreatic carcinoma—Duodenal carcinoma

Introduction

Pancreaticoduodenectomy (PD) is the first treatment choice for pancreatic carcinoma, distal bile duct carcinoma, ampullary carcinoma, and duodenal carcinoma. We reviewed retrospectively a 10-year experience with pancreaticoduodenectomy at China–Japan Friendship Hospital.

Patients and Methods

From 1984 until 1994, 100 patients underwent PD for ampullary carcinoma ($n = 39$), distal bile duct carcinoma ($n = 21$), pancreatic carcinoma ($n = 28$), or duodenal carcinoma ($n = 12$). The 100 patients had a median age of 55 years; 61 were men and 39 were women.

Department of General Surgery, China–Japan Friendship Hospital, Beijing 100029, China.

Jaundice was the most frequent symptom, occurring in 86% of the patients; abdominal or back pain occurred in 40% and weight loss in 35%. The median duration of symptoms before surgery was 10 weeks (range, 1–45 weeks).

Most patients underwent conventional ultrasound (98%), endoscopic retrograde cholangiopancreaticography (75%), computed tomographic scanning (90%), percutaneus transhepatic cholangiography or drainage (41%), or selective angiography (10%).

Before the operation, computed tomographic scanning-guided percutaneous fine-needle aspiration biopsy was performed on 25 patients; the correct diagnosis was obtained in 20 of 25, a diagnostic accuracy of 80%. In ultrasonography-guided percutaneous fine-needle aspiration biopsy performed on 30 patients, the correct diagnosis was obtained in 21 patients, a diagnosis accuracy of 70%. Biopsies performed with fibroendoscopy gave a positive diagnosis of ampullary and duodenal carcinoma in 30 patients (100%). Intraoperative fine-needle aspiration biopsy, performed on 20 patients, provided the correct diagnosis in 18 (90%). Biopsy performed on 8 patients provided the correct diagnosis in all. Before PD, pathological diagnosis was made in 97 patients. After surgery, histological examination was performed on all specimens.

Margins were considered positive if any of the following had infiltrating adenocarcinoma present at careful microscopic analysis of the resected specimen: pancreatic neck margin, uncinate process margin, retroperitoneal soft tissue margin, duodenal margins, or bile duct margin. Patients with negative margins ($n = 85$) had a median survival of 24 months and a 5-year survival of 29%, while those resected with positive margins ($n = 15$) had a median survival of 8 months and a 5-year survival of 6%. Those resected with positive margins had significantly poorer survival ($P < .05$).

Lymph nodes were considered positive if any resected nodes contained adenocarcinoma. Lymph nodes were considered negative if all resected lymph nodes were histologically free of tumor. Patients resected with negative lymph nodes ($n = 45$) had a median survival of 25 months and a 5-year survival of 35%; those resected with positive lymph nodes ($n = 55$) had a median survival of 18 months and 5-year survival of 20%. Those resected with positive lymph nodes had significantly poorer survival ($P < .05$).

Poor tumor differentiation grade ($n = 40$) was associated with lower survival than well-differentiated ($n = 35$) and moderately differentiated ($n = 25$) tumors.

Median intraoperative blood loss was less than 2000 ml in 95 patients and more than 2000 ml in 5 patients. The operative time median was 5 h (<5 h, $n = 52$; >5 h, $n = 48$).

The pylorus-preserving modification of the Whipple procedure was used for 15 patients and the conventional Whipple operation for 85 patients. Patients were followed for survival analysis; 10 patients were lost to follow-up. Prognostic factors were determined using the chi-square test. A P value less than .05 was considered to be significant.

Results

Preoperative biliary drainage was performed with percutaneous transhepatic choledochography drainage ($n = 25$); 30 patients, of whom 20 were jaundiced (bilirubin, $>100 \mu$mol/l), underwent no preoperative drainage. There was no significant difference in survival in these subgroups.

Pancreatic carcinoma ($n = 28$) median diameter was 3.5 cm (<3.5 cm, $n = 15$; >3.5 cm, $n = 13$); ampullary carcinoma ($n = 39$) median diameter was 1.5 cm (<1.5 cm, $n = 15$; >1.5 cm, $n = 24$); duodenal carcinoma ($n = 12$) median diameter was 3 cm (>3 cm, $n = 8$; <3 cm, $n = 4$); and distal bile duct carcinoma ($n = 21$) median diameter was 2 cm (<2 cm, $n = 9$; >2 cm, $n = 12$). Patients with tumors less than 3 cm in diameter had significantly longer median survival ($P < .05$).

In this group, complications occurred in 42 patients. These included 6 patients with pancreatic anastomotic leaks, 5 patients with biliary anastomotic leaks, 4 patients with intraabdominal hemorrhage, 3 patients with wound infections, and 4 patients with acute renal failure. Delayed gastric emptying, defined as no oral intake by postoperative day 15, occurred in 20 patients (pylorus-preserving, 8/15).

The 30-day operative mortality rate was 6%. Two patients died on postoperative day 3 of intraabdominal hemorrhage, four patients died on postoperative day 12 of acute renal failure, and three patients died more than 30 days after their operations during the same hospitalization for an overall hospital mortality rate of 9%; causes of the additional deaths were multiple organ failure: Hospital mortality was not significantly different in patients with ampullary carcinoma (7%), distal bile duct carcinoma (9%), pancreatic carcinoma (10%), or duodenal carcinoma (9%).

The actuarial 1-, 3-, and 5-year survival rates for all 100 patients were 70%, 50%, and 30%, respectively. The 5-year survival for patients with ampullary carcinoma was 55%, for distal bile duct carcinoma, 30%, for duodenal carcinoma, 40%, and for pancreatic carcinoma, 10%.

Discussion

During the 1960s, some authors [1,2] suggested that PD for pancreatic cancer be abandoned because of high complication and mortality rates and low survival rates. In recent years, the surgical treatment of adenocarcinoma of pancreas via PD has been associated with falling postoperative morbidity and mortality rates and improving long-term survival. In this group, mortality of patients after PD was 9% and mortality was not significantly different among the pancreas (10%), ampullary (7%), bile duct (9%), and duodenal (9%) subgroups of carcinoma. In the past decade, others [3,4] reported the average mortality after PD was 10%–12%. Series were recently reported of more than 100 consecutive PDs without mortality. In our group, 5-year survival for patients with ampullary carcinoma was significantly better (55%) than survival for duodenal carcinoma (40%) and for distal bile duct carcinoma (30%); the survival for patients with pancreatic carcinoma (6%) was significantly poorer. In PD series reported recently [5–7], the average 5-year survival was 11% for patients with pancreatic carcinoma, 24% for those with distal bile duct carcinoma, and 38% for those with ampullary carcinoma.

The negative effect of blood transfusion on survival has been reported for patients with periampullary tumors. In our group, blood transfusion of more than 2000 ml was required for five patients; blood transfusion and operative time were not significant in evaluating prognostic factors for survival.

This group study showed a negative association between involvement of resection margins (15 patients), lymph node metastasis (55 patients), and poorly differentiated tumor (40 patients). The diameter of the tumor was an important predictor of survival. Patients with tumors less than 3 cm in diameter had significantly longer median survival time. Long-term survival of patients with periampullary malignant disease following pylorus-preserving PD (15 patients) is similar to that following PD (85 patients).

In conclusion, the results of this study show that in these 100 patients with periampullary malignant disease, 5-year survival was significantly better after PD for patients with ampullary carcinoma than for other subgroups, and negative prognostic factors were positive margins, lymph node metastasis, and tumor size. Gender, age, and preoperative symptoms were not significant.

References

1. Crile G Jr (1970) The advantages of bypass operations over radical pancreatico-duodenectomy in the treatment of pancreatic carcinoms. Surg Gynecol Obstet 130: 1049–1053
2. Trede M (1985) The surgicla treatment of pancreatic carcinoma. Surgery (St Louis) 97:28–35
3. Michelassi F, Erroi F, Dawson PJ, Pietrabissa A, Noda S, Handkock M (1989) Experience with 647 consecutive tumors of the duodenum, ampulla, head of the pancreas and distal common bile duct. Ann Surg 210:544–556
4. Monson JRT, Donohue JH, McEntee GP, Van Heerden JA, Shorter RG (1991) Radical rection for carcinoma of the ampullar of Vater. Arch Surg 128:353–357
5. Connolly MM, Dawson PJ, Michelassi F, Moossa AR, Lowenstein F (1987) Survival in 1001 patients with carcinoma of the pancreas. Ann Surg 206:366–373
6. Trede M, Schwall G, Saeger H-D (1990) Survival after pancreatoduodenectomy. Ann Surg 211:447–458
7. Knox RA, Kingston RD (1986) Carcinoma of the ampulla of Vater. Br J Surg 73:72–73

Pancreaticogastrostomy for Reconstruction of Pancreatic Stump After Pancreaticoduodenectomy in Ampullary Carcinoma: Experience in 125 Cases

B.M.L. Kapur[1] and Neeti Kapur[2]

Summary. Pancreaticogastrostomy was done for reconstruction of the pancreatic stump after pancreaticoduodenectomy in 125 cases of ampullary carcinoma. There were no pancreatic leaks. The 5-year survival rate was excellent for patients who had no pancreatic or lymph node involvement.

Key words. Pancreaticogastrostomy—Pancreaticoduodenectomy—Ampullary carcinoma

Introduction

The major cause of morbidity and mortality after pancreacticoduodenectomy (PD) is the disruption of the pancreaticoenteric anastomosis. Pancreatic leak accounts for 5%–20% of reported morbidity. Several methods including total pancreatectomy have been advocated in the management of the pancreatic stump after PD to decrease morbidity and mortality [1]. The senior author published in 1986 his initial experience of pancreaticogastrostomy (PG) after PD in 31 cases of ampullary carcinoma [2]. This chapter presents our experience with 125 patients with ampullary carcinoma who underwent PG for reconstruction of the pancreatic stump after PD.

Clinical Material

Our 125 patients who had been diagnosed as having ampullary carcinoma underwent surgery in one surgical unit at the All India Institute of Medical Sciences Hospital (1977–1991), Holy Family Hospital, and Mool Chand Hospital, New Delhi (1991–1995). There were 88 male and 37 female patients, most of whom were in the age group of 41–60 years (Table 1). The youngest was a 17-year-old girl and the oldest a 76-year-old man. All patients had a history of jaundice with fluctuation in 40% of the cases; 80% had pruritus while 60% had abdominal pain and weight loss, and 50% gave a

[1] Former Head of Surgery, All India Institute of Medical Sciences, New Delhi 110024, India.
[2] Surgeon, RML Hospital, New Delhi, India

TABLE 1. Age and sex distribution

Age (years)	Men	Women	Total
<20	1	2	3
21–30	6	2	8
31–40	16	4	20
41–50	31	14	45
51–60	21	9	30
61–70	10	4	14
>70	3	2	5
Totals	88	37	125

TABLE 2. Duration of symptoms

Period (months)	Patients (n)
1–3	36
4–6	47
7–12	19
13–18	14
19–24	7
>24	2

TABLE 3. Level of serum bilirubin

Serum bilirubin (mg%)	Patients (n)
≤5	15
6–10	26
11–15	28
16–20	24
21–30	22
>31	10

history of recurrent fever and decreased appetite. The first symptom was jaundice in 50%, fever in 20%, pain in the abdomen in 20%, and anorexia in 10%. The majority of the patients had had symptoms for 1–6 months, while 2 had had symptom for more than 2 years (Table 2).

Investigation revealed that most of these patients had a serum bilirubin of more than 10 mg, and ten had a level of more than 31 mg (Table 3); 40% of the patients had serum albumin of less than 3 gm%. The diagnosis was made by ultrasound and side-viewing duodenoscopy. Ultrasound examination showed the common bile duct dilated up to its lower end and the pancreatic duct dilated up to the ampulla. This was in contrast to the findings in carcinoma of the head of the pancreas, in which the common bile duct was dilated up to the level of the upper border of the pancreatic head and the pancreatic duct was dilated up to 2–4 cm from the ampulla. The side-viewing duodenoscopy showed either a prominent protruding ampulla or an ulcerated or cauliflower lesion. Endoscopic biopsies were positive in only half the cases; most of the cases of protruding ampulla had a negative biopsy. Endoscopy was not repeated after a negative biopsy because reliance was on the endoscopic appearance. There was complete corroboration of endoscopic findings with the histopathological findings of the resected specimens.

Preliminary biliary drainage was not routinely done even with high levels of serum bilirubin. Preoperative biliary drainage was done only in cases of cholangitis that did not respond to conservative treatment or for patients in very poor general condition. This drainage was done for 16 patients, by tube cholecystostomy under local anesthesia in 8 cases and by nasobiliary drainage in 5 cases. Three patients underwent cholecystojejunostomies, which were done in other hospitals.

Operative Procedures

Pancreaticoduodenectomy and reconstruction of the pancreatic stump by pancreaticogastrostomy was done as described earlier [2]. Bilioenteric anastomosis was done by single-layer interrupted 3-0 catgut. The anastomosis was kept about 2 cm wide. In cases in which the common bile duct was not sufficently dilated, it was slit anteriorly. T-tube drainage of the anastomosis was done only in early cases; truncal vagotomy was routinely done and all cases had antrectomy.

Postoperative Course

Postoperatively, three patients had intragastric bleeds. Two patients resolved with conservative treatment; one patient, who had bleeding from the pancreatic stump that required reoperation subsequently recovered. Four cases were reoperated within 24 h for intraperitoneal bleeding. Bile leak was seen in five cases, which settled by conservative treatment in 5–10 days. None had pancreatic leak. Chest infection was seen in eight cases. Mild wound infection was seen in five cases while four had severe wound infection. Postoperative nasogastric aspiration was done for an average of 4 days (range, 3–7 days). The average stay in the hospital was 10 days, with a range of 8–27 days.

There were six deaths. Two patients died of liver failure, two had acute myocardial infarction, and two had septicemia and multiple organ failure. Histopathological examination showed the growth to be confined to the ampulla in 81 cases, and infiltration of the pancreas or involvement of the regional lymph nodes was seen in 44 cases. Follow-up of more than 5 years is available in 83 cases; 46 patients have lived more than 5 years and 37 have died. Those patients who died were dead within 2 years of surgery. None of the patients who had involvement of pancreatic head or regional hymph nodes as shown by histopathology lived more than 2 years.

Discussion

Pancreaticoduodenectomy has become a safe procedure for benign and malignant diseases of the pancreas and malignant disease of the ampulla, duodenum, and lower end of the common bile duct (CBD), with mortality less than 5%. In the present series, the mortality was 4.8%. The finding of pancreaticoenteric fistula is the main factor in morbidity and mortality after PD. Various techniques of reconstruction of the pancreatic stump have been advocated to decrease this complication. Pancreaticogastrostomy has been recommended as one of the methods with minimum incidence of pancreatic leak. The feasibility of PG was demonstrated in canine experiments, and subsquently Waugh and Clagett [3] published in 1946 the first successful clinical report of PG following PD. However, the procedure did not gain widespread popularity despite its numerous technical and theoretical benefits.

The senior author has been using the technique of PG after PD since 1977 and published his initial results in 1986. Various other authors [3–12] have now published their results of PG, with no or minimal pancreatic leak and no pancreatic fistula-related deaths. Various techniques of pancreaticogastrostomy have been described: telescoping the stump [2,4–6], duct-to-mucosa anastomosis [7–9], and single-layer [5,10] or two-layer [4,7,9,10] anastomosis performed with [4,5,9,10] or without stents [2,4,8,11]. The results of all these techniques have been uniformly good. In the present series of 125 patients with ampullary carcinoma who underwent PG after PD, there was no pancreatic leak. With the excellent results of PG as reported by the author, most of the centers in India are performing PG after PD.

References

1. Sikora SS, Posner MC (1995) Management of the pancreatic stump following pancreaticoduodenectomy. Br J Surg 82:1590–1597
2. Kapur BML (1986) Pancreaticogastrostomy in pancreaticoduodenal resection for ampullary carcinoma; experience in thirty-one cases. Surgery (St Louis) 100:489–492
3. Waugh JM, Clagett OT (1946) Resection of the duodenum and the pancreas for carcinoma. An analysis of thirty cases. Surgery (St Louis) 20:224–232
4. Delcore R, Thomas JH, Pierce GE, Hermerck AS (1990) Pancreaticogastrostomy: a safe drainage procedure after pancreaticoduodenectomy. Surgery (St Louis) 108:641–647
5. Myagawa S, Makuuchi M, Lygidakis NJ, et al (1992) A retrospective comparative study of reconstructive methods following pancreaticoduodenectomy—pancreaticojejunostomy vs pancreaticogastrostomy. Hepato-Gastroenterology 39:381–384
6. Arnaud JP, Bergamashi R, Casa C, Serra-Maudet V (1993) Pancreaticogastrostomy following pancreaticoduodenectomy: a safe drainage procedure. Int Surg 78:352–353
7. Mikie JA, Rhoads JE, Park CD (1975) Pancreaticogastrostomy: a further evaluation. Ann Surg 181:541–545
8. Morris DM, Ford RS (1993) Pancreaticogastrostomy: preferred reconstruction for Whipple resection. J Surg Res 54:122–125
9. Bradbeer JW, Johnson CD (1990) Pancreaticogastrostomy after pancreaticoduodenectomy. Ann R Coll Surg Engl 72:266–269
10. Takao S, Shimazu H, Meanohara S, Shinchi H, Aikou T (1993) Modified pancreaticogastrostomy following pancreaticoduodenectomy. Ann Surg 165:317–321
11. Ramesh H, Thomas PG (1990) Pancreaticojejunostomy vs pancreaticogastrostomy in reconstruction following pancreaticoduodenectomy. Aust N Z J Surg 60:973–976
12. Icard P, Dubois F (1988) Pancreaticogastrostomy following pancreaticoduodenectomy. Ann Surg 207:253–256

Pancreatoduodenectomy for Periampullary Carcinoma: Experience with 320 Cases

Yong-Feng Liu, Li-Ming Wang, Jian Liang, Jia-Lin Zhang, Shao-Wei Song, Yu-Lin Tian, Kui Shen, and San-Guang He

Summary. From 1962 to 1994, 1200 patients with periampullary carcinoma had laparotomy in our department. Of these cases, 320 underwent pancreatoduodenectomy (PD); the resection rate was 25.8%. Hospital mortality was 23 cases (7.19%), and hospital morbidity was 69 cases (21.9%). The 320 PD, 214 were men and 106 women, ranging in age from 26 to 73 years, with a median of 52.9 years. The lesions of the 320 cases were carcinoma in the head of pancreas (81 cases), in the common bile duct (85), in the ampulla of Vater (104), and in the duodenum (50). The method of resection we preferred is to follow the order of gallbladder, bile duct, stomach, proximal jejunum, and duodenum initially and leave the pancreas until last; this method provides excellent exposure of the uncinate process and controls bleeding easily. Gastrojejunual anastomosis was the retrocolic procedure. The end of the jejunum is brought into the upper abdomen in a retrocolic position, but anterior to the mesenteric vessels. Pancreatic fistula is a common and serious complication following PD. From 1962 to 1970, 43 PDs with end-to-side anastomosis without pancreatic drainage were performed; the fistula occurred in 10 patients and 6 died; thus, we changed the method to end-to-end anastomosis between the pancreas and jejunum, and in 14 patients with internal drainage by use of a short tube, fistula occurred in 2 cases. We then changed to a long catheter for external drainage for 237 cases, and the fistula occurred only in 3 cases. Our data show that the postoperative survival rate is poor for pancreatic carcinoma. The 1-year survival rate is no more than 50%, and the 3-year rate is only 13.58%. However, for carcinoma of the ampulla of Vater and common bile duct, the result is better; the 5-year survival rate for carcinoma of the ampulla of Vater is 41.54%, which is the best result.

Key words. Pancreatoduodenectomy—Periampullary carcinoma—Pancreatic cancer—Pancreatic fistula

Department of Surgery, First University Hospital China Medical University, Shen Yang 110001, China.

Introduction

Pancreatoduodenectomy (PD) is the major method of treatment for periampullary malignant tumors. Of 1200 patients with periampullary carcinoma who had laparotomy from 1962 to 1994 in our department, 320 underwent PD. The resection rate was 25.8%, hospital mortality was 23 cases, and the mortality rate was 7.19%.

Clinical Material

From 1962 to 1994, 320 patients underwent PD in our department; the 214 men and 106 women ranged from 26 to 73 years in age with a median of 52.9 years. The lesions of these 320 cases are shown in Table 1. The initial 43 patients underwent the Whipple procedure; the others underwent pancreas–bile duct gastrojejunostomy [1,2]. Pylorus-preserving pancreatodenectomy was performed in 28 patients; the reconstruction methods are displayed in Table 2.

To decrease the incidence of pancreatic fistula, different procedures were used for the management of the pancreatic remnant (Table 3). The complications of 320 cases of PD are shown in Table 4, and the results of follow-up are displayed in Table 5.

TABLE 1. Lesions of the 320 cases

Carcinoma	Cases
Head of pancreas	81
Common bile duct	85
Ampulla of Vater	104
Duodenum	50

TABLE 2. Reconstruction method

Reconstruction	Cases
1962–1970, Bile duct, pancreas, gastrojejunostomy (antecolic)	43
1970–1994, Pancreas, bile duct, gastrojejunostomy	277
Antecolic anastomosis	231
Retrocolic anastomosis	46
Pylorus-preserving	28

TABLE 3. Management of pancreatic remnant

Method	Cases	Fistula	Deaths
End-to-side pancreaticojejunostmy			
Without drainage	43	10	6
Pancreatic duct injection	25	1	1
End-to-end invagination			
Internal drainage	14	2	0
External drainage	237	3	1
No drainage	1	1	0
Totals:	320	17 (5.3%)	8 (2.5%)

TABLE 4. Complications of pancreatoduodenectomy

Complication	Cases	Deaths
Pancreatic fistula	17	8
Abdominal infection	17	6
Bile fistula	7	1
Alimentary tract hemorrhage	6	1
Abdominal bleeding	4	2
Intestincal obstruction	4	1
Renal failure	2	1
Portal vein thrombosis	2	1
Cardiac arrest	1	1
Intestinal fistula	2	1
Wound infection	4	—
Biliary tract bleeding	1	—
Pneumonia	2	—
Totals:	69 (21.9%)	23 (7.19%)

TABLE 5. Outpatient follow-up

Carcinoma	Cases	Survival rate (%)		
		>1 yr	>3 yr	>5 yr
Pancreatic carcinoma	81	44.44	13.58	7.14
Ampullary carcinoma	65	73.85	52.31	41.54
Biliary duct carcinoma	33	60.61	48.48	21.21
Averages:		58.1	34.08	22.35

Discussion

The resection range is different in various reports. Our standard is that the pancreatic incision line for carcinoma of the ampulla of Vater and the common bile duct is at the line of the supramesentric vein, and the incision line for pancreatic head carcinoma is at the left margin of the aorta.

The PD procedure has been standardized. Some surgeons used to separate and resect in the order of bile duct, stomach, pancreas, duodenum, and proximal jejunum [3]. We prefer to separate and resect following the order of gallbladder, bile duct, stomach, proximal jejunum, and duodenum initially and leave the pancreas until last. This method provides excellent exposure of the uncinate process and good hemostasis if copious bleeding occurs. We recommend our method in the case of severe pancreatic adhesions.

By pathological examination of 498 nodes of 23 PD cases, 32 lymph nodes were shown to be metastasic in 10 patients. Most of the metastasic nodes were aggregated around the head of the pancreas and the mesentery, but 1 case had metastasis around the aorta.

There are a number of methods for reconstruction of gastrointestinal continuity. We operated on 43 cases using the original Whipple method before 1970 and then changed the order of anastomosis. The end of the jejunum is brought into the upper abdomen in a retrocolic position but anterior to the mesenteric vessels. Reconstruction beings with end-to-end anastomosis between pancreas and jejunum. The second anastomosis is an end-to-side choledochojejunostomy, and the last anastomosis is end-to-side gastrojejunostomy. The distance from the biliary anastomosis to the gastrojejunostomy is about 40–50 cm to prevent the reflux of gastric contents into the bile duct. The gastrojejunostomy was antecolic in the past, but recently we changed the method to the retrocolic manner for 46 cases; this method simplified the procedure, and there have been no complications so far.

Pancreatic fistula is a common and serious complication following PD. The incidence rate is 7%–23%, and once the fistula occurs, the mortality rate may be 50% [4]. Thus, the management of the pancreatic remnant attracts much attention. We initially used end-to-side pancreatojejunostomy in 43 patients from 1962 to 1970, the pancreatic fistula occurrence was as high as 23.2% (10/43), and the mortality rate was 60% (6/ 10). Thus, we changed to the use of end-to-end invagination pancreatojejunostomy later, and a stent was utilized to drain the pancreatic juice. We first used short internal drainage, for 14 cases, but after 2 fistulas occurred we then used long external drainage. We can observe the exocrine function by this method. The occurrence of pancreatic fistula decreased greatly, only 3 cases appearing in 237 patients (1.2%). No stent drainage was applied in 1 patient because we failed to find the pancreatic duct during the operation. The result showed that the method is quite safe and minimizes the occurrence of pancreatic fistula.

The pancreatic duct injection maneuver was performed in 25 cases in our group. The benefit of this method is to avoid the occurrence of fistula and simplfy the operation, but it destroys the exocrinic function of the pancreas. It can also affect the endocrinic function for long-term survival. Thus, we have a prudent attitude toward it.

By the study of the pancreatic exocrine function of 44 PD cases, we found that some of the patients exhibited a different extent of pancreatic exocrine mulfunction. Most of the malfunction occurred within 1 year after operation.

Partial gastric resection was once considered the necessary procedure of PD so as to resect the tumor completely and prevent the occurrence of marginal ulcers. A series of complications, however, appeared after partial gastric resection, such as refluent alkaline gastritis, dumping syndrome, and malnutrition. Traverso and Longmire [5] first reported pylorus-preserving pancreatoduodenectomy (PPPD) in 1978. We performed PPPD in 28 patients recently, including 18 cases of pancreatic head carcinoma and 2 cases of duodenal carcinoma. PPPD can apparently improve digestion and absorption, and it can prevent the occurrence of reflux of gastrointestinal fluid and dumping syndrome. Gastric stasis occurred in 5 patients of 28 PPPD cases and was cured by nasogastric drainage and drugs within 1 week; the prognosis was good. PPPD can be performed in cases without gastroduodenal invasion and lymph node metastasis around the pylorus, but the cut margin of the duodenum must be examined by frozen section during the operation to detect residual carcinoma.

Outpatient Follow-Up

The survival rate of patients with carcinoma of the ampulla of Vater and common bile duct was better than that of those with pancreatic head carcinoma. Our data show that postoperative survival rate is poor for pancreatic carcinoma. The 1-year survival rate is less than 50%, and the 3-year rate is only 13.85%. For carcinoma of the ampulla of Vater and the common bile duct, the result is better. The 5-year survival rate for carcinoma of the ampulla of Vater is 41.54%, which is the best result.

References

1. Whipple AO, Parson WB, Mullins CR (1963) Treatment of carcinoma of the ampulla of Vater. Ann Surg 102:763–779
2. Child CG (1994) Pancreaticojejunostomy and other problems associated with the surgical management of carcinoma involving the head of pancreas. Ann Surg 119:845–855
3. Jordan GL Jr (1989) Pancreatic resection for pancreatic cancer. Surg Clin North Am 69:569–595
4. Trede M, Gunther Schwall BA (1988) The complications of pancreatectomy. Ann Surg 207:39–47
5. Traverso LW, Longmire WP Jr (1978) Preservation of the pylorus in pancreaticodudenectomy. Surg Gynecol Obstet 146:957–962

Pancreatoduodenectomy in Seoul National University Hospital

Kuhn Uk Lee, Eui Gon Youk, and Keon-Young Lee

Summary. We have experienced 328 pancreatoduodenectomies during a 23-year period from January 1972 to December 1994. Recently, about 50 of these operations have been performed annually, and the trend is increasing. The most common diagnosis of resectable cases was ampulla of Vater cancer, followed by distal common bile duct, pancreas head, and duodenal cancer. The overall operative morbidity and mortality were 37.5% and 3.4%, respectively, and the rates are continuing to decrease. In studies conducted to determine the operative methods that can be performed with the lowest morbidity and mortality, no one method has proved to be the best, and the most important thing may be strict adherence to basic surgical principles and the patient's general condition. The indications for pancreatoduodenectomy should be refined when more experience is gained.

Key words. Pancreatoduodenectomy—Periampullary cancer—Prognostic factor

Introduction

As one of the largest surgical oncology centers in Korea, the surgical department of Seoul National University Hospital has performed more pancreatoduodenectomies than any other center in this country. Since the introduction of this surgical modality in Korea in the early 1960s [1], many brilliant and diligent pioneer surgeons have made every effort to establish this surgical technique. By virtue of their memorable self-sacrifice and the increasing number of indicated cases, pancreatoduodenectomy has become a well-established procedure although there still remain some controversial technical details. The annual number of patients undergoing pancreatoduodenectomy has been increasing steadily, partly because of the increased number of cases detected early and partly because of broader indications for this procedure (Fig. 1). The actual number of patients suffering from periampullary malignancies may be increasing as well [1,2].

In recent years we have performed nearly 50 pancreatoduodenectomies per year while the major operative complications and mortality rate have continued to de-

Department of Surgery, Seoul National University College of Medicine, Seoul, Korea.

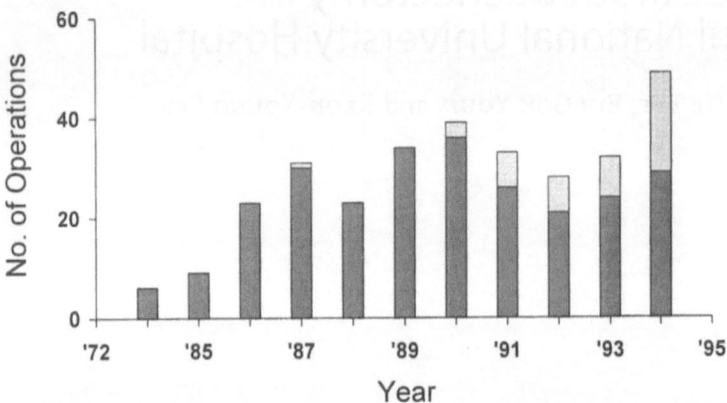

Fig. 1. Annual number of pancreatoduodenectomies (PD) performed in the Department of Surgery, Seoul National University Hospital (SNUH). The annual number is an increasing trend, and the proportion of pylorus-preserving pancreatoduodenectomies (PPPD) is also increasing. *Dotted bars*, PPPD; *shaded bars*, conventional Whipple's operation

crease [1,3]. During the evolution of pancreatoduodenectomy since its first introduction by Whipple et al. [4] in 1935, two major alternatives have been developed. One is the so-called conventional Whipple's operation, and the other is the pylorus-preserving pancreatoduodenectomy (PPPD) introduced by Watson [5] in 1944 and established by Traverso and Longmire [6] in 1978, which was introduced in this country by the late 1980s. These two modalities are now performed complementarily according to the patient's condition.

Indications

Both benign (Table 1) and malignant (Table 2) diseases have been indications for pancreatoduodenectomy. Blunt abdominal trauma cases have been relatively few because our institute is a tertiary referral hospital.

Benign Diseases

Pancreatic cystic neoplasm was the most common indication among benign diseases. Mucinous cystic neoplasms and papillary-cystic neoplasms located in the head of the pancreas have been managed with pancreatoduodenectomy because of the potential malignancy [7,8]. In cases with serous cystadenoma, we usually do not perform pancreatoduodenectomy because this is generally regarded as benign [9], although a malignant variant has been reported [10,11]. We did, however, conduct the operation for macrocystic serous cystadenoma cases [12] and for cystic neoplasm cases having a diagnostic dilemma in that the operative morbidity and mortality have fallen into an acceptable range [13].

For patients with chronic pancreatitis, pancreatoduodenectomy has been performed to relieve medically intractable pain or to manage the accompanying complications [14]. The number of patients who have undergone this operation because of

TABLE 1. Indications: benign diseases[a]

Disease	Whipple	PPPD[b]	Total
Pancreatic cystic neoplasm	2	1	3
Chronic pancreatitis	1	1	2
Duodenal adenoma	2		2
Duodenal leiomyoma	1		1
Duodenal ulcer perforation	1		1
Blunt abdominal trauma	1		1
Common bile duct (CBD) adenomatosis	1		1
Choledochal cyst		1	1
Total:	9	3	12

[a] Seoul National University Hospital (SNUH), January 1972–December 1994.
[b] Pylorus-preserving pancreatoduodenectomy.

TABLE 2. Indications: malignant diseases[a]

Disease	Whipple	PPPD	Total
Ampulla of Vater cancer	90	26	116
Distal CBD cancer	85	16	101
Pancreatic head cancer	58	0	58
Duodenal cancer	25[b]	1	26
Stomach cancer	10		10
Colon cancer	3		3
Gallbladder (GB) cancer	1	1	2
Total:	272	44	316

[a] SNUH, January 1972–December 1994.
[b] Including lymphoma (2) and leiomyosarcoma (2).

chronic pancreatitis has been relatively small, however, compared to that in other countries, probably because we have fewer pancreatitis cases. Benign duodenal tumors received pancreatoduodenectomy to rule out malignancies or because the tumor was too large to excise locally. Other indications included complicated peptic ulcer diseases and choledochal cysts with malignant potential.

Malignant Diseases

Four periampullary cancers have been the major indications for pancreatoduodenectomy. Ampulla of Vater (AOV) cancers and distal common bile duct (CBD) cancers constitute more than two-thirds of all resected cases. Pancreas head cancers are the most common periampullary cancer but were more prone to be unresectable because they become symptomatic relatively later in their natural course and frequently invade the vital structures locally [1,15,16]. The application of PPPD in patients with pancreatic head cancer is somewhat controversial, and there are reports insisting upon its radicality and safety [17,18] while there are still others against its application [19,20]. In our institute, PPPD is not conducted for patients with pancreatic head cancer. Duodenal cancers are rare, and their proportion in the pancreatoduodenectomy cases is accordingly small [1,21,22].

Because stomach cancer is the most common cancer in Korea, we have had ten gastric cancer patients who underwent Whipple's operation. The criteria for resection include absence of distant metastasis, extension to the proximal duodenum beyond the pylorus, or direct pancreatic invasion. Lymph node dissection in those cases was done much the same as in the usual radical gastrectomy cases. Other indications for pancreatoduodenectomy were locally advanced cancers including colon and gallbladder (GB) cancers without evidence of distant metastasis [23].

Preoperative Workup

Preoperative workup procedures depend largely on the presumptive diagnosis, but there are some general guidelines. For periampullary cancers, we usually perform abdominal ultrasonography (US) or computed axial tomography (CT) initially because most of the patients present with obstructive jaundice [1]. When tumor is detected by the imaging studies and the most probable diagnosis can be made, further evaluation is conducted according to the presumptive diagnosis to aid in determining the resectability more precisely or to aid in detailed planning of the operative procedures [24]. These evaluations include celiac angiography followed by portography, mainly to predict involvement of surrounding vascular structures.

Unresectability criteria for angiography include major extrapancreatic arterial involvement (e.g., celiac, splenic, hepatic, gastroduodenal, and superior mesenteric arteries) or venous involvement (e.g., portal, superior mesenteric, and splenic), and the accuracy is greater than 90% in most series [25,26]. Currently, angiography is not indicated for tumors diagnosed as unresectable in high-resolution CT and is usually indicated when the resectability is equivocal on CT [27].

Endoscopic retrograde cholangiopancreatography (ERCP) is performed to evaluate directly gastric and proximal duodenal lesions or to visualize the pancreatic or biliary ductal system. The presumptive margin of tumor infiltration can be obtained and the diagnostic possibility of chronic pancreatitis can be assumed indirectly by the appearance of the pancreatic duct [28]. We do not perform ERCP routinely but use it as an adjunctive modality especially in cases of duodenal, distal CBD, or AOV cancer.

Other optional procedures include endoscopic ultrasonography (EUS), magnetic resonance imaging (MRI), fine-needle aspiration biopsy (FNAB), and positron emission tomography (PET). EUS has the advantage that the ductal and vascular structures can be delineated in detail, and the accuracy for unresectability is reported to be from 75% to 92% [29]. In our institute, EUS is still undergoing clinical trial and the data are unavailable. The MRI criteria for unresectability of pancreatic head cancer are similar to those of CT and include vascular invasion, lymph node or liver metastasis, ascites, etc. Steiner et al. [30] in 1989 compared CT to .6-T MRI and concluded that accuracy for diagnosis of the original lesion and extrapancreatic metastasis was similar and that MRI had no advantage over CT. By using 1.5-T MRI, Warshaw et al. [31] showed that MRI is superior to CT in the diagnosis of vascular invasion and extrapancreatic invasion. MRI has no advantage over CT and is indicated only when the result of CT is equivocal.

Our experience with MRI for periampullary cancers is limited, and we perform the procedure when the diagnosis is unclear by CT. We seldom do FNAB as a routine, but it is indicated when the tissue diagnosis is essential such as in cases with overt unresectable tumors without biliary or enteric obstruction or with poor systemic condition precluding the operation. The reported positive rate of FNAB is between 85% and 95% [32]. The application of PET in patients with suspected pancreatic cancer is under intensive study but the results are inconclusive [33]. We have little experience with this diagnostic modality and are planning a controlled clinical study.

One of the issues under intense discussion may be the preoperative decompression of the biliary tract in patients with obstructive jaundice. It is generally accepted that preoperative percutaneous transhepatic biliary drainage (PTBD) may reduce surgical morbidity, but it has its own complications and does not affect the overall prognosis [34]. Our own series also showed that the overall morbidity of the preoperative PTBD and non-PTBD groups were 39.1% and 28.6%, respectively ($P > .05$), and the PTBD group had a longer hospital stay by about 10 days. Mortality did not differ between the two groups [35]. In spite of all these results, many surgeons still recommend preoperative PTBD in patients with very high serum bilirubin (>20 mg%) or cholangitis.

Operative Procedures

General Preparations of the Patient

At preoperative day 1, the patient is put in NPO and the bowel preparation is begun. On the operative day, bowel preparation is completed with one more glycerin enema and nasogastric intubation is done. Prophylactic antibiotics are given 1 h before the induction of anesthesia with a full dose of first-generation cephalosporin. After the induction of general endotracheal anesthesia, full monitoring is performed with blood pressure via arterial cannulation, electrocardiogram, body temperature, oxygen saturation, urine output via Foley catheter insertion, etc.

Operative Procedures in Detail

Like most other abdominal surgery, pancreatoduodenectomy can be divided into two major components, resection and reconstruction. These procedures are somewhat different depending on whether the planned operation is the conventional Whipple's operation or PPPD. Each procedure is described separately.

Whipple's Operation

When Professor Whipple first described the operation in 1935, it was a two-staged procedure, the first stage being cholecystogastrostomy and the second stage being the partial resection of the duodenum and the head portion of the pancreas [4]. Today, the operative procedure has evolved and the resection includes the distal half of the stomach, the duodenum, the head portion of the pancreas at the right side of the superior mesenteric vein, the distal CBD, and the gallbladder. There have been pessimistic opinions about periampullary cancers, especially pancreatic cancers, that the prognosis is so grave and operative morbidity and mortality are so high that curative surgery has no prognostic benefit over palliative bypass surgery.

On the other hand, there also have been reports that the curative surgery conducted by an expert surgeon has an acceptable complication rate and can provide long-term survival if proper patient selection is made. As an extreme, there are reports concluding that even palliative resection can provide some survival benefit [36]. In the authors' opinion, based on our recent data, carefully performed pancreaticoduodenectomy not only has low morbidity and mortality rates but also provides the only chance for cure [3,37]. With respect to the benefit of lymph node dissection, we have no well-designed case-control study because we have performed radical node dissection as a routine. Our data suggest that lymph node involvement has a tendency toward a poor prognosis.

Reconstruction after pancreatoduodenectomy has some alternatives in each anastomosis, i.e., gastrojejunostomy (G-J), choledochojejunostomy (C-J), and pancreaticoenterostomy (P-E). G-J is done as the Hoffmeister method with closure of the lesser curvature side of gastric stump. Recently, GIA autosuture has sometimes been used but the two-layer hand-sewing technique is prefered. In most cases, loop G-J is used instead of the Roux-en-Y type unless there is a definite reason for reconstructing the latter. To prevent alkaline reflux and augment gastric reservoir function, the addition of jejunojejunostomy (J-J) may be an another option. C-J is usually performed with one-layer interrupted suture using synthetic absorbable material. A silastic tube stent is an option. For P-E, there are more alternatives than for other anastomoses. The pancreatic stump can be anastomosed either to the jejunum (pancreaticojejunostomy, P-J) or to the stomach (pancreaticogastrostomy, P-G); Table 3 shows our preference.

P-J can be divided further into three alternatives according to the exact method of anastomosis, and which method to follow depends entirely on the surgeon's personal experience and preference. Duct-to-mucosa anastomosis, which we prefer, is begun with the pancreatic ductal mucosa anastomosed to the jejunal mucosa with a polyethylene tube stent inside the duct using nonabsorbable fine suture material. Then the outer layer of P-J is completed with nonabsorbable interrupted suture anastomosing the pancreatic capsule to the seromuscular layer of the jejunum. The conventional end-to-side P-J is performed in a similar manner except that the jejunum is anastomosed to the pancreatic parenchyme rather than to the pancreatic duct. In the telescopic type of end-to-end P-J, pancreatic parenchyme is anastomosed to the jejunal free end and then invaginated into the jejunal lumen, again with a tube stent (Fig. 2). Still another method is P-G, in which the pancreatic stump is anastomosed to the posterior wall of the remnant stomach with two-layered sutures (Fig. 3).

Originally, all these methods were designed in an attempt to prevent pancreatic leakage, one of the most serious complications in pancreatoduodenectomy. As is discussed later, however, our data have failed to prove any one method as being superior to the others. Our impression is that the occurrence of complication depends not on which method to follow, but on the strictness with which the operating surgeon adheres to basic and meticulous surgical principles, and, to a lesser degree, the patient's general condition.

When the anastomoses are completed, the peritoneal cavity is irrigated and examined again for possible hidden bleeding. A drain is inserted and the number and site

TABLE 3. Pancreaticoenterostomy methods[a]

Pancreaticojejunostomy	293
Duct-to-mucosa	75
End-to-side	198
Telescopic end-to-end	20
Pancreaticogastrostomy	35

[a] SNUH, January 1972–December 1994; number of cases.

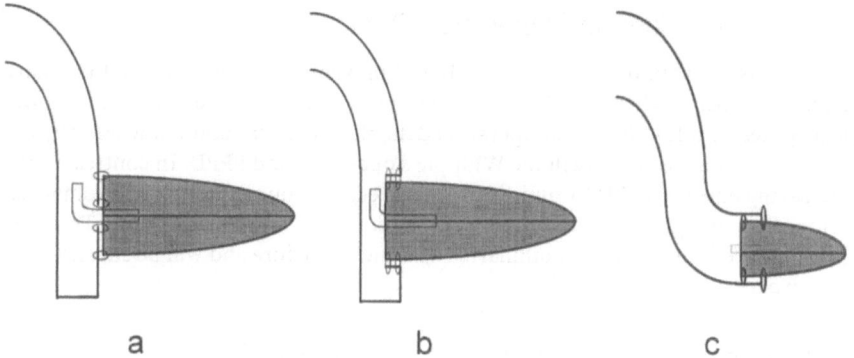

FIG. 2a–c. Schematic presentations of anastomotic methods of pancreaticojejunostomy (P-J). **a** Duct-to-mucosa method. **b** End-to-side invagination method. **c** Telescopic end-to-end P-J

FIG. 3a,b. Schematic presentations of pancreaticogastrostomy (P-G). **a** An overview of P-G. **b** Anastomotic detail of P-G, double-layered invagination method

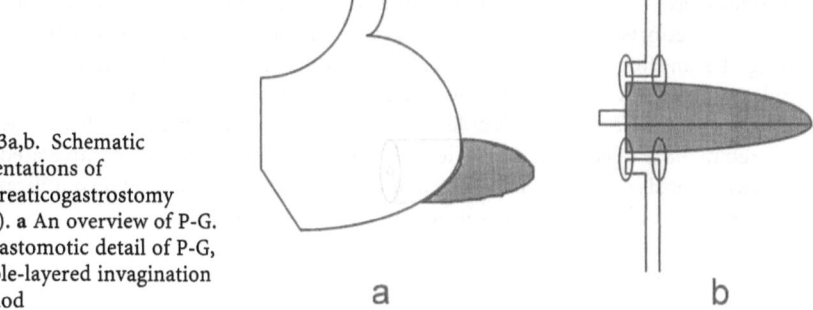

are dependent upon the surgeon's decision. A sump drain is usually located so as to drain a P-J site, while a silastic penrose is used to drain a C-J site. The operation wound is closed layer by layer.

PPPD

The resection of PPPD is similar to that of Whipple's operation except that the distal stomach is preserved along with the proximal duodenum. The theoretical practical advantages and disadvantages have long been controversial issues, and study results have been equivocal as well. We usually preserve the proximal 2 cm of duodenum so that the pacemaker can be saved, which is believed to be located within 1 cm from the pylorus.

There are several options in the order of reconstruction. The pancreatic stump can be anastomosed first, either to the jejunum or to the posterior gastric wall. Then, C-J is usually done in an end-to-side manner. Finally, duodenojejunostomy (D-J) can usually be done in a loop type. When the main procedures are completed, C-J and P-E sites are drained similar to the Whipple procedure, and the operative wound is closed.

454   K.U. Lee et al.

Postoperative Care and Operation Data

The patients are kept on NPO until the bowel movement returns. Surgical intensive care is not routine. When bowel movement returns, oral intake is encouraged without a leakage test. Table 4 shows our operation data; the mean operation time was 7 h, and no difference was seen between the Whipple's operation and PPPD. In contrast to the time-saving effect of PPPD by omitting the gastrectomy, our data showed a somewhat prolonged, although not significantly so, operation time in the PPPD group. This may be the result of our relative unfamiliarity with the procedure and will be shortened as more experience is gained.

Postoperative Complications and Mortality

Complications

The types of complications and their incidence in our institution are summarized in Table 5. The most common and serious complication after pancreatoduodenectomy may be the formation of various types of fistula. In fact, the diverse anastomotic techniques have been designed to prevent or decrease the indicence of fistula. In spite of unceasing efforts, reports worldwide have failed to find any difference in fistula rate among the anastomotic techniques [38], and our data were very much the same (Tables 6, 7). The overall complication rate was about 40%, including minor problems such as wound infection [1] (Table 5). C-J leakage results in biliary fistula, which occurred in 5.8% of cases in our series. Biliary fistula can be further complicated and progress to sepsis and eventually multiple organ failure, but these fatal complications occurred more commonly as a consequence of pancreatic fistula.

TABLE 4. Operation data[a]

	Whipple	PPPD
Blood transfusion (unit)	2.5 (0–7)	3.0 (0–6)
Operation time (h)	6.9 (4.8–10.0)	7.5 (5.3–10.8)
Mean operation time (h)	7.0 (4.8–10.8)	

[a] SNUH, January 1972–December 1994.

TABLE 5. Postoperative complications after pancreatoduodenectomy (PD)

Fistulous complications	45 (14.1%)
Biliary fistula	19
Pancreatic fistula	22
Enterocutaneous fistula	4
Infectious complications	44 (13.8%)
Wound infection	21
Intraabdominal abscess	12
Pneumonia	6
Cholangitis	5
Hemorrhage	13 (4.1%)
Others	21 (6.6%)
Total:	123 (37.5%)

TABLE 6. Comparison of pancreaticojejunostomy leakage[a]

	Duct to mucosa	Telescopic end-to-end	End-to-side
Leakage rate	6/75 (8.0%)	1/20 (5.0%)	3/41 (7.3%)
Operative mortality	0/75 (0.0%)	0/20 (0.0%)	2/41 (4.9%)

[a] SNUH, January 1991–December 1994.

TABLE 7. Comparison of complications for pancreaticojejunostomy and pancreaticogastrostomy[a]

Complication (%)	Pancreaticojejunostomy ($n = 293$)	Pancreaticogastrostomy ($n = 35$)
Pancreatic leakage	21 (7.2)	1 (2.9)
Biliary leakage	19 (6.5)	1 (2.9)
Bleeding	12 (4.1)	1 (2.9)
Abdominal abscess	10 (3.4)	2 (5.7)
Delayed gastric emptying	0	2 (5.7)
Other[b]	48 (16.4)	6 (17.1)
Total:	110 (37.5%)	13 (37%)

[a] SNUH, January 1972–December 1994.
[b] Wound infection, pulmonary complications, cholangitis, etc.

TABLE 8. Consequences of pancreatic fistula[a]

Consequence	Number of patients	Management	End results
Bleeding	5	Reoperation (3)	Expired (2) Improved (1)
		Conservative (2)	Expired (2)
Intraabdominal abscess	3	Drainage (2) Reoperation (1)	Improved (3)
Controlled fistula	6	Conservative (2) Octreotide (4)	Improved (6)
Panperitonitis	1	Reoperation (1)	Expired (1)
Sepsis	3	Conservative (3)	Expired (3)
Total:	22[b]	Reoperation (5) Conservative (13)	Expired (8) Improved (10)

[a] SNUH, January 1972–December 1994.
[b] Unknown consequences (4).

In our series, the incidence of pancreatic fistula was 6.7%, a value similar to that in other reports [1,39,40]. The consequences and results of treatment for pancreatic fistula are depicted in Table 8. Operative treatment was performed in 22.7% of patients with pancreatic fistula and conservative management in 59.1%. The conservatively managed group included those cases managed by interventional radiologic technique such as percutaneous drainage (PCD) and octreotide (Sandostatin). The mortality from P-J leakage was 36.4%. We compared Whipple's operation and PPPD in terms of the incidence of complications (Table 9) and could not find any significant difference between the two procedures.

TABLE 9. Comparison of Whipple and PPPD[a]

Complication (%)	Whipple	PPPD	Total
Pancreatic fistula	20 (7.2)	2 (4.3)	22 (6.7)
Wound abscess	18 (6.5)	3 (6.4)	21 (6.4)
Biliary fistula	17 (6.1)	2 (4.3)	19 (5.8)
Bleeding	11 (3.9)	2 (4.3)	13 (4.0)
Intraabdominal abscess	9 (3.2)	3 (6.4)	12 (3.7)
Pulmonary complication	4 (1.4)	2 (4.3)	6 (1.8)
Cholangitis	4 (1.4)	1 (2.1)	5 (1.5)
Duodenojejunostomy leakage	0	4 (8.5)	4 (1.2)
Delayed gastric emptying	0	2 (4.3)	2 (0.6)
Other	18 (6.5)	1 (2.1)	19 (5.8)
Total:	101 (36.2)	22 (46.8)	123 (37.5)

[a] SNUH, January 1972–December 1994.

TABLE 10. Operative mortality[a] after PD

Cause of death	Number
Hemorrhage	6 (1.9%)
Sepsis	3 (0.9%)
Adult respiratory distress syndrome (ARDS)	2 (0.6%)
Total:	11 (3.4%)

[a] Death within 30 days postoperatively.

Operative Mortality

In the literature, the reported operative mortality of pancreatcoduodenectomy ranges from 1.7% to 5.4% [41]. Defined as death within 30 days postoperatively, the overall operative mortality in our series was 3.4%. Hemorrhage and its consequences were the most common cause of death; four of six cases with hemorrhagic death were caused by pancreatic fistula, again emphasizing the serious nature of this complication (Table 10). As shown in Table 11, mortality did not differ between P-J and P-G groups although the number of cases in the P-G group is too small to provide statistical significance.

Prognosis and Prognostic Factors for Periampullary Cancers

Pancreas Head Cancer

Although pancreas head cancer is the most common periampullary cancer, the resectability is relatively low and the prognosis poor because the proportion of cases already advanced at the time of first diagnosis is high [1,15,41]. In our series, the total number of patients with resectable tumors was 58 and the resectability was 14.4%; the male-to-female ratio was 1.9:1. Pancreas head cancer had the most grave prognosis with a 5-year survival rate of 7.4% and median survival of 16 months. These results are comparable to other reports [36,37,38], but there are still others insisting the survival rate is as high as 26%. In a study based on 31 patients with resectable pancreas head cancer, Lee and Williams in 1984 [16] reported that those with hemoglobin equal to or less than 12 mg/dl and those without diabetes had significantly better survival. To analyze the factors determining prognosis, we performed a univariate and multivariate study and have found the Hermreck stage to be the only significant factor (Table 12). Stage I patients had significantly better prognosis than stage II or III patients (Fig. 4).

Distal Common Bile Duct Cancer

Distal CBD cancer is the second most common periampullary cancer, with 101 resected cases. Resectability was much better than with pancreas head cancers, reaching 34.5%; the male-to-female ratio was 1.4 to 1. The 5-year survival of resectable distal CBD cancers was also better than that of pancreas head cancers, 27.3%. The univariate analysis data of possible prognostic factors are shown in Table 13. Cases with tumor invasion less than the proper muscle (T1) had a better prognosis than more deeply invaded cases (Fig. 5).

Ampulla of Vater Cancers

AOV cancer is known to be the most favorable periampullary cancer [1,41]. Our result was similar to that of other reports. According to our series based on 116 resectable

TABLE 11. Comparison of operative mortality for pancreaticojejunostomy and pancreaticogastrostomy

Cause	Pancreaticojejunostomy (292)	Pancreaticogastrostomy (35)
Bleeding	5	1
Sepsis	3	0
ARDS	1	1
Total:	9 (3.1%)	2 (5.7%)

TABLE 12. Prognostic factors in pancreas head cancer[a]

Factor	Number of patients	Median survival (mo)	P value
Stage (Hermreck)			.0002
I	12	22	
II	4	6	
III	13	12	
Tumor size			.822
<4 cm	14	16	
≥4 cm	15	13	
Vascular invasion			.197
Negative	26	16	
Positive	3	9	
Lymph node involvement			.547
Negative	16	16	
Positive	13	12	
Total:	29	16	

[a] SNUH, January 1988–April 1994.

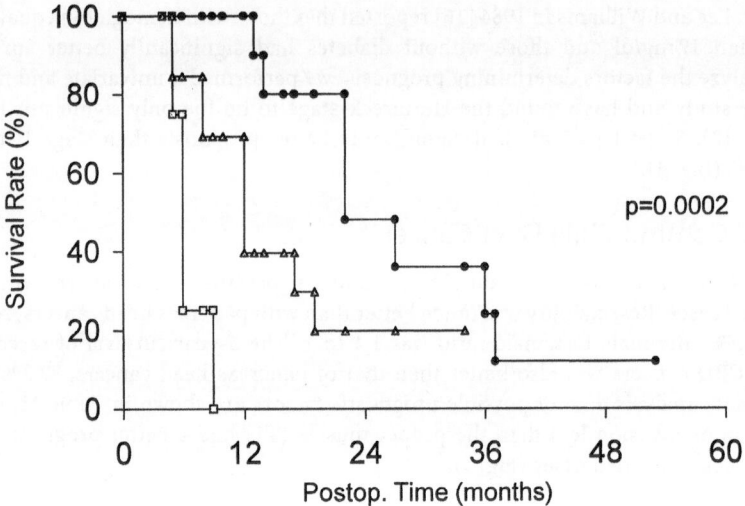

FIG. 4. Survival curves of resected pancreas head cancer cases, January 1988 to April 1995. Hermreck stage I cases had significantly better prognosis than stage II or III cases. *Cirecles*, stage I; *squares*, stage II; *triangles*, stage III

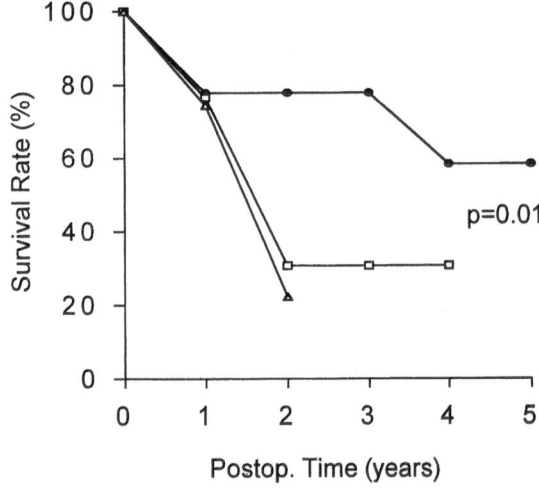

FIG. 5. Survival curves of resected distal common bile duct (CBD) cancer cases, January 1986 to December 1993. Cases with tumor invasion limited to the proper muscle layer had significantly better prognosis than more deeply invaded cases. *Çircles*, invasion limited to proper muscle layer; *square*, perimuscular connective tissue involvement; *triangles*, pancreas, liver, or duodenal invasion

AOV cancer patients, the male-to-female ratio was 1.5:1, resectability reached 78.4%, and the 5-year survival rate was 63.2%. Factor analysis showed that the depth of invasion and lymph node metastasis were the factors determining the prognosis (Table 14; Fig. 6).

TABLE 13. Prognostic factors in distal common bile duct (CBD) cancer[a]

Parameter	Number of patients	5-Year survival rate (%)	P value
Depth of invasion			
Limited to proper muscle layer	14	58.4	.010
Perimuscular connective tissue involvement	9	31.7	
Pancreas, liver, duodenum	23	22.1	
Lymph node metastasis			
Positive	12	12.4	.327
Negative	41	38.1	
Total:	54	27.3	

[a] SNUH, January 1986–December 1993.

TABLE 14. Prognostic factors in ampulla of Vater (AOV) cancer[a]

Parameter	Number of patients	5-Year survival rate (%)	P value
Preoperative bilirubin			
≤5 mg%	39	76.5	.293
>5 mg%	30	51.9	
Depth of invasion			
AOV	28	74.5	.031
Duodenal invasion (+)	18	59.6	
Pancreas invasion (+)	21	37.8	
Lymph node metastasis			
Positive	22	34.9	.005
Negative	52	75.7	
Total:	74	63.2	

[a] SNUH, January 1986–December 1993.

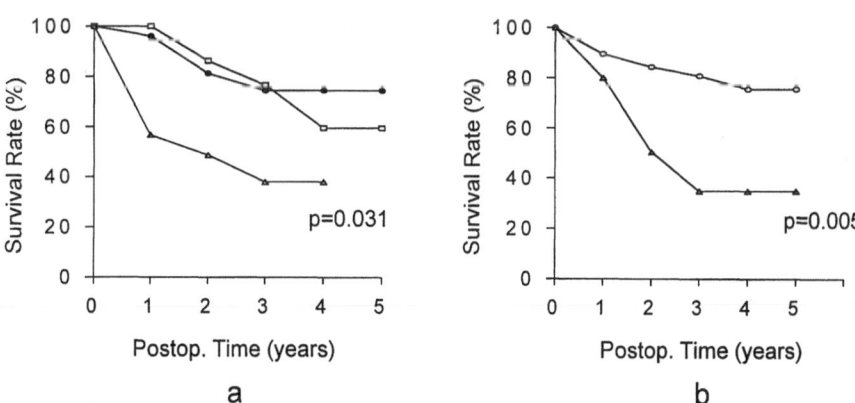

FIG. 6a,b. Survival curves of resected ampulla of Vater (AOV) cancer cases, January 1986 to December 1993. Cases with tumor invasion limited to AOV or duodenum and those without lymph node (LN) metastasis had significantly better prognosis than more advanced cases. a Survival curves according to depth of invasion. *Circles,* tumor invasion confined to AOV; *squares,* duodenal invasion; *triangles,* pancreatic invasion. b Survival curves according to LN metastasis. *Circles,* without LN metastasis; *triangles,* with LN metastasis

Duodenal Cancers

Duodenal cancers are relatively uncommon and reported to be less than 5% among periampullary cancers [22]; our previous report showed the same result [21]. The number of patients with resectable duodenal cancer was 22, resectability was 32.5%, and male-to-female ratio was 1.4:1. The prognosis was somewhat grave, and the 5-year survival rate was 17%. The prognostic factors were difficult to analyze because of the small sample size, but nonparametric analysis revealed that lymph node involvement was the only significant factor. Further study is recommended when more cases are collected (Table 15; Fig. 7).

Gastric Cancers

Gastric cancer patients undergoing Whipple's operation are very limited because the tumors resected only by pancreaticoduodenectomy are usually far advanced diseases. We have experienced ten cases in which tumors could be radically resected by Whipple's operation; the male-to-female ratio was 7:3 and median survival was 33

TABLE 15. Prognostic factors in duodenal cancer[a]

Parameter	Number of patients	Median survival (mo)	P value
Lymph node involvement			.033
Negative	9	41	
Positive	2	4	
Depth of invasion			.885
T1, T2, T3	2	59	
T4	9	35	
Total:	11	35	

[a] SNUH, January 1980–April 1991.

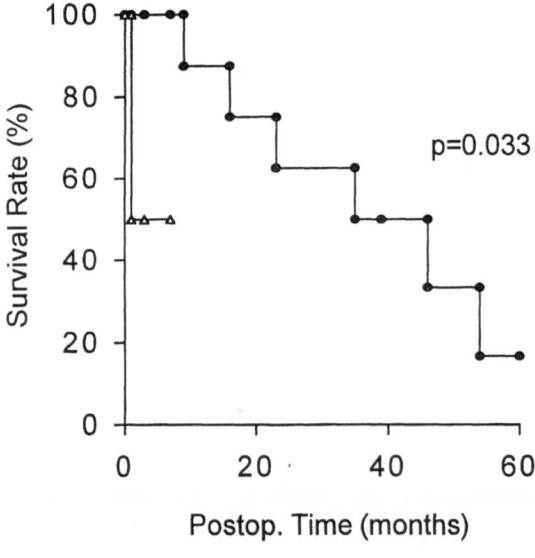

FIG. 7. Survival curves of resected duodenal cancer cases, January 1980 to April 1991. Cases without LN metastasis had significantly better prognosis than those with LN involvement. *Cirlces*, without LN metastasis; *triangles*, with LN metastasis

TABLE 16. Factors predictive for good prognosis

Disease	Indications
Pancreas head cancer	Hermreck stage I
Distal CBD cancer	Tumor confined to mucosa or perimuscular connective tissue
Ampulla of Vater cancer	Tumor confined to duodenum Without lymph node involvement
Duodenal cancer	Without lymph node involvement
Gastric cancer	Without colon or proximal stomach involvement

months. It was worth noting that one patient survived more than 4 years without evidence of recurrence. Again, the sample size was too small to analyze statistically but nonparametric analysis showed that combined resection with stomach or colon were predictive for poor prognosis.

Factors Predictive for Good Prognosis After Pancreatoduodenectomy

Pancreatoduodenectomy is still an operative procedure with high morbidity and mortality. We tried to determine factors that can predict favorable prognosis after pancreatoduodenectomy (Table 16). Of course, these factors cannot be absolute because the data were immature, but we believe that the criteria may provide a guideline in performing pancreatoduodenectomy. We recommend that the indications be refined by further investigations.

Conclusions

In a study based on 328 pancreatoduodenectomies performed during a 23-year period from January 1972 to December 1994, we have tried to suggest the indications, operative methods, and prognostic factors that predict a good prognosis. Recently the annual number of pancreatoduodenectomies has been about 50 cases and the trend is increasing. The most common diagnosis of resectable cases was ampulla of Vater cancer followed by distal CBD, pancreas head, and duodenal cancer. The overall operative morbidity and mortality were 37.5% and 3.4%, respectively, and the rates are continuing to decrease. In studies conducted to identify the operative methods that can be performed with the lowest morbidity and mortality, no one method has proved to be the best, and the most important thing may be the strict adherence to basic surgical principles and the patient's general condition. The indications for pancreatoduodenectomy should be refined when more experience has been gained.

References

1. Min-Gu Oh, Kuhn Uk Lee, Jin-Pok Kim (1986) Surgical management of periampullary cancer (in Korean). J Korean Surg Soc 31:437–444
2. Jin-Pok Kim, Woo-Song Ha (1980) Clinical study of periampullary cancer (in Korean). J Korean Cancer Res Assoc 12:79–85

3. Byung-Sun Cho, Keon-Young Lee, Sun-Whe Kim, Jung-Kee Chung, Kuhn Uk Lee, Yong-Hyun Park, Jin-Pok Kim (1995) The recent experience with pancreatic ductal adenocarcinoma at a single institution (in Korean). J Korean Surg Soc 49:981–988
4. Whipple AO, Parson W, Mullins CR (1935) Treatment of carcinoma of the ampulla of Vater. Ann Surg 102:763–769
5. Watson K (1944) Carcinoma of the ampulla of Vater. Br J Surg 31:368–373
6. Traverso LW, Longmire WP (1978) Preservation of the pylorus in pancreatic-oduodenectomy. Surg Gynecol Obstet 146:959–962
7. Compagno J, Oertel JE (1978) Mucinous cystic neoplasms of the pancreas with overt and latent malignancy (cystadenocarcinoma and cystadenoma): a clinicopathologic study of 41 cases. Am J Clin Pathol 69:573–580
8. Sclafani LM, Reuter VE, Coit DG, Brennan MF (1991) The malignant nature of papillary and cystic neoplasm of the pancreas. Cancer (Phila) 68:153–158
9. Compagno J, Oertel JE (1978) Microcystic adenomas of the pancreas (glycogen-rich cystadenomas): a clinicopathologic study of 34 cases. Am J Clin Pathol 69:289–298
10. Pyke CM, van Heerden JA, Colby TV, Sarr MG, Weaver AL (1992) The spectrum of serous cystadenoma of the pancreas: clinical, pathologic and surgical aspects. Ann Surg 215:132–139
11. Yoshimi N, Sugie S, Tanaka T, Aijin W, Bunai Y, Tatematsu A, Okada T, Mori H (1992) A rare case of serous cystadenocarcinoma of the pancreas. Cancer (Phila) 69:2449–2453
12. Lewandrowski KB, Warshaw AL, Compton CC (1992) Macrocystic serous cystadenoma of the pancreas: a morphologic variant differing from microcystic adenoma. Hum Pathol 23:871–875
13. Keon-Young Lee, Young Min Woo, Kuhn Uk Lee (1995) Pancreatic cystic neoplasms: a clinical review (in Korean). Korean J Gastroenterol 27:110–119
14. Braasch JW, Rossi RL (1993) Partial pancreatoduodenectomy for chronic pancreatitis. In: Trede M, Carter DC (eds) Surgery of the pancreas. Churchill Livingstone, New York, pp 329–338
15. Yamaguchi K, Enjoji M, Tsuneyoshi M (1991) Pancreatoduodenal carcinoma: a clinicopathologic study of 304 patients and immunohistochemical observation for CEA and CA 19-9. J Surg Oncol 47:148–154
16. Lee Y-TN, Williams MD (1984) Clinical and laboratory findings of carcinoma of the pancreas and periampullary structures. J Surg Oncol 25:1–7
17. Grace PA, Pitt HA, Longmire WP (1990) Pylorus-preserving pancreatoduodenectomy: an overview. Br J Surg 77:968–974
18. Klinkenbijl JHG, van der Schelling GP, Hop WCJ, van Pel R, Bruning HA, Jeekel J (1992) The advantage of pylorus-preserving pancreatoduodenectomy in malignant disease of the pancreas and periampullary region. Ann Surg 216(2):142–145
19. Roder JD, Stein HJ, Hutti W, Siewert JR (1992) Pylorus-preserving versus standard pancreatoduodenectomy: an analysis of 110 pancreatic and periampullary carcinoma. Br J Surg 79:152–155
20. Patel AG, Toyama MT, Kusske AM, Alexander P, Ashley SW, Reber HA (1995) Pylorus-preserving Whipple resection for pancreatic cancer: is it any better? Arch Surg 130:838–842
21. Wan Suk Park, Sun-Whe Kim, Kuhn Uk Lee, Yong-Hyun Park, Kuk Jin Choe, Jin-Pok Kim (1992) A clinical analysis of primary malignant tumors of duodenum (in Korean). J Korean Surg Soc 43:211–219
22. Zollinger RM Jr, Sternfeld WC, Schreiver H (1986) Primary neoplasm of the small intestine. Am J Surg 151:654–658
23. Nakamura S, Nishiyama R, Yokoi Y, Serizawa A, Nishiwaki Y, Konno H, Baba S, Muro H (1994) Hepatopancreatoduodenectomy for advanced gallbladder carcinoma. Arch Surg 129:625–629
24. Andersen HB, Effersoe H, Tjalve E, Burcharth F (1993) CT for assessment of pancreatic and periampullary cancer. Acta Radiol (Stockh) 34:569–572
25. Aspestrand F, Kolmannskog F (1992) CT compared to angiography for staging of tumors of the pancreatic head. Acta Radiol (Stockh) 33:556–560

26. Rosch T, Braig C, Gain T, Feuerbach S, Siewert JR, Schusdziarra V, Classen M (1992) Staging of pancreatic and ampullary carcinoma by endoscopic ultrasonography. Comparison with conventional sonography, computed tomography, and angiography. Gastroenterology 102:188–199

27. Trede M, Schwall G, Saeger HD (1990) Survival after pancreatoduodenectomy. 118 consecutive resections without an operative mortality. Ann Surg 211:447–458

28. Pasanen PA, Partanen KP, Pikkarainen PH, Alhava EM, Janatuinen EK, Pirinen AE (1993) A comparison of ultrasound, computed tomography and endoscopic retrograde cholangiopancreatography in the differential diagnosis of bengin and malignant jaundice and cholestasis. Eur J Surg 159:23–29

29. Nakaizumi A, Uehara H, Iishi H, Tatsuta M, Kitamura T, Kuroda C, Ohigashi H, Ishikawa O, Okuda S (1995) Endoscopic ultrasonography in diagnosis and staging of pancreatic cancer. Dig Dis Sci 40:696–700

30. Steiner E, Stark DD, Hahn PF, Saini S, Simeone JF, Mueller PR, Wittenberg J, Ferrucci JT (1989) Imaging of pancreatic neoplasms: comparison of MR and CT. AJR 152:487–491

31. Warshaw AL, Gu ZY, Wittenberg J, Waltman AC (1990) Preoperative staging and assessment of resectability of pancreatic cancer. Arch Surg 125:230–233

32. Bakkevold KE, Arnesjo B, Kambestad B (1992) Carcinoma of the pancreas and papilla of Vater: presenting symptoms, signs, and diagnosis related to stage and tumor site. A prospective multicentre trial in 472 patients. Norwegian Pancreatic Cancer Trial. Scand J Gastroenterol 27:317–325

33. Kato T, Fukatsu H, Ito K, Tadokoro M, Ota T, Ikeda M, Isomura T, Ito S, Nishino M, Ishigaki T (1995) Fluorodeoxyglucose positron emission tomography in pancreatic cancer: an unsolved problem. Eur J Nucl Med 22:32–39

34. Smith RC, Pooley M, George CRP, Faithful GR (1985) Preoperative percutaneous transhepatic internal drainage in obstructive jaundice: a randomized controlled trial examining renal function. Surgery (St Louis) 97:641–648

35. Jae Sik Joo, Kuhn Uk Lee, Jae Hyung Park (1987) Preoperative percutaneous transhepatic biliary drainage in patients with malignant obstructive jaundice (in Korean). J Korean Surg Soc 32:661–668

36. Klinkenbijl JHG, Jeekel J, Schmitz PIM, Rombout PAR, Nix GAJJ, Bruining HA, van Blankenstein M (1993) Carcinoma of the pancreas and periampullary region: palliation versus cure. Br J Surg 80:1575–1578

37. Kuhn Uk Lee, Il Dong Kim, Jin Cheon Kim, Jin Pok Kim (1989) Prognostic factors and adequate surgical management of pancreatic cancer: clinical analysis of 12 years from 1976 to 1987 (in Korean). Korean J Gastroenterol 21:404–413

38. Grace PA, Pill HA, Tomkins RK, Den Boston L, Longmire WP Jr (1986) Decreased morbidity and mortality after pancreatoduodenectomy. Am J Surg 151:141–149

39. Trede M, Carter DC (1993) The complications of pancreatoduodenectomy and their management. In: Trede M, Carter DC (eds) Surgery of the pancreas. Churchill Livingstone, New York, pp 629–644

40. Madiba TE, Thomson SR (1995) Restoration of continuity following pancreaticoduodenectomy. Br J Surg 82:158–165

41. Trede M (1994) Periampullary and pancreatic cancer. In: Blumgart LH (eds) Surgery of the liver and biliary tract. Churchill Livingstone, New York, pp 997–1008

Pancreaticoduodenectomy in Hong Kong: An Audit of the Queen Mary Hospital Experience

Edward C.S. Lai, Chung-Yau Lo, Alexander Chu, Kent-Man Chu, Sheung-Tat Fan, Chung-Mau Lo, and Chi-Leung Liu

Summary. Pancreaticoduodenectomy is an established procedure for various periampullary cancers in Hong Kong. During the past decade, tumors at the head of the pancreas (27 patients), the ampulla (23 patients), and the distal bile duct (11 patients) constituted about 90% of the 68 patients who underwent the procedure at the Queen Mary Hospital. Preoperative biliary decompression was used selectively as analysis of the postoperative outcome of the 38 jaundiced patients who failed to demonstrate any benefit. During the past 2 years, diagnostic laparoscopy and a laparoscopic ultrasound examination were conducted routinely before laparotomy. In the absence of gastric outlet obstruction, patients with unresectable disease would be managed by nonoperative measures. While the techniques chosen by an individual surgeon varied, the majority of patients had an antrectomy (58 patients) and a pancreaticojejunostomy (66 patients). None of our patients had concomitant resection of the portal vein and superior mesenteric artery. Similar to recent reports, results of surgery improved over the years. In contrast to the overall hospital death rate of 5.8% the rate has dropped to 2.6% since 1990. Adjunctive therapies, including perioperative radiotherapy and systemic chemotherapy, were not given. The median survival of the 57 patients who were discharged from hospital after resection of their tumors was 26%, 16%, and 16% for patients with cancer of the ampulla (26 patients), head of the pancreas (17 patients), and distal bile duct (10 patients), respectively. Further studies are necessary to elucidate an effective means to improve the prognosis of these patients.

Key words. Pancreatic resection—Pancreatic cancer

Introduction

Pancreaticoduodenectomy is an accepted procedure for a number of conditions, but the procedure is frequently performed for malignancies in the periampullary region. According to the statistics from the Hong Kong Cancer Registry, pancreatic carcinoma, including cancer of the ampulla of Vater and the distal common bile duct,

Department of Surgery, The University of Hong Kong, Queen Mary Hospital, Hong Kong.

ranks as the 16th most common for men and 17th most common for women of new cancers diagnosed in 1991. The incidence rates per 100 000 were 3.7 for men and 2.6 for women [1]. The disease has a slightly male predominance, affecting individuals in their late sixties onward, and claims close to 250 lives yearly. The present retrospective report summarizes the results and practice of Whipple's operation at the Queen Mary Hospital, Hong Kong, in recent years.

Patients and Methods

The clinical records of all patients who had undergone a pancreaticoduodenectomy (Whipple's operation) in the Department of Surgery, the University of Hong Kong at Queen Mary Hospital, were retrospectively reviewed. Between January 1985 and October 1995, there were 68 patients, 40 men and 28 women, of a mean age of 64 ± 10 years (range, 35–86 years); 19 patients were 70 years or older at the time of their operation.

The routine preoperative evaluation began with a percutaneous ultrasound examination. For patients who presented with suspected periampullary carcinoma, an endoscopic retrograde cholangiopancreatography (ERCP) was performed to delineate both the pancreatic and bile ducts, and an ampullary biopsy or brush cytology of the lesion taken whenever feasible. However, cytological examination of the pancreatic juice was not performed. In the presence of biliary obstruction, biliary decompression was used selectively depending on the general condition of the patient, evidence of concomitant biliary sepsis, and the probable timing of surgery. When indicated, internal biliary drainage using a straight endoscopic stent of the largest possible size was the preferred mode. Percutaneous biliary drainage was used when endoscopic drainage failed. Once the biliary obstruction had been relieved, the operation was usually deferred for 2–3 weeks until the jaundice subsided (to a serum total bilirubin level less than 100 μmol/l). In the presence of dehydration or malnutrition, parenteral nutritional support was also given.

Computed tomography, supplemented by intravenous contrast medium injection, has been used with increasing frequency over the years to determine the relationship between the lesion and the portal vein and superior mesenteric artery. When encasement or invasion of the major vessels was suspected, a superior mesenteric angiogram was conducted. Since the beginning of 1994, a diagnostic laparoscopy and laparoscopic ultrasound examination of the liver has been conducted immediately before the laparotomy. If disseminated disease was detected, the operation was abandoned unless there was evidence of gastric outlet obstruction. The malignant biliary stricture was managed by long-term stenting using either a plastic or self-expandable metallic stent. Peritoneal lavage for cytology examination has never been practiced.

All explorations were done via a bilateral subcostal incision. After an intraoperative ultrasound examination of the liver, an extensive kocherization, including the peritoneum and the soft tissue anterior to the right renal hilus, was performed. If a distinct pulsation of the superior mesenteric artery could not be felt, an intraoperative ultrasound examination of the head of the pancreas was repeated to determine the extent of the disease by noting the changes of echogenic pattern, and the site of interruption of the pancreatic duct in relationship to the superior mesenteric vessels. All connective tissues in front of the aorta and inferior vena cava, including the intervening lymph nodes, were resected.

For those patients with a borderline general condition, the procedure was abandoned if the lymph nodes between the great vessels were positive for metastatic disease. The portal vein at the inferior border of the pancreas was mobilized to exclude infiltration at the neck of the pancreas. If the portal vein was free, the common bile duct was then transected above the insertion of the cystic duct after a cholecystectomy. Both portal vein and common hepatic artery were skeletonized. If the pylorus-preserving variant was chosen for reconstruction, about 3 cm of the first part of the duodenum was preserved by dividing the vascular arcades at the level of the pyloric ring. Duodenectomy was then completed in the usual manner before division of the neck of the pancreas between stay stitches. The uncinate process was detached from the superior mesenteric artery between multiple ligatures.

The usual sequence of reconstruction was a retrocolic pancreaticojejunostomy, then a choledochojejunostomy, and last a gastro- or duodenojejunostomy in an antecolic fashion. Depending on the diameter of the pancreatic duct, and the preference of the individual surgeon, a mucosa-to-mucosa or a dunking anastomosis was constructed over a stent. Recently, all pancreatic stents have been left short within the jejunal loop lumen and allowed to pass spontaneously. The choledochojejunostomy was performed using one layer of interrupted absorbable sutures, and a T-tube was inserted if the diameter of the common duct was less than 1 cm. Both gastro- and duodenojejunostomy were done in two layers and splinted by a nasogastric tube. Gastrostomy and feeding jejunostomy were not done. Soft silastic drains were left in front of and behind the pancreaticojejunostomy before closure for all patients.

Tissue glue and somatostatin, or its analog, were not routinely used to protect the pancreaticoenteric anastomosis. When parenteral nutrition was started before operation, it was continued into the postoperative period until oral feeding was resumed. The nasogastric tube was removed if the output measured less than 100 ml per day. In the absence of the ileus, a diagnosis of gastric stasis was made if there was persistent output for more than 14 days. Serial amylase assay of the drain fluid was commenced at about day 4 after surgery. A pancreatic fistula was considered present if the drain fluid amylase level exceeded 1000 IU/ml, irrespective of the clinical manifestations. If the amount of amylase present in the drain fluid was low, the anterior drain was first removed, and assay of the drain fluid amylase content was repeated, before the posterior drain was taken off.

The statistical tests used included Student's *t*-test, the Mann–Whitney U test, the chi-square test with Yates' correction, and Fisher's exact test. The survival rate was estimated according to the Kaplan–Meier method and compared with the log rank test after all hospital deaths were excluded [2]. Statistical significance was considered at $P < .05$. All statistical calculations were conducted with standardized biomedical statistical programs (SPSS/PC+, SPSS, Chicago, IL, U.S.A.).

Results

Clinical Features and Preoperative Evaluation

The operation was elected by 65 of 68 patients; the remaining 3 patients had an emergency Whipple's operation. One patient has persistent bleeding from a tumor that had infiltrated the duodenum. One young male patient had pancreatic duct leakage following an enucleation of insulinoma. The last patient was an 89-year-old man who had a previous Billroth II gastrectomy reconstructed in a retrocolic manner.

The duodenum herniated internally behind the superior mesenteric vessels and became infarcted as the vessels were severely kinked. All 3 patients survived their operations without major complication. The operative diagnoses of the 68 patients are listed in Table 1.

The majority of patients (59 of 68) had a percutaneous ultrasound examination; 58 patients (85%) had an ERCP, and 10 patients had a percutaneous transhepatic cholangiography, with or without stenting, when ERCP failed. Computed tomography was performed in 36 patients in our series. In fact, this investigation was done with increasing frequency over the years and has become virtually a routine preoperative evaluation except for patients with ampullary carcinoma. Hepatic and superior mesenteric angiography was performed in 24 patients (35%) only.

A history of cholangitis was present in 11 patients, 1 of whom had hypotension, and 38 of the 65 patients (58%) were jaundiced (serum total bilirubin level more than $100 \mu mol/l$) at the time of presentation. Biliary drainage was established in 18 of them using either the endoscopic (14 patients) or the percutaneous (4 patients) approach. Jaundice was invariably relieved effectively with no complications related to these nonoperative interventions.

Operative Diagnosis and Procedure

Four surgeons were responsible primarily for all patients reported. All except three patients had a curative resection performed according to intraoperative evaluation given by the surgeon. One of these three had an emergency procedure for continuous bleeding from the tumor. The second patient had extensive disease at the uncinate process and the surrounding superior mesenteric artery; the operative finding was noted only after the neck of pancreas had been transected. The third patient had marked infiltration of both superior mesenteric vessels at the inferior border of the pancreas. Torrential bleeding was encountered when the surgeon tried to free the vessels from the lesions. A Whipple's operation had to be carried out to provide the necessary exposure for hemostasis. All three patients who had a palliative operation for their carcinoma of pancreas survived the procedure uneventfully.

TABLE 1. Operative diagnosis in 68 patients after pancreaticoduodenectomy at Queen Mary Hospital

Operative diagnosis	Number of patients
Carcinoma of pancreas	20 (3)[a]
Carcinoma of ampulla	26
Carcinoma of bile duct	11 (1)[a]
Carcinoma of duodenum	1
Chronic pancreatitis	3
Duodenal leiomyosarcoma	2
Telangiectasia of ampulla	1
Infarcted duodenum	1
Recurrent renal cell carcinoma	1
Nonfunctioning islet cell tumor	1
Insulinoma	1
Total:	68

[a] Numbers in parentheses are hospital deaths.

A pylorus-preserving variant was performed for 10 patients for lesions other than carcinoma of the head of the pancreas; all of these were performed over the past 3 years. The pancreatic tissue was considered firm in 21 of the 66 patients with available information. The pancreatic duct was anastomosed to the jejunal loop in 68 patients, and 2 patients had a pancreaticogastrostomy instead. Mucosa-to-mucosa anastomosis (59%) was used slightly more frequently than the dunking type. A pancreatic stent was left to splint the pancreatic duct in 46 patients, especially in those who had a mucosa-to-mucosa anastomosis. A T-tube was used to splint the choledochoenteric anastomosis in 56 of the 68 patients. No patient in the present series had a concomitant portal vein resection. The overall average operative blood loss was $1.6 \pm .861$.

Morbidity and Mortality

Of these patients, 23 (35%) patients developed various complications (Table 2), and 8 patients required a reexploration. A leakage at the pancreaticojejunostomy was the most common complication; 4 of the 12 patients eventually required reexploration despite active conservative measures. Attempts to repair the pancreaticojejunostomy leakage using the detached round ligament were made on two occasions. One patient was successfully managed but the other had a persistent fistula that eventually resolved with conservative measures. One patient required a completed total pancreatectomy.

The use of preoperative biliary drainage had no demonstrable benefit on the postoperative outcome of our patients; 2 of 4 patients with percutaneous drainage, 4 of 14 patients with endoscopic drainage, and 5 of 15 patients with no drainage had complications. One patient with jaundice suffered an accidental ligation of the common hepatic artery at surgery. Despite a patent portal venous system, segment VII of his liver became infarcted. Debridement and drainage was performed and the patient survived.

There were four hospital deaths (5.8%) in the current series. Since 1990, 1 patient (2.6%) was lost of the most recent 39 patients. Experience of the surgeon was probably a determinant of the outcome of these patients, although our number was too small to draw any meaningful statistical conclusion. While the senior author had 1 death in 38 consecutive patients, the mortality rates for the others ranged from 11% to 17%.

TABLE 2. Postoperative complications in 68 patients after pancreaticoduodenectomy at Queen Mary Hospital

Complications	Number of patients
Chest infection	8
Wound infection	6
Gastrointestinal bleeding	4 (1)[a]
Pancreaticojejunostomy leakage	12 (4)[a]
Choledochojejunostomy leakage	2 (2)[a]
Postinfarction liver abscess	1 (1)[a]
Gastric stasis	4
Total:	23 (8)[a]

[a] Numbers in parentheses are numbers of patients who had a reexploration for their complications.

TABLE 3. Survival rates of 58 patients after pancreaticoduodenectomy for periampullary cancers at Queen Mary
Hospital

Survival rate	Ampulla cancer ($n = 26$)	Pancreas cancer ($n = 17$)	Bile duct cancer ($n = 10$)
1 year	91%	61%	55%
3 years	39%	20%	44%
5 years	33%	20%	44%
Median (months)	33	16	16

Survival

Analysis of survival was made with reference to different periampullary tumors only.
The 1-, 3-, and 5-year survival rates and the respective median survival are listed in
Table 3. Given the limitation of the small sample size, there were no statistical differences in the survival rates between patients with lesions located at the ampulla, the
distal common duct, or the head of the pancreas in the present series. Excluding
the hospital deaths, the number of 3-year and 5-year survivors in the 57 patients
with periampullary tumors, after surgery, were carcinoma of ampulla, 6 patients and
4 patients, respectively; with carcinoma of the head of the pancreas, 3 patients and 1
patient, respectively; and with carcinoma of the distal bile duct, 4 patients and 1
patient, respectively.

Discussion

Over the years, the resectability of patients who presented with tumors at the
periampullary cancers had remained low. The number of suitable surgical candidates
in Hong Kong was approximately 20%–30%, as reported elsewhere. In recent literature, different centers had reported a remarkable reduction in the mortality rate for
patients undergoing a pancreaticoduodenectomy [3–7]. Despite our limited experience, the results at the Queen Mary Hospital also demonstrated an improvement in
recent years and were comparable with those of others. Our hospital death rate has
dropped from 10.3% to 2.6% in the past 5 years. The number of patients in the present
series is too small for isolating the probable contributing factors to the better results
observed. As in our own practice, the techniques adopted by individual surgeons
varied, and clinical trials that evaluated different technical details, such as anastomosing the pancreatic remnant to either the stomach or the jejunal loop, showed similar
results [8]. Conceivably, the technical experience of the operating surgeon is more
important than the fine technical details in determining the outcome of patients
undergoing a pancreaticoduodenectomy.

Since the introduction of parenteral nutrition, somatostatin, and its analog [9,10],
surgeons are better equipped to handle the complications associated with a pancreaticoduodenectomy. With the accepted mortality rate associated with the procedure dropping to 5% or less, further efforts should focus on perioperative measures
that could lower the complication rate instead. Attempts to reduce hyperbilirubinemia by various nonoperative measures have been widely practiced de-

spite inconclusive clinical evidence. Data from previous reported randomized controlled trials with percutaneous biliary drainage may not be applicable to patients undergoing a pancreaticoduodenectomy. First, patients of all levels of ductal obstruction have been included. Second, the number of patients who had a major pancreatectomy was small. Third, the incidence of procedure-related complications of percutaneous drainage had offset any theoretical advantage derived in most studies [11–13].

Data on the use of endoscopic drainage have been conflicting [3,14]. A controlled trial on preoperative endoscopic biliary drainage reported from the Queen Mary Hospital failed to demonstrate any significant benefit although the study shared many of the shortcomings just mentioned [15]. In the present retrospective analysis of 38 patients with jaundice before their pancreaticoduodenectomy, a clear advantage of preoperative biliary decompression was also absent. While we would not recommend a routine preoperative biliary drainage, we prefer an internal biliary decompression via the endoscopic route if the procedure is necessary.

The extent of resection of the tumors and its associated lymph nodes for patients with periampullary cancers to achieve a cure remains an open question. According to different studies, resection of the portal vein when involved [16,17], taking the regional nerve plexus and lymph node routinely [18,19], and, for patients with cancer at the head of the pancreas, intraoperative irradiation [20,21] or postoperative chemoradiotherapy [22,23] given in the perioperative period, had all claimed good results. With increasing experience, recent data showed that the long-term outcome of patients with an involved portal vein remained unsatisfactory despite aggressive resection [16,17]. After intraoperative irradiation, serious postoperative complications had also been reported [21]. Although we had assumed a more conservative attitude in resecting these tumors, the overall survival figures were acceptable, In our experience, the incidence of gastric stasis rises with the increased extent of lymph node resection. In addition, the finding of nodal metastases outside the confine of the head of the pancreas was taken by us as a relative contraindication for a major pancreatic resection. In the few patients we had with positive disease in their regional lymph nodes, all of them presented with early recurrences despite vigorous chemotherapy started in the early postoperative period. Clearly, the value of extensive intervention must be weighed against the risk of incapacitating morbidity in these patients with an already guarded prognosis. Further clinical studies are required to resolve the dilemma.

References

1. Hong Kong Cancer Registry Annual Report 1991, appendixes 4 and 5
2. Kaplan EL, Meier P (1958) Non-parametric estimation from incomplete observation. JAMA 53:457–481
3. Trede M, Schwall G, Saeger H (1990) Survival after pancreatoduodenectomy: 118 consecutive resections without an operative mortality. Ann Surg 447–458
4. Bakkevold KE, Kambestad B (1993) Morbidity and mortality after radical and palliative pancreatic cancer surgery. Risk factors influencing the short-term results. Ann Surg 217:356–368
5. Klinkenbijl JHG, Jeekel J, Schmitz PI, Rombout PA, Nix GA, Bruining HA, van Blankenstein M (1993) Carcinoma of the pancreas and periampullary region: palliation versus cure. Br J Surg 80:1575–1578

6. Cameron JL, Pitt HA, Yeo CJ, Lillemoe KD, Kaufman HS, Coleman J (1993) One hundred and forty-five consecutive pancreatoduodenectomies without mortalities. Ann Surg 217:430–438
7. Castillo CF, Rattner DW, Warshaw AL (1995) Standards for pancreatic resection in the 1990s. Arch Surg 130:295–300
8. Yeo CJ, Cameron JL, Maher MM, Sauter PK, Zahurak ML, Talamini MA, Lillemoe KD, Pitt HA (1995) A prospective randomized trial of pancreaticogastrostomy *versus* pancreaticojejunostomy after pancreaticoduodenectomy. Ann Surg 222:580–592
9. Buchler M, Friess H, Klempa I, et al (1992) Role of octreotide in the prevention of postoperative complications following pancreatic resection. Am J Surg 163:125–130
10. Montorsi M, Zago M, Mosca F, et al (1995) Efficacy of octreotide in the prevention of pancreatic fistula after elective pancreatic resections: a prospective, controlled, randomized clinical trial. Surgery (St Louis) 117:26–31
11. Hatfield ARW, Terblanche J, Fataar S, Kernoff L, Tobias R, Girwood AH, et al (1982) Preoperative external biliary drainage in obstructive jaundice. A prospective controlled clinical trial. Lancet ii:896–899
12. McPherson GAD, Benjamin IS, Hodgson HJF, Bowley NB, Allison DJ, Blumgart LH (1984) Preoperative percutaneous transhepatic biliary drainage: the results of a controlled trial. Br J Surg 71:371–375
13. Pitt HA, Gomes AS, Lois JF, Mann LL, Deutsch LS, Longmire WP Jr (1985) Does preoperative percutaneous biliary drainage reduce operative risk or increase hospital cost? Ann Surg 201:545–553
14. Ceuterick M, Gelin M, Rickaert F, Van de Stadt J, Deviere J, Cremer M, Lambilliotte JP (1989) Pancreaticoduodenal resection for pancreatic or periampullary tumors—a ten-year experience. Hepato-Gastroenterology 36:467–473
15. Lai ECS, Mok FPT, Fan ST, Lo CM, Chu KM, Liu CL, Wong J (1994) Preoperative endoscopic drainage for malignant obstructive jaundice. Br J Surg 81:1195–1198
16. Ishikawa O, Ohigashi H, Imaoka S, Furukawa H, Sasaki Y, Fujita M, Kuroda C, Iwanaga T (1992) Preoperative indications for extended pancreatectomy for locally advanced pancreas cancer involving the portal vein. Ann Surg 215:231–236
17. Nakao A, Harada A, Nonami T, Kaneko T, Inoue S, Takagi H (1995) Clinical significance of portal invasion by pancreatic head carcinoma. Surgery (St Louis) 117:50–55
18. Nakao A, Harada A, Nonami T, Kaneko T, Murakami H, Inoue S, Takeuchi Y, Takagi H (1995) Lymph node metastases in carcinoma of the head of the pancreas region. Br J Surg 82:399–402
19. Kayahara M, Nagakawa T, Ueno K, Ohta T, Tsukioka Y, Miyazaki I (1995) Surgical strategy for carcinoma of the pancreas head area based on clinicopathologic analysis of nodal involvement and plexus invasion. Surgery (St Louis) 117:616–623
20. Evans DB, Termuhlen PM, Byrd DR, Ames FC, Ochran TG, Rich TA (1993) Intraoperative radiation therapy following pancreaticoduodenectomy. Ann Surg 218:54–60
21. Zerbi A, Fossati V, Parolini D, Carlucci M, Balzano G, Bordogna G, Staudacher C, Di Carlo V (1994) Intraoperative radiation therapy adjuvant to resection in the treatment of pancreatic cancer. Cancer (Phila) 73:2930–2935
22. Kasperk R, Klever P, Andreopoulos D, Schumpelick V (1995) Intraoperative radiotherapy for pancreatic carcinoma. Br J Surg 82:1259–1261
23. Gastrointestinal Tumor Study Group (1987) Further evidence of effective adjuvant combined radiation and chemotherapy following curative resection of pancreatic cancer. Cancer 59:2006–2010

Epidemiology and Experience in Pancreatic Cancer in Chile

Jose Klinger-Roitman[1], B. Manuel Novajas[2], and P. Carlos Chavez[2]

Summary. Although many advances have been made in the management of pancreatic cancer, especially in diagnosis, surgical techniques, and control of morbidity and mortality, the survival rate is still very poor according to the series reported by referral centers. These groups have reported a mortality rate that ranges between 0.2% and 5% and survival of 3%–10% at 5 years. The only curative procedure is radical resection, extended to the vessels invaded by tumor, and because of this attitude the resectability rate has increased to about 30%. Unfortunately, pancreatic cancer is still a dreadful disease, except in types such as ampullary, distal common bile duct, and duodenum cancer, in which the survival rate has been reported to be as high as 50%–60%.

Key words. Pancreatic cancer—Epidemiology—Pancreatoduodenectomy—Periampullar tumor—Palliative treatment

Introduction

It is a well-known fact that neoplastic lesions of the pancreas are a dreadful disease, with a mortality rate of 20%–40% as of 20 years ago, and with a survival rate that is practically nil, with a range of 1% to 3% at 5 years. During recent years this has changed, especially in referral centers, because of progress in diagnostic techniques by imaging, which has allowed an earlier diagnosis with lesions of 2 cm or less, with patients in better condition and surgically treated by experienced surgeons with excellent postoperative ICU care.

At the present time, series reported by different groups show a mortality rate of 0%–2% and a mortality at 30 days of 5%–10%, a morbidity rate of 20%–30%, and survival rates accordingly, with the types of periampullary carcinoma in the range of 20%–60%. Among these, papillary cancer, distal common bile duct (DCBD) cancer, and duodenal cancer have a survival rate at 5 years of about 60%. No matter how

---

[1] Service of Surgery at Dr. Gustavo Fricke Hospital, Viña del Mar, Chile.
[2] Department of Surgery and Gastroenterology, School of Medicine, University of Valparaiso, Chile.

much progress is made, morbidity is still high, and the most common postoperative complications are leaking at the pancreatojejunal anastomosis, a high digestive hemorrhage (HDH), sepsis, pancreatic abscess, pancreatitis of the pancreatic stump, and peritoneal abscess [1–8].

With the intention of an up-to-date summary of the results of pancreatoduodenectomy (PD), Professor Fujio Hanyu of the Tokyo Women's Hospital Center invited surgeons from all over the world to participate in a symposium to celebrate the treatment of 1067 patients by PD at that center and to compare experiences. We were invited to present the Chilean epidemiology and treatment of periampullary carcinomas of the pancreas. Unfortunately, there are no collective series of the different groups handling these cases, and so I refer to the experience published by five groups, including our own experience.

De Aretxabala et al. [9,10] presented their experience of 24 patients treated by PD without mortality; 16 were papillary cancer, 5 cancer of the head of the pancreas, and 3 cancer of the DCBD. In cases in which the diameter of the pancreatic duct was less than 4 mm, they used the intussusception method, and in 11 patients the mucomucosal end-to-lateral pancreatojejunal anastomosis, with a stent exteriorized by gastrostomy. Complications appeared in 7 patients, and 3 patients needed a reoperation.

Burmeister et al. [11] presented a series of seven patients who underwent PD, none of whom had a tumor of the head of the pancreas. They employed the technique of PD with pyloric preservation (PDPP); three patients developed complications, but none died.

The largest series was presented by Caracci et al. [12], who treated 40 patients in the period 1973–1993. They performed a PDPP in 33 of their patients, a standard Whipple operation in 7 patients, total pancreatectomy in 8, and an en bloc resection of the portal–superior mesenteric confluence in 5 patients; 50% presented complications, with anastomotic fistulas in 20% and a mortality of 7.5% (3 patients). Survival at 1 years was 61.3%, at 2 years 35.5%, at 3 years 19.4%, and at 4 years 6.5%, with an average survival of 19 months.

Guzman et al. [13] reported a series of 34 patients, 50% with ampullary cancer, 35% with cancer of the pancreatic head, and 15% with cancer of the DCBD, with a global mortality of 11.8%. In the last 17 patients, however, only 1 died (5.8%).

In 1995 we reviewed the pancreatic cancer experience at Viña del Mar Hospital, Chile, from January 1989 to March 1995, with a total of 30 patients; 18 men and 12 women with a mean age of 62.6 years (range, 38–86 years). When 28 patients were submitted to surgical exploration, operative findings confirmed that 16 had cancer located at the pancreatic head, 6 had ampullary cancer, and 6 had DCBD tumor. Of the total number, 3 patients were treated by PD without anastomosis, 14 with a biliary-enteric by pass with a T-tube left in the jejunum, 4 with gastrojejunoanastomosis and cholecystojejunoanastomosis, 1 a cholecystostomy, and with 1 a partial resection of the CBD with a hepatic jejunostomy; 4 had exploratory laparotomy only. During 1990–1995, with M.D. Chavez we reported the endoscopic experience with biliary endoprosthesis; indications were periampullary carcinoma and DCBD, for a total of 114 patients treated. Morbidity was cholangitis in 5 patients, hemorrhage after endoscopic sphincterotomy in 3, acute pancreatitis in 2, and duodenal perforation and migration of the stent in 1 patient. Mortality for the series was 6 patients, 5 of cholangitis and 1 of duodenal perforation. Failure of the cannulation of the CBD occurred in 14 cases (12.3%), which included the cholangitis patients and the patient with perforation.

Discussion

Periampullary carcinoma (PC) is a relatively frequent disease in Chile, with an overall survival rate of less than 1% at 5 years. Every year 300–500 patients die of pancreatic cancer, and the national rate is 3.1 per 100000 inhabitants; it is the sixth most common cause of death by cancer. The resection rate is very low (20%), diagnosis is late, and the disease is advanced at presentation. There is a difference in gender, 2:1, men to women, and the highest incidence is in the fifth and sixth decades of life. Ampullary cancer is more frequent in younger patients [2–7].

In contrast, in the United States pancreatic cancer is the fourth or fifth most common cause of death related to cancer in both men and women, with 24000 to 28000 deaths yearly [3–5]; the most frequent type is ductal adenocarcinoma, and 90% are exocrine pancreatic tumors. Pancreatic cancer ranks ninth in cancer incidence, and survival is poor, 8% at 2 years [8]. Pancreatic cancer has increased threefold in the 1980–1990 decade, but appears to have stopped increasing and even to have declined in recent years [8].

Mortality from pancreatic cancer is more pronounced in the black than in the white population; 80% of the cases occur between 60 and 80 years of age, and it is extremely rare under 40 years of age [1,2,8]. Environmental factors are involved. Incidence is higher in Jews, low socioeconomic groups, Western industrialized countries, Hawaiian women, and Korean-Americans. Immigrants from Japan are at about threefold higher risk than Nisei (those born in the United States of Japanese parents). At diagnosis, 40% of lesions are confined to the pancreatic gland, 40% are locally advanced, and 50% present as disseminated disease [3]. After resection for cure, patients have a median survival rate of about 10% at 5 years; resectability has increased to 25%–30% because of better selection of the patients [1,3,11–21].

Lillimoe [1] has reported that the overall survival rate at 5 years is 3%, similar to the data reported by others [8–21], but Pitt [14], Cameron [6], and Yeo et al. [17] show better survival rates, from 5% to 10% at 5 years.

During recent years, diagnosis has tended to be made 6 months earlier than was possible a decade ago as the result of diagnostic imaging with computed tomography (CT) scan, both standard and enhanced with contrast medium, ultrasonography (US), endoscopic retrograde cholangiopancreatography (ERCP), intraoperative US, endoscopic US, angiography, magnetic resonance imaging (MRI), tumor markers, and laparoscopy [1,4,8].

Lillimoe insists that early diagnosis requires a low threshold of suspicion and appropriate aggressiveness. Every jaundiced patient should be submitted to a study protocol that should include chemical tests, a CT scan, and US in its different types; recently others have advocated the use of intravenous and oral contrast-enhanced spiral CT as offering the best imagery. Percutaneous fine-needle aspiration in selected patients is safe and reliable but there are arguments against its use [1]. The known delay in diagnosis is partly the fault of the patients, as well as the physicians' lack of suspicion and delay in gaining access to both the diagnostic protocol and the tools [21].

Screening of asymptomatic patients is not an option because no high-risk group has been identified; 100000 individuals would have to be fully investigated to detect 1 early cancer, and there is no single, cost-effective, noninvasive and higly sensitive test that can be applied on such a large scale [21]. In preoperative and operative staging, the goal is to determine preoperatively the feasibility of surgery and the optimal treatment for each individual. With the means available nowadays it is possible to determine location, extension, liver metastasis, lymph node status, or major vascular invasion, and the extent of further staging is dependent on the patient and surgeon's preference. If the philosophy is to pursue surgical treatment for all patients, either resection or surgical palliation, further staging is unnecessary, but if the findings preclude an operation and lead to nonoperative palliation, these efforts are worthwhile [8].

MRI has been of limited use because it is deficient in visualization of the pancreas, but the speed of MRI, with oral contrast and the technique of fat suppression and intravenous gadolinium, has shown advantages over CT [8]. Warshaw [15] has stated that pancreatography might be useful, although X-ray cannot differentiate between pseudocysts and neoplastic cysts; however, the analysis of cyst liquid may help, as may also the technique of carcino embryonic antigen (CEA).

It is a generally accepted fact that the only possibility of cure for pancreatic cancer is surgery, and since Whipple and associates first performed the radical excision of a periampullary carcinoma in 1934 the original technique has undergone multiple modifications. For 40 years the morbidity and mortality rates were prohibitive, but in the past decade a number of reports have documented improvement both in operative mortality and in the long-term survival rate at 5 years [1,16–24].

Longmire and Traverso introduced a modification in relation to the antral resection during PD and proposed the PD with pyloric preservation, which is a modification of the standard Whipple operation employed by many surgeons; there are no significant differences in the results. One of the major modifications has been block resection of the vessels invaded by tumor, which is not a contraindication to an extended operation like the one mentioned. There are different ways to handle reconstruction after major vessel resection; this modification and other technical aspects, such as extended resection with extended lymphadenectomy and total pancreatectomy, are not yet proven as to the benefit for the patient. Thus, there is need of sound and good surgical judgment to submit a patient with these advanced diseases to extended operations that have a high cost in morbidity and mortality [16–18].

According to Kayahara et al. [16], the extent of lymphadenectomy varies among the periampullary carcinomas, and they concluded that it is necessary for cancers at the head of the pancreas to resect lymph nodes 13a, 13b, 14, 16, and 17a; in DCBD cancer, lymph nodes 12, 13a, and 14; and in ampullary cancer, lymph nodes 13b and 14, based in the Japanese classification of the lymphatic drainage. There are no randomized studies to support conclusively this agressive approach.

Figures about survival are controversial, depending on whether they are for real survival or actuarial survival. In the experience of the Mayo Clinic [24], on the basis of 186 patients the hospital mortality was 3%; the overall actuarial 5-year survival rate was 6.8% in patients submitted to curative resection and was greater in the subset of patients with negative lymph nodes and no perineural or duodenal invasion; also, the rate was better for ampullary, DCBD and duodenal cancers, with ranges of 30% to 60%.

Unfortunately, up to the present time only 20%–25% of these patients have been resectable, and thus the remaining 80% need to be treated by palliative methods, the goal of which is basically to relieve jaundice, pruritus, and pain. For this goal, there are surgical, percutaneous, and endoscopic methods that in addition to palliation of the obstructive jaundice can alleviate obstruction of the gastrointestinal tract [26–28].

The goals of surgical palliation should be a low morbidity and mortality rate and long survival with adequate quality of life. At Johns Hopkins, this type of palliation has been obtained with a mortality of 2.5% and with morbidity related to the bilioenteric bypass and gastrojejunostomy of about 37%; however, mostly these were minor complications [26].

Percutaneous palliative drainage is obtained with different means but can be achieved in 90% of cases, with a complication rate of 5%–26% and mortality in the range of 0.7%–1.5%. This type of drainage has an occlusion rate of 6%–23% in cases with cholangitis. The availability of new devices such as metallic expandable stents has resulted, in a success rate of 77%–100%, with patency lasting 6–7 months and occlusions in about 7%–24%. The main indication is a lesion of DCBD cancer and periampullary cancer.

Endoscopic palliation was introduced by Soehendra in 1980, and at present the success rate is in the 85%–90% range, with 0%–35% morbidity that is serious only in 10% of cases. Comparing surgical with endoscopic palliation, some randomized studies show that the control of jaundice is similar but the hospital stay is shorter and also complications are less frequent; with the expandable metallic stents, results are even better [28].

Last but not least, a few words about adjuvant therapy. Chemotherapy and radiation therapy are used after surgery when there is no evidence of residual disease and the failure of PD to provide a cure is the result of subclinical residual disease, positive lymph nodes, etc. [29]. The use of chemo- and radiotherapy in unresectable cases is controversial because the results are not reliable and the data differ in the series reported. Usually the number of cases treated is small, the staging is not accurate, and the drugs used and the radiotherapy dosages are different in every study. From some studies it appears that the combination of both methods is likely to obtain better results, and from others that to determine the exact role of adjuvant therapy we need randomized studies based on the same protocols.

Abrams and Grochow [29] concluded that combined therapy prolonged survival substantially (40–42 weeks vs. 23 when only radiotherapy was used). Chemotherapy alone with different drugs is not as successful as the use of both therapies combined (41% vs. 19% when only chemotherapy was used), and they recommended that the adjuvant therapy to be used in nonresectable patients should be the combination of radiotherapy with chemotherapy with 5-FU (fluorouracil) [30].

References

1. Lillimoe KD (1995) Current management of pancreatic cancer. Ann Surg 221(2):133–148
2. Klinger J (1994) Cancer pancreatico. Temas de cirugia. BM publicidad. Grafica AL, Universidad de Valparaiso, pp 259–267
3. Reber HA, Ashley SW, McFadden W (1995) Curative treatment for pancreatic neoplasm, radical resection. Surg Clin North Am 75(5):905–912
4. Schwartz I (1995) Textbook of surgery—exocrine pancreatic cancer. Ed. Internacional, Philadelphia, Saunders, pp 1091–1121
5. Gold EB (1995) Epidemiology of and risk factors for pancreatic Cancer. Surg Clin North Am 75(5):819–837
6. Cameron JL (1995) Long-term survival following PD for adenocarcinoma of the pancreas. Surg Clin North Am 75(5):939–951
7. Altschiller H (1990) Cancer de pancreas. Recalcine, Laboratory, pp 227–234

8. Moosa AR, Gamagami RA (1995) Diagnosis and staging of pancreatic neoplasms. Surg Clin North Am 75(5):871–890
9. De Aretxabala X, et al (1992) Cancer de la ampolla de Vater. Rev Chil Cir 44(1):89–96
10. De Aretxabala X, et al (1994) Experiencia en 24 PD sin mortalidad. Rev Chil Cir 46(4):342–347
11. Burmeister R, et al (1993) Pancreatoduodenectomia con preservacion pilorica. Rev Chil Cir 45(6):551–556
12. Caracci M, et al (1994) PD en el cancer de la cabeza del pancreas. Rev Chil Cir 46(5):470–476
13. Guzman S, et al (1992) PD, mortalidad y morbilidad. Analisis de 20 años. Rev Chil Cir 44(1):23–28
14. Pitt HA (1995) Curative treatment for pancreatic cancer; standard resection. Surg Clin North Am 75(5):891–904
15. Warshaw A (1995) Tumores quísticos de pancreas no neoplasicos. Experiencia del Massachusetts General Hospital, Boston, USA. In: Curso patología digestiva, Director Dr. E. Moreno González. Madrid, España, Mayo 1995
16. Kayahara M, et al (1995) Surgical strategy for pancreatic cancer of the head, based on clinicopathological analysis of nodal involvement and plexus invasion. Surgery (St Louis) 117:616–623
17. Yeo CJ, Cameron JL, Lillimoe KD, Sitzmann JB, Hruban RH (1995) Pancreatoduodenectomy for cancer of the head of the pancreas; 201 patients. Ann Surg 221(6):721–733
18. Cusack JC, Evans DB (1995) Pancreato-dudenectomy. Unsuspected tumor invasion of SM—portal vein confluence. Chir Int 4
19. Williamson T (1995) Ampullary cancer. In: Symposium on pancreato-biliary diseases, Berne, Switzerland, May 1995
20. Carboni M (1995) Ampullomas in Italy. In: Symposium on pancreato-biliary diseases, Berne, Switzerland, May 1995
21. Williamson T (1995) Pancreato-duodenectomy as elective treatment of Pca. In: Symposium on pancreato-biliary diseases, Berne, Switzerland, May 1995
22. Reissman P, Perry Y, Cuenca A, Bloom A, Eid A, Shiloni E, Rivkind A, Durst A (1995) Pancreatojejunostomy vs. controlled pancreatocutaneous fistula in PD for periampullary cancer. Am J Surg 169:585–588
23. Hein SJ, Reinders ME, Van Gulik TM, Van Lewuwen DJ, Verbeek PCM, de Wit LT, Gouma DJ (1995) Results of PD for ampullary cancer and analysis of prognostic factors for survival. Surgery (St Louis) 117:247–253
24. Nitecki SS, Sarr AG, Colby TV, Van Heerden JA (1995) Long-term survival after resection for ductal carcinoma of the pancreas: is it really improving. Ann Surg 221(1):59–66
25. Yeo CJ (1995) Management of complications following PD. Surg Clin North Am 75(5):913–924
26. Lillimoe KD, Barnes SA (1995) Surgical palliation in non resectable Pca. Surg Clin North Am 75(5):953–968
27. Aufman SL (1995) Percutaneous palliation of unresectable Pca. Surg Clin North Am 75(5):989–999
28. Lichtenstein DR, Carr-Locke DL (1995) Endoscopic palliation for unresectable Pca. Surg Clin North Am 75(5):969–988
29. Abrams MA, Grochow LS (1995) Adjuvant therapy with chemotherapy and radiation therapy in the management of cancer of the head of the pancreas. Surg Clin North Am 75(5):925–938

Multimodality Treatment of Pancreatic Duct Carcinoma: A Prospective Randomized Study

N.J. Lygidakis and K. Stringaris

Summary. The poor prognosis for pancreatic duct carcinoma requires researchers to continue searching for a therapy or therapies that can provide some hope for patients. Traditional systemic chemotherapy has been proven ineffective, mainly because to deliver sufficient drug concentration to the site of the disease risks severe, toxic side effects. Systemic immunotherapy also suffers the same handicap. Surgery alone may successfully remove a tumor, but the rate of recurrence is very high. One exciting new technique is the use of a targeting method to deliver anticancer drugs directly to the affected organ. Immunochemotherapeutic drugs are suspended in an emulsion which is then injected into the splenic artery and superior mesenteric artery via two arterial catheters. The drugs are delivered directly to the organ space occupied by the tumor, and the nature of the emulsion ensures that the drugs are retained in the region for extended periods. The results of this therapy are detailed in this chapter.

Introduction

Pancreatic duct carcinoma remains a challenging disease, with a dismal prognosis [1]. Even after application of ever more aggressive surgical techniques, overall long-term survival remains limited, with poor quality of life [2]. This has led to much interest in alternate treatment modalities to improve survival.

As a prospective study, we randomly assigned a number of patients undergoing pancreatic resection for pancreatic ductal carcinoma into two groups. Group A ($n = 30$) patients were treated by pancreatic resection alone; group B ($n = 30$) patients received pancreatic resection plus adjuvant locoregional immunochemotherapy. Patients with extended subtotal pancreatic resection were included in the study, while patients undergoing total pancreatectomy were excluded. This chapter presents our results and discusses the pros and cons of adjuvant locoregional immunochemotherapy as a supplementary procedure to pancreatic resection for pancreatic ductal carcinoma.

[1] Department of Surgery, Atheneon Hospital, GR-116 34, Athens, Greece.
[2] Department of Radiology, Athens General Hospital, GR-154 52, Athens, Greece.

Material and Methods

From February 1992 to March 1996, 60 patients with a diagnosis of pancreatic duct carcinoma underwent pancreatic resection at the Greek National Cancer Institute and the Atheneon Hospital in Athens. On admission, all patients underwent a screening investigation that included chest X-rays, upper-abdominal computed tomography, endoscopic retrograde cholangiopancreatography (ERCP), and blood tests for hematocrit (Ht), hemoglobin (Hb), white blood cell count (WBC), glucose, urea-creatinine, serum glutamic oxaloacetic transaminase (SGOT), serum glutamic pyruvic transaminase (SGPT), gamma-glucose transaminase (γ-GT), alkaline phosphatase, bilirubin, total serum protein albumin, globulin ratio, and serum levels of carcinoembryonic antigen (CEA), CA 19-9, and CA50.

A standard operative procedure was carried out in all patients. The method of choice was extended subtotal pancreatectomy with regional lymphodenectomy of the celiac axis, the hepatoduodenal ligament, and the superior mesenteric vessels [1]. Patients were assigned randomly into two groups by the anesthetist, who drew an envelope immediately after the operation.

The clinical characteristics, sex and age ratios, disease stage, pathological findings, and presence of multi-drug resistance protein per patient and per group are shown in Tables 1 and 2. Group A ($n = 30$) patients were to receive only pancreatic resection, while group B ($n = 30$) patients were treated with pancreatic resection supplemented with combined locoregional immunochemotherapy. Group B patients had two arterial catheters implanted: one via the splenic artery, after its ligation near the origin at the celiac axis and directed toward the spleen, and the second catheter into a side arterial branch of the middle colic artery into the superior mesenteric artery. The specially designed catheters (Jet Port Arterial Catheter, PFM, Germany) were placed under angiographic control using selective digital angiography (Fig. 1). The locoregional immunostimulation regime was given 5 days transplenically via the splenic artery catheter and 5 days transarterially via the superior messenteric artery catheter into the region of the resected pancreatic head and the ancinate process.

TABLE 1. Clinical characteristics of 60 pancreatic resection patients with pancreatic duct carcinoma

Characteristic	Group A ($n = 30$)	Group B ($n = 30$)
Age (years)		
Range	30–81	35–80
Median	61	60
Male	17	18
Female	13	12
Pain	11	10
Previous surgery	8	9
A-Glycoprotein		
MDRG (+)	21	22
MDRG (−)	9	8
Jaundice	6	8
Malaise	17	18
Weight loss	21	22

MDRG, multi-drug resistance protein.

TABLE 2. Operative and pathological findings

Finding	Group A ($n = 30$)	Group B ($n = 30$)
Stage		
I	2	1
II	7	9
III	21	20
Grade differentiation		
Well	5	6
Middle	7	8
Poor	18	16
Vascular involvement	5	7
Lymph nodes (+)	21	24
Tumor size		
>4 cm	18	20
<4 cm	12	10

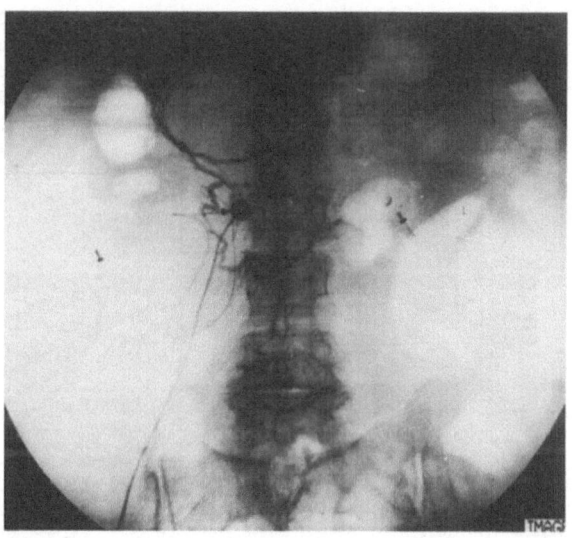

FIG. 1. Placement of arterial catheters under selective digital angiography

Fifteen days after pancreatic resection, all group B patients underwent 10 daily courses of locoregional targeting immunostimulation using a standard immunostimulation regimen (Table 3) emulsified in Lipiodol-Urografin. Fifteen days later, a bolus locoregional chemotherapeutical regimen (Table 4) was administered, again suspended in a Lipiodol-Urografin emulsion. Locoregional immunotherapy was administered only by way of the splenic artery; however, during the late venous phase the immunotherapeutical drug also reached the liver (Fig. 2). Two days later an upper-abdominal computed tomography was performed together with blood screening tests for Ht, Hb, WBC, glucose, urea-creatinine, SGOT, SGPT, γ-GT, alkaline phosphatase, bilirubin, total serum protein albumin, globulin ratio, and serum levels of CEA, CA 19-9, and CA50, in all group B patients.

This sequence of combined locoregional immunochemotherapy was carried out every 3 months during the first postoperative year and every 4 months during the

TABLE 3. Standard immunochemotherapeutical regimen

Therapy	Component	Dosage
Immunostimulation	18×10^6 Proleukin IL-2 emulsified in 2 ml Lipiodol	1 ml
	Urografin 58%	0.5 ml
Chemotherapy	Mitomycin-C	0.2 mg/kg body weight
	cis-Platinum	50 mg/m^2 body surface area
	5-Fluorouracil	10 mg/kg body weight
	Leukovorin	3 mg/kg body weight

TABLE 4. Side effects and sequelae from immunochemotherapy and from use of arterial catheters in group B patients ($n = 30$)

Symptoms	Number of patients
Fever	28
Chills	26
Malaise	14
Anemia	3
Port infection	2
Catheter obstruction	1

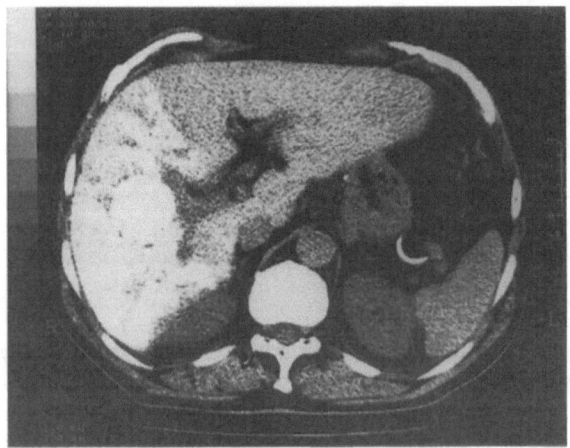

FIG. 2. Immunotherapeutic drug reaches the liver during the late venous phase

second and third postoperative years. The therapy was then given twice during the fifth postoperative year. Treatment was interrupted in cases of serious side effects. All patient data from both groups were controlled at every sixth month. Findings of this checkup were recorded. Statistical analysis was carried out using the χ^2 test, and Kaplan–Meier survival curves were calculated.

Results

Operative deaths, two patients in group A and one patient in group B, were excluded. Surviving patients did well, and there was no difference in terms of postoperative quality of life between patients of group A and those of group B. Sequelae and side effects from the clinical application of locoregional targeting immunochemotherapy were mild, and complications from use of arterial catheters were minimal see (Table 4).

Group B patients had a significantly longer time of survival (27 months) compared to group A patients (17 months) (Tables 5 and 6; $P < .001$). It is interesting that at the time of this writing more patients from group B are alive than from group A (90% of group B versus 60% of group A). Furthermore, a striking difference is seen in stage III patients. Only 10 group A patients of 21 (48%) are still alive, versus 17 of 20 (85%) group B patients (Tables 5 and 6). Additionally, median survival for patients who are still living was 16 months for group A patients versus 28 months for group B patients ($P < .001$). For patients who have already died, median postoperative survival time was 11 months for group A versus 22 months for group B ($P < .001$).

In addition, the presence of the multi-drug resistance gene (MDRG), detected in all patients, was associated with a poorer prognosis for patients of Group A. Indeed, only 8 of 21 patients of group A tested positive for the MDRG are currently alive, with a median survival of 14 months. Patients who have already died had a median survival of 12 months. In contrast, of the 22 group B patients with a positive test for MDRG, 19 are alive with a median survival of 27 months ($P < .001$); the 3 patients who have died had a median survival time of 24 months.

Grading of the tumor, size of the tumor, and presence of positive lymph nodes were seen to be very important factors affecting overall survival in group A patients but not in group B patients (see Tables 5 and 6). It is impressive that of 21 group A patients

TABLE 5. Postoperative survival of group A patients with pancreatic duct carcinoma

| | Patients who are still alive | | Patients who have died | | |
Characteristic	n	Survival in months	n	Survival in months	Total (n)
Stage					
I	2	28	—	—	2
II	5	21	2	14	7
III	10	16	11	11	21
MRDG					
(+)	8	14	22	12	30
(−)	8	20	1	16	9
Differentiation					
Well	5	19	—	—	5
Medium	5	16	2	12	7
Poor	7	14	11	12	18
Tumor size					
<4 cm	7	17	11	14	18
>4 cm	10	14	2	14	12
Lymph nodes					
(+)	8	13	13	11	21
(−)	9	18	—	—	9

(−) Means negative.

TABLE 6. Postoperative survival of group B patients with pancreatic duct carcinoma

	Patients who are still alive		Patients who have died		
Characteristic	n	Survival in months	n	Survival in months	Total (n)
Stage					
I	1	40	—	—	1
II	9	30	2	14	9
III	17	28	3	22	20
MRDG					
(+)	19	27	3	24	22
(−)	8	28	—	—	8
Differentiation					
Well	6	28	—	—	6
Medium	8	27	—	—	8
Poor	13	28	3	24	16
Tumor size					
<4 cm	17	28	3	24	20
>4 cm	10	28	—	—	10
Lymph nodes					
(+)	21	29	3	24	24
(−)	6	31	—	—	6

with lymph node involvement, only 8 are alive at present, versus 21 alive of a total of 24 group B patients with positive lymph nodes ($P < .001$). Of the 13 patients of group A who have died, 11 had local recurrence of their tumor; in the other 2 patients, the disease was disseminated (lung metastasis, peritoneal carcinomatosis, and liver secondaries). Of the 3 patients of group B who have died, 1 had local recurrence and the 2 remaining patients had lung metastases.

Discussion

This study revealed clearly that locoregional immunochemotherapy as an adjuvant therapy for patients undergoing subtotal pancreatectomy for pancreatic duct carcinoma is desirable, useful, effective, and safe. A number of recent publications demonstrate the feasibility of locoregional combined immunochemotherapy using a Lipidiol-Urografin emulsion as a carrier for both the immuno- and chemotherapeutical drugs [2–4]. The fact that Lipiodol-Urografin droplets are an ideal carrier of fat- and water-soluble substances and are retained exclusively in the vascular network of the organ space occupied by the tumor has been clearly demonstrated [5]. This therapy is desirable because, as shown by the current data, it is associated with optimal results for patients with advanced pancreatic duct carcinoma, a large proportion of whom (70%) are found in stage III of their disease. For these patients resectional pancreatic surgery offers only limited survival even after the most aggressive, radical, and extensive types of surgical resection [1,2].

The therapy is useful because it is, at least at the time of this writing, the most effective way of controlling the high incidence of locoregional disease recurrence of advanced pancreatic duct carcinoma. It is also effective because, as shown from the results of this prospective randomized study, the therapy is associated with significantly higher and longer survival times compared to conventional resectional pancreatic surgery for patients suffering from stage III pancreatic duct carcinoma, including those patients seen with the multi-drug resistance gene, positive lymph nodes, and tumors more than 4 cm in diameter. By using locoregional combined immunochemotherapy, we could achieve impressive results regarding survival even for patients with positive lymph nodes, or with poorly differentiated adenocarcinomas, or for tumor sizes greater than 4 cm. Further, locoregional combined immunochemotherapy is safe because it has been carried out with a minimum of side effects and complications as well as with a good quality of posttreatment life.

Pancreatic cancer is a disease diagnosed almost universally at an advanced stage [1]. Unquestionably, patients with an advanced stage (stage III) have limited chances for long-term survival even after the most extensive surgical resections [6]. With regard to today's accepted treatment possibilities, this study opens new horizons of hope for patients with advanced disease. Combined locoregional targeting immunochemotherapy should therefore be considered a new therapeutical adjuvant treatment to resectional pancreatic surgery. The therapy is safe, effective, useful, and desirable.

References

1. Lygidakis NJ, Ziras N, Kyparidou E, Parissis J, et al (1995) Combined immuno-pharmaceutical therapy of patients with unresectable pancreatic carcinoma. Hepato-Gastroenterology 42:1039–1052
2. Lygidakis NJ (1995) New frontiers in oncology. Hepato-Gastroenterology 42:432–437
3. Lygidakis NJ, et al (1995) Resection versus resection combined with adjuvant pre- and post-operative chemotherapy immunotherapy for metastatic colorectal liver cancer. A new look to an old problem. Hepato-Gastroenterology 42:155–161
4. Johnson R (1995) Pancreatic cancer. Hepato-Gastroenterology 42:294–297
5. Lygidakis NJ, et al (1996) Locoregional chemotherapy versus locoregional combined immunochemotherapy for patients with advanced metastatic liver disease of colorectal origin. A prospective randomized study. Hepato-Gastroenterology 43:212–220
6. Lygidakis NJ, et al (1995) Pancreatic head carcinoma: is pancreatic resection indicated for patients with stage III pancreatic duct cancer? Hepato-Gastroenterology 42:587–596

Experience and Problems of Pylorus-Preserving Pancreatoduodenectomy

Zhao Yupei, Cai Lixing, Zhong Shouxian, and Zhu Yu

Summary. Seventy-eight patients with neoplasm (74 cases) or pancreatitis (4 cases) were treated with pylorus-preserving pancreatoduodenectomy (PPPD) from 1984 to 1994. One postoperative death occurred. Follow-up studies were performed in 35 patients who had been treated by PPPD or the standard Whipple procedure beyond 1 year post operation; they were questioned carefully concerning clinical symptoms. Further studies were performed in 20 patients with or without pylorus preservation (10 patients each). Nutritional status and gastrointestinal digestive and absorptive function were evaluated by determination of serum components, gastric analysis, barium emptying time, D-xylose absorptive test, CO_2 breath test, p-aminobenzoic acid (PABA), and other methods. The results demonstrated malnutrition and postgastrectomy syndromes in some patients after the conventional Whipple procedure, but not in those with PPPD; the quality of life was better in the latter. Pylorus preservation may be the main reason for this difference. Delayed gastric emptying in the early postoperative period was a complication in some patients (22%). We recommend PPPD for pancreatoduodenectomy.

Key words. Pylorus-preserving—Pancreatoduodenectomy—Delayed gastric emptying—Quality of life—Digestive function

Introduction

As a component of pancreatoduodenectomy (Whipple's procedure), partial gastrectomy was designed to prevent postoperative jejunal ulceration and to contribute to the radical cure of cancer [1], although it may induce a series of complications. In 1978, a method of pylorus-preserving pancreatoduodenectomy (PPPD) was invented by Traverse and Longmire [2] to preserve the normal physiological function of the stomach and pylorus, avoid postoperative complications, reduce operative trauma, and help the patient to recover. During the past 14 years, this method has been increasingly adopted [3].

Department of Surgery, Peking Union Medical College Hospital, Beijing 100730, China.

It is important to evaluate this variation in pancreatoduodenectomy to determine whether its promise of improved gastrointestinal function is realized and to document its effect on cancer survival and postoperative morbidity and mortality, as well as the incidence of jejunal ulceration, a complication that has plagued the standard Whipple procedure. In an earlier report [4], we documented our preliminary results with this operation. We report here on more patients and a systematic follow-up study.

Materials and Methods

From 1984 through 1994, 78 patients underwent PPPD in our hospital, including 43 men and 35 women. Their ages ranged from 32 to 78 years, with a median of 59 years. The diagnosis was neoplasm in 74 patients and chronic pancreatitis in 4 (Table 1).

Patients with chronic pancreatitis selected for operation had lateralization of advanced disease to the head of the pancreas, had appreciable alteration of life-style because of the disease, required narcotic agents to control pain, and had masses undistinguishable from cancer. In patients with adenocarcinoma of the pancreas and ampullar region, PPPD, like the standard pancreatoduodenectomy, was carried out if the initial dissection and preoperative selected angiography (SAG) of celiac and superior mesenteric artery demonstrated no serious invasion of the portal vein, superior mesenteric vein, or hepatic artery, and if the result of fine-needle aspiration cytodiagnosis from the mass was positive. On anastomosis of the pancreas stump and jejunum, we improved on the routine end-to-end pancreaticojejunostomy or end-to-side pancreaticojejunostomy to pancreaticojejunostomy with the invagination of the pancreatic stump, by invaginating the end-to-end anastomotic stoma into the jejunum (Fig. 1). For duodenojejunostomy below the pylorus, we adopted the improved Zheng's mode of Roux-en-Y-type anastomosis (Fig. 2).

Follow-up studies were performed in 35 patients treated by PPPD or the standard Whipple procedure after 1 year post operation (18 and 17 patients, respectively). Patients were questioned carefully concerning weight loss, nausea and vomiting, postprandial satiety, diarrhea, and food intake. Further studies were performed in 20 patients with or without pylorus preservation (10 patients each). Nutritional status was evaluated by determination of serum iron protein, albumin, iron, vitamin A, and vitamin D. Gastric secretion was evaluated by gastric analysis and serum gastrin determination. Gastrointestinal motility was assessed by barium emptying time, while

TABLE 1. Diagnosis in 78 patients with pylorus-preserving pancreaticoduodenectomy (PPPD) (1984–1994)

Diagnosis	Number	Percentage
Ampullar adenocarcinoma	56	72
Pancreatic head adenocarcinoma	9	12
Bile duct adenocarcinoma	4	5
Duodenal adenocarcinoma	5	6
Chronic pancreatitis	4	5
Total	78	100

Patients included 43 men and 35 women, aged 32–78 years (average, 59 years).

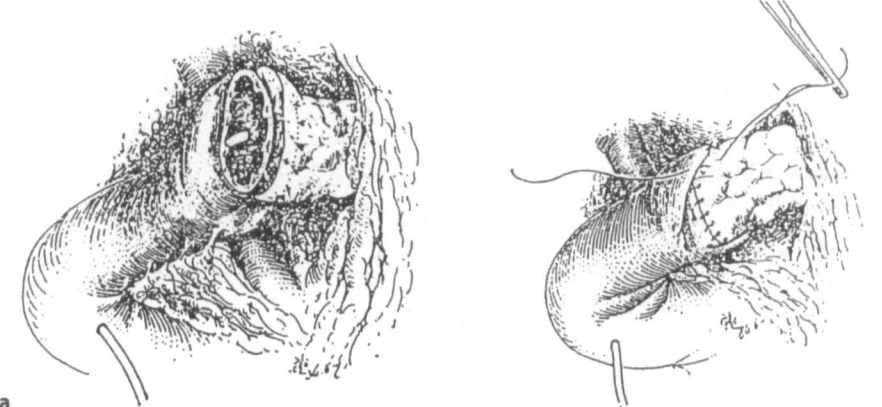

a   b

FIG. 1. **a** Lateral anastomosis between broken pancreatic end and jejunal side wall. An opening was made on the jejunal wall and anastomosed with pancreatic duct. **b** End-to-end anastomosis between broken pancreatic and jejunal end; the anterior lip was sutured to the anterior border of the broken surface of the pancreas and then encased into the intestinal cavity

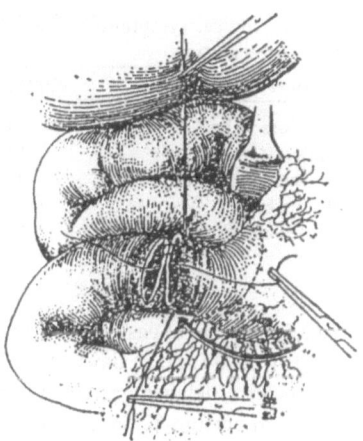

FIG. 2. Improved duodenojejunostomy of Roux-en-Y type

intestinal absorption was assessed by the D-xylose absorptive test. Fat absorption and exocrine function of the pancreas were studied by the $^{14}CO_2$ breath test, p-aminobenzoic acid (PABA), and fecal fat evaluation.

Results

Seventy-eight pancreatoduodenectomy procedures with pylorus and gastric preservation were accomplished. One patient died of postoperative complications as the result of massive brain embolism on the tenth postoperative day. Postoperative complications are detailed in Table 2. By far the commonest was transient delayed gastric emptying, defined as requiring gastric suction for more than 10 days after operation. This delay in gastric emptying was experienced by about 22% of patients in whom the

TABLE 2. Postoperative complications after PPPD

Complication	Number	Percentage
Pneumonitis with fever	3	3.8
Pancreatic fistula	1	1.3
Biliary fistula	1	1.3
Abdominal abscess	1	1.3
Brain embolism (dead)	1	1.3
Delayed gastric emptying (average, 16 days; longest, 41 days)[a]	17	22.0
Total	24	29.0

[a] Gastric suction required for more than 10 days.

TABLE 3. X-Ray manifestation in 15 of 17 patients with delayed gastric emptying

X-Ray manifestations	Number	Percentage
Increase in gastric volume	3	17
Slow barium passing the anastomosis	3	17
Gastric hypoperistalsis with fluid level	9	66

TABLE 4. Clinical symptoms beyond 1 year post operation in 35 patients with or without pylorus preservation

Symptoms	PPPD (18 cases)	Standard Whipple's (17 cases)	P value
Weight loss >5 kg	1 (6%)	9 (53%)	<.01
Postprandial satiety	1 (6%)	2 (12%)	>.05
Postprandial diarrhea	0 (0)	6 (35%)	<.01
Vomiting bile	0 (0)	5 (29%)	<.01
Increased bowel movements	1 (6%)	8 (47%)	<.01

median duration of gastric suction was to the sixteenth postoperative day; the longest periods were 39 and 41 days. Gastric emptying and pylorus function in 15 (88%) of 17 patients with delayed gastric emptying were observed via an upper gastrointestinal series with barium 10 days post operation (Table 3). The problems were successfully resolved in all patients by fasting, gastrointestinal decompression, and intravenous feeding; 13 with jejunostomy were fed with a mixture of milk and bean powder 1 week after operation, and maintained ideal nutritional status. The clinical symptoms are listed in Table 4. A systematic comparison of nutrition and digestive function between the 10 patients with PPPD and the 10 patients with routine pancreatoduodenectomy is presented in Table 5.

The following test results were obtained an average of 15 and 17 months post operation (range, 12–27 and 14–31 months), respectively. The results showed that gastrointestinal emptying during a gastrointestinal series using barium were normal in all patients with PPPD, but that patients treated by routine methods showed rapid gastrointestinal emptying ($P < .01$). Gastric analysis yielded normal achlorhydria results in all patients with PPPD, with a basal acid mean output and maximum acid mean output (BAO/MAO) of 2.57/8.25 mEq/h; however, in those patients treated by routine methods BAO/MAO was .25/1.62 mEq/h ($P < .01$). The concentrations of serum gastrin and iron protein were normal in all patients with PPPD, but in patients

TABLE 5. Analysis of gastrointestinal functions in 20 patients with or without pylorus preservation

Examination	PPPD (10 cases)	Standard Whipple's (10 cases)	P value
Gastric analysis			
BAO (mEq/h)	2.57	0.25	<.01
MAO (mEq/h)	8.28	1.62	<.01
Serum gastrin (pg/ml)	115.2	29.7	<.01
Gastric emptying (min)	50.5	10.7	<.01
Intestinal transit (min)	284	161	<.01
Serum iron (µg/100 ml)	179.9	155.4	>.05
Serum iron protein (ng/ml)	39.09	16.6	<.05
Vitamin A (µg/dl)	48.9	42.9	>.05
Vitamin E (µg/dl)	492.4	474.2	>.05
D-Xylose absorptive test (g/5 h)	1.3	1.4	>.05
Urine PABA (%)	55.6	57.4	>.05
CO breath test	0.43	0.21	<.05

BAO, Basal acid mean output; MAO, maximum acid mean output; PABA, p-ammobenzoic acid.

with standard pancreatoduodenectomy the results were 29.7 pg/ml and 16.6 ng/ml, significantly lower than normal ($P < .01$). The results obtained from gastroscopy demonstrated that three patients (30%) with routine pancreatoduodenectomy suffered from enterogastric reflux gastritis.

Pancreatic exocrine function was found to be abnormal in all patients, with or without pylorus preservation. Although the results of PABA and the $^{14}CO_2$ breath test were markedly abnormal in both groups of patients, the extent of fat malabsorption was more evident in those patients with routine pancreatoduodenectomy. The results of the D-xylose absorptive test were normal in all patients.

Discussion

Traverse and Longmire initially performed PPPD in two patients. Of 400 PPPD operations reported by overseas experts since 1978, 49% suffered from chronic pancreatitis, while 54% had malignant tumors of the pancreas or ampulla. Doubts have been raised as to the advisability of performing the PPPD for malignant diseases in the periampullary area, as the field of resection may be reduced and survival thereby compromised [5,6]. Moossa [7] has argued that the pylorus preservation procedure is not applicable to cancer of the head of the pancreas or distal common bile duct tumors because it may compromise the only chance of cure in these patients. Sharp and his colleagues [5] have also reported tumor recurrence at the duodenal suture line. However, Newsman and associates [8] have observed that the other resection margins in pancreatoduodenectomy are much closer to the tumor than to the duodenum and antrum. Performing frozen section of the duodenal resection margin should help minimize this problem. Therefore, leaving the antrum, pylorus, and first few centimeters of the duodenum is not likely to compromise the field of resection.

Of 78 PPPD operations conducted in our hospital since 1984, 95% were for malignant diseases and 5% were for chronic pancreatitis (see Table 1). The pathological report showed that all duodenal samples cut from the incisal margin were negative. Research on the samples of 64 cases of carcinoma of the head of the pancreas treated by standard pancreatoduodenectomy showed no neoplastic invasion of the nearby pylorus and lymph nodes. However, considering the high tendency of malignancy of pancreatic head cancer and the possibility of easy transfer to lymph nodes, pylorus preservation would affect radical clearing of lymph nodes around the pylorus. Therefore, we only administered the PPPD method to patients with smaller carcinoma of the pancreatic head.

As with routine pancreatoduodenectomy, the possibility of excision was evaluated first to determine whether large vessels were invaded by preoperative selective angiography (SAG) of the celiac artery and superior mesenteric artery. Nerves and vessels to the pylorus and first part of the duodenum and right gastric artery, especially the gastroepiploic vessels to the greater curvature of the stomach and branches of the vagus nerve to the gastric antrum and pylorus, were imaged; injuries of these nervous branches would induce postoperative functional disorder of gastric emptying.

In 1980, we replaced the routine end-to-end pancreaticojejunostomy or end-to-side pancreaticojejunostomy with invagination of the pancreatic stump, namely by invaginating the end-to-end anastomotic stoma into the jejunum. This improvement reduced the incidence of pancreatic fistula to 2.5% from 15.2%. Another advantage of this method is that it ensures an unobstructed pancreatic duct and serous coats coat (Fig. 1).

For duodenojejunostomy below the pylorus, we adopted the improved Zheng's mode of Roux-en-Y type, making a transverse incision on the jejunal wall, expanding the sphincter before anastomosis, and setting the anastomotic stoma beneath the transverse mesocolon. Preservation of the jejunal circular muscle and its contractive function decreased the occurrence of gastric emptying disorder and anastomotic ulceration. The valve formed by this method could prevent chyme from returning to the jejunal cavity above the anastomotic stoma, thus avoiding infection of the bile duct (Fig. 2).

It is important to note that operative time is shortened with pyloric and gastric preservation because gastric resection and a large gastrojejunal anastomosis need not be carried out. Anastomosis of the duodenum to the jejunum is relatively simple and quickly accomplished. Pancreatoduodenectomy with preservation of the pylorus simplifies the operation, reduces the chance of operative trauma, and saves at least 30 min of operative time.

Routine pancreatoduodenectomy can result in the sequelae of bile regurgitational gastritis, dumping syndrome, diarrhea, and loss of body weight, because it removes most of the stomach, affects the function of the pylorus, and decreases the storage volume of the stomach. Preserving the pylorus maintains the integrity of the stomach and pylorus and the normal functions of gastric secretion and emptying, greatly decreasing the occurrence of complications and helping to maintain nutrition. The follow-up results in our study demonstrated that patients treated by the routine method had significantly lower gastrin, iron, basal acid output (BAO), and maximum acid output (MAO), and faster gastrointestinal emptying, with 30% suffering from enterogastric reflux gastritis and anastomotic inflammation. Patients treated by the PPPD method had normal secretion of gastrin, iron, BAO/MAO, and gastrointestinal emptying, and no regurgitational gastritis was found in these patients. Patients with and without pylorus preservation in our study achieved a median of 99% and 88% of pre-illness weight and 106% and 97% of preoperative weight, respectively. Unfortunately, all these patients suffered from decreased external secretion of the pancreas, and therefore treatment of pancreatic dysfunction is very important.

The main complication of the improved method was delayed gastric emptying in the early period after the operation; the patients could not eat liquid meals within 10 days after the operation. In 1990, Grace et al. [3] reviewed 288 cases of PPPD patients and concluded that the incidence of transient delayed gastric emptying was 27.1%. There was no satisfactory explanation for this delayed emptying. It was considered that poor blood supply to the preserved duodenum, trauma of the pylorus and Latarjet nerve, and removal of the duodenal pacemaker might contribute to delayed gastric emptying.

Of the 78 cases with preserved pylorus in our study, the incidence of delayed gastric emptying was 22%. With fasting, gastrointestinal decompression, and intravenous feeding, all the patients recovered successfully. Of these, 13 with jejunostomy were fed a mixture of milk and eggs or homogenate 1 week after operation and maintained an ideal nutrition condition. The patients who received an artificial gastric fistula also recovered satisfactorily, although they suffered delayed gastric emptying.

Considering the disadvantages of the artificial gastric fistula such as increase of operative time, operative trauma, complications, and delayed gastric emptying in one-fifth of patients, we recently have used only an artificial jejunal fistula in patients with preserved pylorus. If the gastric drainage was required more than 1 week after operation, a flexible silica gel tube with a diameter of .3 cm was used for gastrointestinal decompression instead of the common gastric tube. Experimental application of the silica gel tube in 14 patients showed satisfactory decompression. Combined with artificial jejunostomy, gastrointestinal feeding helped the patients overcome gastric emptying. Therefore, dysfunction of the stomach was recoverable if properly treated.

Delayed gastric emptying was prevented by the following: (1) preservation of the nerves and nervous branches of Lartarjet and blood supply to the lesser curvature of the stomach; (2) preservation of the duodenum 1.5 cm below the pylorus and expansion of the pylorus by hand; and (3) avoidance of damage to the pylorus sphincter during anastomosis.

In brief, we recommend PPPD for pancreatoduodenectomy, because the prognosis of the patient is not liable to be negatively affected.

References

1. Whipple AO, et al (1935) Treatment of carcinoma of the ampulla of Vater. Ann Surg 102:763
2. Traverso LW, Longmire WP Jr (1978) Preservation of the pylorus in pancreatoduodenectomy. Surg Gynecol Obstet 146:959
3. Grace PA, et al (1990) Pylorus-preserving pancreatoduodenectomy: an overview. Br J Surg 77:968
4. Zhao YP, et al (1988) Effect of pylorus preservation on nutrition and digestive function after pancreaticoduodenectomy: a follow-up observation. Clin J Surg 12:725
5. Sharp KW, et al (1989) Pancreatoduodenectomy with pyloric preservation for carcinoma of the pancreas: a cautionary note. Surgery (St Louis) 105:645
6. Hayes DH, et al (1987) Carcinoma of the ampulla of Vater. Ann Surg 2:572
7. Moossa AR, et al (1982) Pancreatic cancer. Approach to diagnosis, selection for surgery and choice of operation. Cancer (Phila) 50:2689
8. Newsman KD, et al (1983) Pyloric and gastric preservation with pancreatoduodenectomy. Am J Surg 145:152

Three Decades of Progress in Surgery for Primary Liver Cancer

Xin-Da Zhou, Zhao-You Tang, and Ye-Qin Yu

Summary. This chapter reports the progress of surgery in the treatment of 2388 patients with pathologically proven primary liver cancer (PLC) during the past three decades. The 5- and 10-year survival rates after resection of PLC were 39.3% and 29.2%, respectively, for the whole series ($n = 1650$), and 61.9% and 45.4%, respectively, for patients with small PLC ($\leq$ 5cm). The 5-year survival rate after cryosurgery was 37.9% for the whole series ($n = 191$) and 53.1% for patients with small PLC ($n = 56$). The 5-year survival of 71 patients receiving sequential resection after cytoreduction therapy was 66.0%, and the 5-year survival after reresection for recurrence of tumor ($n = 147$) was 34.5%. Of 214 patients who survived more than 5 years, 113 patients (52.8%) had a small PLC, and 57 patients survived more than 10 years. Encouraging changes in the prognostic pattern were observed when the PLC data of 1958–1970 ($n = 178$), 1971–1982 ($n = 582$), and 1983–1994 ($n = 1628$) were compared, the 5-year survival rates being 4.8%, 11.2%, and 45.7%, respectively, and the 10-year survival rates being 4.2%, 7.5%, and 33.0%, respectively. Some aspects to prolong survival further are discussed.

Key words. Liver tumor—Resection—Cryosurgery

Introduction

Primary liver cancer (PLC) is one of the world's commonest malignant neoplasms. It is most prevalent in southeast Asia and portions of Africa, and is a relatively rare malignancy in the Western world. Parkin et al. (1993) reported that in 1985 the total number of new PLC patients in the world was 315 000; among them, 137 500 (43.7%) occurred in China [1]. In China, PLC was the leading cancer killer in rural areas and has ranked second in the cities since the 1990s [2]. PLC has been considered an incurable disease for several decades. In 1974, 3254 cases of PLC in China were analyzed: the proportion of late-stage patients with jaundice or ascites was extremely high (52.6%), the resection rate was extremely low (5.3%), and ultimate outcome (1-

Liver Cancer Institute, Shanghai Medical University, Shanghai 200032, China.

year survival, 8.6%) was dismal [3]. During the past 20 years, however, rapid progress has been made in clinical research of PLC. Based on the advances of early detection of subclinical PLC, the growing knowledge regarding the biological basis of surgical oncology, and the introduction of new surgical techniques and development of new surgical modalities, the role of surgery for PLC has become more important [4–6]. The only effective treatment for PLC is surgical resection. Furthermore, reoperation for subclinical liver recurrence or solitary pulmonary metastasis after a radical resection seems acceptable with further prolongation of survival [7,8]. Moreover, multi-modality palliative surgery and new modality treatment have provided an opportunity to convert nonresectable to resectable PLC [9–11]. Thus, overall PLC prognosis has progressed. In this chapter, the analysis of 2388 patients with pathologically proven PLC in the period 1958–1994 will help to reflect the progress of surgery in the treatment of PLC. Some aspects to improve long-term survival are discussed.

Materials and Methods

Between January 1958 and December 1994, a total of 2388 patients with pathologically proven PLC were admitted to the Zhong Shan Hospital of Shanghai Medical University. The median age of the entire series was 48 years (range, 12–82 years), and the male:female ratio was 8.1:1. Criteria for clinical staging were arbitrarily defined as follows: stage I (subclinical), without obvious PLC symptoms or signs; stage II (moderate), between the criteria for stages I and III; and stage III (late), with obvious cachexia, jaundice, ascites, or distant metastases). In this series, the subclinical stage accounted for 29.1% (695/2388), moderate stage for 61.7% (1473/2388), and the late stage, 9.2% (220/2388). There were 613 cases with small PLC (≤5 cm). Histological findings revealed that hepatocellular carcinoma (HCC) amounted to 97.4% (2327/2388), cholangiocarcinoma, 1.3% (31/2388), and mixed type, 1.3% (30/2388). Single-nodule tumors amounted to 61.3%.

Liver disease background was noted as follows. Patients with hepatitis history were 48.6% (1155/2377); of these, 87.7% (1013/1155) had a hepatitis history of more than 5 years; those with coexistent liver cirrhosis, 87.5% (2037/2327); those with macronodular cirrhosis, 74.6% (1519/2037); and those patients with micronodular cirrhosis, 25.4% (518/2037). Positivity of serum hepatitis B surface antigen (HBsAg) was 78.7% (1825/2319). However, positivity of serum anti-HCV was only 8.3% (31/376).

The serum concentration of alpha-fetoprotein (AFP) was abnormal (>20 ng/ml, by immunoassay) in 67.2% (794/1181) of the patients tested. Of the entire series, resection was done in 1650 patients (69.1%), and curative resection in 1361 patients (82.5%). Curative resection refers to complete removal of the tumor, with no macroscopically identified tumor emboli in the portal vein, and no tumor residue in the remaining liver tissue or in the cut surface. Palliative surgery other than resection, including cryosurgery, hepatic artery ligation (HAL), hepatic artery cannulation and infusion (HAI), laser vaporization, or microwave coagulation, etc., was performed for 620 patients (26.0%). Conservative treatment was given to 73 patients (3.1%), and no treatment was given to 45 patients (1.9%) in early years.

Reresection for recurrent or metastatic lesions (mainly for subclinical recurrence or solitary pulmonary metastasis) after an initial curative resection was performed in 155 patients.

"Cytoreduction and sequential resection" was arbitrary defined as surgically verified, unresectable, huge PLC; this was treated with palliative surgery such as hepatic artery ligation and infusion chemotherapy with or without radiotherapy as the first step; resection was done as the second step after marked tumor regression had occurred. In this series, 71 patients received sequential resection.

A microcomputer was used for the storage, analysis, and statistical treatment of clinical data. Survival rates were calculated according to the life table method. Statistical differences were tested by the log rank method.

Results

Comparison Between Small PLC and Large PLC

When compared with large PLC ($n = 1775$), patients with small PLC ($n = 613$) had a higher resection rate (92.8% versus 60.9%; $P < .01$) and a lower operative mortality (1.9% versus 7.9%; $P < .05$). A limited resection (any kind of nonsegment resection) was performed more frequently for patients with small PLC (84.2% versus 56.2%; $P < .05$) (Table 1).

In comparison with those with large PLC, patients with small PLC had a better differentiation of cancer cells (Edmondson's grade III, 9.7% versus 16.0%; $P < .01$), a higher incidence of single-nodule tumor (79.1% versus 53.9%; $P < .01$), a higher

TABLE 1. Type of resection in small PLC and large PLC

Resection	Small PLC (%)	Large PLC (%)
Limited resection[a]	84.2 (479/569)	56.2 (607/1081)
Left lateral segmentectomy	9.5 (54/569)	15.0 (162/1081)
Left hemihepatectomy	5.4 (31/569)	21.8 (236/1081)
Extended left hemihepatectomy	0.2 (1/569)	1.7 (18/1081)
Right hemihepatectomy	0.7 (4/569)	5.0 (54/1081)
Extended right hemihepatectomy	0	0.4 (4/1081)
Resection rate	92.8 (569/613)	60.9 (1081/1775)
Operative mortality	1.9 (11/569)	7.9 (85/1081)

[a] Limited resection is any kind of nonsegment resection.
PLC, primary liver cancer.

TABLE 2. Pathological findings in small PLC and large PLC

Characteristics	Small PLC (%)	Large PLC (%)
Edmondson's grade:		
I	5.8 (28/483)	5.5 (58/1050)
II	84.5 (408/483)	77.8 (817/1050)
III	9.7 (47/483)	16.0 (168/1050)
IV	0	0.7 (7/1050)
Single nodule	79.1 (485/613)	53.9 (795/1474)
Well-encapsulated tumor	73.9 (425/575)	35.8 (451/1260)
Tumor emboli in portal vein	30.0 (157/523)	44.1 (449/1017)

proportion of well-encapsulated tumor (73.9% versus 35.8%; $P < .01$), and fewer tumor emboli in the portal vein (30.0% versus 44.1%; $P < .01$) (Table 2).

The 1-, 3-, 5-, and 10-year survival rates after resection were 87.8%, 73.2%, 61.9%, and 45.5%, respectively, for patients with small PLC ($n = 569$), and 55.1%, 33.8%, 20.4%, and 20.0%, respectively, for the patients who had resection of large PLC ($n = 1081$; $P < .01$).

Hepatic Cryosurgery

Cryosurgery with liquid nitrogen (−196°C) was performed in 191 PLC patients. Hepatic cryosurgery proved to be a safe procedure, involving no deaths or significant complications such as rupture of tumor, secondary bleeding, or bile leakage in this series.

The 1-, 3-, and 5-year survival rates were 74.8%, 50.8%, and 37.9%, respectively, for the 191 PLC patients, and 90.7%, 71.8% and 53.1%, respectively, for the 56 patients with small PLC.

Cytoreduction and Sequential Resection

In this series, 71 patients with surgically verified unresectable PLC received cytoreduction therapy and sequential resection. The median tumor size was 10 cm in diameter at the first operation and 6 cm in diameter at the second operation. The median interval between the first and second operation was 5 months. The 1-, 3-, and 5-year survival rates of these 71 patients were 87.2%, 76.6%, and 66.0%, respectively.

Reresection for Recurrence of PLC

Of the 1650 patients undergoing resection, 147 patients received reresection for recurrent PLC. The 1-, 3-, and 5-year survival rates were 82.6%, 41.1%, and 34.5%, respectively, calculated from the reresection, and 96.9%, 70.8%, and 51.4%, respectively, calculated from the first resection. Eight patients underwent reresection for solitary lung metastasis, the average survival being 9 years (8 months to 17 years and 6 months), calculated from the reresection of metastatic lung cancer, and 11 years and 11 months (1 year and 4 months to 20 years and 7 months), from the first resection. Four patients who underwent reresection of solitary lung metastasis have still survived for 20 years and 7 months, 20 years and 3 months, 20 years and 2 months, and 6 years and 6 months, respectively, after the first operation. One patient has received six operations at different times and is still in good condition (Fig. 1).

Long-Term Survivors

In this series, by the end of December 1994, 214 patients had survived for more than 5 years, 57 of them surviving for more than 10 years. Analysis of treatment modalities of the 214 patients with a 5-year survival revealed that small PLC resection was 53.7% (115/214) and large PLC resection 33.2% (71/214), cytoreduction and sequential resection of unresectable PLC were 7.5% (16/214), and palliative therapy other than resection was 5.6% (12/214). The majority of long-term survivors have returned to their original work, four young patients were married after resection, and some can even play football again.

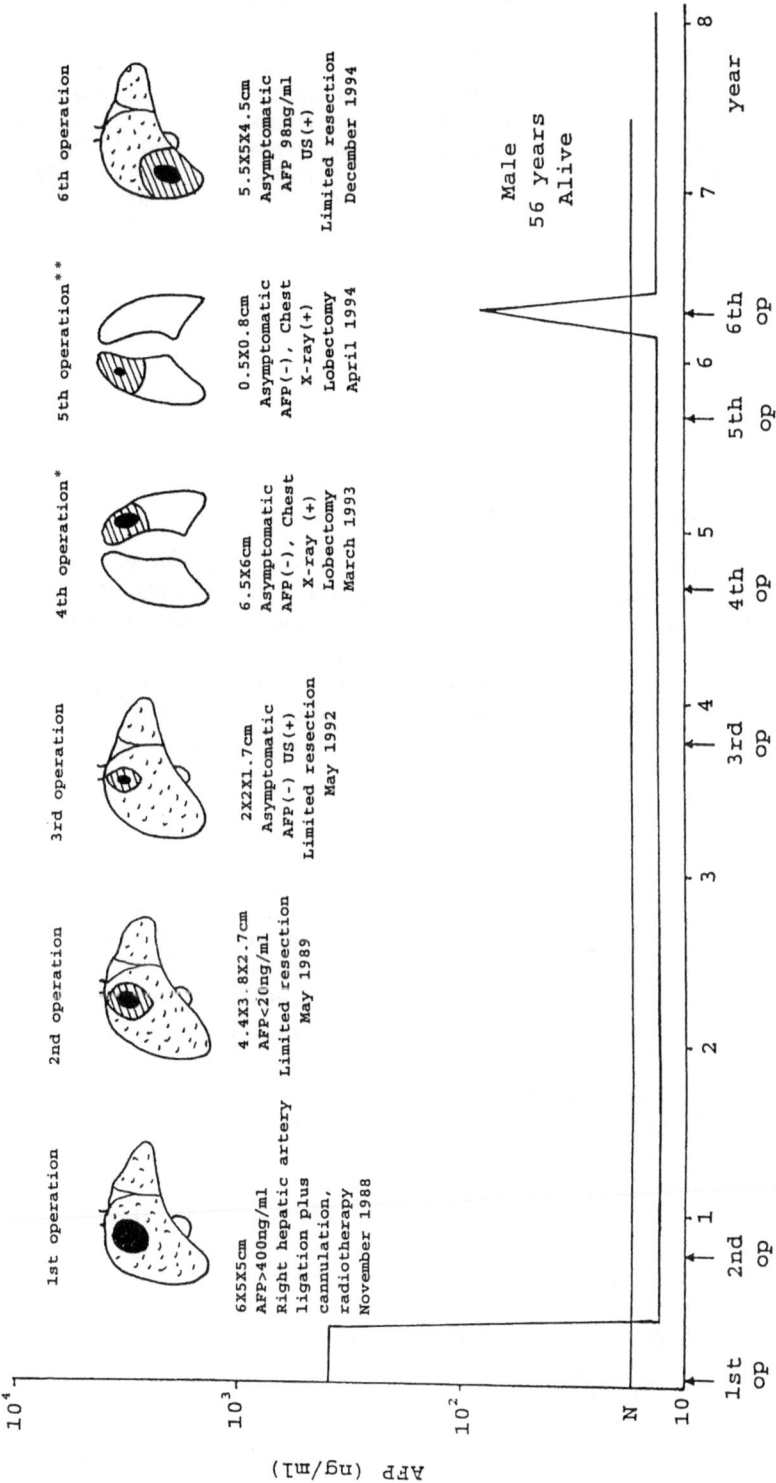

FIG. 1. Cytoreduction and sequential resection and reresection of subclinical recurrence in the liver and solitary pulmonary metastasis. *, Pathologicallly proven primary pulmonary adenocarcinoma; **, pathologically proven secondary pulmonary adenocarcinoma from PLC. *AFP*, alpha-fetoprotein

TABLE 3. Summation data of 2388 PLC patients in three chronological periods

Factor	1958–1970 (n = 178)	1971–1982 (n = 582)	1983–1994 (n = 1628)
Tumor 5 cm or less (%)	2.2 (4/178)	11.5 (67/582)	33.3 (542/1628)
Resection rate (%)	53.9 (96/178)	62.2 (362/582)	73.2 (1192/1628)
Limited resection (%)	37.5 (36/96)	66.0 (239/362)	77.8 (927/1192)
Operative mortality (%)	39.6 (38/96)	7.7 (28/362)	2.5 (30/1192)
Cytoreduction and sequential resection (cases)	0	4	67
Reresection (cases)	0	27	120
Survival (%):			
1 year	13.8	31.4	76.0
3 year	6.6	15.2	55.6
5 year	4.8	11.2	45.7
10 year	4.2	7.5	33.0

Comparing Three Decades of Data

As summarized in Table 3, encouraging changes in the prognostic pattern were observed on comparing the data for 1958–1970, 1971–1982, and 1983–1994. Obviously, the major factor that related to these encouraging results was the markedly increased proportion of small PLC and resection. The markedly increased proportion of limited resections has resulted in decreasing operative mortality. The employment of reresection for recurrent or metastatic lesions and cytoreduction and sequential resection for initially unresectable huge PLC has further improved survival.

Discussion

Patients with small PLC were seldom encountered in symptomatic clinical cases. During 1958–1970, a total of 178 cases with pathologically proven PLC were admitted to our hospital, only 4 (2.2%) being incidentally found to be cases of small PLC. However, the discovery of AFP in 1956 and its detection in the serum of PLC patients has opened a new era for the early detection and early diagnosis of PLC [12,13]. In China, an AFP serosurvey in the natural population was carried out in 1971. In this series, during 1971–1982 the number of cases of small PLC increased to 67, the incidence being 11.5% (67/582). As a result of screening in the high-risk population or regular health checkups for middle-aged persons, using an AFP serosurvey and real-time ultrasonography, the number of cases of small PLC during 1983–1994 remarkably increased to 542, the incidence being 33.3% (542/1628).

Cryosurgery is a treatment in which tumors are frozen and then left in situ to be reabsorbed. We have previously demonstrated the pilot results of cryosurgery as a regional treatment for PLC in experimental systems and in humans [14–18]. Cryosurgery has certain merits in the treatment of PLC [19]: (1) it does not require the resection of large volumes of normal surrounding liver parenchyma; (2) because large blood vessels tolerate freezing extremely well without rupture or occlusion, tumors close to the large blood vessels can be safely treated; (3) because freezing can be applied focally, multiple cancer nodules of the liver can be treated successively; (4) in recurrent cases in which a major liver resection had been performed previously and remaining liver tissue is to small to be resected, cryosurgery allows retreatment of recurrent lesions; (5) cryosurgery is a safe procedure involving no blood loss during operation; and (6) there is some evidence that cryosurgery of a tumor has an added immunological benefit by possibly sensitizing the patient to tumor antigens. It has been reported that 4 of 33 patients treated with cryosurgery for lung metastases showed contralateral regression of tumor. The current study demonstrated that long-term control of liver cancer could be achievable by cryosurgery, the 5-year survival rate being 37.9% for the 191 patients with PLC and 53.1% for the 56 patients with small PLC.

In patients with a huge tumor that is technically difficult to resect, the best way might be to decrease the tumor size as the first step and resect the tumor as the second step. Effective approaches for successful cytoreduction might include hepatic artery ligation and infusion chemotherapy, hepatic arterial chemoembolization, radiotherapy, and radioimmunotherapy. In this series, 71 patients underwent sequential resection after marked regression of the tumor, 5-year survival being 66.0% after resection, which approach may provide hope for the prolongation of survival in some patients with initially unresectable PLC.

At present, the long-term results after resection of PLC are not yet satisfactory, the main reason being the high recurrence rate. As we reported previously, the 1-, 3-, and 5-year recurrence rates after curative resection of PLC were 17.1%, 32.5%, and 61.5%, respectively, reoperation for subclinical recurrence or solitary pulmonary metastasis resulted in a 19.1%, increase (from 47.7% to 66.8%) in 5-year survival after curative resection of PLC [20]. In this series, 155 patients underwent reresection for recurrent PLC or solitary pulmonary metastasis with encouraging results, and this seems to be an important approach for further prolonging survival after curative resection of PLC.

Conclusion

The changing concepts of surgical oncology and innovations of surgical treatment have improved the scope of surgical therapy in the last decade. The remarkable advances seen here in the prognostic patterns appear to result from early detection and resection of smaller asymptomatic PLC, reresection of subclinical recurrence and metastasis, and cytoreduction and sequential resection for originally unresectable tumors.

Cryosurgery is a promising procedure, which may be an effective alternative to liver resection in patients having severe cirrhosis with marginal hepatic function reserve in whom liver resection would be contraindicated. The development of new cryosurgery instrumentation to treat larger and deeper lesions and to treat multiple lesions simultaneously will further extend the role of hepatic cryosurgery. Problems to be studied include the development of more specific treatment for unresectable PLC with uncompensated cirrhosis, and an effective approach for preventing recurrence and metastasis after curative resection.

References

1. Parkin DM, Pisani P, Ferlay J (1993) Estimates of worldwide incidence of eighteen major cancers in 1985. Int J Cancer 54:594–606
2. Center of Health Statistics Information, Ministry of Public Health, Peoples Republic of China (1991) Selected edition on health statistics of China (1978–1990) (in Chinese). Ministry of Public Health, P. R. China, Beijing, pp 78–79

3. Tang ZY, Yang BH (1974) Primary liver cancer—clinical analysis of 3254 cases (from 11 provinces, 21 hospitals, in China) (in Chinese). Cancer Res Prev Treat 2:207–215
4. Tang ZY, Yu YQ, Zhou XD (1986) The changing role of surgery in the treatment of primary liver cancer. Semin Surg Oncol 2:103–112
5. Zhou XD, Yu YQ, Tang ZY, Ma ZC (1994) Results of liver resection for primary liver cancer. J Hepato Biliary Pancr Surg 2:118–122
6. Zhou XD, Yu YQ, Tang ZY (1994) Advances in surgery for hepatocellular carcinoma. Asian J Surg 17:34–39
7. Zhou XD, Tang ZY, Yu YQ, Yang BH, Lu JZ, Lin ZY, Ma ZC, Zhang BH (1994) Recurrence after resection of alpha fetoprotein-positive hepatocellular carcinoma. J Cancer Res Clin Oncol 120:369–373
8. Zhou XD, Yu YQ, Tang ZY, Yang BH, Lu JZ, Lin ZY, Ma ZC, Xu DB, Zhang BH, Zheng YX, Tang CL (1993) Surgical treatment of recurrent hepatocellular carcinoma. Hepato-Gastroenterology 40:333–336
9. Tang ZY, Yu YQ, Zhou XD, Ma ZC, Yang BH, Lin ZY, Lu JZ, Liu KD, Fan Zeng, Zeng ZC (1995) Treatment of unresectable primary liver cancer: with reference to cytoreduction and sequential resection. World J Surg 19:47–52
10. Zhou XD, Tang ZY, Yu YQ (1996) Ablative approach for primary liver cancer. Surg Oncol Clin North Am 5:379–390
11. Zhou XD, Tang ZY, Yu YQ, Yang BH, Lu JZ, Lin ZY, Ma ZC (1995) Multimodality treatment in advanced primary liver cancer. Jpn J Cancer Chemother 22 (suppl III):286–289
12. Tang ZY, Yu YQ, Zhou XD, Yang BH, Ma ZC, Lin ZY (1993) Subclinical hepatocellular carcinoma: an analysis of 391 patients. J Surg Oncol 3:55–58
13. Zhou XD, Tang ZY, Yu YQ, Yang BH, Lin ZY, Lu JZ, Ma ZC (1996) Long-term results of surgery for small primary liver cancer in 514 adults. J Cancer Res Clin Oncol 121:59–62
14. Zhou XD, Tang ZY, Yu YQ, Lu HX, Jiang ZG, Jiang YM, Shu RT (1979) Cryosurgery for liver cancer—experimental and clinical study (in Chinese). Chin J Surg 17:480–483
15. Zhou XD, Tang ZY, Yu YQ (1985) Cryosurgery for hepatocellular carcinoma. In: Tang ZY (ed) Subclinical hepatocellular carcinoma. China Academic Publishers/Springer, Beijing/Berlin, pp 107–119
16. Zhou XD, Tang ZY, Yu YQ, Ma ZC (1988) Clinical evaluation of cryosurgery in the treatment of primary liver cancer. Report of 60 cases. Cancer (Phila) 61:1889–1892
17. Zhou XD, Yu YQ, Tang ZY, Weng JM, Ma ZC, Xu DB (1992) An 18-year study of cryosurgery in the treatment of primary liver cancer. Asian J Surg 15:43–47
18. Zhou XD, Tang ZY, Yu YQ, Weng JM, Ma ZC, Zhang BH, Zheng XY (1993) The role of cryosurgery in the treatment of hepatic cancer: a report of 113 cases. Cancer Res Clin Oncol 120:100–102
19. Zhou XD, Tang ZY, Yu YQ (1995) Cryosurgery for liver tumors. In: Kawasaki S, Makuuchi M (eds) Novel regional therapies for liver tumors. Landes, Austin, pp 187–196
20. Tang ZY, Yu YQ, Zhou XD (1984) An important approach to prolonging survival further after radical resection of AFP-positive hepatocellular carcinoma. J Exp Clin Cancer Res 3:359–368

Keyword Index